Guides to Clinical
Aspiration Biopsy

Thyroid

Guides to Clinical Aspiration Biopsy

Series Editor: Tilde S. Kline, M.D.

Prostate
Tilde S. Kline, M.D.

Retroperitoneum and Intestine
Kenneth C. Suen, M.B., B.S., F.R.C.P.(C)

Thyroid
Sudha R. Kini, M.D.

Guides to Clinical Aspiration Biopsy
Thyroid

Sudha R. Kini, M.D.

Director, Cytopathology Laboratory
Senior Staff Pathologist
Henry Ford Hospital
Detroit, Michigan

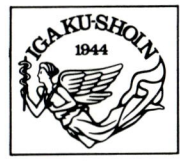

IGAKU-SHOIN   New York   •   Tokyo

Interior Design by Lila G. Maron
Cover Design by Paul Agule Design
Typesetting by Braun-Brumfield, Inc. in Garamond
Printing and Binding by Braun-Brumfield, Inc.

Published and distributed by

IGAKU-SHOIN Medical Publishers, Inc.
1140 Avenue of the Americas, New York, N.Y. 10036

IGAKU-SHOIN Ltd.,
5-24-3 Hongo, Bunkyo-ku, Tokyo

Library of Congress Cataloging-in-Publication Data

Kini, Sudha R.
  Thyroid.

  (Guides to clinical aspiration biopsy)
  Includes bibliographies and index.
  1. Thyroid gland—Biopsy, Needle. 2. Thyroid
gland—Diseases—Diagnosis. I. Title. II. Series.
[DNLM: 1. Biopsy, Needle. 2. Thyroid Neoplasms—
diagnosis.   WK 270 K55t]
RC655.5.K56   1987   616.4′40758   86-19988

ISBN: 0-89640-124-3 (New York)
ISBN: 4-260-14124-4 (Tokyo)

Printed and bound in U.S.A.

10 9 8 7 6 5 4 3 2 1

To

*Ratnaker, for his patience, encouragement,
moral support, and pride in everything I do,*

and to

Sarita and Sunita

Preface

When Dr. Tilde Kline asked me to contribute to the series "Guides to Clinical Apsiration Biopsy," my initial reaction was, "No, not again!" I had already coauthored an atlas and a textbook on needle biopsy of the thyroid. I felt I could not—and should not—repeat what I had already said. Dr. Kline, however, convinced me otherwise, and I undertook the task of writing this work on the cytopathology of thyroid, oriented to pathologists and cytotechnologists. The earlier atlas[3] and textbook[5] on which I had worked were clinically oriented.

I started interpreting thyroid aspirates 10 years ago after a request from Dr. J. Martin Miller to "get educated in something new." My qualifications at that time consisted of 6 years experience in managing a cytopathology laboratory, a basic knowledge of thyroid histopathology, and minimal experience in aspiration biopsy cytology limited to liver aspirates only.

Interpretation of the first few hundred cases was a struggle. No detailed descriptions or illustrations of Papanicolaou-stained materials were available, and there were no guidelines on the adequacy of specimens, reporting systems, or diagnostic pitfalls. No attempt had been made to provide diagnostic criteria for follicular lesions with any staining technique. My relative inexperience in thyroid histopathology was also a handicap.

Cases at the Henry Ford Hospital were augmented by triple the number from Associated Endocrinologists of Southfield, Michigan, and I began my cytohistologic correlations by comparing these studies with large needle biopsy specimens and surgically removed specimens. The inevitable early diagnostic errors served as a stimulus for improving my skills.

My bias for Papanicolaou stain stems from my primary interest in cytopathology. I have had no experience in evaluating aspiration biopsy material stained by Romanowsky technique. Hence, this book conspicuously lacks illustrations of material stained by Romanowsky method, with one exception—a case of medullary thyroid carcinoma. In my opinion, Papanicolaou stain brings out superb details in architectural patterns as well as cytomorphology.

This guide does not follow the conventional system of describing benign non-neoplastic conditions followed by neoplasia, benign and malignant; neither have I adhered to the generally accepted classification of thyroid neoplasms.[4] The format chosen—the one that has helped our clinicians—is geared toward practical application. This format is also the one that I have used while giving workshops over the years. Hashimoto's disease is covered last, not only because it is the greatest imitator, but also because it is often associated with neoplasms. One must, therefore, be familiar with cytopathology of neoplasms to understand the diagnostic pitfalls.

Throughout this monograph, I have tried to illustrate diagnostic pitfalls, overlapping patterns, and differential diagnoses. Errors in interpretation are an inevitable part of any self-taught learning process. I have tried to focus attention on these more than on the successes because I learned from them and hope the readers will too. The available literature on thyroid cytopathology is grossly lacking in information on adequacy, differential diagnosis, and diagnostic pitfalls. However, I hope that nonbelievers in thyroid cytopathology[2] do not use these examples to discourage needle biopsy as a diagnostic procedure for evaluating cold nodules of the thyroid. As a thyroidologist colleague has pointed out, fine needle biopsy need not be perfect, only better than the diagnostic system it replaces.

An entire chapter is devoted to concepts basic to thyroid cytopathology. The idea of concepts was borrowed from Dr. J. K. Frost.[1] The 2 valuable weeks I spent in his postgraduate institute of cytopathology enabled me to correlate thyroid cytopathology and histopathology.

I have modified the concepts to suit thyroid histo- and cytopathology. The reason for devoting the entire chapter to this area was my conversation with an eminent surgical pathologist who remarked that the language of cytopathology is quite often not understood by surgical pathologists. When one is used to sections of uniform thickness that have been stained by hematoxylin and eosin, it is difficult to appreciate architectural configurations in smears of uneven thickness. Thus, I have introduced cytopathology in this monograph by defining the various types of tissue fragments, followed by descriptions of their applications. I have attempted to explain various structural patterns of tissue fragments of papillary carcinoma by pointing out the similarities to an ear of corn viewed in different planes. From my exposure to British and Canadian writings, I have long realized that gross pathology is best described by calling attention to similarities with edibles or other things that are familiar from everyday life. Descriptive terms such as "bread-and-butter effect" for pericarditis, "sugar frosting" for perisplenitis, "sago spleen" for amyloidosis, and "nutmeg liver" are easily remembered. When its similarity to something as commonly encountered as an ear of corn is highlighted, the concept of papillary carcinoma may be better appreciated.

The importance of adequate cellular material, optimal cytopreparatory techniques (fixation, processing, and staining), and good communication with the clinicians managing thyroid nodules cannot be overemphasized. Expertise in cytopathology is useless for interpreting inadequate, poorly fixed, or poorly prepared and stained smears. If the cytopathologist does not do the biopsy, it is essential to have an adequate liaison with understanding clinicians who are not offended or discouraged by inadequate specimens or indeterminate diagnoses (eg, a few atypical cells seen). I have been extremely fortunate in having had the best of all worlds. First, I encountered a large volume of cases that sustained my interest and provided a tremendous learning experience; I have had experience with over 8,000 needle aspirates, 1,400 large-needle biopsy specimens, and 1,100 surgical specimens. Second, I was associated with J. Martin Miller, M.D., a nationally renown thyroidologist who was susceptible to my indoctrination in the discipline of cytopathology and, thus, was able to provide the necessary liaison between the patients and me to ensure the necessary follow-up. Third, and of equal importance, I was blessed with a laboratory supervisor who excelled in cytopreparatory techniques and staining.

Writing this monograph has been an enjoyable experience, and I do hope it will be an enjoyable reading experience for others.

My special thanks to Drs. Charles Taylor, Michael Garcia, and Don Meier of Associated Endocrinologists, and to Joel L. Hamburger and Sheldon Stoffer, all of the Detroit Metropolitan area, for sending me biopsy material and for having confidence in my interpretations; and to the many pathologists in the Detroit, Michigan, metropolitan area and across the country who provided the histologic material, for without cytohistologic correlation, thyroid cytopathology would have been extremely difficult. I appreciate Dr. Jean Riddle's generosity in granting unlimited access to the use of her photomicroscope and to her staff for technical assistance. I gratefully acknowledge the photographic assistance of Art Bowden, Nancy Peshkin, and Jim Latif; artwork by Jessica Goodwin, Robert Mohr, and Jay Knipstein; and typing assistance of Sherryl McCray and Pat Schwartzman. Acknowledgment also goes to my secretary, Grace Furca, for her relentless typing of the manuscript; Dr. Patricia Cornett for editorial assistance; and Dr. Tilde Kline for advice. My heartfelt thanks are due to Walter Harlan for printing hundreds of black-and-white illustrations from color transparencies and for their excellent quality. I am forever grateful to Jane Smith-Purslow for providing me with superbly stained slides, for taking hundreds and thousands of Kodachromes of unsurpassable quality, for making the composites, and for her enthusiasm. Her contribution was invaluable. I am indebted to J. Martin Miller, M.D., for his contribution to the book, for his moral support throughout our association as a biopsy team, and for his contribution to needle biopsy of the thyroid. Without his assistance, this work would not have been possible. I also acknowledge the support of Dr. Kenneth A. Greenawald, Chairman of the Department of Pathology at Henry Ford Hospital, where I work, and my professional colleagues for their understanding while I was writing this book.

This monograph has truly been a combined effort of all the people listed.

Sudha R. Kini, M.D.

REFERENCES

1. Frost JK: *Concepts Basic to General Cytopathology*. Baltimore, The Johns Hopkins Press, 1972.

2. Hajdu SI, Melamed MR: Limitations of aspiration cytology in the diagnosis of primary neoplasms. *Acta Cytol* 28:337–345, 1984.

3. Hamburger JI, Miller JM, Kini SR: Clinical-pathological evaluation of thyroid nodules. In: *Handbook and Atlas*, Southfield, MI, published privately, 1979, p. 15.

4. Heddinger CHR, Sobin LH: Histologic typing of thyroid tumors. In: *International Histologic Classification of Tumors*, NR 11, Geneva, WHO, 1974.

5. Miller JM, Kini SR, Hamburger JI: *Needle Biopsy of the Thyroid*. New York, Praeger Publishers, 1983.

Permission to reproduce the following is gratefully acknowledged: From Miller JM, Kini SR, Hamburger JI: *Needle Biopsy of the Thyroid*, Praeger Publishers, New York, 1983, Figs. 2.2, 2.3, 2.4, and 2.5. From Kini SR, Miller JM, Hamburger JI, Smith-Purslow MJ: Cytopathology of follicular lesions of the thyroid gland, *Diagn Cytopathol* 1:123–132, 1985, published by Igaku-Shoin, New York, Figs. 4.3, 4.6, 6.9A and B, 6.14, 6.20, 6.22, 6.23, 6.30, and 8.60, and Tables 6.4, 6.5, 6.6, 6.7, 6.8, and 6.9.

From Cervino JM, Paseyro P, Grosso O, Maggioto S: *La exploration citologic de la glandula tirodes y sus correlaciones anatomoclinicas, An Facultad Med* 47:128–143, 1962, Fig. 6.29.

From Boon ME, Löwhagen T, Williams JS: Planimetric studies on fine needle aspirates from follicular adenoma and follicular carcinoma of the thyroid, *Acta Cytol* 24:145–148, 1980, published by Science Printers & Publishers Inc., St. Louis, Table 6.10.

From Kini SR, Miller JM, Hamburger JI: Problems in the cytologic diagnosis of the "cold" thyroid nodule in patients with lymphocytic thyroiditis, *Acta Cytol* 25:506–512, 1981, published by Science Printers & Publishers Inc., St. Louis, Table 11.4.

From Sajal Choudary, M.D., Associate Pathologist, Mt. Carmel Mercy Hospital, Detroit, MI, Fig. 13.11.

Contributors

J. Martin Miller, M.D.
Consultant, Division of Endocrinology
Department of Internal Medicine
Henry Ford Hospital
Detroit, Michigan
and
Endocrinologist
Associated Endocrinologists
Southfield, Michigan
and
Emeritas Clinical Associate Professor
University of Michigan, Ann Arbor, Michigan

M. Jane Smith-Purslow, B.S., CT(ASCP) CMIAC
Supervisor, Cytopathology Laboratory
Department of Pathology
Henry Ford Hospital
Detroit, Michigan

Contents

1

Introduction

J. Martin Miller, M.D.

Shortly after World War II, articles appeared in the medical literature stating the incidence of thyroid cancer in surgically removed thyroid nodules to be 20–30%. These articles also suggested that these findings were representative of the entire nodular goiter population.[2,3] Opponents of this point of view cited the low incidence of cancer of thyroid as a cause of death in autopsy material,[12] and a controversy was born as to the true risk of a thyroid nodule to the patient. By the 1950s, it was generally agreed that the morbidity and mortality of thyroid cancer did not justify removal of all thyroid nodules,[7] so today the controversy focuses on the means of selection of patient nodules for surgical biopsy, ie, the method of determining the risk of a given thyroid nodule.

During the 1960s and 1970s, it became evident to physicians in the United States that radionuclide or ultrasound images of the thyroid were successful in eliminating consideration of thyroid surgery for no more than 10–20% of thyroid nodules. However, as early as 1950 in the Scandinavian countries, attention was focused on the use of a fine needle to aspirate a cytologic sample from thyroid nodules[13] and, thus, determine from it the probable pathologic diagnosis. For 25 years, such reports evoked little interest in North America. The reasons for this are speculative and include dissatisfaction with the variable reported sensitivity of the European studies, failure of authors to provide direction for use of biopsy data in avoiding thyroid surgery, and the "sure knowledge" that cytology would not provide a diagnosis of a lesion often requiring many histologic sections for identification. Overreaction to one reported case of subcutaneous tumor implant by needle biopsy[4] was also a factor, as was the use of Giemsa stain by the Europeans, a cytologic stain not popular among American cytopathologists accustomed to Papanicolaou staining techniques.

By the late 1970s, the Canadians had reported experience with fine-needle biopsy,[5] and groups in Cleveland and Boston had evaluated large-needle biopsy.[4,14] The first American study combining both was reported in 1979 by our group.[11] Since that

1

time numerous reports have appeared in the English literature on the diagnosis of thyroid nodules by needle biopsy, mostly by the cytologic specimens obtained by fine-needle aspiration. In spite of limited but definite advantages to the combined use of large- and fine-needle biopsy in a biopsy program,[9] the universal application, simplicity, safety, ease of performance, and patient acceptance of fine-needle biopsy account for its exclusive use in most reported studies.[1]

Our experience with over 4,500 satisfactory biopsies spans the 10 years from 1975 to 1985, and has provided us with over 1,100 correlations with surgical specimens. Our purpose has been twofold: (1) to provide diagnostic information for the management of our patients and those of our referring doctors; and (2) to record our experience in obtaining and diagnosing thyroid needle biopsy specimens in such a way that others might profit from our trials and errors. This book is our third attempt to make available to our colleagues our total needle biopsy experience. Unlike the first two attempts,[6,8] we have limited this work to fine-needle biopsy. Its purpose is to assist the cytopathologist in the proper interpretation of cytologic samples from the thyroid gland. Therefore, most of the text is concerned with our experience in obtaining these samples by fine needle and interpreting them. If cytologic diagnosis was an exact science, and if there was a predictable correlation between a particular diagnosis and tumor behavior, this information would suffice. Such is not the case, and certain ancillary information is of value to the interpreter of thyroid cyto- pathology. This includes the gross and histologic anatomy of the lesion subjected to biopsy, the life history of benign and malignant thyroid nodules, and the manage- ment of thyroid nodules with and without biopsy.

IMPORTANCE OF NEEDLE BIOPSY

The morbidity and mortality of thyroid cancer do not qualify it as an important public health problem. The number of noninvasive diagnostic tests and surgical lobectomies done to establish or exclude its presence, however, make it a disease of economic importance. Living in a society concerned with containment of medical costs, we should carefully select the most cost-effective diagnostic tests. The experience of our group is that needle biopsy is far more accurate for the selection of patients with nodules for diagnostic lobectomy and is much cheaper than any combination of noninvasive tests. Its use has halved the number of operations prescribed and has doubled the number of cancers identified per 100 surgical removals.[10] Cutting surgical and hospital bills for nodule management in half is a worthwhile achievement. Our figures also suggest that we are now identifying cancers that were diagnosed as benign nodules, or we are making the diagnosis of cancer at an earlier stage. Determining whether this too is advantageous and will favorably influence the morbidity and mortality of thyroid cancer will require many years of study.

In summary, most physicians agree that neither removing all thyroid nodules nor removing no thyroid nodules is a sensible management approach. Therefore, they employ some process of selection in prescribing surgical lobectomy. The most cost-effective method of selection is needle biopsy.

REFERENCES

1. Ashcraft MW, Van Herle AJ: Management of thyroid nodules II, scanning techniques, thyroid suppression therapy and fine needle aspiration. *Head Neck Surg* 3:297, 1981.

2. Cerise EJ, Ranoall S, Ochsner A: Carcinoma of the thyroid and nontoxic nodular goiter. *Surgery* 31:552, 1952.

3. Cole WH, Majarakis JO, Slaughter OP: Incidence of carcinoma of the thyroid in nodular goiter. *J Clin Endocrinol* 9:1007, 1949.

4. Crile G Jr, Hawk WA Jr: Aspiration biopsy of thyroid nodules. *Surg Gynecol Obstet* 136:241–245, 1973.

5. Crockford PM, Bain GO: Fine-needle aspiration biopsy of the thyroid. *Can Med Assoc J* 110:1029–1032, 1974.

6. Hamburger JI, Miller JM, Kini SR: Clinical-Pathological Evaluation of Thyroid Nodules. In: *Handbook & Atlas*. Southfield, MI, 1979. p. 15.

7. Miller JM: Carcinoma and thyroid nodules. Problem in endemic goiter, *N Engl J Med* 252:247–251, 1955.

8. Miller JM, Kini SR, Hamburger JI: *Needle Biopsy of Thyroid*. New York, Praeger Publishers, 1983.

9. Miller JM, Hamburger JI, Kini SR: Fine needle aspiration cytology, cutting biopsy or both in the evaluation of thyroid nodules? In Thompson NW, Vinik AI: *Endocrine Surgery Update*. New York, Grune & Stratton, 1983, p. 23.

10. Miller JM, Hamburger JI, Kini SR: The impact of needle biopsy on the preoperative diagnosis of thyroid nodules. *Henry Ford Hosp Med J* 28:145, 1980.

11. Miller JM, Hamburger JI, Kini SR: Diagnosis of thyroid nodules by fine needle aspiration and needle biopsy. *JAMA* 241:481–486, 1979.

12. Rogers WF, Asper SP, Williams RH: Clinical significance of malignant neoplasms of the thyroid gland. *N Engl J Med* 237:569, 1947.

13. Söderström N: Puncture of goiters for aspiration biopsy. A preliminary report. *Acta Med Scand* 144:235–244, 1952.

14. Wang C, Vickery AL Jr, Maloof F: Needle biopsy of the thyroid. *Surg Gynecol Obstet* 143:365–368, 1976.

2

Techniques of Fine-Needle Aspiration Biopsy

J. Martin Miller, M.D.

It is axiomatic that a pathologist must have an adequate biopsy specimen to make a satisfactory interpretation. Obtaining an adequate cellular sample requires enough capillary blood or tissue fluid to serve as a vehicle, but not so much as to cause a problem by dilution. The sample must then be fixed and stained in such a way as to permit the most accurate interpretation possible. Obtaining an adequate cytologic sample from the thyroid is a simple procedure. However, the number of failures by physicians of little experience suggests that matters of technique, although simple, are indeed essential.

Before beginning the discussion of "how to do it," we acknowledge the prerequisite of experience in palpating thyroid nodules for the biopsy physician. Little experience is needed to palpate a nodule of 4–5 cm in the greatest dimension, but the 1-cm nodule on the posterior aspect of a lobe requires skillful palpation. Nodules felt by single-digit palpation with the patient erect can always be felt with the patient in the recumbent biopsy position. Most nodules felt by bidigital examination with the patient seated can at least be localized with the patient supine.

PREPARATION—MENTAL

Proper mental preparation is the first step in the performance of a thyroid biopsy. Most of the pain experienced by patients is minor discomfort magnified by anxiety. The patient should be reassured as to the simplicity, painlessness, and brevity of the procedure. The prick of the anesthetic needle and the sting of the local anesthetic should be described immediately before they are felt by the patient. The patient

5

should be asked not to swallow while the needle is in the nodule and should be assured that this represents a small fraction of the total time involved in doing a biopsy, ie, swallowing is minimally restricted. (Pain and even serious vascular injury may result if the patient swallows when the needle has passed through the nodule). We find that anxiety is lessened by maintaining pleasant conversation with the patient during the procedure.

PREPARATION—PHYSICAL

With a few exceptions (we have performed biopsies on a few patients while they were sitting), the patient assumes a supine position, with the head and neck extended over a pillow. The degree of extension should not produce a skin tension that interferes with nodule palpation or partially obstructs the vertebral artery blood flow in the elderly. The site of needle puncture is cleaned by firm application of an alcohol swab. We attribute the total absence of infection in over 7,000 biopsy attempts to the adequacy of normal body defense mechanisms, rather than to the excellence of our sterile technique.

ANESTHETIC—TO USE OR NOT TO USE

If the operator can be certain that only one needle will be necessary, a local anesthetic is superfluous. This assumes no bloody aspirates, no degenerated nodules, no cystic lesions, and no grossly unsatisfactory specimens. It also assumes adequate sampling by multiple passes of the same needle, as recommended by some Swedish physicians.[3] We make none of these assumptions, so to limit patient discomfort to one needle, we use lidocaine. The possible disadvantages to the use of an anesthetic are two-fold. First, the patient may be allergic to lidocaine and not aware of it. We have had several patients with known allergies to lidocaine for whom we have used either mepivacaine (Carbocaine) or nothing, but we have not encountered a patient with a lidocaine allergy of which he or she was unaware. Second, the anesthetic may obscure the nodule. In such a situation, a little local massage will disperse the fluid.

Many physicians consider local anesthetic to be superfluous even when three or four needles are used. We agree that most patients can tolerate this discomfort, but why should they?

We use 1–2 ml of 1% lidocaine for the skin and subcutaneous tissues. Care is exercised not to infiltrate the nodule, which might cause a "lidocaine aspirate."

SYRINGE

A 10-ml syringe provides ample negative pressure for obtaining cytologic specimens.

NEEDLES

The larger the needle, the larger the tissue sample and the greater the possibility of an unwanted volume of blood. We have found the 25-gauge, 1.5-in. needle to be suitable for the majority of nodules. With less vascular nodules, a 22-gauge or even a 20-gauge needle gives better results. When we use a mechanical suction device, we prefer the greater rigidity of a 22-gauge needle.

NEEDLE PLACEMENT

The right-handed physician fixes right-sided nodules between the second and third digit of the left hand, and inserts the needle with the right hand while standing behind the patient. For left-sided nodules, it is more comfortable to perform the nodule immobilization while standing on the right side of the patient. For nodules 1.5 cm or smaller, simply inserting the needle into the nodule is a reasonable goal. With larger nodules, peripheral subcapsular parts of the nodule should be sampled, rather than the center. The periphery is more apt to be predictive of histologic behavior. The center often is undergoing degenerative change.

SUCTION—HOW AND HOW MUCH

Suction is applied once, repetitively, or during maneuvers designed to further disrupt the follicular epithelium. The total procedure should be sufficient to make aspirate appear in the hub of the needle, but not in the barrel of the syringe. Aspirate within the syringe must be removed by a washing procedure followed by a concentrating one, both of which tend to distort cytologic features and add to the complexity and cost of the procedure.

Many of the pioneers in needle biopsy consider a mechanical suction device for producing suction as absolutely essential for this procedure[2] (Fig. 2.1). Producing suction with this device and maintaining it requires only one hand and allows the operator to continuously fix nodules by the left hand while suction is maintained by the right (Fig. 2.2). It also allows the maximum possible suction from a 10-ml syringe.

We performed our first 3,000 satisfactory biopsies without recourse to, or even knowledge of the existence of, this mechanical device. We find it simple to maintain suction with one hand with no mechanical assistance once suction has been achieved and the needle is in the nodule (Fig. 2.3). This requires reestablishing fixation, which seems to be a disadvantage only in very small nodules. Among the disadvantages of the mechanical suction device are its one-time expense of approximately $150, the more remote "touch" occasioned by the hand being a greater distance from the needle, and the fact that the needle cannot be twirled while suction is being applied (see section below on Tissue Disruption).

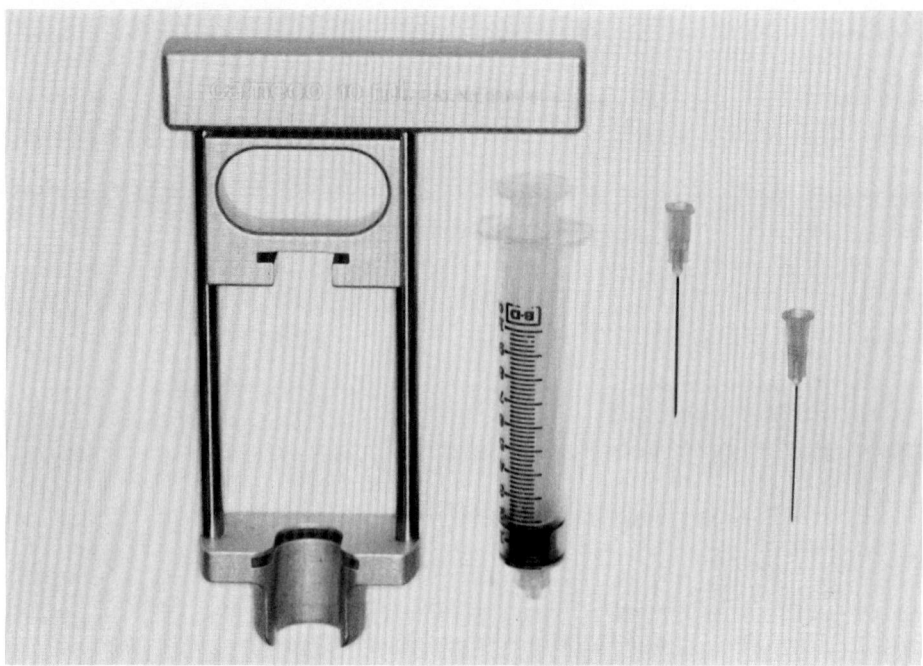

Fig. 2.1. Mechanical syringe holder, 10-ml plastic B–D syringe, 22-gauge, 1.5-in. needle, and 25-gauge, 1.5 in. needle.

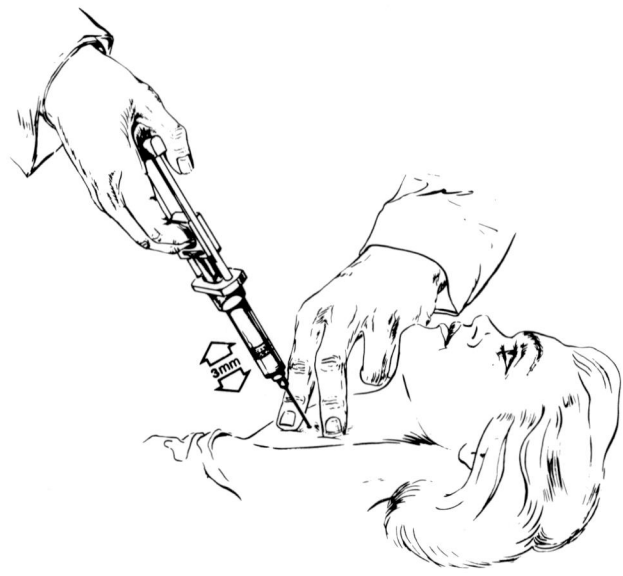

Fig. 2.2. Aspiration using the mechanical device to produce suction. Tissue disrupted by vertical movement.

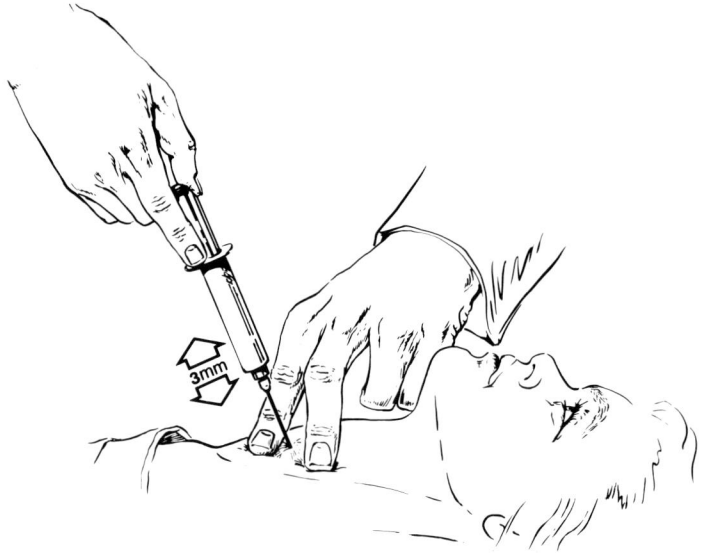

Fig. 2.3. Same maneuver as shown in Fig. 2.2, but without mechanical holder.

TISSUE DISRUPTION

Simple application of suction by pulling the plunger of the syringe back to 6 or 7 ml is often unsatisfactory. Results may be improved if a pumping action is used, and improved even more if the barrel of the syringe is rotated rapidly while the plunger is held stationary as suction is maintained (Fig. 2.4). Moving the needle in and out (but with the tip in the nodule) has much the same effect (Figs. 2.2 and 2.3) The nodule must be fixed during this maneuver to prevent a small nodule from moving with the needle, thus eliminating the motion of the needle within the nodule.

The cutting action of any needle motion is improved by speed. It is our practice that if nothing appears in the needle hub from maintained suction, we twirl and then move the needle in and out until something appears.

SMEARS

After the suction, the needle is removed and the plunger is withdrawn a couple of milliliters. The needle is re-affixed and the specimen is expressed onto the slide. This procedure is the same with or without the use of a mechanical suction device. At this point, an estimate is made as to whether or not the volume of the aspirate is suitable for smearing on the slide. If it is not excessive, it may be either smeared with the edge of another slide, as is usual with a blood smear (Fig. 2.5—1); or, if particulate matter or colloid is visibly present, the material may be compressed between two slides and smeared (Fig. 2.5—2). If the volume of the specimen seems too great for the slide, tilt it and remove the blood that flows to the low side by the use of an absorbent tissue (Fig. 2.6). Smearing is then done as described above. Another recommended

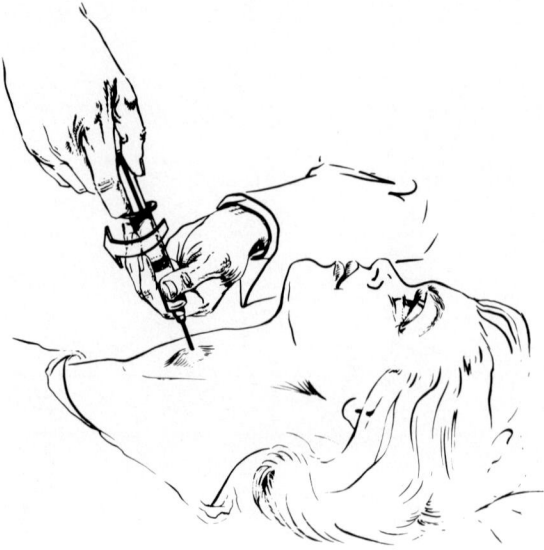

Fig. 2.4. Rotation technique for fine-needle biopsy. Note that the index finger of the right hand maintains suction while the left hand rotates the barrel of the syringe.

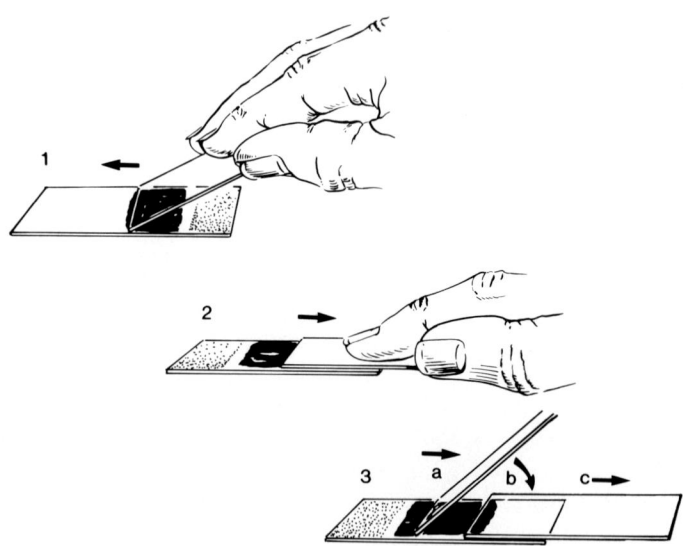

Fig. 2.5. Three methods of smearing the fine-needle aspirate. See text for details.

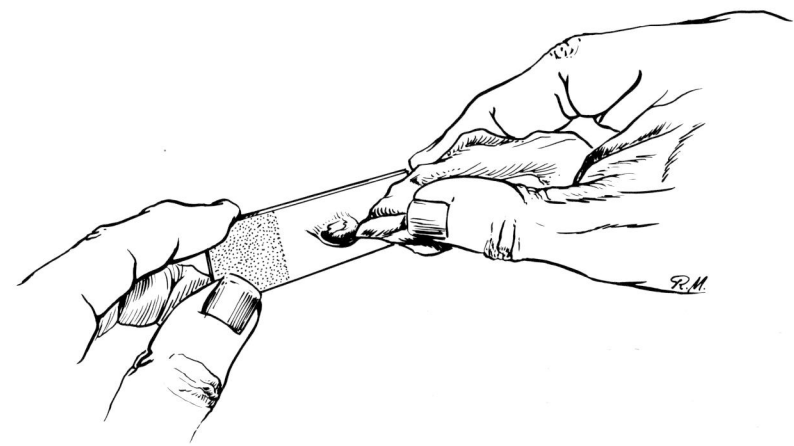

Fig. 2.6. To remove excess blood or fluid, the slide is tilted and a tongue of absorbing tissue is touched to the dependent portion of the drop.

technique for concentrating cellular material is shown in Fig. 2.5—3. The slide with the specimen may be tilted frosted-end down to enlist the aid of gravity while the edge of the smearing slide is drawn upward. After the blood has been separated, the smearing slide is flattened, and the smear is completed.

There have been elegant treatises on the exact hand and slide maneuvers necessary for producing the best smears.[1] It is sometimes difficult to identify the experiences of those who perform biopsies only of the thyroid with those who perform biopsies on many types of more cellular tumors. As 70% of thyroid specimens will be from benign disease and will have minimal cell density, the procedures suggested for transferring material to two or more slides are probably unnecessary. Be that as it may, the simple instructions given here have served us very well in a fairly large experience.

SMEARS—NUMBER

If a smear looks unsatisfactory, it usually is. If it looks satisfactory, it may be so. We take six smears to ensure three good ones and adequate sampling.

FIXATION

Fixation must be matched to the staining technique employed. We use a modified Papanicolaou staining technique and, therfore, fix immediately with alcohol as part of a spray. If May–Grünwald Giemsa stain is used, the smear is air-dried and no prompt fixation is necessary.

POSTBIOPSY CARE

If there has been no intranodular bleeding, we apply an elastic bandage and keep the patient under surveillance for about 15 minutes. If there has been some bleeding into the nodule, we ask the patient to maintain pressure for about one-half hour. In either instance, removal of the bandage after 1 hour is authorized.

REFERENCES

1. Abele JS, Miller TR, King EB, Löwhagen T: Smearing techniques for the concentration of particles from fine needle aspiration biopsy. *Diagn Cytopathol* 1:59, 1985.
2. Löwhagen T, Willems JS, Lundell G, et al: Aspiration biopsy cytology in diagnosis of cancer. *World J Surg* 5:61–73, 1981.
3. Willems JS, Löwhagen T: Fine needle aspiration cytology in thyroid disease. In Williams: *Clinics in Endocrinology and Metabolism*, vol 10. Philadelphia, Saunders, 1981, pp. 247–266.

3

Adequacy, Reporting System, and Cytopreparatory Technique

The ultimate result of an aspiration biopsy procedure should be a smear prepared and stained in such a way as to enable a cytopathologist to give an accurate and meaningful cytopathologic evaluation, one that is in the best interest of the patient. The specimen must be adequate in terms of cellularity, and the smear must be satisfactory in terms of quality, ie, thickness, fixation, and staining. This chapter will deal with adequacy of the specimen, the reporting system, unsatisfactory and inadequate diagnoses, and cytopreparatory technique as well as staining.

ADEQUACY

It is very difficult to define an adequate cytologic specimen of a thyroid aspirate, as there are no clear-cut established criteria. The criteria used tend to be subjective and differ among pathologists. Adequacy of the thyroid aspirate must always be judged in a clinical context. The clinician, whether an endocrinologist, internist, or a surgeon, must be familiar with the reporting system of the cytopathology laboratory and must work closely with the cytopathologist.

An adequate specimen is one in which the cytologic material is sufficient to render a diagnosis, benign or otherwise. A rare group of benign follicular cells should not be considered as indicative of a benign disease. Poor cellular yield can be due to several reasons (Table. 3.1). As conservative management is generally indicated for benign non-neoplastic diseases, the pathologist must feel comfortable in rendering such a diagnosis. To avoid false-negative results, a benign diagnosis should never be attempted based on a few unremarkable cells.

An argument can be made against reporting aspirates as "unsatisfactory" or "inadequate" in the following cases of colloid nodules that yield abundant colloid

13

TABLE 3.1. Probable Reasons for Inadequate Specimens

1. Sclerotic lesions
   Fibrous variant of Hashimoto's thyroiditis
   Reidel's thyroiditis
   Neoplasms with marked desmoplasia
2. Thick, fibrous, sclerotic and calcified capsule
3. Large lesions with cystic degeneration
4. Long-standing cysts
5. Necrotic lesions
   Abscess
   Infarct
   Necrosis of the tumor
6. Very vascular neoplasms
7. Sampling error—needle not in the lesion
8. Faulty technique—too much or too little suction

with few (Fig. 3.1) or without any follicular cells; a long-standing cyst of an adenomatous goiter that yields only histiocytes (Fig. 3.2); or a few lymphocytes and stromal cells with no epithelial cells in clinically documented cases of Hashimoto's thyroiditis (Figs. 3.3 and 3.4).

Abundant colloid is often considered a feature of benign condition.[3] Although this impression most often holds true, it is not unusual to find abundant colloid in a differentiated cancer (Fig. 3.5). By the same token, a large number of histiocytes and degenerated follicular cells from a cystic lesion do not rule out a neoplasm. Therefore, such specimens are considered unsatisfactory for cytologic evaluation despite the cellularity, although they are benign in clinical context.

Just as reporting a benign diagnosis based on a scanty aspirate is not recommended, a diagnostic interpretation must not be attempted on few atypically appearing cells (Fig. 3.6). The aspiration biopsy must be repeated in such instances.

Through experience we have laid out the criteria for adequacy of a specimen. Guidelines for ensuring a satisfactory and adequate sample are presented in Table 3.2.

Our minimal requirement of 8–10 tissue fragments of well-preserved follicular epithelium on at least two slides (Fig. 3.7) may seem very rigid. It raises the percentage of unsatisfactory results; eg, because of this requirement, the rate of unsatisfactory results in our series is 20%.[7] But such rigid criteria minimize the risk of false-negative diagnoses. Most of our errors in terms of false-negative diagnoses were encountered during the first few years and, on retrospective review, the majority were based on inadequate specimens.[8] Besides the cellularity, preservation of epithelial cells is also very critical in Papanicolaou-stained material (Fig. 3.8).

An adequate aspirate must also be a satisfactory aspirate for cytopathologic evaluation. Too much blood, cellular and necrotic debris, thick smears, poor fixation, and suboptimal stain can all influence the final product (Fig. 3.9).[2] An adequately cellular specimen can be unsatisfactory for cytopathologic evaluation due to any of these causes. Situations in which an unsatisfactory diagnosis may result are listed in Table 3.3.

TABLE 3.2. Recommended Guidelines for Ensuring Adequate and Satisfactory Specimens

1. Multiple punctures of the nodule in question, so that several areas are sampled (easily done if aspiration biopsy is performed under a local anesthetic)
2. At least six properly prepared, thin cell spreads
3. Immediate wet fixation for Papanicolaou staining technique and a good staining procedure
4. A minimum of 8–10 tissue fragments of *well preserved* follicular epithelium on each of two slides

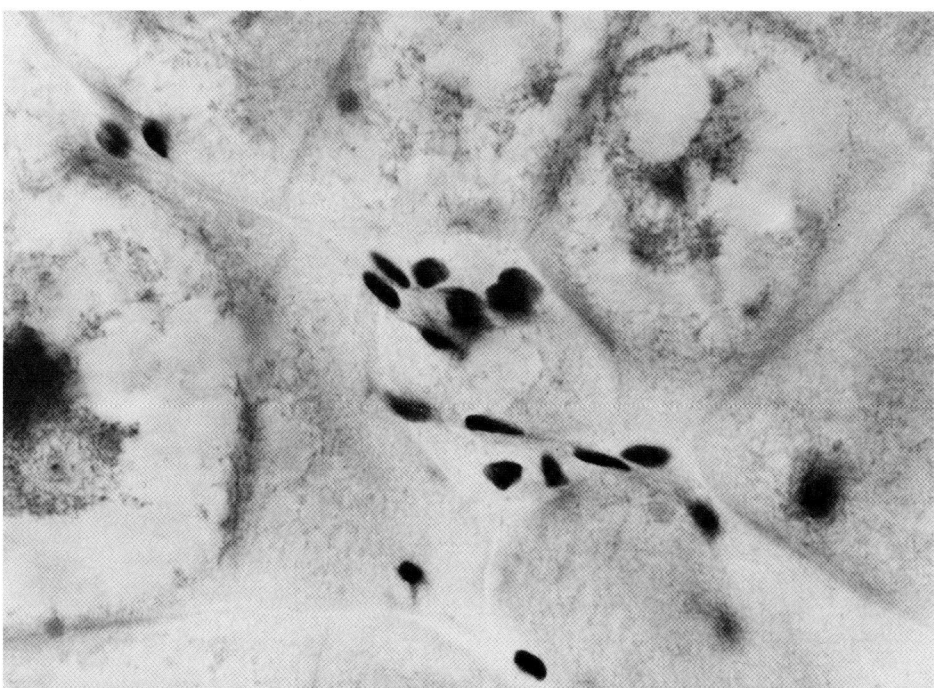

Fig. 3.1. Abundant colloid, very few follicular cells with indistinct cell borders, and pyknotic nuclei. This aspirate is cytologically unsatisfactory, but may be benign in clinical context. Papanicolaou preparation. × 630.

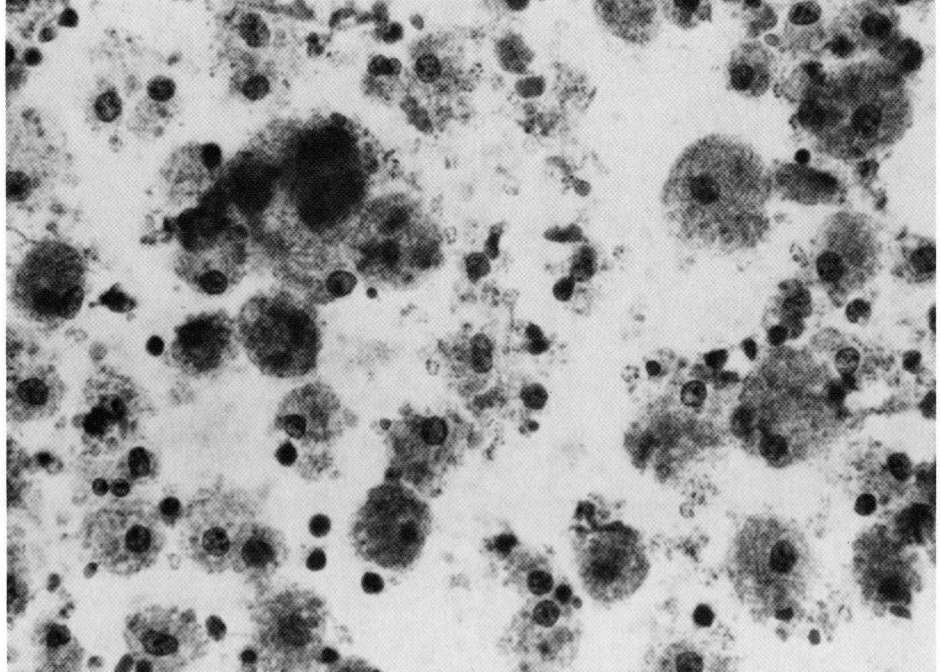

Fig. 3.2. Fluid from cystic nodular goiter showing degenerated follicular cells, and hemosiderin-containing macrophages. In spite of adequate cellularity, this aspirate is unsatisfactory because of the absence of well-preserved follicular epithelium. Papanicolaou preparation. × 630.

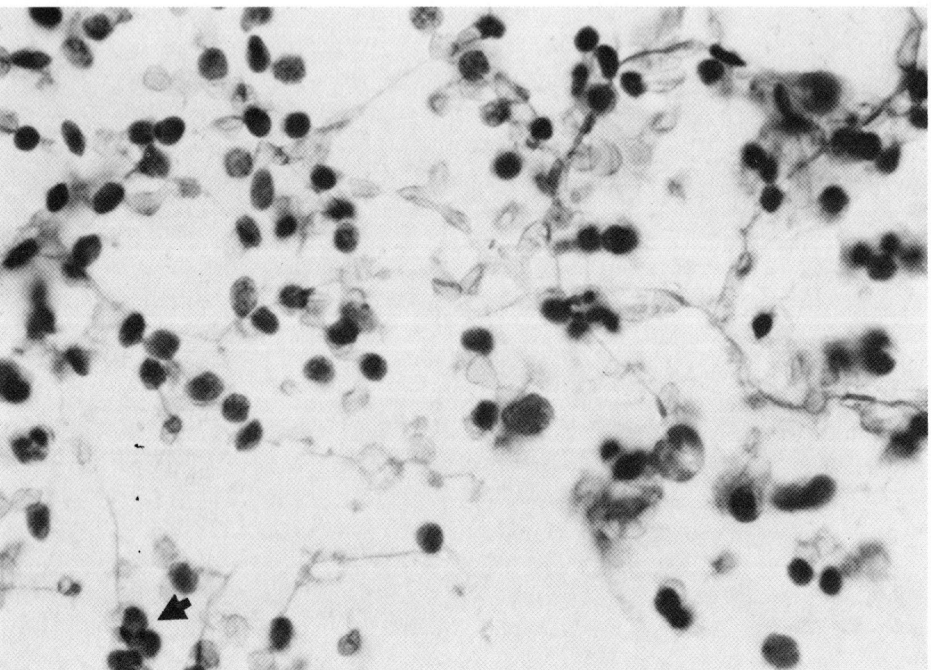

Fig. 3.3. Repeated attempts at aspiration biopsy in a patient with a nodularity of the thyroid and documented history of Hashimoto's thyroiditis showed only a few lymphocytes and no follicular or Hürthle cells. This aspirate is cytologically unsatisfactory, but may be benign in clinical context. Papanicolaou preparation. × 630.

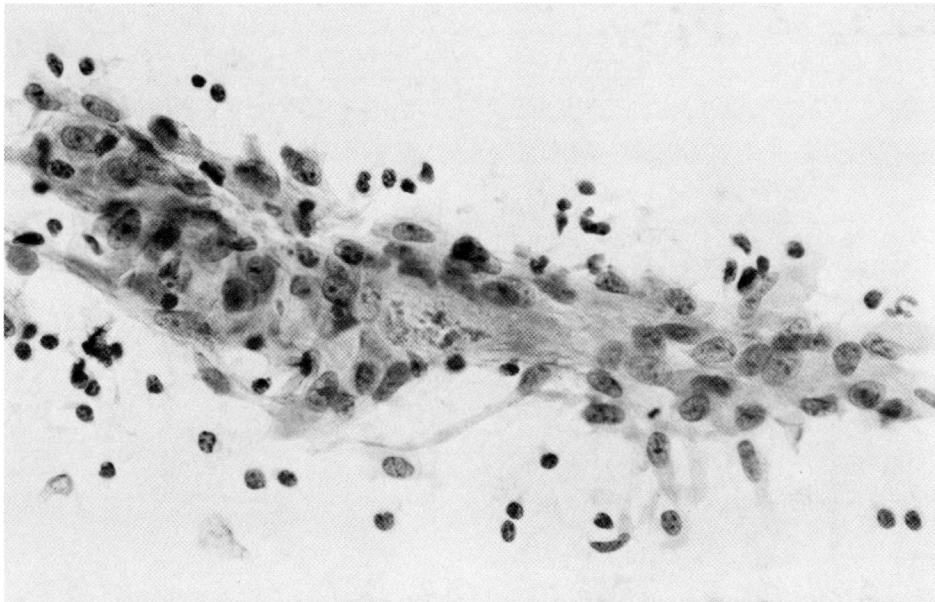

Fig. 3.4. Few lymphocytes and stromal cells may be the only features seen in aspirates of a fibrous variant of Hashimoto's thyroiditis. This aspirate is cytologically unsatisfactory. Papanicolaou preparation. × 400.

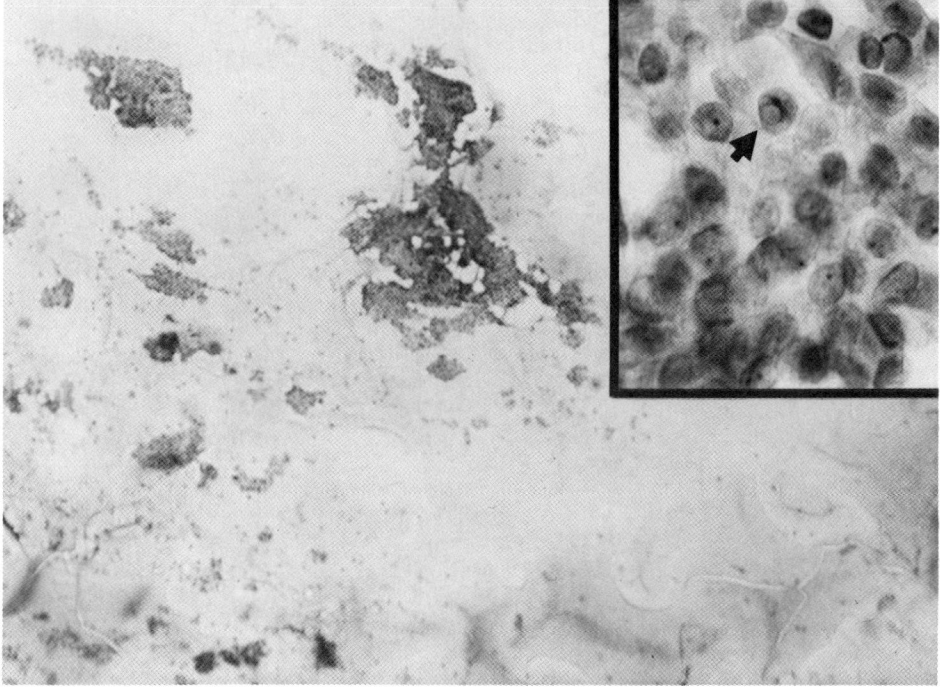

Fig. 3.5. Aspirate of a cold nodule showing abundant colloid and few tissue fragments. Papanicolaou preparation. × 63. *Inset:* Higher magnification showing a typical nuclear morphology of papillary carcinoma, including intranuclear cytoplasmic inclusion (arrow). Papanicolaou preparation. × 630.

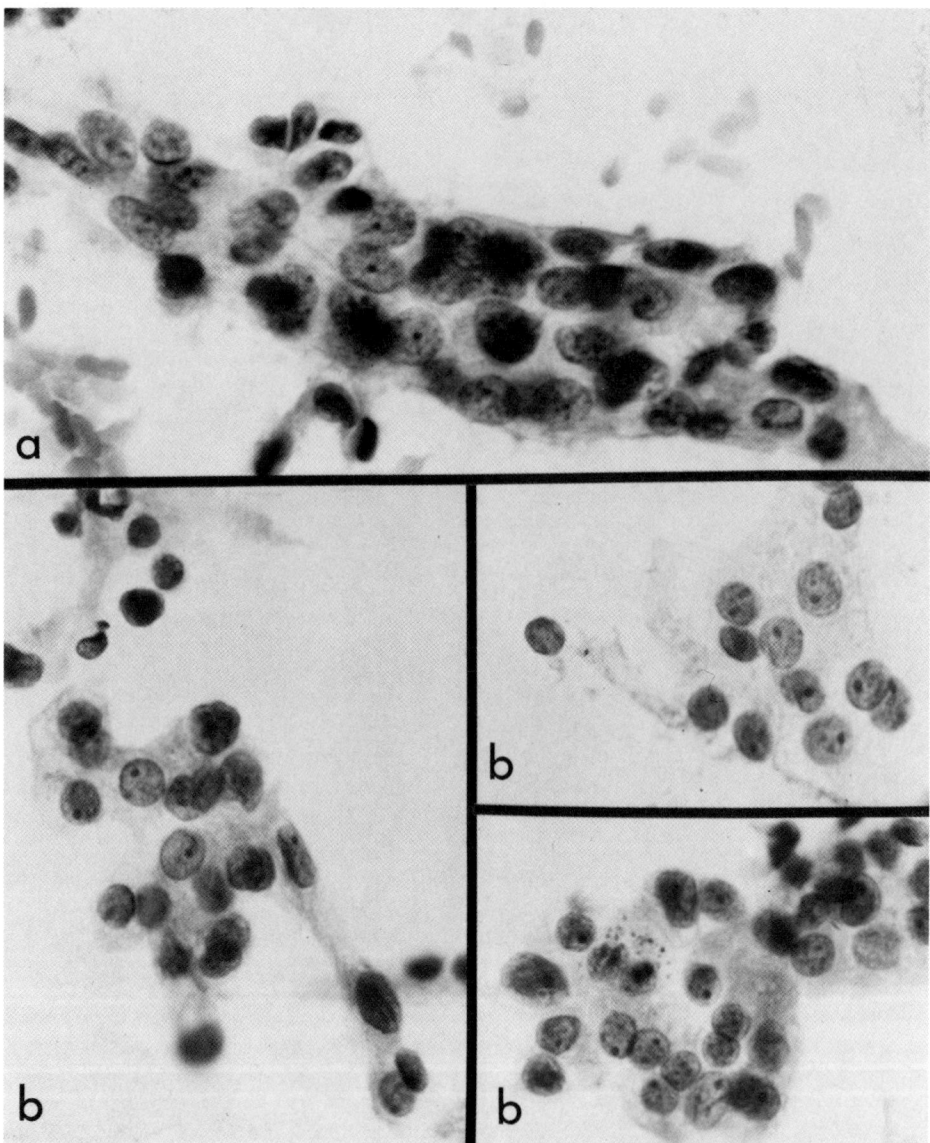

Fig. 3.6. A. Almost acellular aspirate with only one group of markedly atypical follicular cells. Inadequate but suspicious; the biopsy must be repeated. (A repeat biopsy in this case showed follicular carcinoma.) Papanicolaou preparation. × 630. **B.** Multiple punctures of a cold nodule showing only three tissue fragments of follicular epithelium. Unsatisfactory due to inadequate cellular material, but suggestive of a neoplasm due to syncytial arrangement and large nuclei. (Thyroidectomy showed follicular variant of papillary carcinoma.) Papanicolaou preparation. × 630.

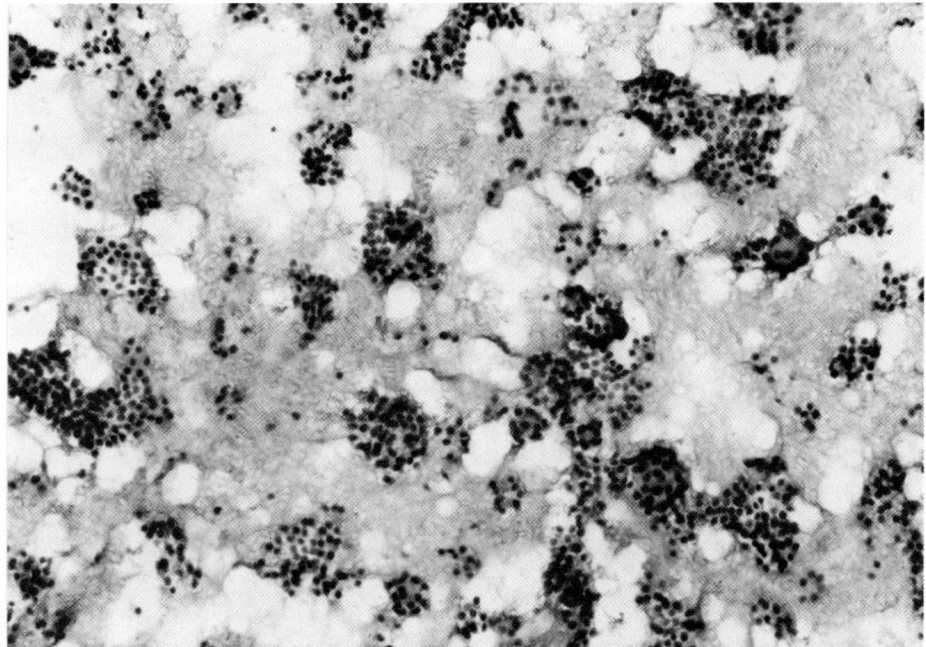

Fig. 3.7. An adequate and satisfactory specimen of thyroid aspirate showing several tissue fragments of well-preserved follicular epithelium. Papanicolaou preparation. × 160.

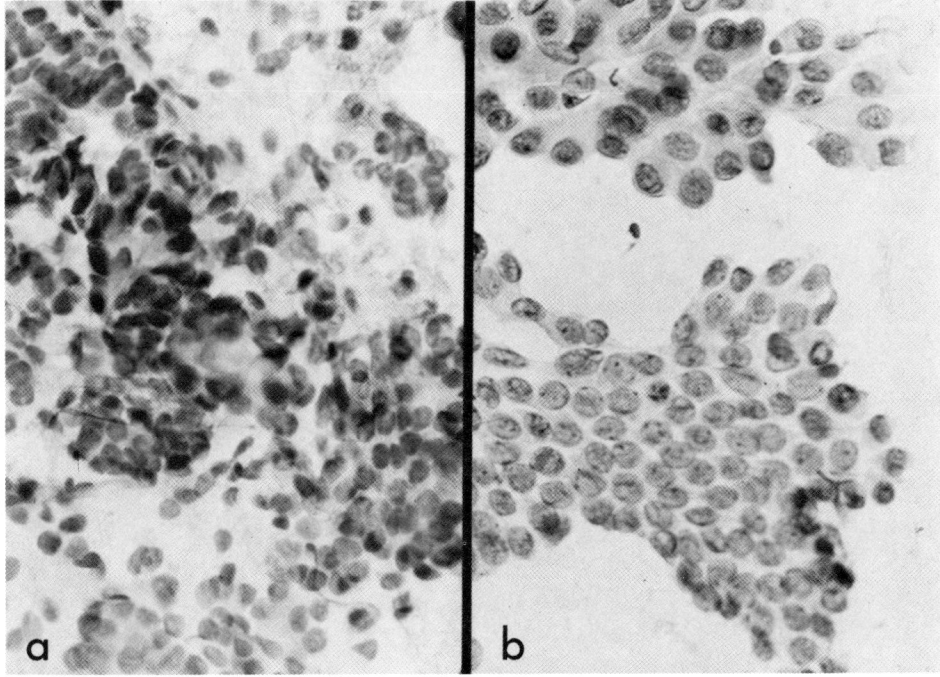

a   b

Fig. 3.8. **A.** This cellular aspirate from a papillary carcinoma is considered unsatisfactory due to the lack of morphologic details as a result of partial air-drying. Papanicolaou preparation. × 630. **B.** An aspirate of papillary carcinoma with monolayered tissue fragment showing typical cytomorphology in a well preserved specimen. Papanicolaou preparation. × 630.

19

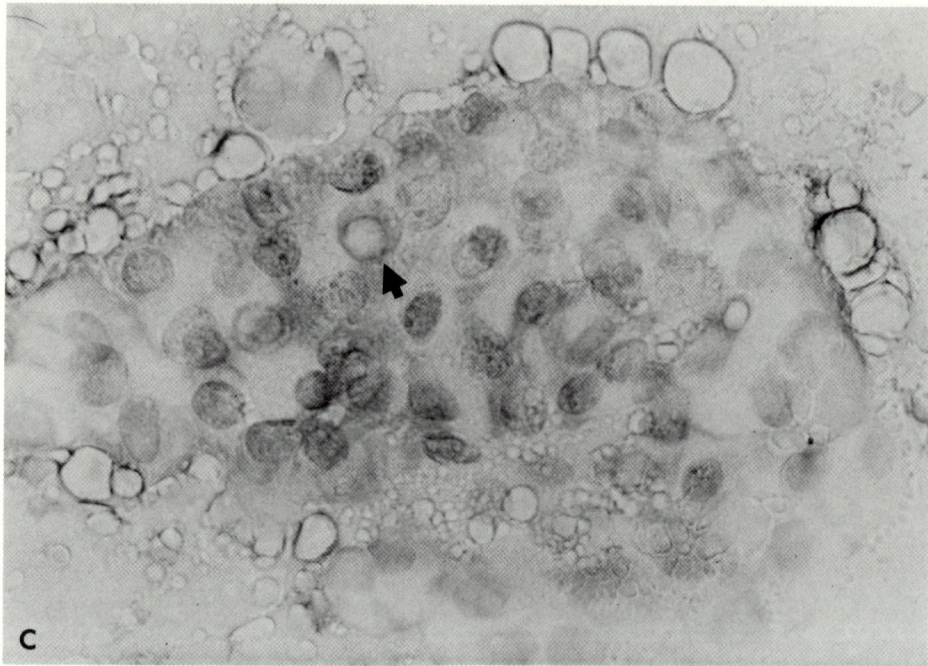

Fig. 3.8. C. Papanicolaou-stained aspirate of papillary carcinoma. Unsatisfactory for cytologic evaluation due to air-drying. Note intranuclear cytoplasmic inclusion (*arrow*). Papanicolaou preparation. × 630.

TABLE 3.3. Situations Resulting in Unsatisfactory Diagnoses

ABC	Explanation and Recommendation
Acellular, bloody	Can be due to multiple reasons (see Table 3.1). Repeat biopsy.
Poor fixation, air-drying (specimen may be adequate in terms of cellularity) (see Fig. 3.8)	Repeat if cells appear atypical.
Only histiocytes and inflammatory cells; no follicular epithelium (nondiagnostic) (see Fig. 3.2)	Most probably cystic nodular goiter; malignancy cannot be ruled out. Reaspirate if recurs. Try aspiration biopsy on residual if palpable. *Clinical correlation essential.*
Only lymphocytes present (see Fig. 3.3)	Confirm that needle was in thyroid, not adjacent lymph node. If sample is from thyroid and if Hashimoto's thyroiditis is suspected, may be consistent with the fibrous variant. *Clinical correlation essential.*
Only colloid present	May represent colloid cyst or colloid nodule. Cytologically unsatisfactory, clinically benign. *Clinical correlation essential.*
Abundant colloid, few follicular cells (see Fig. 3.1)	May represent colloid nodule. If the lesion is over 2 cm, low cellularity can be due to sampling (degeneration and necrosis is common in large lesions). Repeat biopsy recommended.
Few well-preserved follicular cells, colloid absent or scant	Two possibilities if follicular cells are of normal size: (1) nodular goiter; (2) needle in the adjacent normal parenchyma. Repeat biopsy.
Few atypical follicular cells (see Fig. 3.6)	Repeat biopsy.
Stromal cells only (see Fig. 3.4)	Granulation tissue, healing phase of granulomatous thyroiditis, fibrous variant of Hashimoto's thyroiditis. Repeat biopsy.

GENERAL GUIDELINES FOR EVALUATION OF A SMEAR AND REPORTING SYSTEM

A prepared and stained smear of a thyroid aspirate is usually evaluated in three steps. The initial step consists of examination using a 4× objective. This allows evaluation of the following:

1. Assessment of cellularity, ie, adequacy
2. Information regarding concentration of the cellular material in any particular areas of the slide
3. Architectural pattern of the tissue fragments
4. Background features, eg, absence or presence of colloid and its amount, blood, diathesis, calcific debris, inflammatory infiltrate, granuloma, etc

The next step involves examination using a 10× objective to assess the architectural pattern of the tissue fragments, eg, sheet versus syncytium, regular or irregular follicular patterns, and cytomorphology. Most often, a diagnosis can be made after this second step.

The last step involves examination under a 40× objective for assessment of the nuclear size of follicular cells as compared with intact red blood cells, which are the best indicators of size. This helpful feature is lost if the smear is wet fixed in ethyl alcohol or Carbowax, which results in hemolysis of red blood cells.

Once the smear is evaluated, the findings are reported as per the reporting system presented in Table 3.4.

CYTOPREPARATORY TECHNIQUE

Sudha R. Kini, M.D. and M. Jane Smith-Purslow, B.S., CT., ASCP, CMIAC

The importance of optimal cytopreparatory technique and staining cannot be overemphasized. An inferior cytologic preparation will not allow an adequate cytopathologic evaluation.

Several methods exist for specimen collection, fixation, processing, and staining. The cytomorphology varies according to the mode of fixation, type of fixative, and choice of staining technique. Because of familiarity, convenience, or personal preference, every cytopathology laboratory has its own guidelines for specimen collection, cytopreparation, and staining. Cytologic criteria applicable to one preparation may not always apply to other types of preparation. The diagnostic criteria for various thyroid lesions described in this monograph are based on cellular details seen in the preparations from the Cytopathology Laboratory at Henry Ford Hospital in Detroit, Michigan. The cytologic criteria in differentiating certain thyroid neoplasms are very subtle and are dependent on the cellular details that are

TABLE 3.4. Reporting System for Thyroid Aspirates

Category	Observations
Unsatisfactory	I. Acellular
	II. Inadequate specimen
	III. Cellularity adequate, but air-drying or poor fixation*; too thick and bloody, obscuring cell details
Negative for cancer cells	I. Benign follicular cells consistent with nodular goiter
	II. Lymphoid cells and follicular and/or Hürthle cells consistent with lymphocytic thyroiditis[†]
	III. Lymphoid cells and large multinucleated giant cells consistent with granulomatous thyroiditis
Abnormal (also includes suspicious[‡] diagnosis)	I. Follicular cells with syncytial-type tissue fragments, suggestive of cellular adenoma
	II. Hürthle cell tumors
Positive—cancer cells present	Type the carcinoma

*For Papanicolaou-stained material.

[†]Presence of lymphocytes in an aspiration biopsy specimen may be nonspecific and may not necessarily represent Hashimoto's thyroiditis. Hence, the aspirate is reported as "lymphocytic thyroiditis."

[‡]A suspicious diagnosis is given when (1) cellular material is inadequate but suggestive of cancer; or (2) diagnostic criteria are insufficient for a definite diagnosis of malignancy.

best demonstrated in smears fixed with spray fixative and stained by Papanicolaou method. The architecture of the tissue fragments, relationship of one cell to the other, cytoplasmic quality, cell borders, nuclear chromatin, and nucleoli can all be appreciated very well in spray-fixed smears. The pros and cons of different methods of collection, fixation, and staining will be discussed.

Specimen Collection

Specimens obtained by an aspiration biopsy procedure can be submitted in the following ways:

1. Specimen expelled on the slides and smears prepared
2. Specimen collected in a preservative, eg, Saccamano fixative[5]
3. Rinsings of the needle in balanced salt solution after smears have been made
4. Cyst fluid with or without fixative

Smear Preparation

There are several different techniques of smear preparation (see Chapter 2, on Techniques of Fine-Needle Aspiration Biopsy). These techniques include:

1. Peripheral blood smear technique (Fig. 2.5, Fig. 3.9D–G)
2. Squeezing the tissue particles between the glass slide and pulling them apart (Fig. 3.9B)

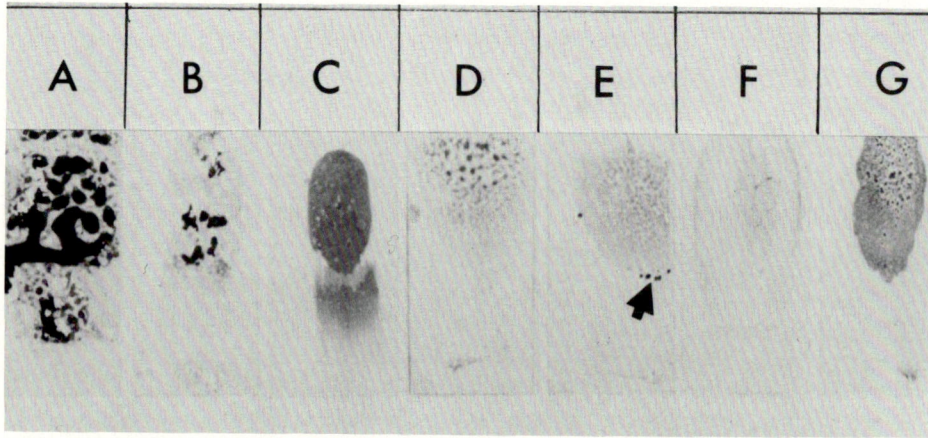

Fig. 3.9. Preparation of aspirate smears. **A.** Too thick—unsatisfactory due to too much blood. **B.** Large crushed particles. Unsatisfactory due to excessive thickness. **C.** Abundant colloid. **D–G.** Ideally prepared, thin cell spreads. Note concentration of the cellular material at the advancing edge of the smeal (*arrow*) (in peripheral blood smear technique). Also note granular particles—a pattern often noted in aspirates of papillary carcinoma.

We prefer and recommend using plain glass slides with frosted ends. In our experience, cellular distortion is seen on smears prepared using fully frosted slides.

Fixation

Smears may be air-dried if Romanowsky stains are used, but wet fixation is necessary for Papanicolaou stains. The methods of wet fixation include:

1. Spray fixative
2. 95% ethyl alcohol—universally accepted as best fixative for Papanicolaou stain
3. Isopropyl alcohol
4. Specimen collected in Saccamano fixative

Several spray fixatives are commercially available. The smears must be immediately flooded with the spray fixative. The spray can should be held at least 12 in. from the slide. Once sprayed, the fixative must be completely dried.* It is removed by soaking in 95% ethyl alcohol before staining. The advantages of spray fixatives are several.

---

*Do not enclose the wet slides in a cardboard folder, as cellular material will adhere to the cardboard folder and be lost forever.

They are inexpensive, less messy than other fixatives, and easy to store. Cellular details are well preserved and are easy to interpret, and the red blood cells in the background are not hemolyzed. The intact red blood cells serve as a guide in judging the follicular nuclear size. The cytoplasm and the cell borders are preserved, and nuclear chromatin and nucleoli are beautifully displayed. *There are no disadvantages to using spray fixatives.*

The universally accepted, ideal fixative for Papanicolaou stain is 95% ethyl alcohol. Also, 80% isopropyl alcohol is sometimes used as a fixative. These fixatives have the following disadvantages:

1. Alcohol hemolyzes the red blood cells, ie, it is cytolytic and it also destroys the cytoplasm of epithelial cells. The relationship of one cell to the other is often lost. This can be avoided if the specimen is collected in a preservative such as heparinized balanced salt solution. Aspiration biopsy specimens are often bloody. The precipitate after hemolysis of red blood cells interferes with the staining quality giving the eosinophilia.
2. The nuclei are also affected to some extent. They shrink, stain dark and compact, and the nucleoli are not often visualized unless a preservative (such as heparin) is used.
3. The thyroid aspirates generally do not adhere to the slides. There seems to be a "fall off" of cellular material when smears are dropped in the fixative. Precoating the slides with egg albumin to prevent the fall off will impart diffuse eosinophilia to the slide and the cells.
4. Ribbing effect is seen if the smears are not dropped swiftly into the alcohol container.
5. Finally, alcohol is flammable.

Saccamano fixative (2% Carbowax in 50% ethyl alcohol) has been recommended by some[5] as an ideal method of collecting aspirates. The specimen can be collected at any site away from the cytopathology laboratory. There is no fear of cell deterioration or air-drying, and there is no need for others to make thin cell spreads. A cell block can be prepared, if necessary. Saccomono fixative has these disadvantages:

1. Longer time needed for cytopreparation
2. Hemolysis of red cells will precipitate in background and cause nuclear shrinkage

Rinsing of the needle in balanced salt solution is used as an adjunct after the smears are made.

Procedure for Cyst Fluids

The gross quality of the cyst fluid determines the method for cytopreparation.

If the specimen is clear, centrifuge it at 2,000 rpm for 10 minutes. If the sediment is visible, make a wet-film preparation (see below). If the specimen is poorly cellular, process it by membrane-filter technique.[6]

If the specimen or sediment is grossly bloody, saponin technique may be used to hemolyze red cells[1,4], with one exception: If the wet film shows adequate cellularity, this technique is not required.

Toluidine Blue Wet-Film Preparation

The wet-film preparation of a sediment from the centrifuged specimen* allows rapid assessment as to its cellularity as well cell type, ie, benign or malignant. This examination guides cytotechnologists to follow a suitable method for processing the specimens and helps prevent cross-contamination. The method consists of the following steps:

1. Place a drop of centrifuged sediment on the slide.
2. Place one drop of toluidine blue solution* on the slide, and mix.
3. Coverslip and examine.

Saponin Technique[1,4]

Saponin is an enzyme that lyses red blood cells. A saponin solution†is extremely useful in processing grossly bloody specimens. Caution must be exercised not to use an excess of saponin, which may destroy the cellular component of the specimen. When saponin technique is controlled, it selectively lyses red blood cells. The technique used consists of the following steps:

1. Resuspend the sediment in 30 ml of balanced salt solution.
2. Add 5 drops of saponin solution and agitate gently for 1 minute.
3. Add 15 drops of calcium gluconate solution‡ to stop the action of saponin enzyme and mix well.
4. Centrifuge 10 minutes at 2,000 rpm.
5. If no sediment is visible, prepare by membrane-filter technique.
6. If the sediment is visible and clear of blood, prepare direct smears, spray fix, and stain. If the sediment is still very bloody, repeat above precedure. Saponin technique is not recommended more than twice, as it may lyse the cells of diagnostic importance. Any leftover sediment is further processed for a cell block (see below).

Agar Method for Cell Block[9]

The agar method for a cell block consists of the following steps[9]:

---

*Toluidine blue solution: 0.5 gm toluidine blue; 20 ml 95% ethyl alcohol; and 30 ml distilled water. Dissolve toluidine blue in alcohol, add distilled water, and store in a dark bottle. Refrigerate when not in use.

†Saponin solution: 1.0 gm saponin; 0.2 gm P-hydroxybenzoic acid sodium salt; and 100 ml distilled water. Mix thoroughly, filter through no. 8 μm membrane filter. Fungi grow very rapidly in this medium; saponin solution must be filtered on a weekly basis. Saponin (toxic, powder) is available from Fisher Scientific, cat. #S-672, 100 gm/bottle. (Fair Lawn, New Jersey 07410)

‡Calcium gluconate solution: 3.0 gm calcium gluconate; 0.02 gm P-hydroxybenzoic acid sodium salt; and 100 ml distilled water. Mix thoroughly, filter through no. 8 μm membrane filter. Calcium gluconate (powder, U.S.P.) is available from J.T. Baker Chemical Company, cat. #1272-1, 500 gm/bottle. (Phillipsburg, New Jersey 08865)

1. Agitate the tube containing the sediment remaining after smears have been prepared.

2. Add 4 ml of 6% melted agar to the sediment, and mix well.

3. Centrifuge for 10 minutes at 2,000 rpm to make a cell button.

4. Refrigerate the tube until the agar is completely solidified (approximately 30 minutes).

5. Gently pry the agar clot from the tube. Slice the visible material in thin sections, and process for paraffin embedding.

Papanicolaou Staining Procedure for Thyroid Aspirates

Papanicolaou stain is generally used for thyroid aspirates in our laboratory.

1.	95% ethyl alcohol	15 minutes
2.	Deionized water	20 dips
3.	Lerner hematoxylin*	1–3 minutes
4.	Deionized water	20 dips
5.	Deionized water	20 dips
6.	Lerner bluing†	1 minute
7.	Deionized water	20 dips
8.	95% ethyl alcohol	10 dips
9.	Cyto-Stain‡	1–3 minutes
10.	95% ethyl alcohol	10 dips
11.	95% ethyl alcohol	10 dips
12.	Absolute alcohol	1 minute
13.	Xylene	1 minute

REFERENCES

1. Coughlin D, Lukeman JM: The use of saponin for hemolysis in effusion cytology. *Acta Cytol* 26:739,1982.

2. Droese M: *Cytological Aspiration Biopsy of the Thyroid.* Stuttgart, F.K. Schattauer-Verlag, 1980, pp. 10–11.

3. Frable WJ: *Thin Needle Aspiration Biopsy.* Philadelphia, Saunders, 1983, p. 153.

4. Gill G: Personal communication.

5. Jennings AS, Atkinson BF: Thyroid needle aspiration: collecting and handling the specimen. *N Engl J Med* 308:1602–1603, 1983.

6. Kini SR, Smith MJ: Diagnostic cytology by membrane filter. *Application Bulletin 100.* Ann Arbor, Gelman Sciences, 1978.

*Lerner hematoxylin is available from American Scientific Products, McGaw, IL, #53140-2.
†Lerner bluing is available from American Scientific Products, McGaw, IL, #57737-41.
‡Cyto-Stain is available from Richard Allen Medical Industries, Richland, MI.

7. Kini SR, Miller JM, Hamburger JI, Smith-Purslow MJ: Cytopathology of follicular lesions of the thyroid gland. *Diagn Cytopathol* 1:123–132, 1985.

8. Miller JM, Kini SR, Hamburger JI: *Needle Biopsy of the Thyroid.* New York, Praeger Publishers, 1983, p. 177.

9. Smith-Purslow MJ, Kini SR: 1985 *Cytopathology Laboratory Manual*, Henry Ford Hospital, Detroit, Michigan.

4

Concepts Basic to Thyroid Cytopathology

Aspiration biopsy is essentially a microbiopsy. The aspirated material contains minute tissue fragments that retain the architectural pattern of the lesion even when smeared on the slide, and is very similar to that seen in paraffin-embedded hematoxylin-and- eosin–stained sections. The only difference is that the thickness of the cellular material is not uniform as in a section cut by a microtome. What makes the aspiration biopsy specimen so interesting is that the nuclear morphology and cytoplasmic differentiation can be appreciated in great detail, especially in Papanicolaou-stained preparations. Thus, ABC is a blend of histopathology and cytopathology, and interpretation of architectural configuration of the tissue fragments (pattern diagnosis) as well as cytomorphology of their component cells and isolated cells (exfoliative cytopathology) are both integral parts of the evaluation. Mere pattern diagnosis or cytomorphologic evaluation is inadequate. A sound knowledge of surgical pathology and expertise in cytopathology are essential.

How does one evaluate the architectural pattern of tissue fragments in cytologic preparations and why is a given tissue fragment papillary or follicular? To appreciate these patterns, certain expressions frequently used in cytopathology are described here.

A tissue fragment[1] (Plate 4.1) is a multicellular tissue formation.

A sheet[2] (Plate 4.2) is a tissue fragment in which the component cells are regularly arranged in relation to one another and possess distinct cell boundaries. The nuclear polarity is maintained, eg, mesothelium with its single layer.

A syncytium[2] (Plate 4.3) is a tissue fragment consisting of cells that are irregularly arranged with respect to one another and have indistinct cell borders. The nuclear polarity is altered.

A cluster[2] (Plate 4.4) is a tissue fragment with a three-dimensional grouping of cells; eg, a thyroid follicle seen in its entirety, a tip of the papilla in papillary carcinoma.

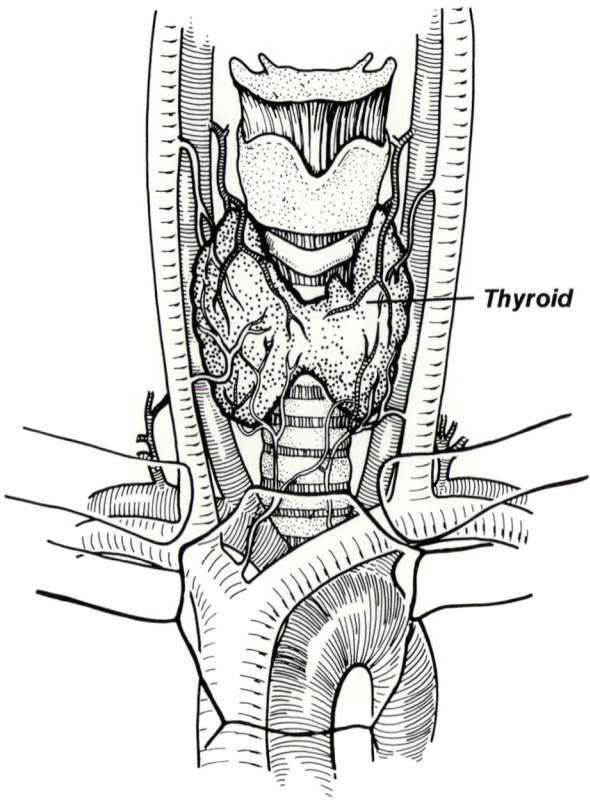

Thyroid

Fig. 4.1. Anatomy of the thyroid.

Most thyroid cancers are differentiated carcinomas. Unlike the diagnosis of anaplastic carcinoma, which can easily be made from bizarre pleomorphic cells presenting glaring malignant criteria (Plate 4.5), differentiated cancers are identified from (1) the architectural patterns of the tissue fragments, eg, papillary (Plate 4.6) or follicular (Plate 4.7); and (2) the cytomorphology of the component cells, which is equally important. The nuclear changes are generally very subtle. These include nuclear size more than shape, chromatin pattern, and presence or absence of nucleoli (Plate 4.8).

The various different structural aberrations presented in aspirated specimens of thyroid lesions can be best appreciated when anatomy and histology of the thyroid, as well as the basic concept of the thyroid follicle, are understood.

The normal thyroid gland is located in front of the neck, straddling across the trachea. It consists of two lobes joined by an isthmus (Fig. 4.1) and weighs approximately 15 gm. Each lobe consists of multiple lobules, and each lobule in turn is composed of several follicles (Fig. 4.2) supported by a delicate but very vascular connective tissue stroma. A follicle represents a unit of thyroid parenchyma. It is a three-dimensional closed sac (Fig. 4.3A) filled with colloid and lined by a single layer of cuboidal epithelium resting on a basement membrane. The nuclei of these cells are centrally located and round to oval with finely granular chromatin. The cell borders

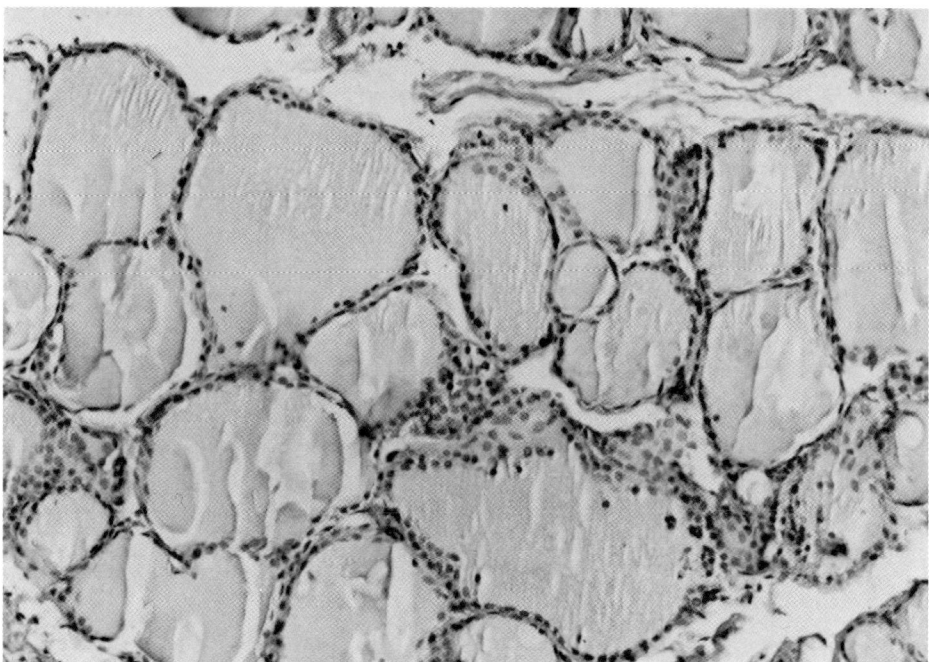

Fig. 4.2. Histologic section of the thyroid showing follicles containing colloid. The lining epithelium is low cuboidal. Hematoxylin and eosin preparation. × 250.

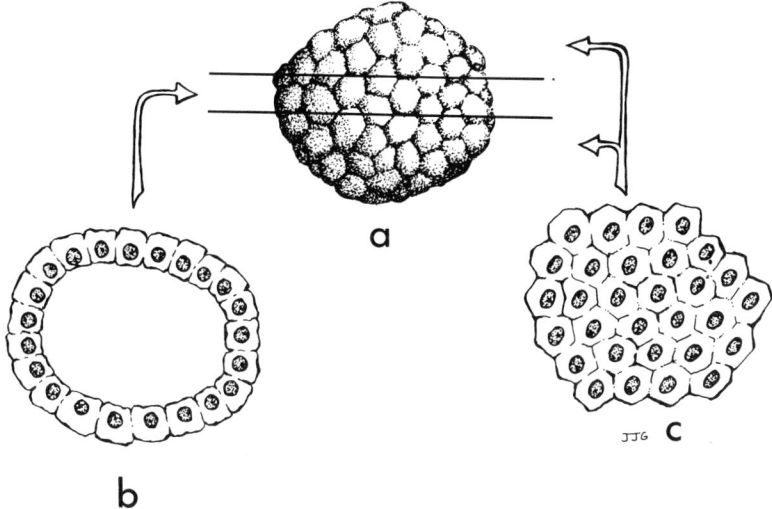

Fig. 4.3. A. Concept of normal thyroid follicle. **B.** Cross- section of the follicle. **C.** Follicle seen en face presenting a honeycomb pattern.

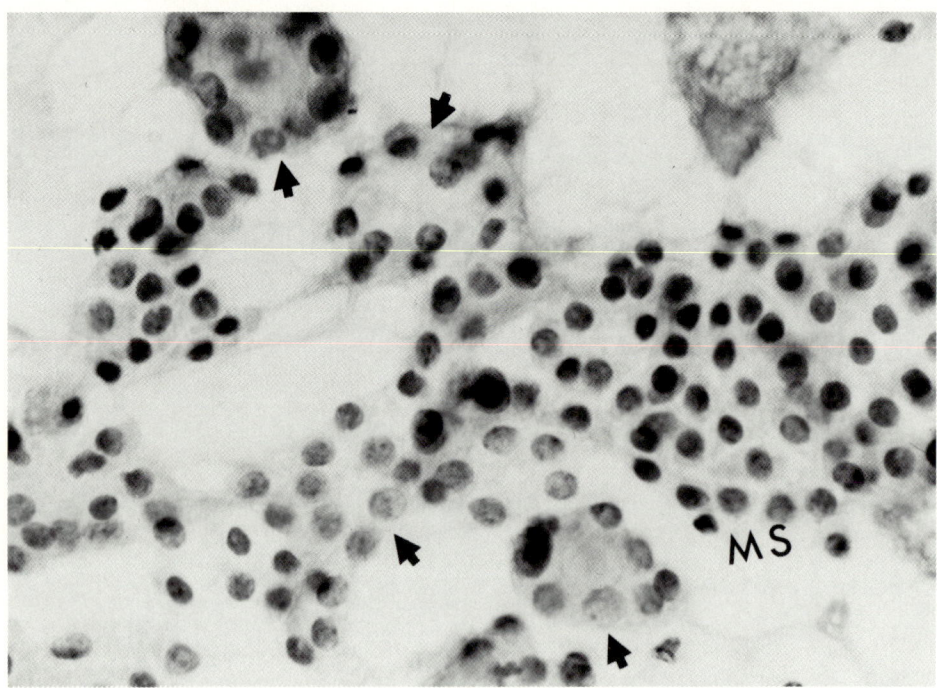

Fig. 4.4. Aspiration biopsy specimen of nodular goiter with regular follicles *(arrows)* and monolayered sheets *(MS)* of cells with honeycomb pattern similar to that in Fig. 4.5. Papanicolaou preparation. × 630.

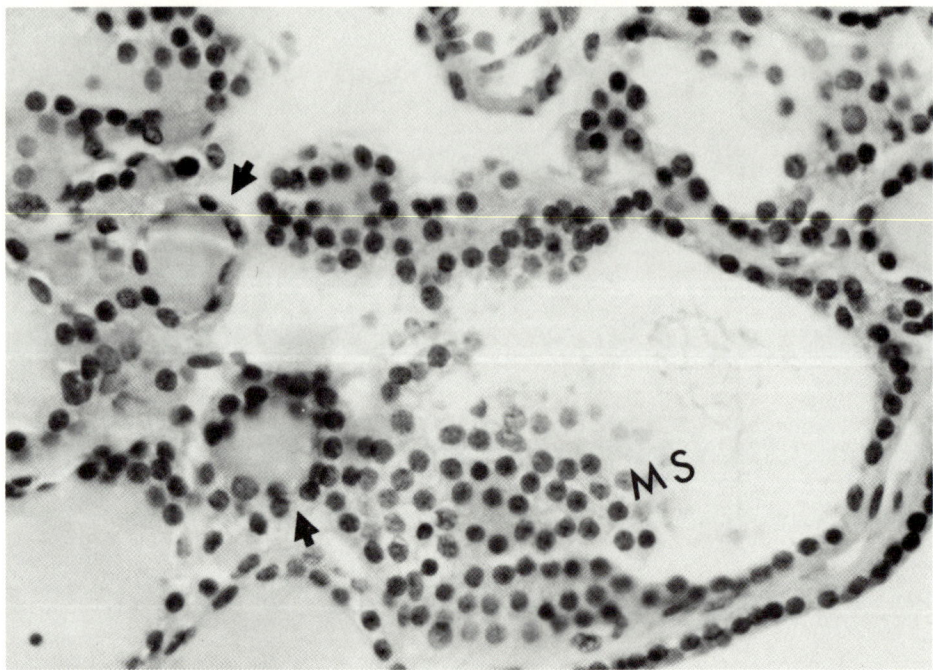

Fig. 4.5. Histologic section of nodular goiter with regular follicles *(arrows)* and monolayered sheet *(MS)* with honeycomb pattern. Note similarity to Fig. 4.4. Hematoxylin and eosin preparation. × 160.

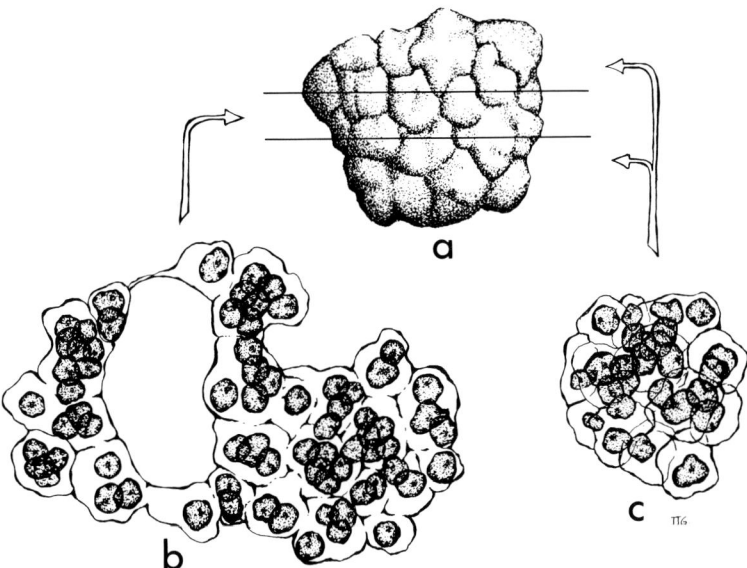

Fig. 4.6. **A.** Concept of neoplastic thyroid follicle. **B.** Cross-section of the neoplastic follicle. A lumen may or may not be present. **C.** Neoplastic follicle seen en face (control) showing syncytial-type tissue fragments with crowded and overlapped nuclei.

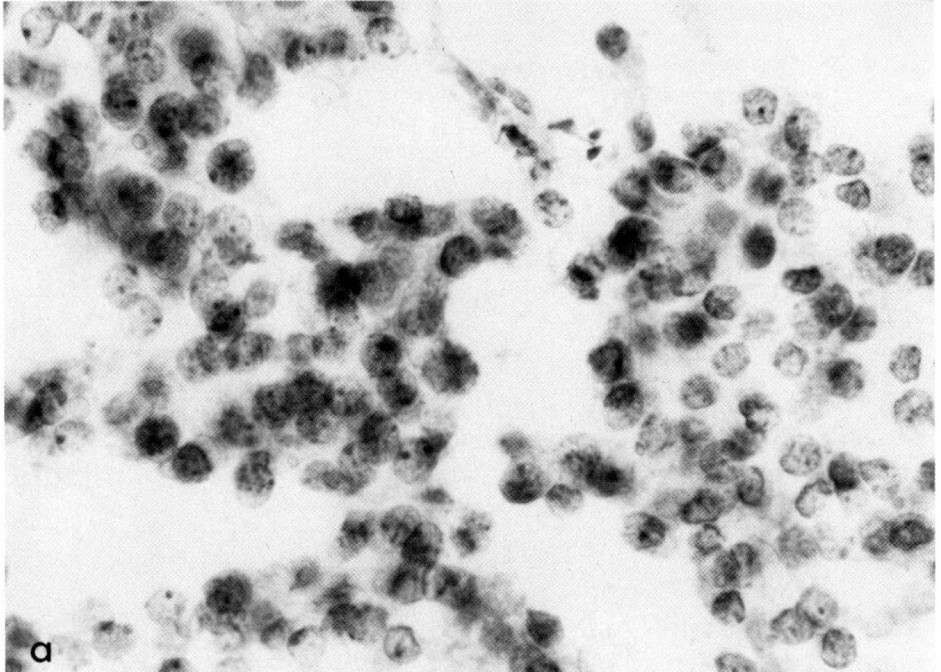

Fig. 4.7. **A.** A cellular follicular neoplasm showing syncytial type tissue fragments with and without follicular pattern. Compare the disturbed architecture to the uniform pattern of Fig. 4.4. Papanicolaou preparation. × 630.

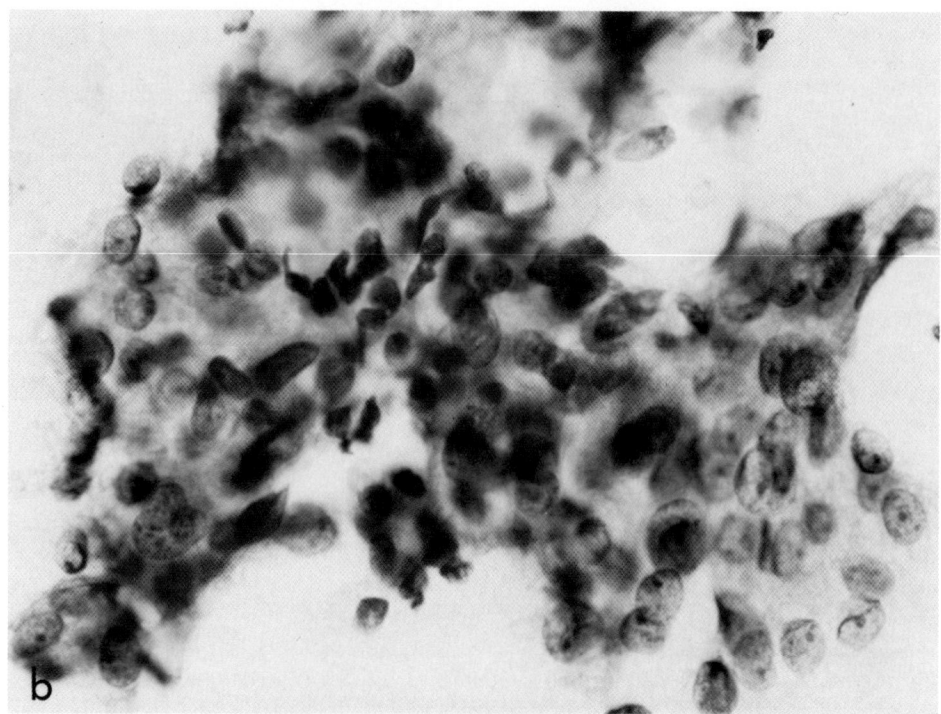

Fig. 4.7. B. Syncytial-type tissue fragments of follicular carcinoma. Note lack of two-dimensional configuration, i.e., monolayered sheet and uniform spacing of nuclei. Papanicolaou preparation. × 630.

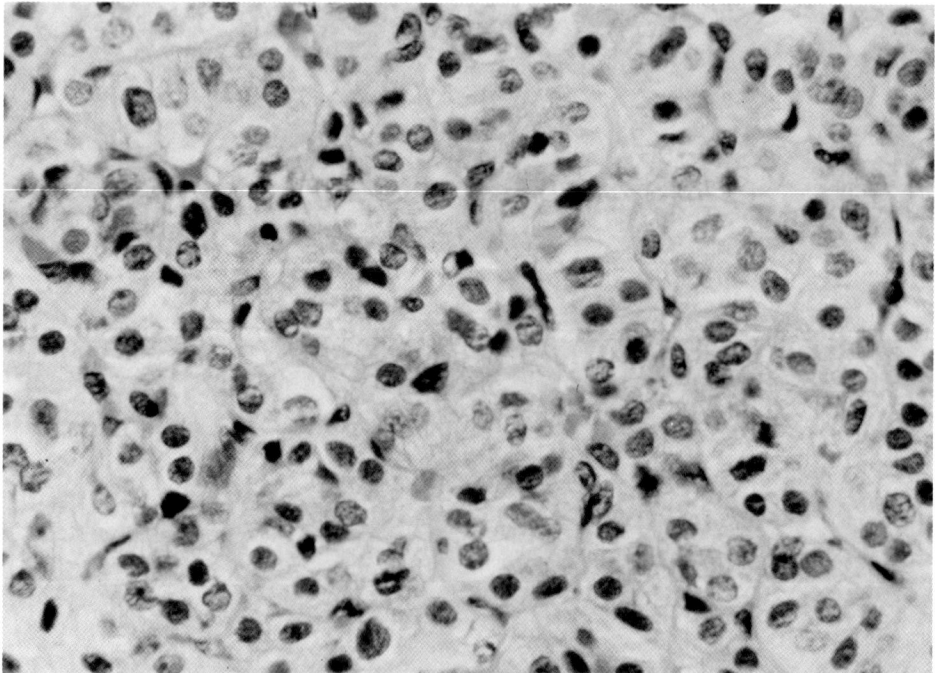

Fig. 4.8. Follicular carcinoma. Note hypercellularity of the neoplasm with poorly developed follicles and trabeculae. Hematoxylin and eosin preparation. × 400.

are well defined, and the cytoplasm is moderate. A follicle seen in cross-section appears as a ringlet of cuboidal cells, with regularly spaced nuclei and an appreciable amount of cytoplasm, around a central lumen (Fig. 4.3B). Viewed en face, it appears as a monolayered sheet of cells with well-defined cell borders and centrally spaced nuclei, giving a honeycomb pattern (Fig. 4.3C). This two-dimensional architecture results from the follicle being lined by a single layer of cells. Thus, depending on how the thyroid follicles are sectioned or smeared, they may appear as regular follicles or honeycomb sheets. Such a pattern is seen in non-neoplastic thyroid lesions, namely nodular goiter, both cytologically and histologically (Figs. 4.4 and 4.5). This regular arrangement of cells of a normal follicle is usually not seen in neoplastic lesions, be they benign or malignant. A neoplastic follicle is irregular (Fig. 4.6A), and whether seen in en face or in a cross-section, appears as a syncytial-type tissue fragment with poorly defined cell borders and crowded and overlapped nuclei (Figs. 4.6B and C). These structural aberrations are easily appreciated in aspirates of follicular neoplasms, both cytologically and histologically (Figs. 4.7 and 4.8).

With this understanding of the follicular structure, we can now focus on the papillary architecture of the tissue fragments, both in papillary hyperplasia and in papillary carcinoma of the thyroid. Papillary hyperplasia of the thyroid follicules involves an infolding of the lining epithelium composed of tall, columnar cells with basally located uniform nuclei (Fig. 4.9A). There is usually no central core of fibrovascular tissue.[3] In contrast, papillary carcinoma has a central core of fibrovascular tissue covered usually by one, and sometimes by more than one, layer of cells with crowded nuclei at all levels. It demonstrates altered polarity (Figs. 4.9B and 4.10).

Consider a papilla to be a three-dimensional structure, and an ear of corn best fits its description (Fig. 4.11). The central fibrovascular core is represented by the cob, and the lining cells are represented by a single layer of kernels. As most papillary carcinomas show a single layer of cells covering the stalk, the patterns of tissue fragments of papillary carcinoma in cytologic samples can be reproduced by sections of the corn in different planes (Figs. 4.12–4.15). A similar analogy can be made for a hyperplastic papilla, although it lacks the central stromal core.

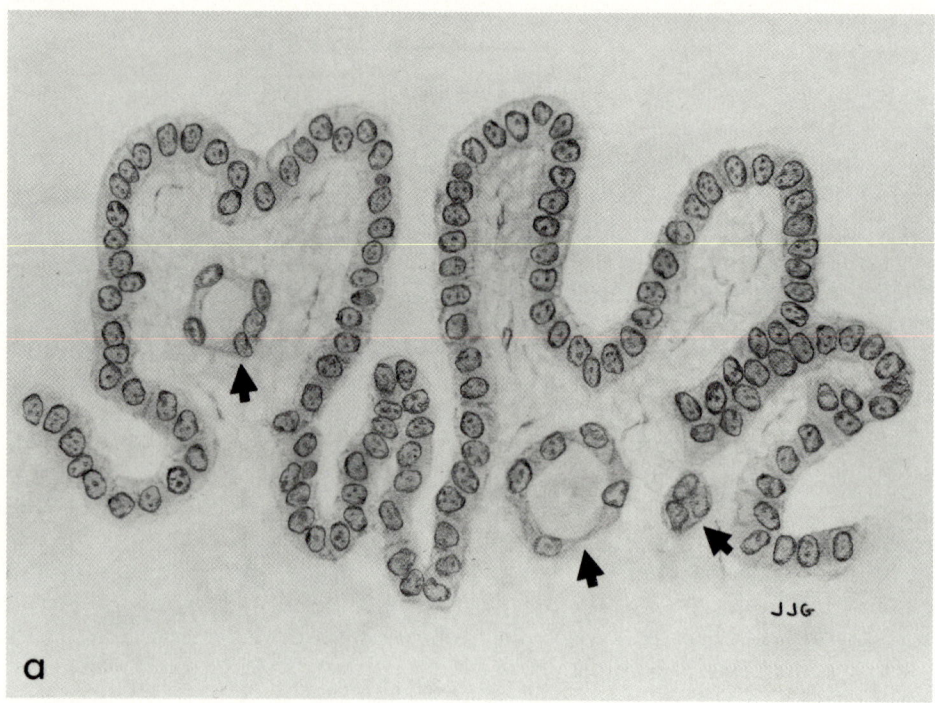

Fig. 4.9. A. Concept of hyperplastic papillae; uniform epithelium with basally located nuclei covering fibrous tissue stroma, containing follicular elements *(arrows)*.

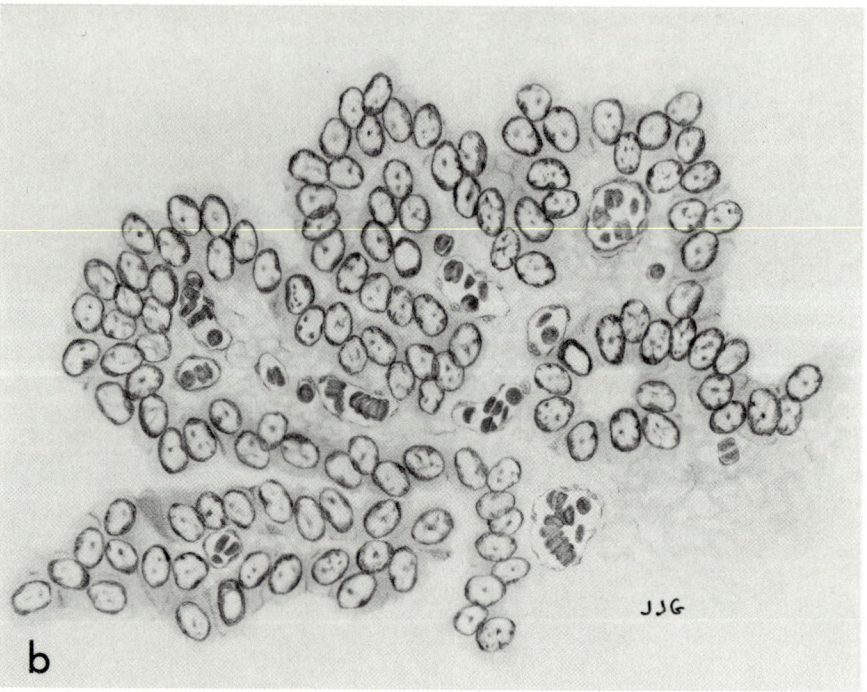

Fig. 4.9. B. Concept of papillae of papillary carcinoma; with central fibrovascular connective tissue stromal core covered by epithelium with crowded and overlapped nuclei at all levels.

36

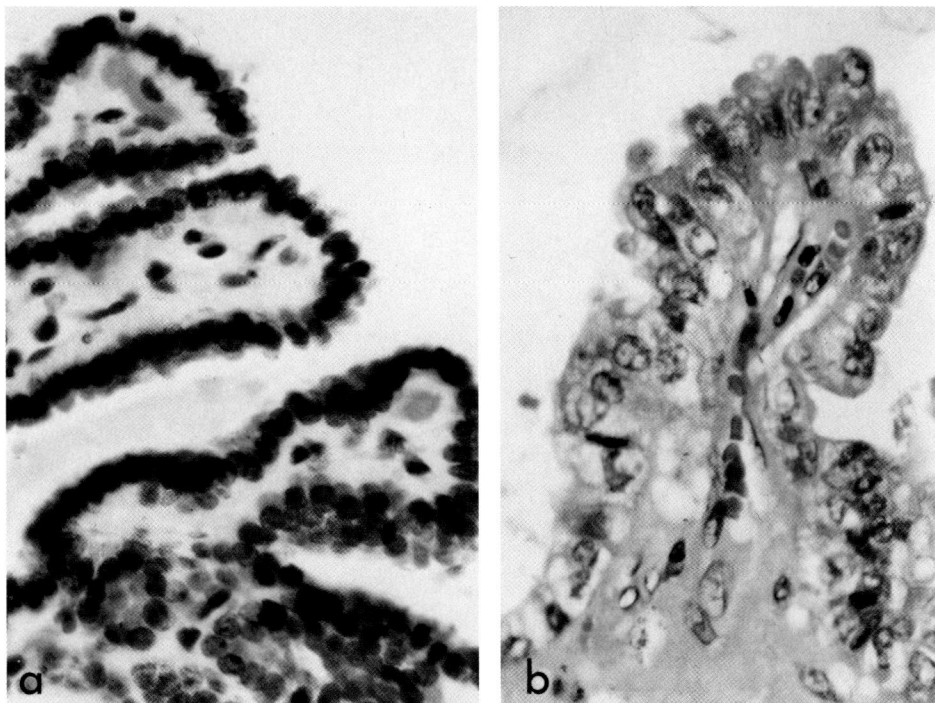

Fig. 4.10. A. Papillary hyperplasia. Hematoxylin and eosin preparation. × 400. B. Papillary carcinoma. Note similarity to Fig. 4.9A and B. Hematoxylin and eosin preparation. × 400.

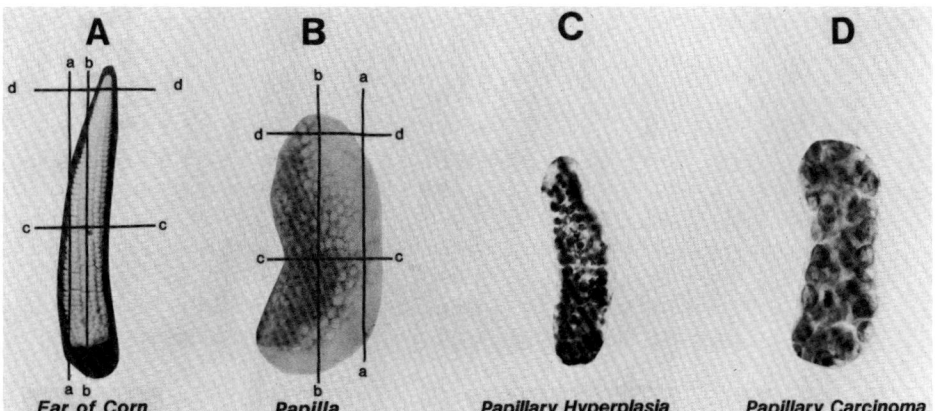

Fig. 4.11. A. Corn on the cob seen en face best fits the description of the three-dimensional nature of a papilla of papillary carcinoma. B. Concept of papilla with a three-dimensional form. C. Hyperplastic papilla seen en face. Papanicolaou preparation. × 630. D. Papilla of carcinoma seen en face. Papanicolaou preparation. × 630. Note smooth external contour and peripheral palisading of nuclei. The similarity to an ear of corn is very apparent. Sections through different planes—*aa*, sagital through superficial area; *bb*, sagital section through the core; *cc*, transverse section; *dd*, transverse section through the tip—are illustrated in Figs. 4.12–4.15.

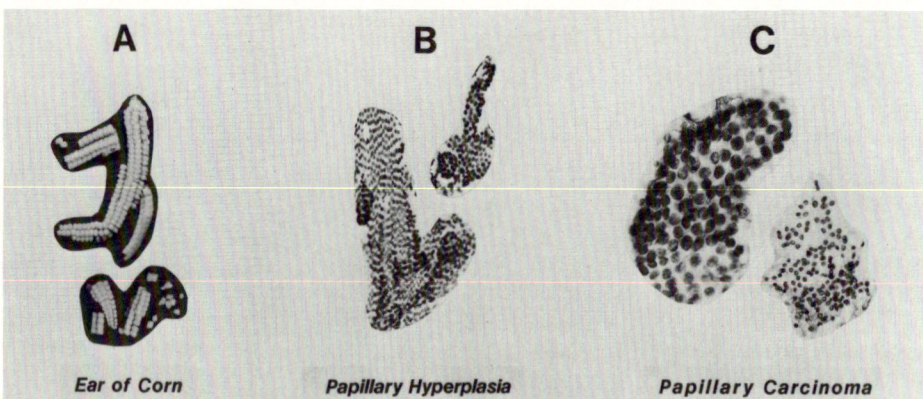

Fig. 4.12. A. Sagital section of corn on the cob through the superficial plane *aa* in Fig. 4.11.
B. Note monolayered configuration with a honeycomb pattern in hyperplasia. Papanicolaou
preparation. × 630. **C.** Note monolayered configuration but syncytial pattern in carcinoma
(left). Papanicolaou preparation. × 630. The cells may also appear isolated *(right)*.
Papanicolaou preparation. × 160. A branching papillary fragment may show monolayered
fragments with sweeping curves.

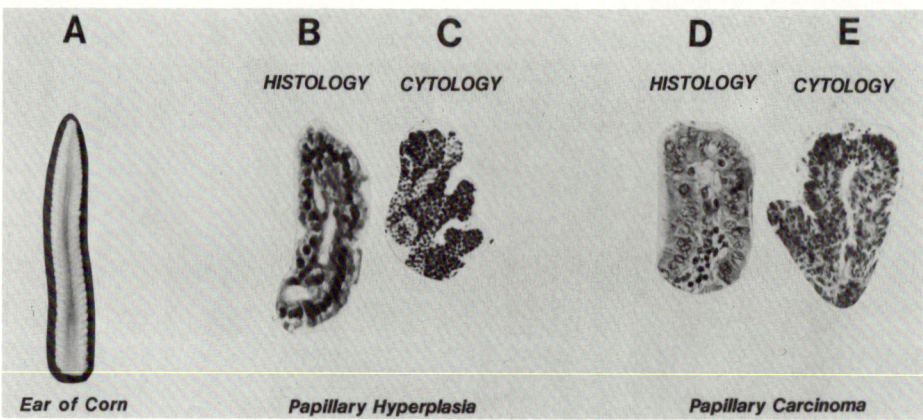

Fig. 4.13. A. Sagital section through the core *bb* in Fig. 4.11. **B.** Hyperplastic papilla
lacking central stromal core. Hematoxylin and eosin preparation. × 400. **C.** Without a
stromal core, the hyperplastic papilla will collapse in the process of smearing, thus appearing
monolayered with a honeycomb pattern. Papanicolaou preparation. × 160. **D.** Papilla of
carcinoma with central stromal core. Hematoxylin and eosin preparation. × 400. **E.** Papilla
of carcinoma demonstrating central stromal core and lining cells with a feathery pattern.
Papanicolaou preparation. × 400.

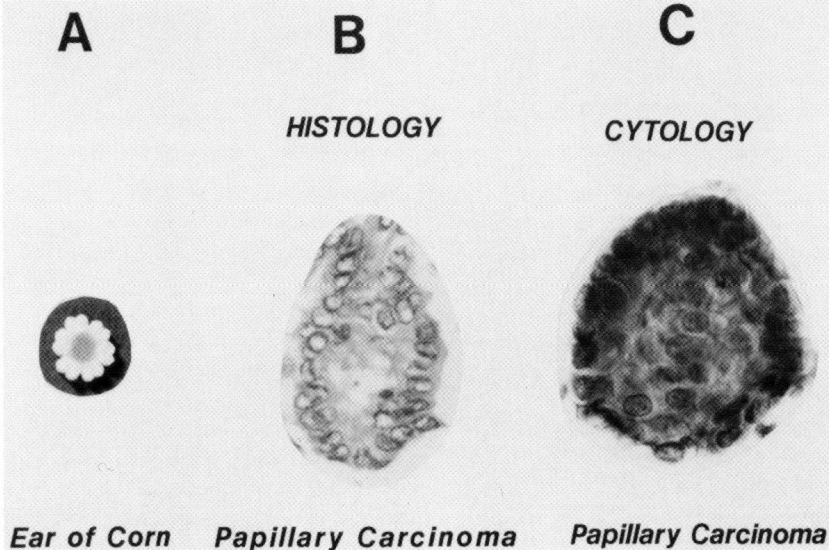

Fig. 4.14. A. Transverse section *cc* in Fig. 4.11. Note central stromal core presenting an alveolar pattern. The stromal core is difficult to visualize in cytologic preparations. **B.** Hematoxylin and eosin preparation. × 400. **C.** Papanicolaou preparation. × 630.

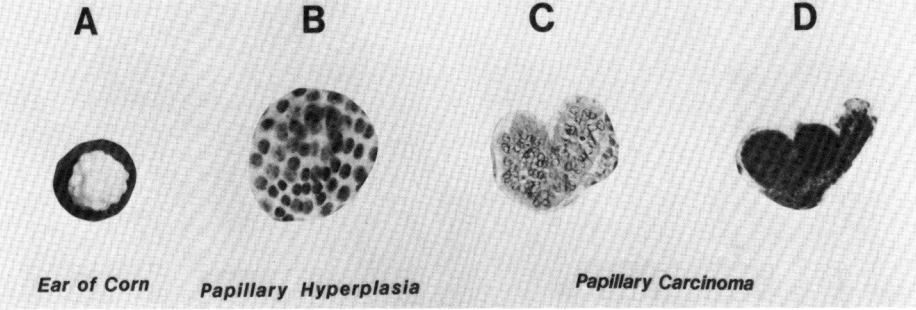

Fig. 4.15. A. Transverse section *dd* through the tip in Fig. 4.11. **B.** As the stromal core may be absent at the tip, a cross-section at this level shows only a ball of cells, with a whirled pattern in nodular goiter. Papanicolaou preparation. × 630. It may also show a three-dimensional pattern with marked crowding and overlapping in carcinoma. **C.** Hematoxylin and eosin preparation. × 400. **D.** Papanicolaou preparation. × 630.

COLOR PLATE

Plate 4.1. Tissue fragment—a multicellular formation. Papanicolaou preparation. × 630.

Plate 4.2. Sheet of cells with well-defined cell borders and nuclei maintaining their polarity. Papanicolaou preparation. × 630.

Plate 4.3. Syncytium of cells with poorly defined cell borders and crowded overlapping nuclei with altered polarity. Papanicolaou preparation. × 630.

Plate 4.4. Cluster with three-dimensional grouping of cells. Papanicolaou preparation. × 630.

Plate 4.5. Anaplastic carcinoma with bizarre nuclei displaying criteria of malignancy. Papanicolaou preparation. × 630.

Plate 4.6. Papillary carcinoma with papillary tissue fragments. Papanicolaou preparation. × 630.

Plate 4.7. Follicular carcinoma with tissue fragments exhibiting follicular pattern. Papanicolaou preparation. × 630.

Plate 4.8. A tissue fragment from papillary carcinoma showing typical nuclear cytomorphology. Papanicolaou preparation. × 630.

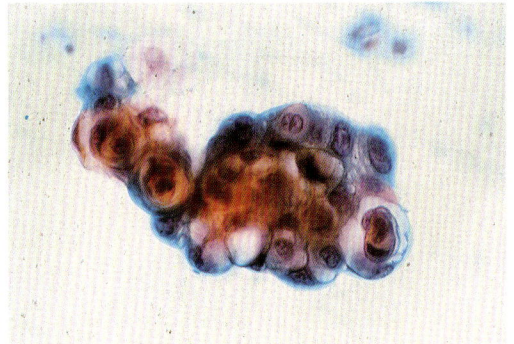

Plate 4.1.

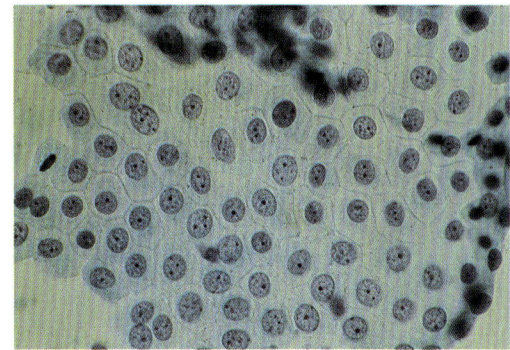

Plate 4.2.

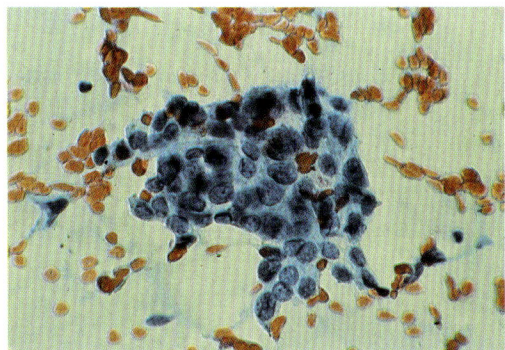

Plate 4.3.

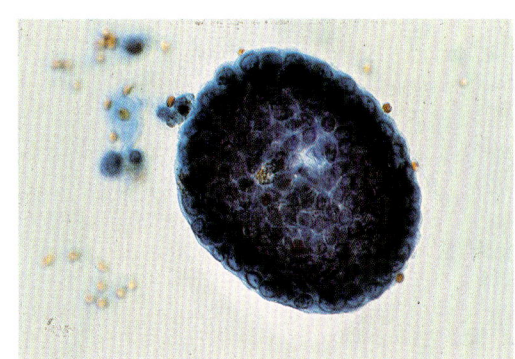

Plate 4.4.

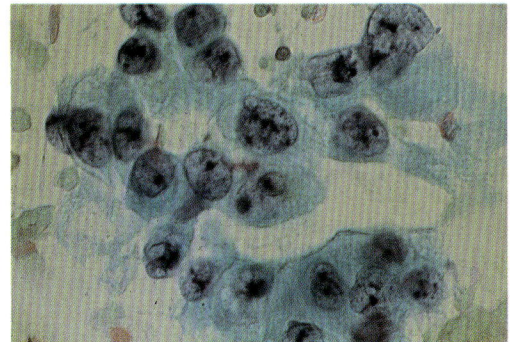

Plate 4.5.

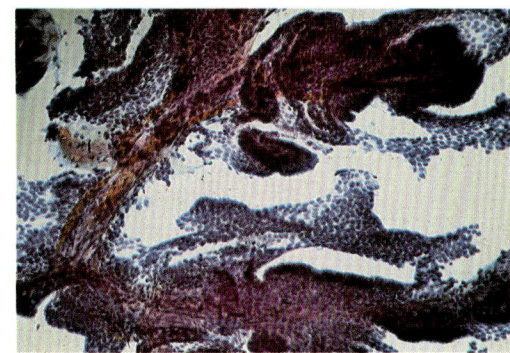

Plate 4.6.

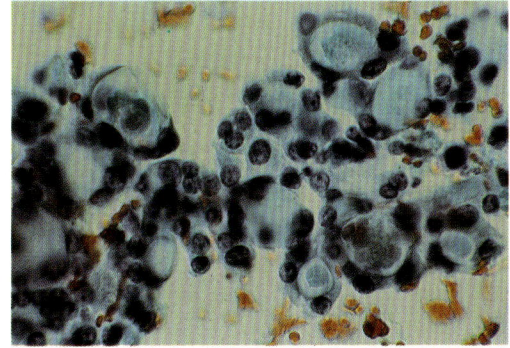

Plate 4.7.

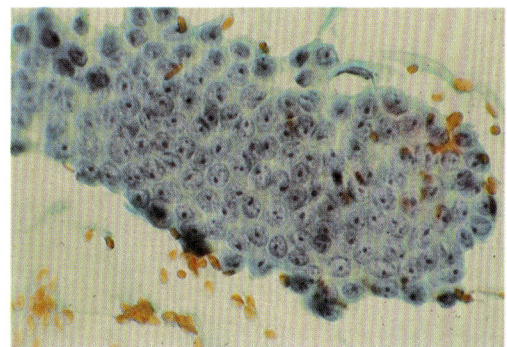

Plate 4.8.

COLOR PLATE

Plate 6.1. Cytologic patterns of follicular lesions of thyroid. **A.** Hyperplastic goiter showing mono-layered tissue fragments with honeycomb pattern and uniform, small nuclei. Papanicolaou preparation. × 630. **B.** Cellular adenoma with syncytial-type tissue fragments with uniformly enlarged and crowded nuclei. Papanicolaou preparation. × 630. **C.** Follicular carcinoma with syncytial-type tissue fragments with considerably enlarged pleomorphic nuclei that are crowded and overlapped. Papanicolaou preparation. × 630. **D.** Follicular variant of papillary carcinoma. Syncytial-type tissue fragments with mildly enlarged, but crowded and overlapped, nuclei. Note powdery chromatin and intranuclear cytoplasmic inclusions (*arrow*). Papanicolaou preparation. × 630.

Plate 6.2. **A.** Nodular goiter. Papanicolaou preparation. × 630. **B.** Simple adenoma. Papanicolaou preparation. × 630. Both **A** and **B** show tissue fragments of follicular epithelium with follicular pattern. The nuclei are small and uniform. Note the morphologic similarities between **A** and **B**.

Plate 6.3. **A.** Hyperplastic nodular goiter. Papanicolaou preparation. × 630. **B.** Cellular adenoma. Papanicolaou preparation. × 630. There is a distinct difference in architectural patterns of tissue fragments—honeycomb in **A**, and syncytial type in **B**. Also the nuclei are larger in cellular adenoma compared with nodular goiter.

Plate 6.4. **A.** Hyperplastic goiter. Papanicolaou preparation. × 630. **B.** Follicular carcinoma. Papanicolaou preparation. × 630. Although both aspirates are cellular, the architectural pattern in follicular carcinoma is syncytial type, with marked crowding and overlapping of enlarged nuclei containing nucleoli. This is in contrast to the honeycomb pattern with uniform, small nuclei in hyperplastic goiter.

Plate 6.5. **A.** Macrofollicular adenoma. Mono-layered tissue fragments with honeycomb pattern and abundant colloid in the background are characteristic of hyperinvoluted goiter or macrofollicular adenoma. Papanicolaou preparation. × 630. **B.** Follicular carcinoma. A syncytial-type tissue fragment with extreme crowding and overlapping of enlarged nuclei. The difference between **A** and **B** is striking. Papanicolaou preparation. × 630.

Plate 6.6. **A.** Cellular adenoma. Papanicolaou preparation. × 630. **B.** Follicular carcinoma. Papanicolaou preparation. × 630. The architectural pattern of tissue fragments in both is similar. The nuclei in **B** are larger and have coarser chromatin than those in **A.** These differences are very subtle.

Plate 6.7. **A.** Cellular adenoma. Papanicolaou preparation. × 630. **B.** Follicular carcinoma. Papanicolaou preparation. × 630. The cytologic patterns in both **A** and **B** are almost identical.

Plate 6.8. **A.** Atypical adenoma. Papanicolaou preparation. × 630. **B.** Follicular carcinoma. Papanicolaou preparation. × 630. The cytomorphology in atypical adenoma may be more striking than in follicular carcinoma.

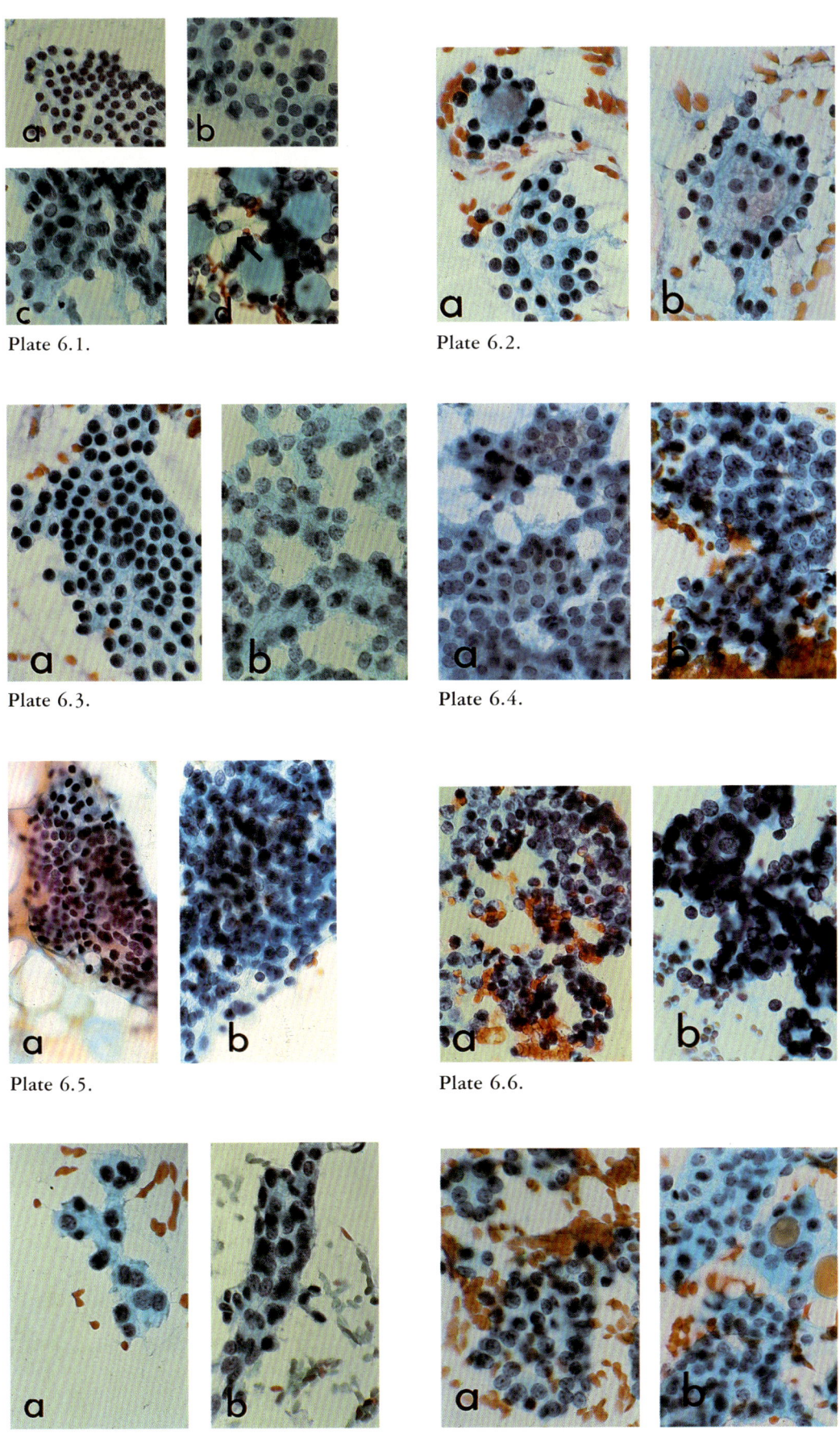

Plate 6.1.

Plate 6.2.

Plate 6.3.

Plate 6.4.

Plate 6.5.

Plate 6.6.

Plate 6.7.

Plate 6.8.

Plate 7.1. Three Hürthle cell tumors with different staining reactions of the cytoplasm. Note that the morphology is similar. **A.** Amphophilic. Papanicolaou preparation. × 630. **B.** Cyanophilic. Papanicolaou preparation. × 630. **C.** Oxyphilic. Papanicolaou preparation. × 630.

Plate 7.2. Hürthle cell tumor. **A.** Smear fixed with spray fixative showing diagnostic cytomorphology with finely granular chromatin and cherry-red macronucleolus. Papanicolaou preparation. × 630. **B.** Smear prepared on albuminized slide and fixed in 95% ethyl alcohol. Note loss of granular cytoplasm, compact chromatin. Nucleoli are seen infrequently. Papanicolaou preparation. × 630.

Plate 7.3. Various Hürthle cell lesions. **A.** Hürthle cell nodule of Hashimoto's thyroiditis. Tissue fragments of Hürthle cells, pleomorphic nuclei, and compact chromatin. Note lack of cherry-red macronucleoli. Papanicolaou preparation. × 630. **B.** Hürthle cell tumor with large polygonal cells, abundant granular cytoplasm, and uniform nuclei with cherry-red macronucleoli. Papanicolaou preparation. × 630. **C.** Sheet of Hürthle cells from nodular goiter nuclei. Note lack of macronucleoli. Papanicolaou preparation. × 630.

Plate 8.1. Papillary carcinoma. A papillary tissue fragment with central fibrovascular core demonstrating capillary loops. Papanicolaou preparation. × 630.

Plate 8.2. Papillary carcinoma. Multiple psammoma bodies exhibiting varied staining reaction. Papanicolaou preparation. × 630.

Plate 8.3. Follicular variant of papillary carcinoma with dense-staining colloid. Papanicolaou preparation. × 400.

Plate 8.5. **A.** Psammoma bodies in papillary carcinoma. Note typical nuclear cytomorphology. Papanicolaou preparation × 630. **B.** Psammoma bodies in nodular goiter. Note lack of typical nuclear cytomorphology of papillary carcinoma. Papanicolaou preparation. × 630.

Plate 8.4. Cystic papillary carcinoma. Papillary tissue fragment is obscured by blood and cellular debris. Papanicolaou preparation. × 630.

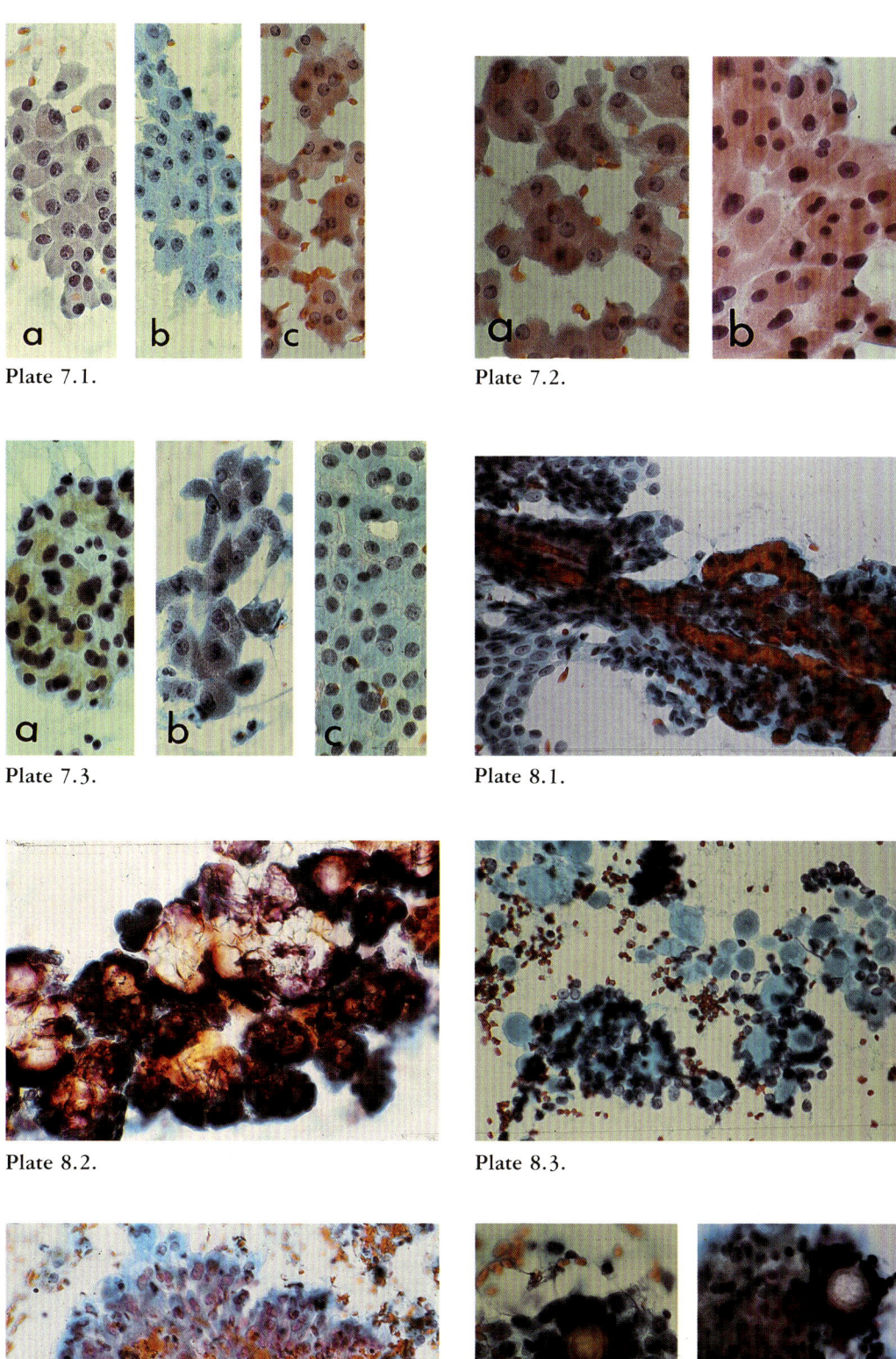

Plate 7.1.

Plate 7.2.

Plate 7.3.

Plate 8.1.

Plate 8.2.

Plate 8.3.

Plate 8.4.

Plate 8.5.

COLOR PLATE

Plate 10.1. Medullary carcinoma cells showing characteristic azurophilic granules in cytoplasm. Giemsa preparation. × 1000.

Plate 10.2. Medullary carcinoma cells showing calcitonin granules stained by immunoperoxidase technique. Avidin Biotin Complex method and Hematoxylin preparation. **A., B.** × 630.

Plate 10.3. Amyloid in aspiration biopsy specimens. **A.** Dense acellular material in background cannot be differentiated from colloid by Papanicolaou stain. Papanicolaou preparation. × 630. **B.** Same smear as in **A** stained by thioflavin T showing bright green fluorescence under ultraviolet light. thioflavin T preparation. × 630.

Plate 11.1. A. Hürthle cell nodule of Hashimoto's thyroiditis. Papanicolaou preparation. × 400. **B.** Hürthle cell tumor. Papanicolaou preparation. × 400. Note compact nuclear chromatin and lack of macronucleoli in **A**, and finely granular chromatin with nucleoli in **B**.

Plate 11.2. A. Follicular cells from Hashimoto's thyroiditis. Papanicolaou preparation. × 400. **B.** Cells of a cellular ademoma. Papanicolaou preparation. × 400. Note the morphologic similarity between **A** and **B**. Presence of lymphocytes in the background of **A** suggests the diagnosis of thyroiditis.

Plate 11.3. A. Marked atypia in follicular cells. As seen here, nuclei in Hashimoto's thyroiditis can be easily mistaken for carcinoma, but for the lymphocytes in the background. Papanicolaou preparation. × 630. **B.** Cells of follicular carcinoma appear bland compared with those in **A**. Papanicolaou preparation. × 630.

Plate 11.4. A. Aspirate of "lymphoid" variety of Hashimoto's thyroiditis which may be mistaken for malignant lymphoma. Papanicolaou preparation. × 1000. **B.** Malignant lymphoma. Papanicolaou preparation. × 1000.

Plate 14.1. A., B. Cyst fluid from nodular goiter. The follicular cells are clustered together and contain degenerating nuclei, which appear very atypical. The hemorrhagic debris obscures the cell details. This was interpreted as suspected papillary carcinoma. Papanicolaou preparation. × 630.

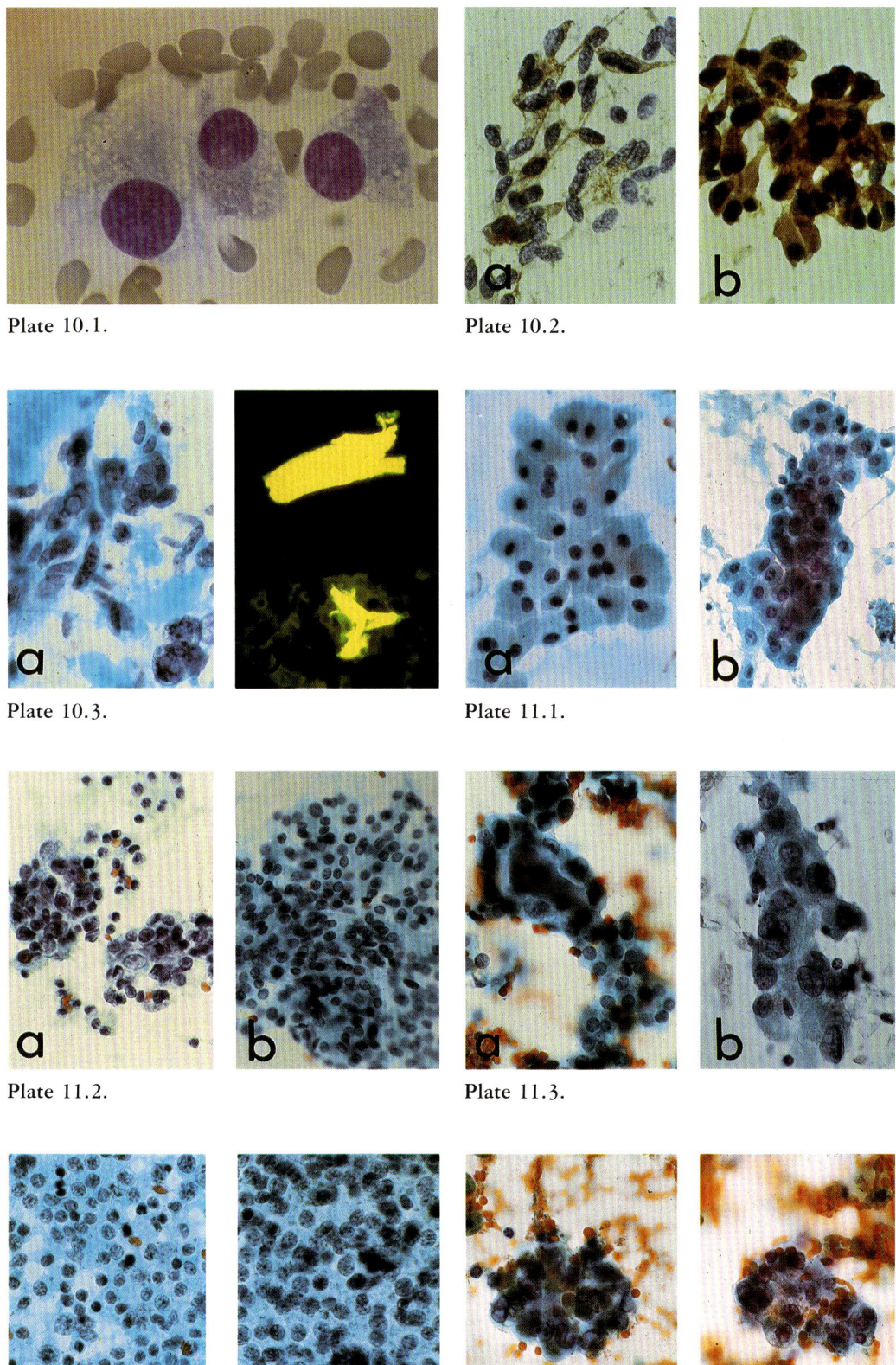

Plate 10.1.

Plate 10.2.

Plate 10.3.

Plate 11.1.

Plate 11.2.

Plate 11.3.

Plate 11.4.

Plate 14.1.

REFERENCES

1. Frost JK: *Concepts Basic to General Cytopathology*. Baltimore, The Johns Hopkins Press, 1972.

2. Patten SF Jr: Diagnostic cytology of the uterine cervix. In Weld GC (ed): *Monographs in Clinical Cytology*, vol. 3 New York, Karger, 1969, p. 5.

3. Vickery AL Jr: Thyroid papillary carcinoma: pathological and philosophical controversies. *Am J Surg Pathol* 7:797–807, 1983.

5

Nodular Goiter

Nodular goiter—synonyms of which include adenomatous goiter, colloid goiter, nontoxic nodular goiter, and multinodular goiter—is an enlargement of the thyroid caused by intermittent or persistent hyperplasia in response to thyroid-stimulating hormone or thyroid-growth immunoglobulin. These hormones are stimulated by hypothyroxinemia related to iodine deficiency, environmental goitrogens, or unknown factors. Nodular goiter is the most common benign condition mistaken for a thyroid tumor.[8]

PATHOLOGY

The gross pathology of nodular goiter depends on the developmental stage. In the initial phases of hyperplasia and involution, the gland is diffusely enlarged. As all the lobules do not react to the cyclic changes of hyperplasia and involution in a uniform fashion, nodularity eventually develops. These nodules vary considerably in size (Fig. 5.1); some are appreciated only microscopically, whereas others are large enough to cause clinical enlargement and pressure symptoms. One or more may be dominant, and clinically they cannot be differentiated from a neoplasm. Retrogressive changes due to a compromise of blood supply are frequent, characterized by infarction, hemorrhage, necrosis, cyst formation, fibrosis, and calcification.

The microscopic pathology is varied (Figs. 5.2–5.6). It includes small follicles without colloid that are lined by tall, columnar epithelium, sometimes with papillary changes during the hyperplastic phase; accumulation of colloid; and low cuboidal epithelium in the involution phase. Hyperinvolution is characterized by overdistention of the follicles with flattening of the lining epithelium. Hürthle cell metaplasia of follicular cells is common, either focal or diffuse.

41

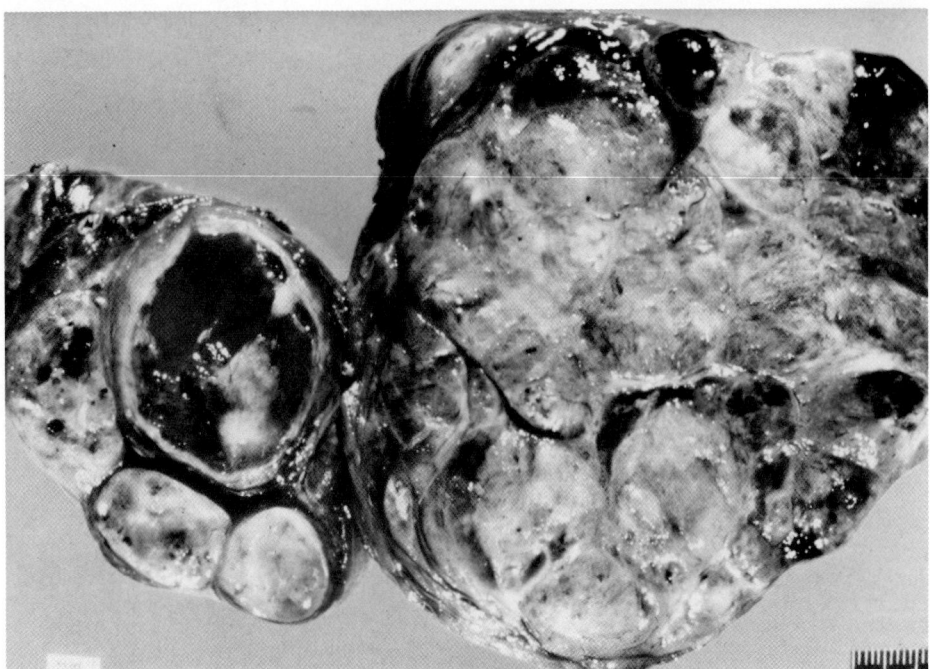

Fig. 5.1. Multinodular goiter. Both lobes of the thyroid show asymmetric enlargement due to multiple nodules, some with cystic changes and hemorrhage.

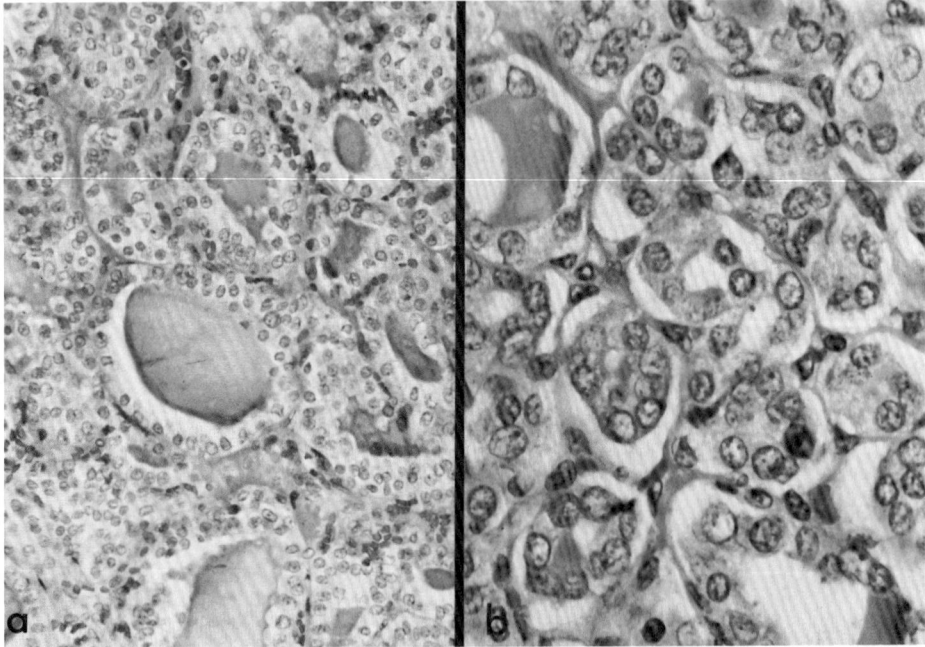

Fig. 5.2. Hyperplastic phase of nodular goiter. **A.** The follicles are crowded and lined by tall columnar epithelium. Very few follicles contain colloid. Hematoxylin and eosin preparation. × 400. **B.** Higher magnification of Fig. 5.2A showing large nuclei. Hematoxylin and eosin preparation. × 630. Aspirates from such nodules may be mistaken for follicular neoplasms or papillary carcinoma.

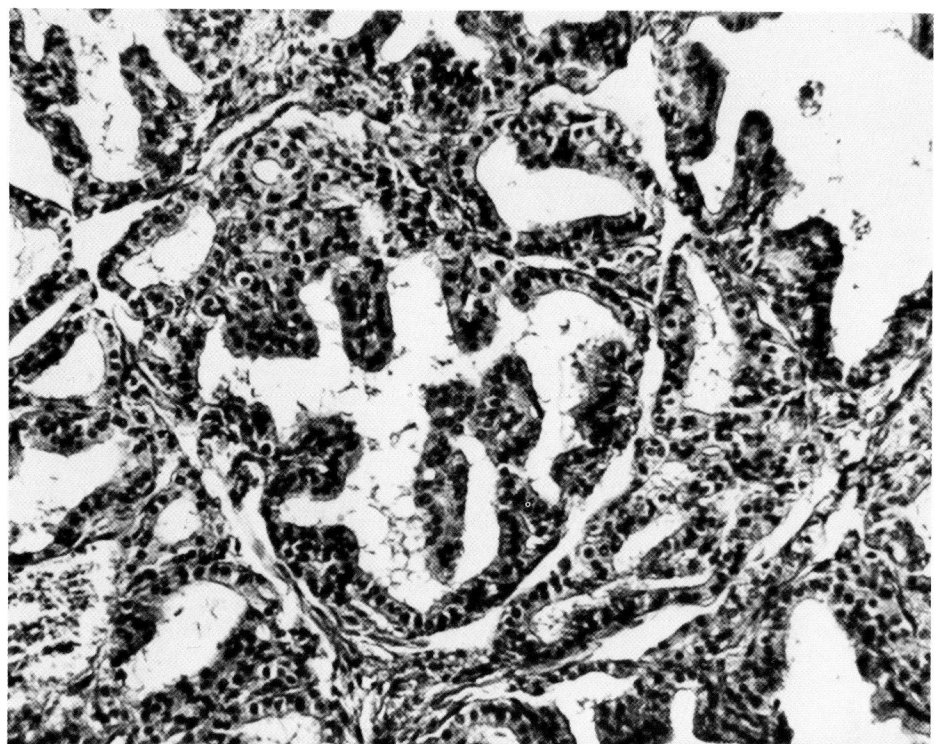

Fig. 5.3. Hyperplastic nodular goiter showing papillary hyperplasia. Aspirates from such nodules may be misinterpreted as papillary carcinoma. Hematoxylin and eosin preparation. × 160.

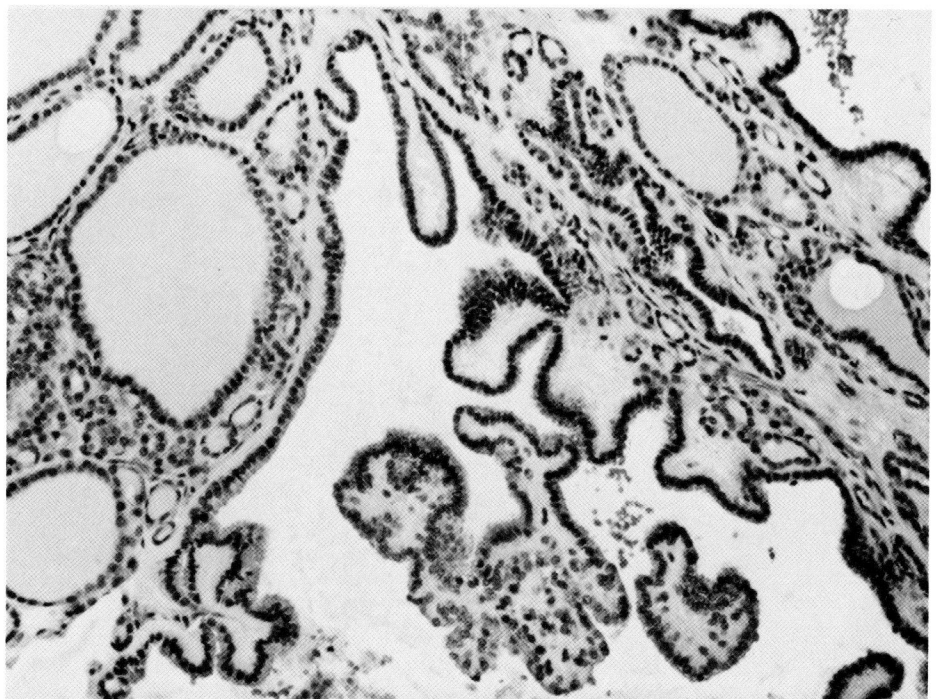

Fig. 5.4. Involution—some follicles are distended with colloid and some exhibit papillary change. The lining epithelium is low cuboidal. Hematoxylin and eosin preparation. × 160.

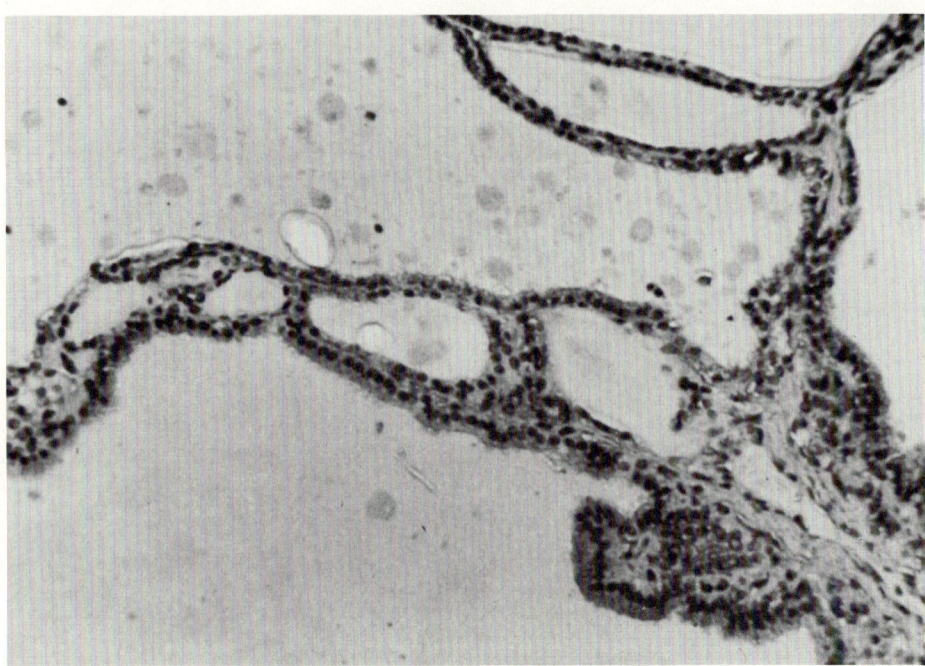

Fig. 5.5. Hyperinvolution. Overdistended follicles with flattened epithelium. Hematoxylin and eosin preparation. × 160.

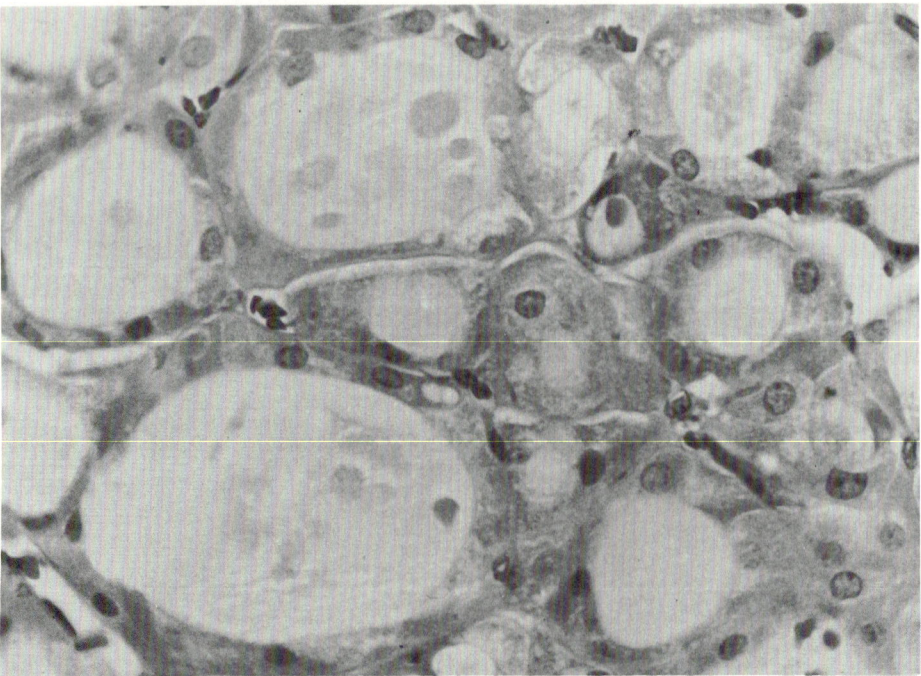

Fig. 5.6. Hürthle cell metaplasia. The follicles are linked by large cells with abundant granular cytoplasm. Hematoxylin and eosin preparations. × 400.

CYTOPATHOLOGY

The cytologic presentation of nodular goiter (Figs. 5.7–5.21; Table 5.1) corresponds to the stage of the disease as well as to secondary changes, such as hemorrhage, degeneration, necrosis, fibrosis, and calcification. Fine-needle aspirates generally show an admixture of colloid and benign follicular cells. The colloid is abundant in hyperinvoluted goiters and scant or absent during the hyperplastic stage. The converse is true of the follicular cells, which are abundant in the hyperplastic stages and scarce in hyperinvoluted goiters. These two patterns represent ends of the spectrum of cytopathologic changes of nodular goiter, with most cases exhibiting a pattern somewhere betweeen, modified by secondary changes.

The appearance of the colloid in Papanicolaou-stained preparations varies. In its pure form, the colloid appears as a thin film of acellular homogeneous material staining pink or greenish-blue and/or orange when mixed with blood. The colloid, after it has been smeared, retracts from the slide. When stained, it appears, as Abele and Miller[1] have stated, like a "crumpled plastic wrap." The inspissated colloid stains dense, appearing as droplets suggestive of follicular luminal casts. Colloid also shows a tendency to crack in a linear fashion, occasionally simulating a psammoma body. Large lakes of colloid with multiple fissures tend to give a mosaic pattern.[7] The presence of colloid is taken by some as presumptive evidence that the mass is benign

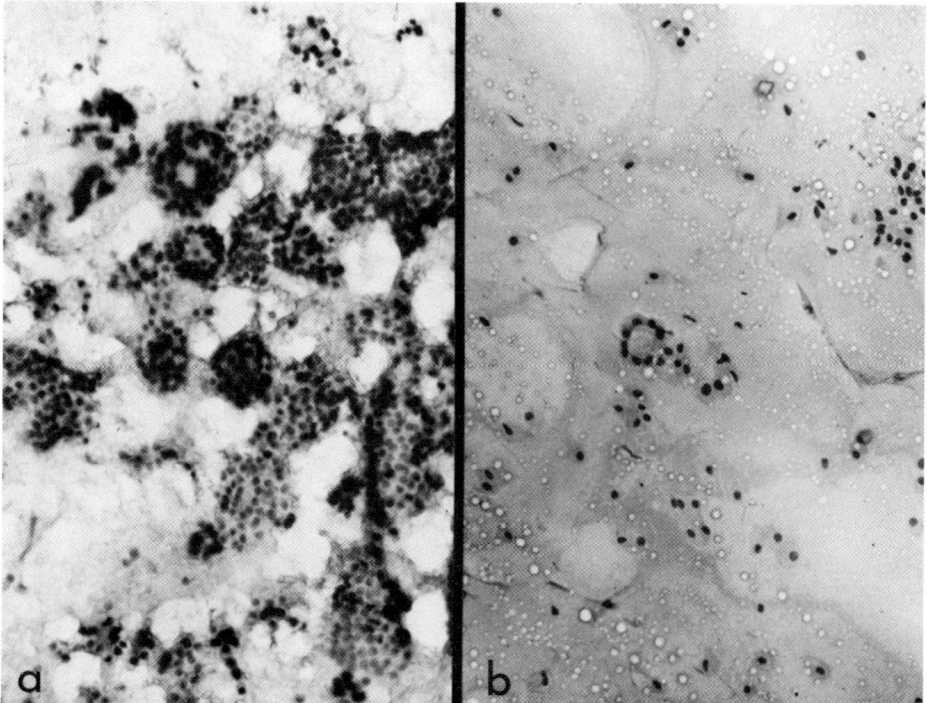

Fig. 5.7. Nodular goiter. **A.** Hypercellular aspirate with scant colloid. Papanicolaou preparation. × 160. **B.** Abundant colloid and sparse cellular component. Papanicolaou preparation. × 160.

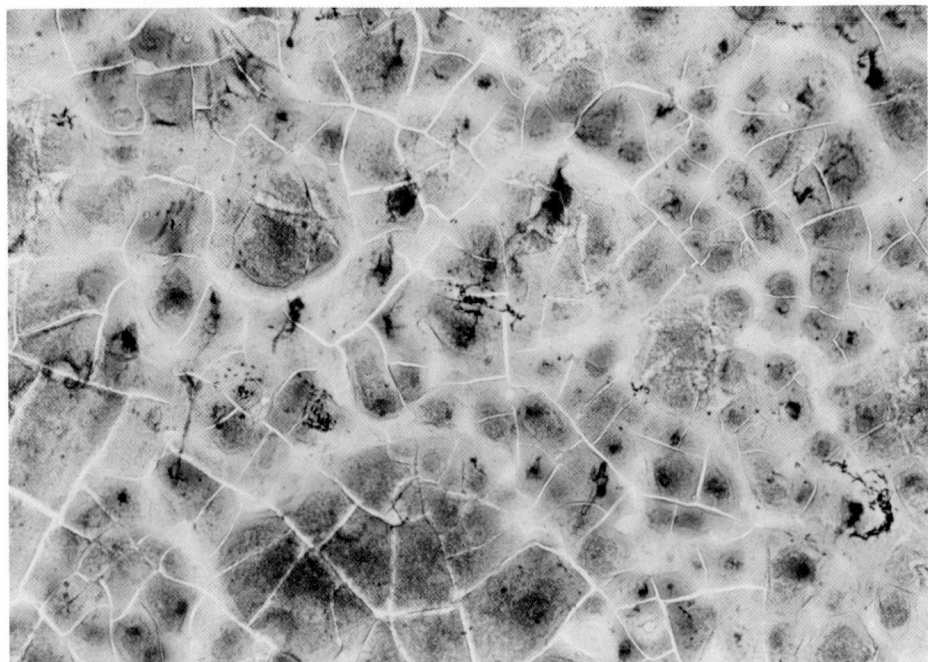

Fig. 5.8. Abundant colloid with linear cracks forming a mosaic pattern. Papanicolaou preparation. × 63.

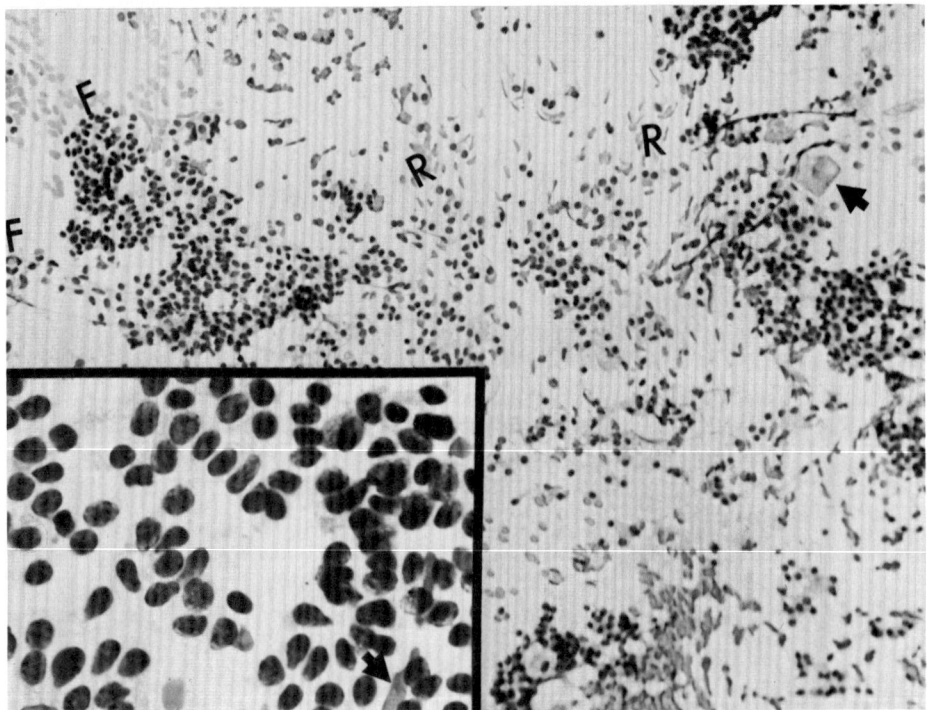

Fig. 5.9. Nodular goiter. Cellular aspirate with minimal colloid *(arrow)* in the background. The follicular cells are isolated or forming small, regular follicles *(F)*. The nuclei are small, compare with the red blood cell *(R)* for the size. Papanicolaou preparation. × 160. *Inset:* Follicular cells with uniform, small nuclei with compact chromatin. Papanicolaou preparation. × 630.

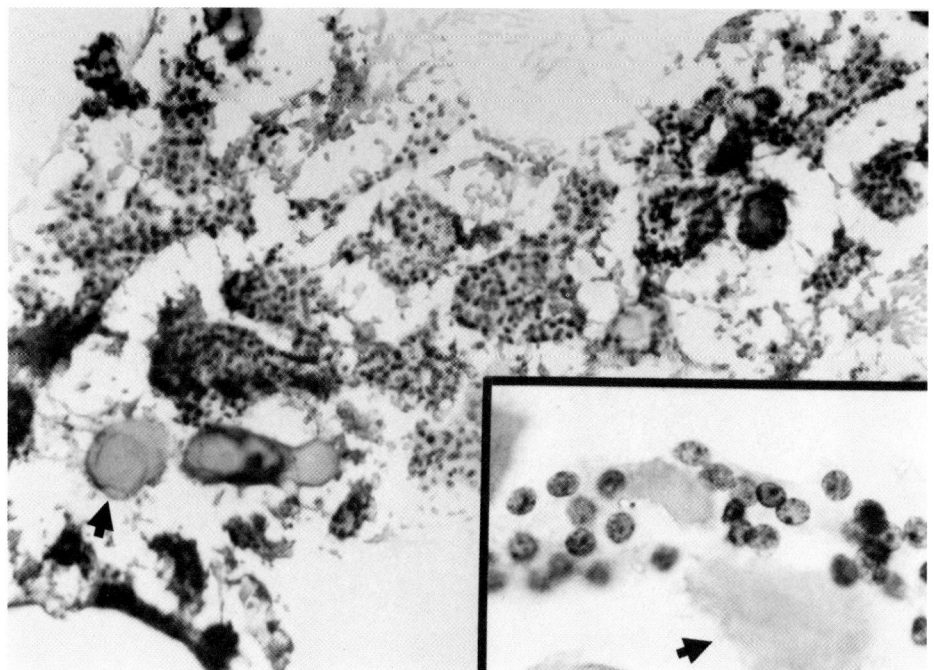

Fig. 5.10. Nodular goiter. Multiple tissue fragments of follicular epithelium with large droplets of colloid *(arrow)*. Papanicolaou preparation. × 160. *Inset:* The nuclei are uniform, with some containing nucleoli. Papanicolaou preparation. × 630.

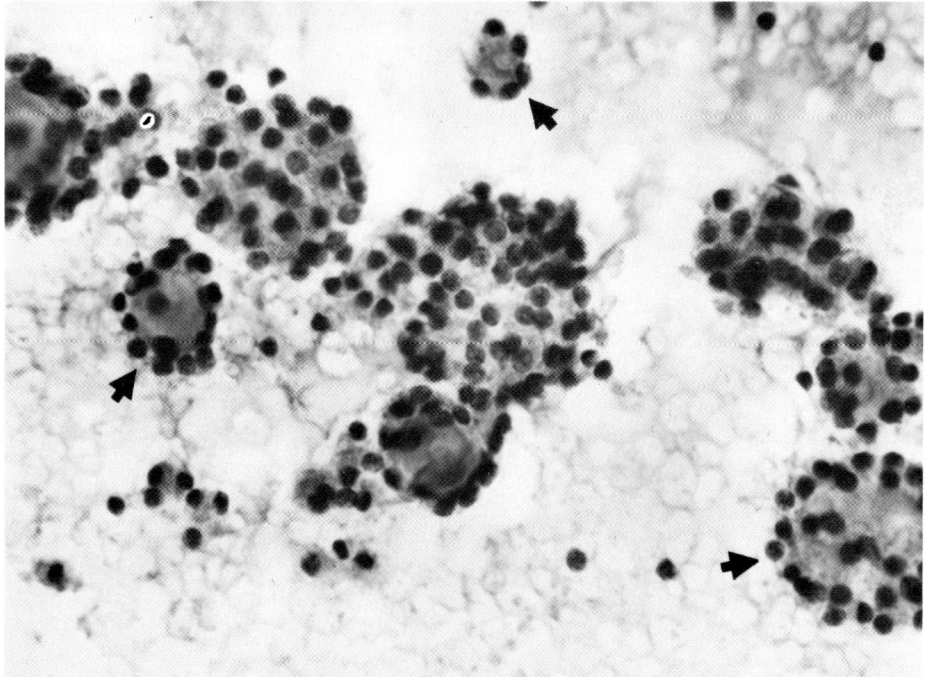

Fig. 5.11. Nodular goiter. Tissue fragments of follicular epithelium presenting a follicular pattern *(arrow)*. The nuclei are uniform, with evenly distributed chromatin. Papanicolaou preparation. × 630.

47

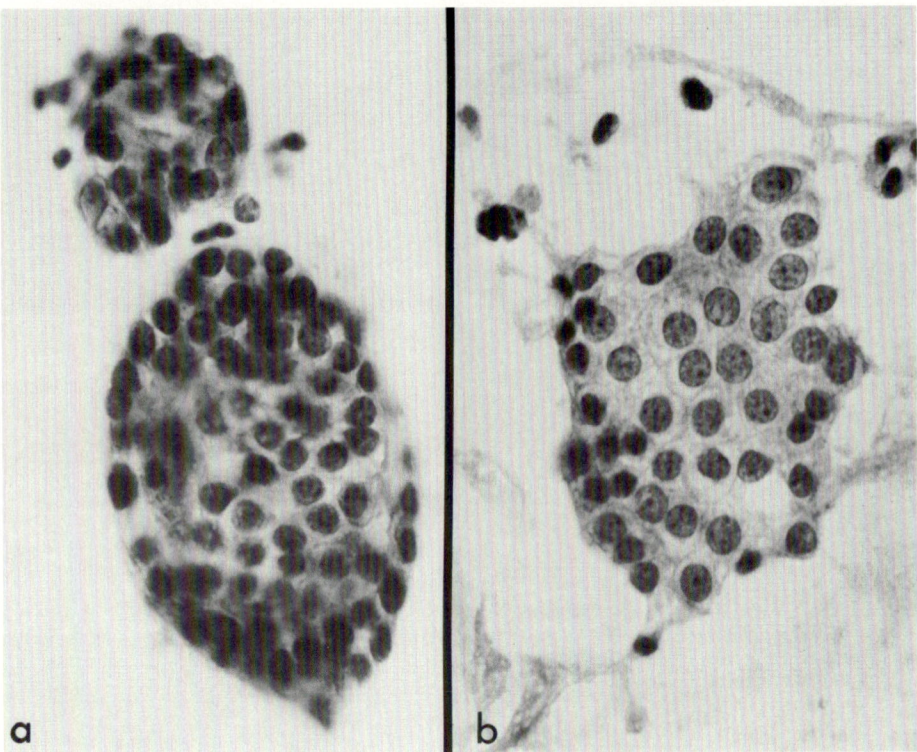

Fig. 5.12. Nodular goiter. **A.** Two follicles seen in their entirety and presenting a three-dimensional pattern. Note uniform, small nuclei with compact chromatin and well-defined cell borders. Papanicolaou preparation. × 630. **B.** A monolayered sheet of follicular epithelium with well-defined cell borders and centrally located, uniform nuclei. The honeycomb pattern is well demonstrated. Papanicolaou preparation. × 630.

and not a true neoplasm.[4–6] Although this rule proves useful and practical, it is not absolute, for aspirates of well-differentiated follicular carcinoma or follicular variant of papillary carcinoma may yield large amounts of colloid (see Chapter 3, Adequacy, Reporting Systems, and Cytopreparatory Technique).

The follicular cells are seen isolated or in tissue fragments with and without a follicular pattern. The follicles are generally small, showing a central lumen bordered by cuboidal cells with regularly spaced, small, uniform nuclei. Colloid may be present within their lumina. Occasionally, a follicle is seen in its entirety in a three-dimensional form. The tissue fragments without a follicular pattern appear monolayered, with a resemblance to a honeycomb (see Chapter 4, Concepts Basic to Thyroid Cytopathology). The component cells have well-defined cytoplasmic borders and contain regularly spaced, uniform nuclei that maintain their polarity. There is an appreciable amount of clear to pale cytoplasm. The follicular cell nuclei are round to oval, with diameters ranging from 7–9 μm.[2] The nuclear chromatin is finely granular and uniformly distributed. Nucleoli are generally not seen, but are present only in hyperplastic cells. Small pyknotic, dense-staining nuclei are characteristic of hyper-involuted goiters where the follicular cells are seen singly or in small groups, floating in large lakes of colloid. Their scanty, pale cytoplasm fades away against the background of the colloid, and their pyknotic nuclei appear bare and are difficult to

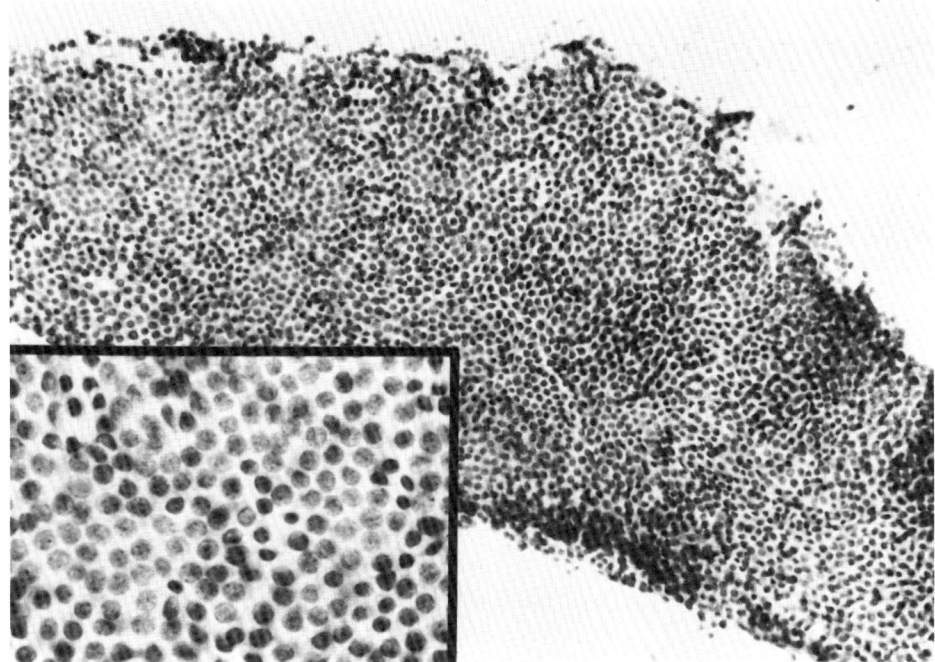

Fig. 5.13. Nodular goiter. Large monolayered tissue fragment of follicular epithelium. The honeycomb pattern is evident, even at low magnification. Papanicolaou preparation. × 160. *Inset:* Small, uniform nuclei with compact chromatin. Papanicolaou preparation. × 630.

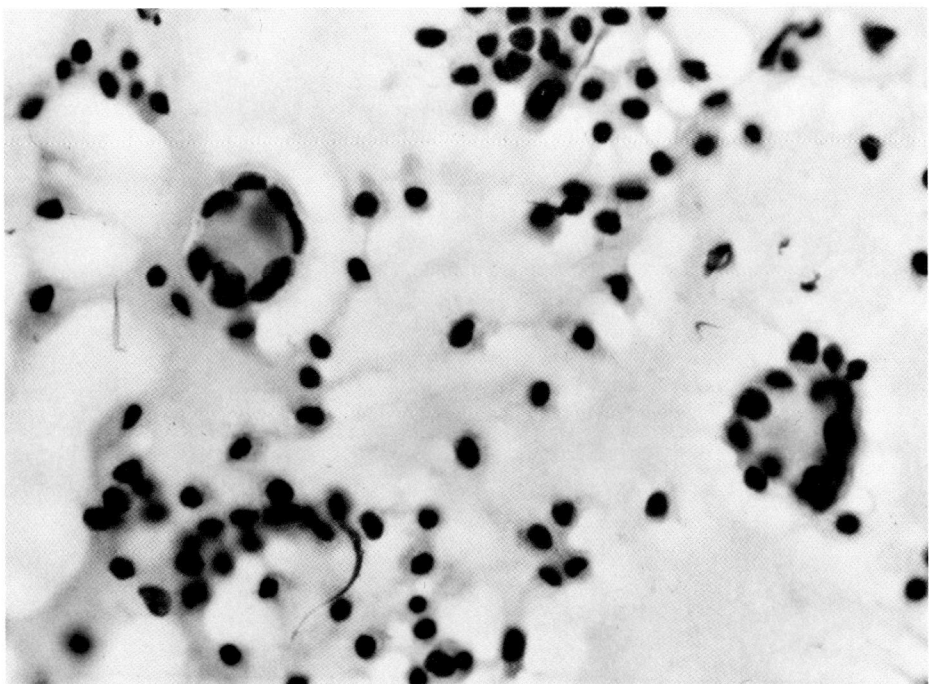

Fig. 5.14. Hyperinvoluted goiter. Sparse epithelial component in the background of abundant colloid. The follicles are small and uniform, and the nuclei appear pyknotic. The cytoplasm fades away and the nuclei appear "naked," resembling lymphocytes. Papanicolaou preparation. × 630.

49

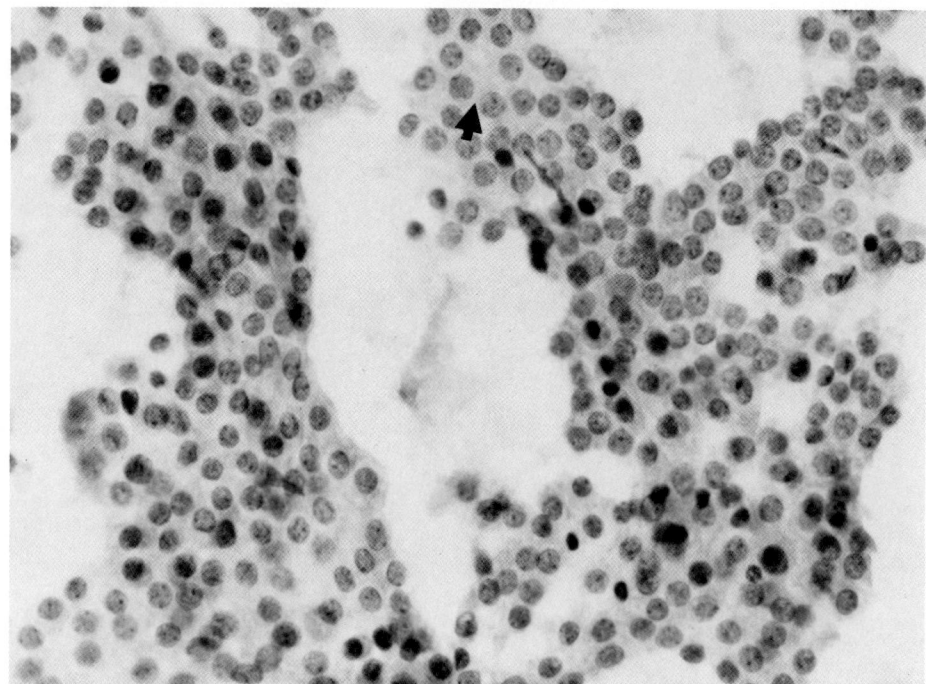

Fig. 5.15. Hyperplastic goiter. Abundant cellular material and lack of colloid in the background may suggest a diagnosis of a follicular neoplasm. However, the uniformity of the follicles *(arrow)*, monolayered tissue fragments with honeycomb pattern, and small, uniform nuclei suggest the diagnosis of nodular goiter. Papanicolaou preparation. × 400.

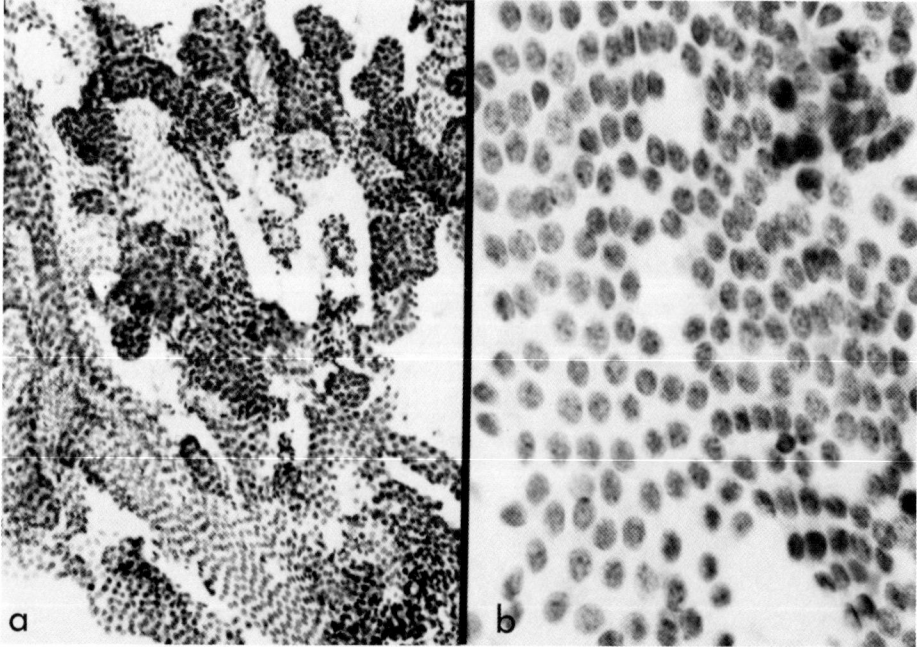

Fig. 5.16. Hyperplastic goiter. **A.** Papillary and monolayered tissue fragments. Under low magnification, this may be mistaken for papillary carcinoma. Papanicolaou preparation. × 63. **B.** Higher magnification showing uniform, small nuclei and a honeycomb pattern, ruling out neoplasia. Papanicolaou preparation. × 630.

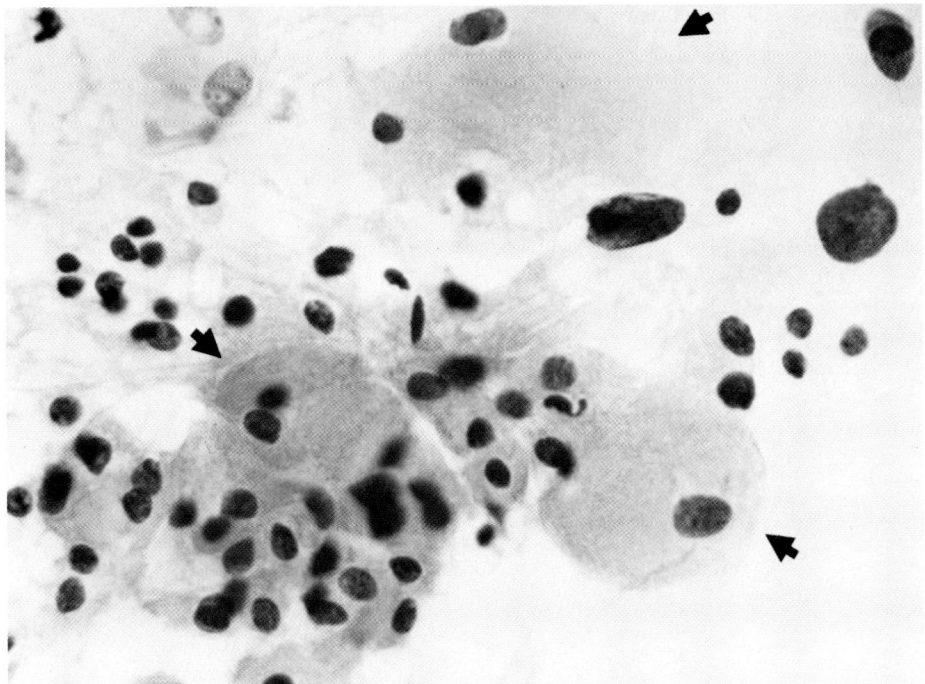

Fig. 5.17. Hürthle cell metaplasia. Benign follicular cells mixed with Hürthle cells *(arrow)* containing abundant granular cytoplasm and pyknotic, varying sized nuclei. Papanicolaou preparation. × 630.

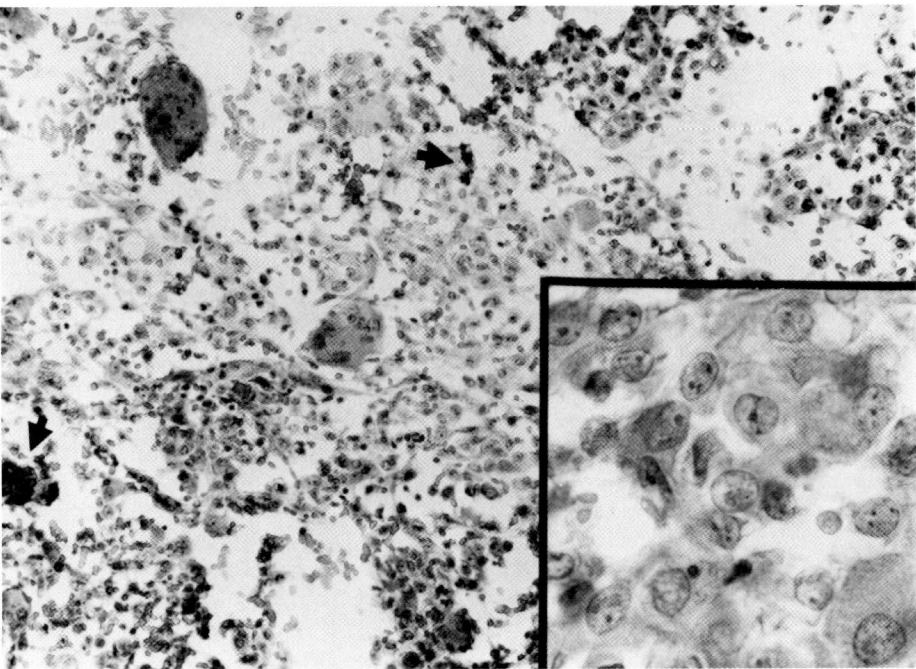

Fig. 5.18. Nodular goiter. Large numbers of discrete enlarged follicular cells, multinucleated foreign-body–type giant cells, and calcific debris *(arrow)*. Papanicolaou preparation. × 160. *Inset:* Higher magnification showing follicular cells with abundant foamy cytoplasm and enlarged nuclei with nucleoli, suggesting retrogressive changes. Papanicolaou preparation. × 630.

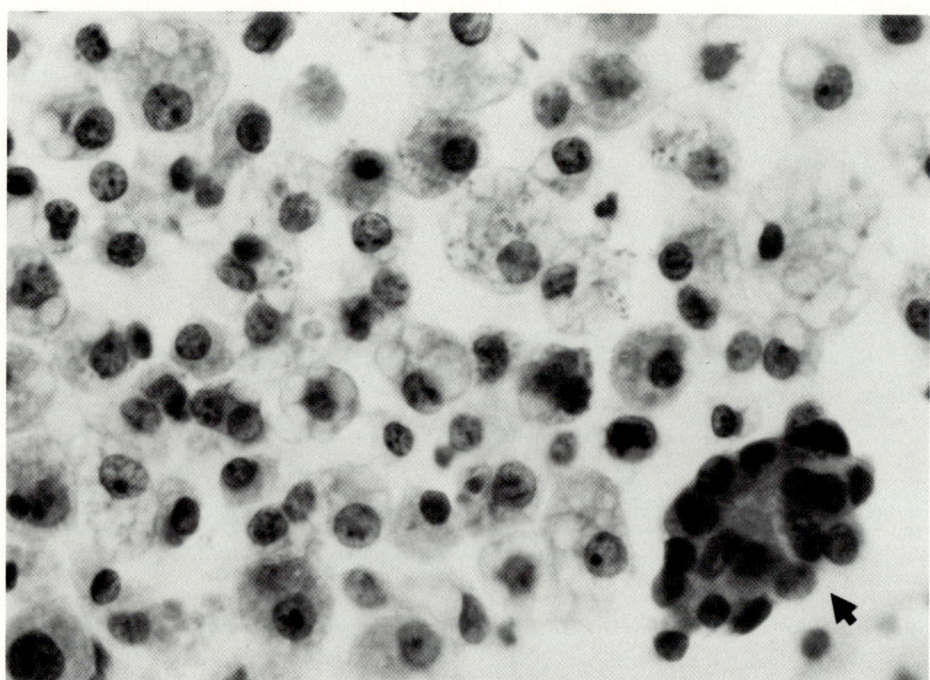

Fig. 5.19. A large population of discrete cells with foamy vacuolated cytoplasm. The nuclei have a uniform chromatin pattern and contain nucleoli. These cells may represent either degenerating follicular cells or histiocytes. Note a tissue fragment of follicular epithelium with pyknotic nuclei (*arrow*). Papanicolaou preparation. × 630.

differentiate from lymphocytes. The aspirates of hyperplastic goiters show abundant cellular material with tissue fragments with and without follicular pattern. The cellularity can be overwhelming. The papillary hyperplasia yields papillary tissue fragments with a branching pattern and smooth external contour, with component cells showing well-defined borders in a honeycomb pattern.

Hürthle cell metaplasia of the follicular cells is a frequent occurrence in nodular goiters. These Hürthle cells are large, oval to polygonal, with abundant granular or sometimes dense cytoplasm, and slightly eccentric nuclei. Transitional forms from regular follicular cells to Hürthle cells may be noted. The metaplastic Hürthle cells often have large, single or multiple pyknotic nuclei.

Hemorrhage and degeneration in a nodular goiter are frequent events initiating regressive changes in follicular cells. They appear enlarged with abundant granular, foamy, or vacuolated cytoplasm, and sometimes with phagocytized hemosiderin pigment.[3] The nuclei remain small, but may contain prominent nucleoli. These cells with prominent nucleoli often cause concern[3] and may be misinterpreted as neoplastic.

Variable numbers of histiocytes are often seen in aspirates from a nodular goiter. Their cytoplasm contains large, coarse, greenish-brown granules of hemosiderin pigment, indicating old hemorrhage in the nodule. Accompanying the histiocytes are multinucleated histiocytic foreign-body–type giant cells. The presence of such cells

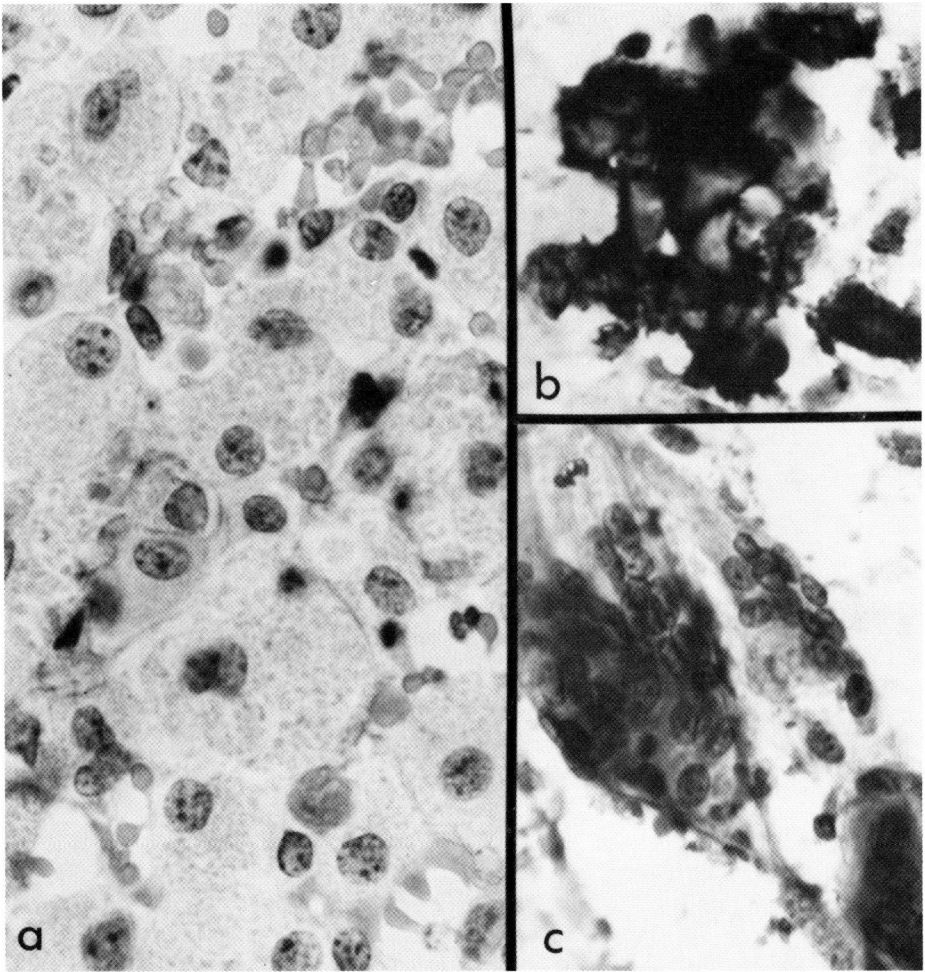

Fig. 5.20. Nodular goiter. **A.** Large cells with abundant foamy cytoplasm, representing either follicular cells or histiocytes. Papanicolaou preparation. × 630. **B.** Calcific debris. Papanicolaou preparation. × 630. **C.** Multinucleated foreign-body–type giant cells. Papanicolaou preparation. × 630.

has no practical significance. The same is true for calcific debris. Rarely, aspirates of nodular goiter may show psammoma bodies (see Chapter 8, Papillary Carcinoma).

Because of old hemorrhage, granulation tissue, and fibrosis, the aspirates of nodular goiter may also show stromal cells, either isolated or in fragments. Isolated stromal cells have large nuclei with nucleoli. Their uniform size and bland chromatin suggest their benign nature.

The usual pattern of nodular goiter thus consists of benign follicular cells and colloid in variable proportions, along with inflammatory cell components suggesting secondary changes. All the listed features may not be present in aspirates of every nodular goiter, and it is not necessary to fulfill all the criteria to make a cytologic diagnosis of nodular goiter.

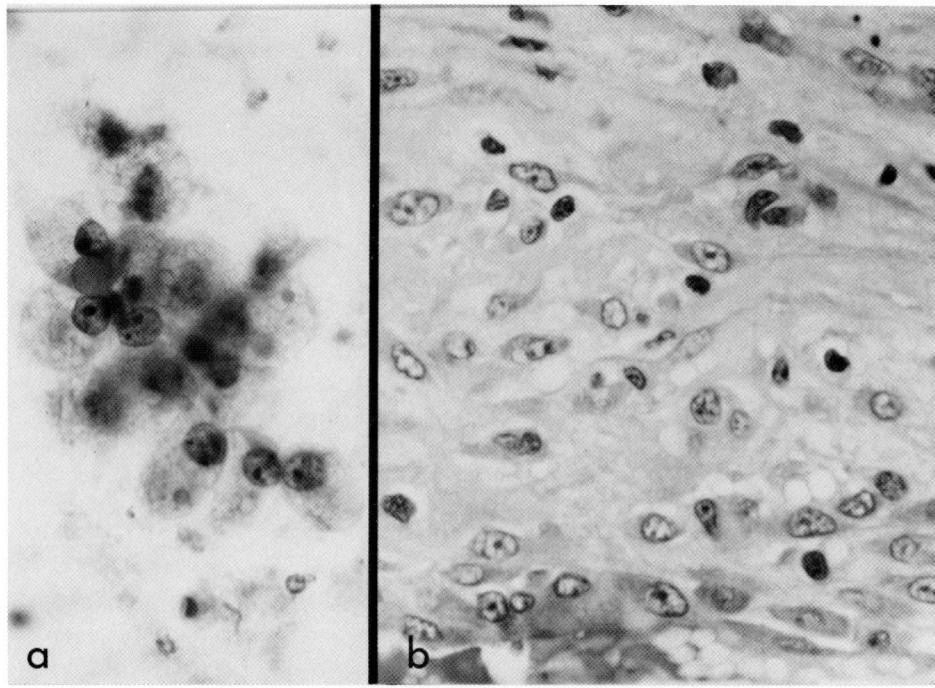

Fig. 5.21. Nodular goiter. **A.** These group of ovoid cells with eccentric nuclei containing nucleoli were present in the background of nodular goiter, and were suspected of malignancy. Papanicolaou preparation. × 630. **B.** Large-needle biopsy specimen of the nodule, showing granulation tissue. Hematoxylin and eosin preparation. × 400. The cells in the aspirate perhaps represent histiocytes. Note similarity in the morphology.

TABLE 5.1. Cytopathologic Features of Nodular Goiter

Pattern	Admixture of benign follicular epithelium and colloid. Cells isolated or in tissue fragments—small, regular follicles or monolayered sheets with a honeycomb pattern, rarely with papillary configuration.
Cells	Small cuboidal, well-defined cell borders; Hürthle cell metaplasia frequent.
Nuclei	About 7–9 μm in diameter, round to oval, finely dispersed chromatin. Nucleoli rare.
Cytoplasm	Moderate, pale.
Background	Degenerative changes common—histiocytes with or without hemosiderin pigment, multinucleated giant cells, calcific debris, stromal cells.

POTENTIAL ERRORS

Variations in the usual pattern described above create settings for potential errors that may lead to false-positive results. Some of the listed criteria of nodular goiter, if present in excess and to the exclusion of other features, may lead to interpretative traps, and the nodular goiter be mistaken for a neoplasm.[9] Such cases with unusual presentations of nodular goiter are infrequent, but they constitute important diagnostic pitfalls. They are best understood when one is familiar with the cytopathologic features of various different thyroid neoplasms. The cytopathologic features of nodular goiter that may be confused with those of neoplasms are listed in Table 5.2 and discussed in detail in other chapters.

TABLE 5.2. Unusual Cytopathologic Patterns of Nodular Goiter—Diagnostic Pitfalls

Cytopathologic Features of Nodular Goiter	Possible Erroneous Interpretations	See Chapter
1. Hyperplastic goiter with cell-rich aspirate, fragments of follicular epithelium with or without follicular pattern. Nuclei uniformly, but slightly enlarged. No colloid.	Cellular follicular adenoma	6, Follicular Adenoma and Carcinoma
2. Hyperplastic goiter with cell-rich aspirate, abundant monolayered sheets and/or papillary tissue fragments. No colloid or no other features of nodular goiter.	Papillary carcinoma	8, Papillary Carcinoma
3. Features of nodular goiter plus occasional true psammoma body or inspissated colloid within follicles, simulating a psammoma body.	Papillary carcinoma	8, Papillary Carcinoma
4. Features of nodular goiter with or without cystic change, follicular cells with nuclear and cytoplasmic pleomorphism, retrogressive changes.	Papillary carcinoma; metastatic carcinoma	8, Papillary Carcinoma; 13, Metastatic Carcinoma to Thyroid
5. Extensive Hürthle cell metaplasia	Hürthle cell tumor	7, Hürthle Cell Lesions
6. Markedly pleomorphic follicular cells, ^{131}I therapy.	Anaplastic carcinoma	9, Anaplastic Carcinoma
7. Spindle-shaped cells, either of stromal origin or from granulation tissue.	Anaplastic carcinoma; medullary carcinoma	9, Anaplastic Carcinoma; 10, Medullary Carcinoma

REFERENCES

1. Abele JS, Miller TR: Fine needle aspiration of the thyroid nodule: clinical application. In Clark OH: *Endocrine Surgery of the Thyroid and Parathyroid Glands*. St. Louis, Mosby, 1985, pp. 293–335.

2. Cervino JM, Pasegro P, Grosso OT, Maggiolo J: La exploration citologic de la glandula tiroides y sus correlaciones anatomoclinices. *An Facultad Med* 47:1728–1743, 1962.

3. Droese M: Cytologic Aspiration Biopsy of the Thyroid Gland. Stuttgart, F.R. Schattauer Verlag, 1980, pp. 55–57.

4. Frable WJ: *Thin Needle Aspiration Biopsy*. Philadelphia, Saunders, 1983, pp. 152–182.

5. Friedman M, Shimaoka KC, Getaz P: Needle aspiration of 310 thyroid lesions. *Acta Cytol* 23:196–203, 1979.

6. Löwhagen T: Thyroid. In Zajicek J: *Aspiration Biopsy Cytology, Part 1. Cytology of supradiaphragmatic organs*. New York, Karger, 1974, pp. 67–89.

7. Löwhagen T, Linsk JA: Aspiration biopsy cytology of the thyroid gland. In *Clinical Aspiration Cytology*. Linsk JA, Sixteen F: Philadelphia, Lippincott, 1983, pp. 67–69.

8. Meissner WA, Warren S: *Tumors of the Thyroid Gland*. Fascicle 4, Second Series, *Atlas of Tumor Pathology*. Washington, DC, Armed Forces Institute of Pathology, 1969.

9. Miller JM, Kini SR, Hamburger JI: Needle Biopsy of the Thyroid Gland—Current Concepts. New York, Praeger Publishers, 1983, pp. 220–223, 247–250.

6

Follicular Adenoma and Carcinoma

FOLLICULAR ADENOMA

Follicular adenomas are benign neoplasms of the thyroid. They are a common occurrence, especially in women. After nodular goiter, they are the most common cause of nonfunctioning nodules. Frequently of great size, they may undergo degeneration, hemorrhage, necrosis, and infarction. Whether adenomas undergo malignant change is a matter of dispute.[20]

Pathology

Grossly, follicular adenomas are sharply circumscribed, discrete, solitary, expansile lesions with a bulging cut surface (Fig. 6.1). Areas of degeneration and hemorrhage may be seen. Microscopically, this tumor is encapsulated, a feature that differentiates it from a non-neoplastic nodule of adenomatous goiter (Fig. 6.2). The thyroid parenchyma adjacent to the capsule is compressed.

Follicular adenomas are subclassified[20] according to the architectural and functional differentiation of the thyroid follicles within the neoplasm, eg, colloid or macrofollicular, simple, microfollicular, and trabecular. The subclassification of Meissner and Warren[20] also includes oxyphil cell (Hürthle cell) and atypical adenomas, but we have chosen to group oxyphil adenomas separately (see Chapter 7, Hürthle Cell Lesions). And because atypical adenoma is a histologic and not a cytologic diagnosis, it is not included here (see this chapter, section on Follicular Carcinoma).

Although subclassifying follicular adenomas may seem superfluous and of dubious value, it helps tremendously in cytohistologic correlation as well as in understanding overlapping cytopathologic patterns. The questions as to why some nodular goiters cannot be differentiated from follicular adenomas, and why some follicular adenomas

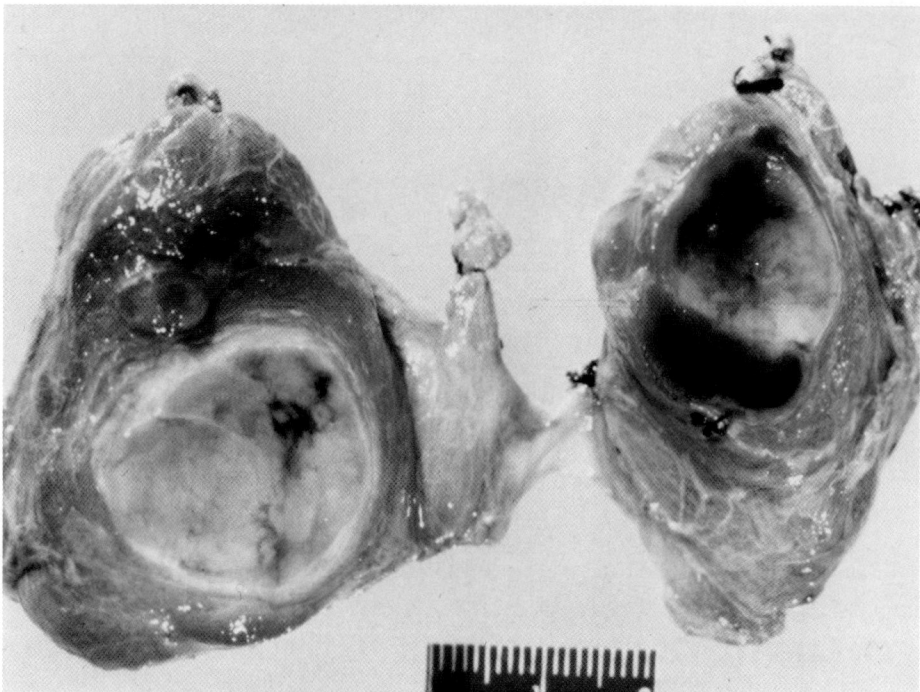

Fig. 6.1. Thyroid with two encapsulated follicular adenomas involving each lobe.

have cytopathologic as well as histopathologic patterns similar to follicular carcinomas, can only be appreciated if one is familiar with the spectrum of morphologic patterns described below.

Colloid adenoma (macrofollicular adenoma) represents the most differentiated of follicular adenomas, with overdistended follicles containing abundant colloid (Fig. 6.2). The lining epithelium is flattened with pyknotic nuclei. This type of adenoma may virtually replicate the pattern of hyperinvoluted goiter, except for the encapsulation.

Simple adenoma consists of well-developed follicles of approximately normal size (Figs. 6.3 and 6.4). The lining epithelium is low cuboidal, with either normal-sized or slightly enlarged nuclei. The amount of colloid within the follicles varies. Cellular areas of less-differentiated follicles may be mixed with more-differentiated follicles.

Microfollicular adenoma (or fetal adenoma), as the name implies, is composed of poorly or maldeveloped follicles with little or no colloid, denoting poor architectural as well as functional differentiation (Fig. 6.5). The lining epithelium is cuboidal, with nuclei that may be slightly increased in size (Fig. 6.6A).

Trabecular adenoma (or embryonal adenoma) displays a trabecular pattern with anastomosing ribbons of follicular epithelium (Fig. 6.6B). There is neither a follicular pattern nor the presence of colloid, indicating a lack of both architectural and functional differentiation at the light-microscopy level in ordinary stained material.

Because microfollicular and trabecular adenomas are cellular neoplasms, they will henceforward be referred to as cellular adenomas.

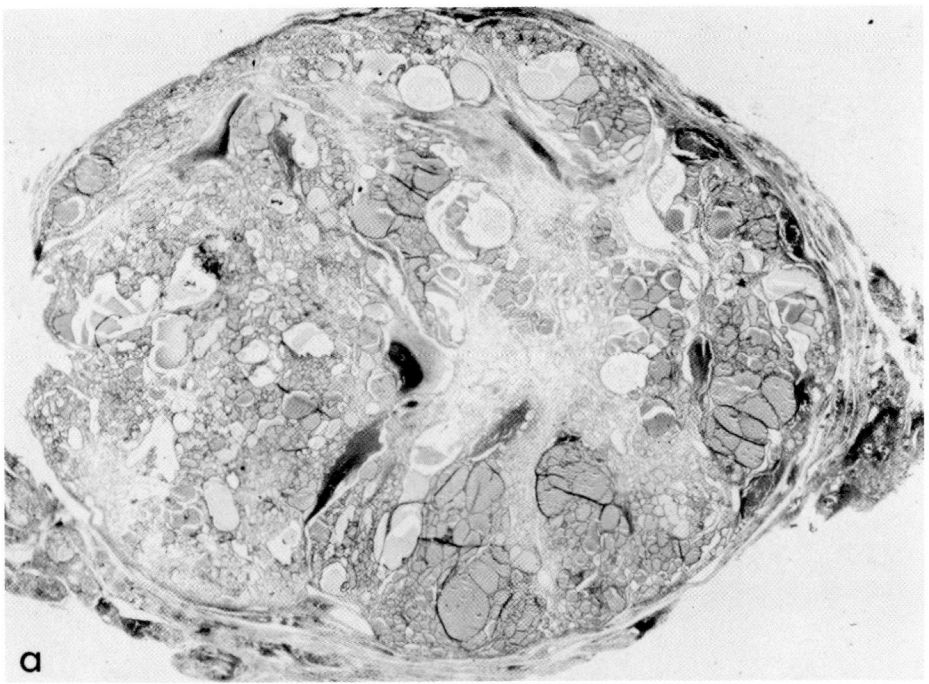

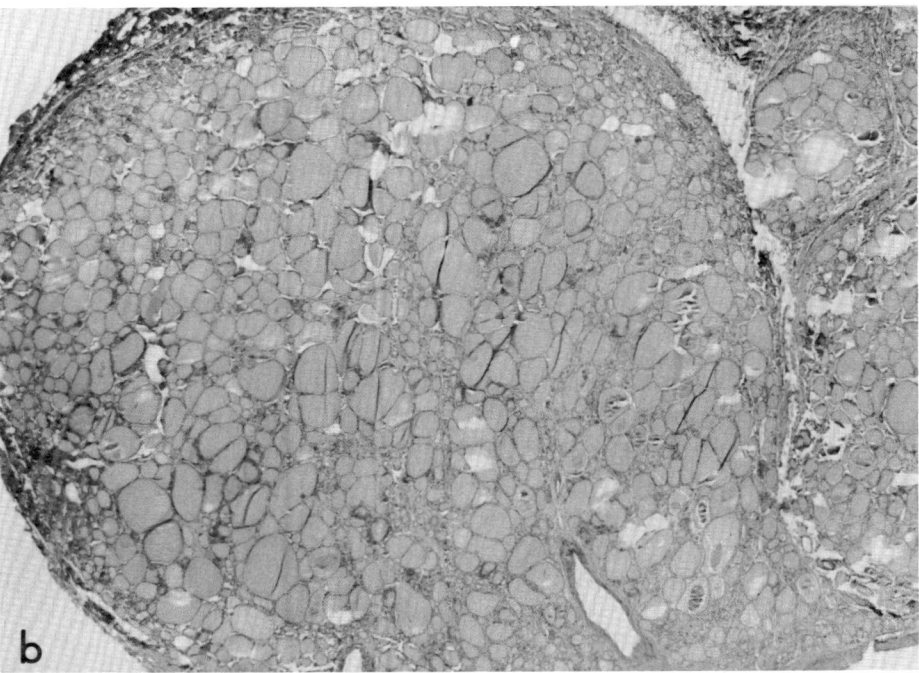

Fig. 6.2. **A.** Macrofollicular adenoma, an encapsulated nodule. The histologic pattern of large, colloid-filled follicles is similar to that seen in hyperinvoluted goiter. Cytologically, this type of adenoma cannot be differentiated from nodular goiter. Hematoxylin and eosin preparation. × 16. **B.** A non-encapsulated nodule of nodular goiter. Hematoxylin and eosin preparation. × 16.

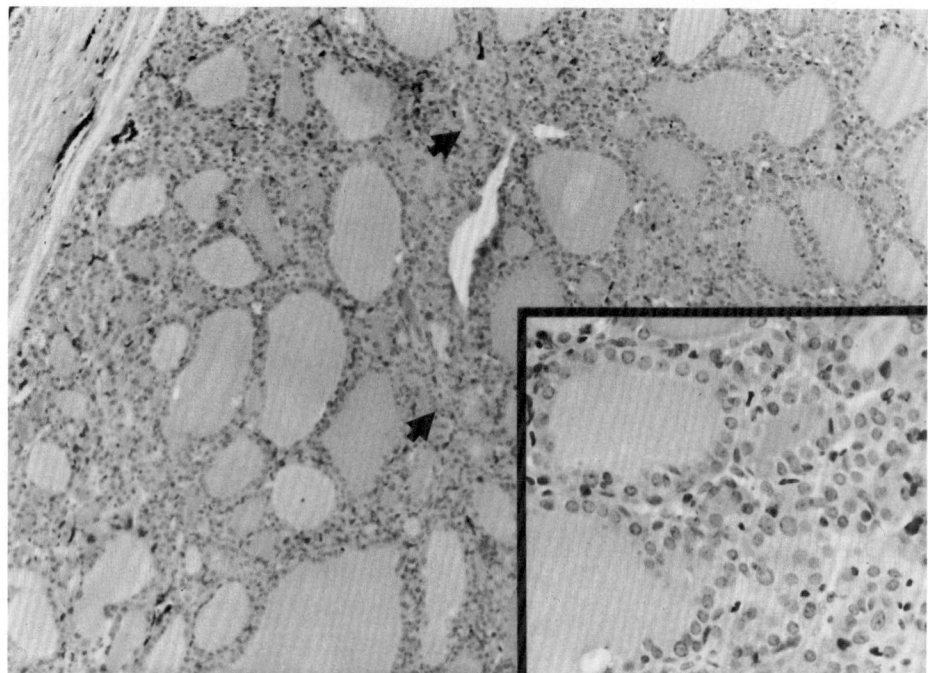

Fig. 6.3. Follicular adenoma, simple type, consisting of follicles of approximately normal size. Note large distended follicles mixed with cellular areas. Hematoxylin and eosin preparation. × 63. *Inset:* Higher magnification of a cellular area showing a microfollicular pattern. Hematoxylin and eosin preparation. × 400.

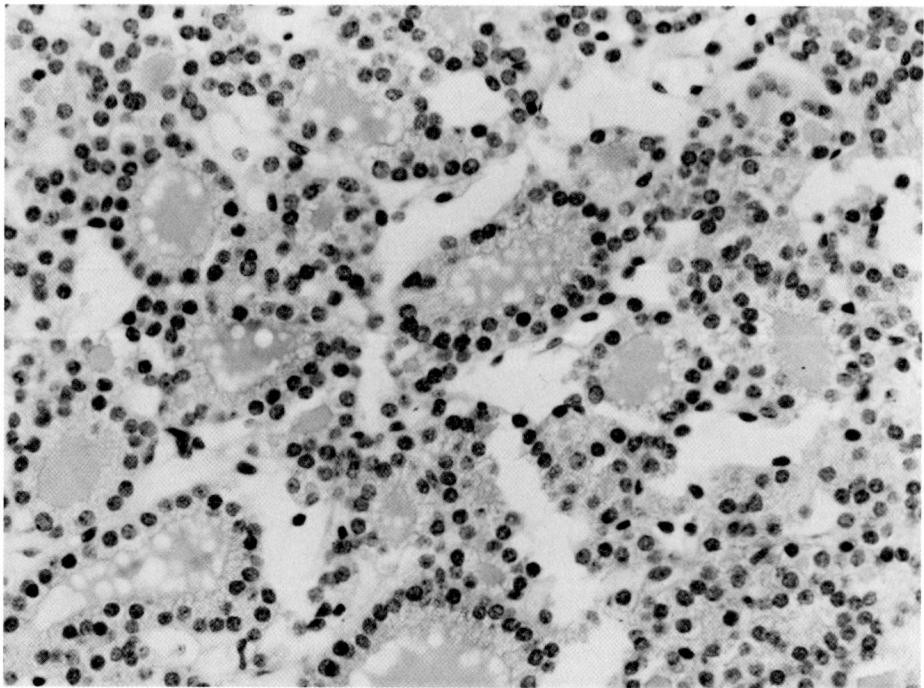

Fig. 6.4. Simple adenoma, showing more cellularity and less colloid than Fig. 6.3. Hematoxylin and eosin preparation. × 160.

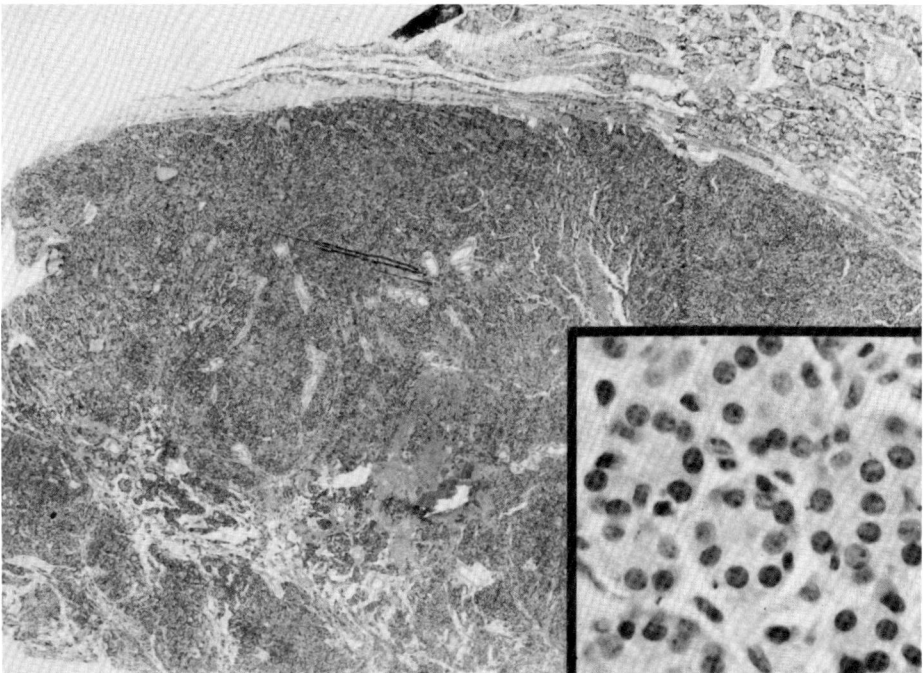

Fig. 6.5. Cellular follicular adenoma with encapsulation. Hematoxylin and eosin preparation. × 16. *Inset:* Microfollicles without colloid. Hematoxylin and eosin preparation. × 400.

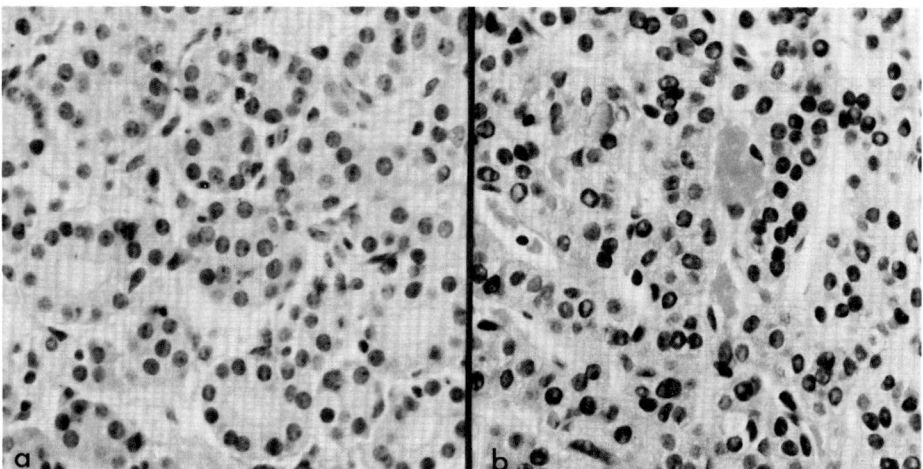

Fig. 6.6. Cellular follicular adenomas. **A.** Microfollicular pattern. Hematoxylin and eosin preparation. × 400. **B.** Trabecular pattern. Hematoxylin and eosin preparation. × 400.

Cytopathology

Colloid Adenoma

Aspirates of colloid adenoma show abundant colloid and have a sparse cellular component, with tissue fragments of follicular epithelium showing small follicles or a honeycomb pattern. Nuclei are small and stain dark. This pattern is indistinguishable from that of hyperinvoluted goiter. Tumors with such a cytologic pattern are rarely, if ever, malignant.[1]

Simple Adenoma

The cytopathologic pattern of simple adenoma (Fig. 6.7) depends on the histologic differentiation. If the histologic differentiation approaches that of a normal gland, the aspirates will show cytopathologic features of a nodular goiter. If cellular areas are sampled, syncytial-type tissue fragments will be present, along with those that appear non-neoplastic. Colloid is variable. Such a varied pattern is more often seen in a large adenoma, due to samples obtained from different areas of the nodule.

Cellular Adenoma

Unlike the aspirates of macrofollicular and simple adenomas, aspirates of cellular adenomas (Figs. 6.8–6.14) show a distinctly different cytopathologic pattern (Table 6.1). The aspirate is usually very cellular and consists of syncytial-type tissue fragments of follicular epithelium with or without a follicular pattern. A follicular pattern is more commonly seen in a microfollicular adenoma, whereas in trabecular type, syncytial-type tissue fragments with broad trabeculae are often seen. The nuclei are uniformly enlarged, crowded, and overlapped. Cell borders are ill-defined, and the nuclei exhibit altered polarity. The nuclear chromatin is granular and rather coarse but evenly distributed. Nucleoli are infrequent and the cytoplasm is variable but scanty, colorless to pale. Colloid is rarely present in the background, but may be seen within the lumina of the follicles.

TABLE 6.1. Cytopathologic Features of Cellular Adenomas

Pattern
Syncytial-type tissue fragments with and without follicular pattern
Nuclei
Round to oval, uniformly increased in size
Coarsely granular chromatin, evenly dispersed
Nucleoli not consistent
Altered polarity
Cytoplasm
Variable but scant
Colorless to pale
Colloid
Scanty, usually absent in background, but may be in follicle lumina

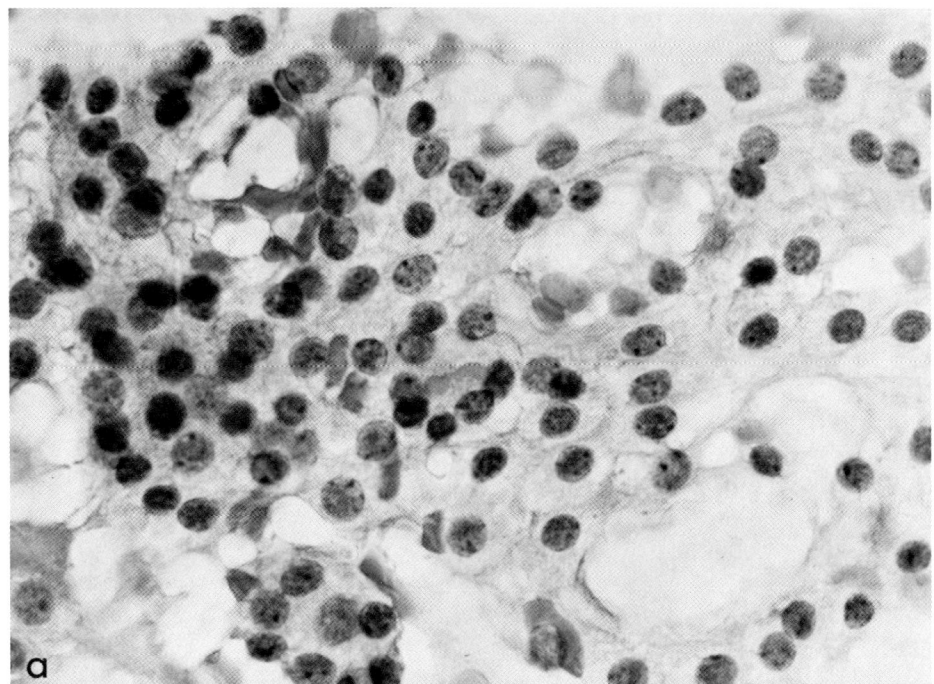

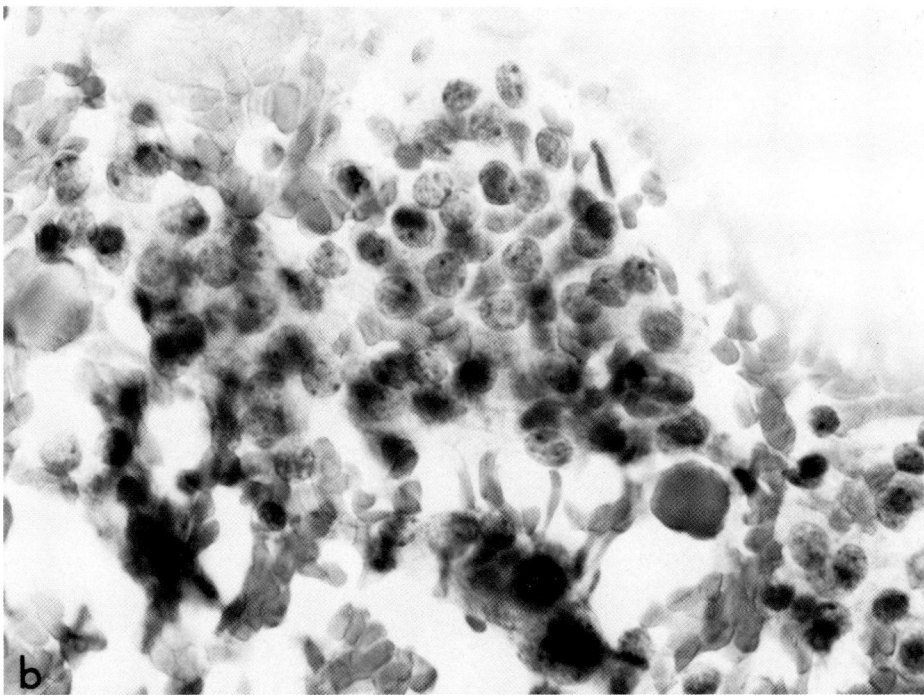

Fig. 6.7. Simple adenoma with mixed cytologic pattern. **A.** Regular follicles, honeycomb sheets, and uniform but slightly enlarged nuclei with compact chromatin. This pattern is consistent with nodular goiter. Papanicolaou preparation. × 630. **B.** Another field from same case as **A** showing a syncytial-type tissue fragment with crowded, overlapped, uniformly enlarged nuclei. This pattern is consistent with cellular adenoma. Papanicolaou preparation. × 630.

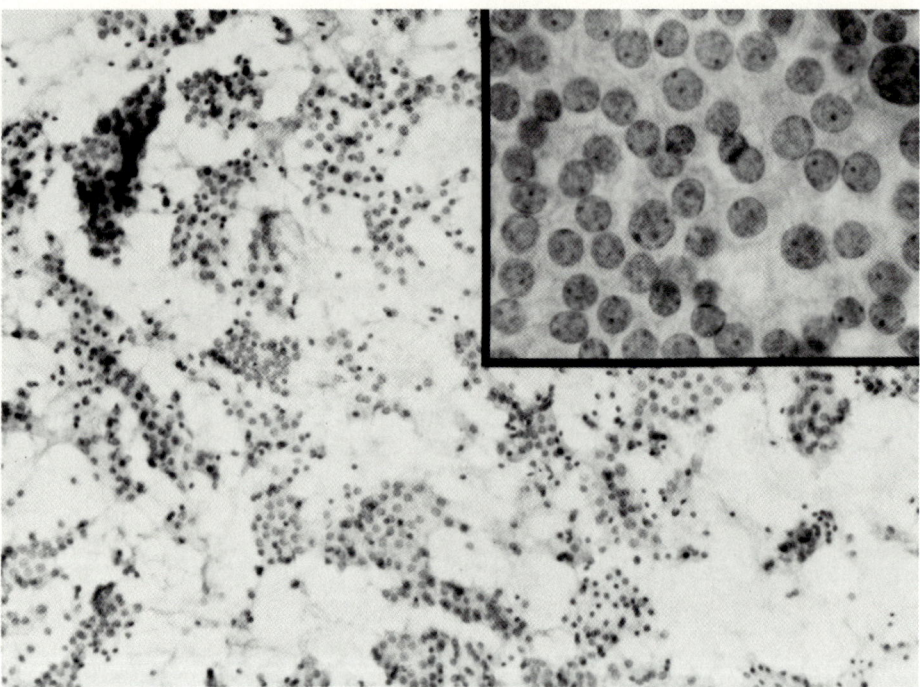

Fig. 6.8. Cellular adenoma. A cellular aspirate with several syncytial- type tissue fragments of follicular epithelium. There is no colloid in the background. Papanicolaou preparation. × 160. *Inset:* The nuclei are pleomorphic in size, with finely granular chromatin. Some contain nuclei. Papanicolaou preparation. × 630.

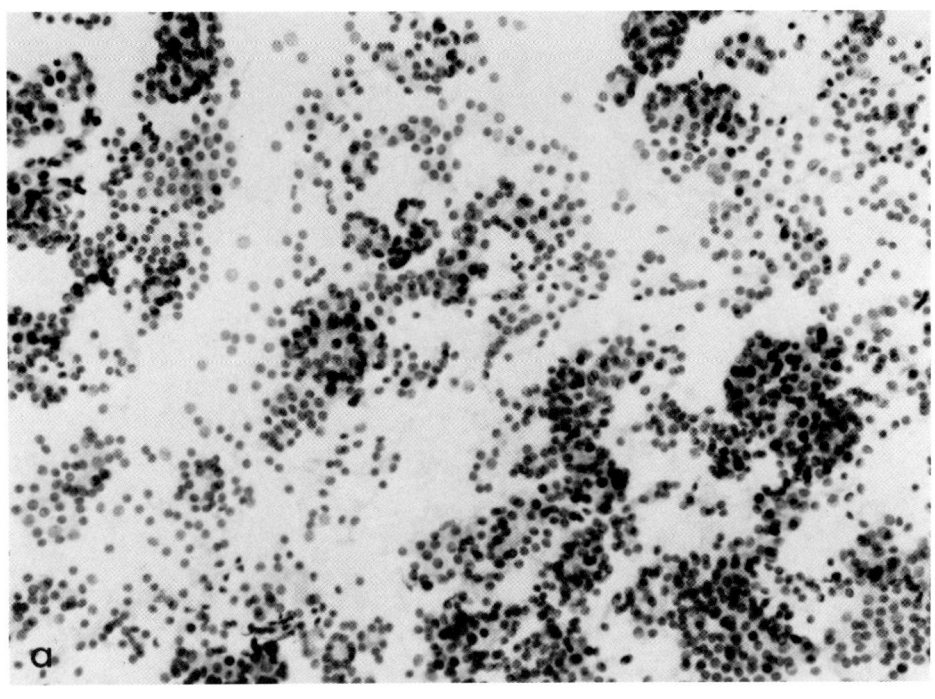

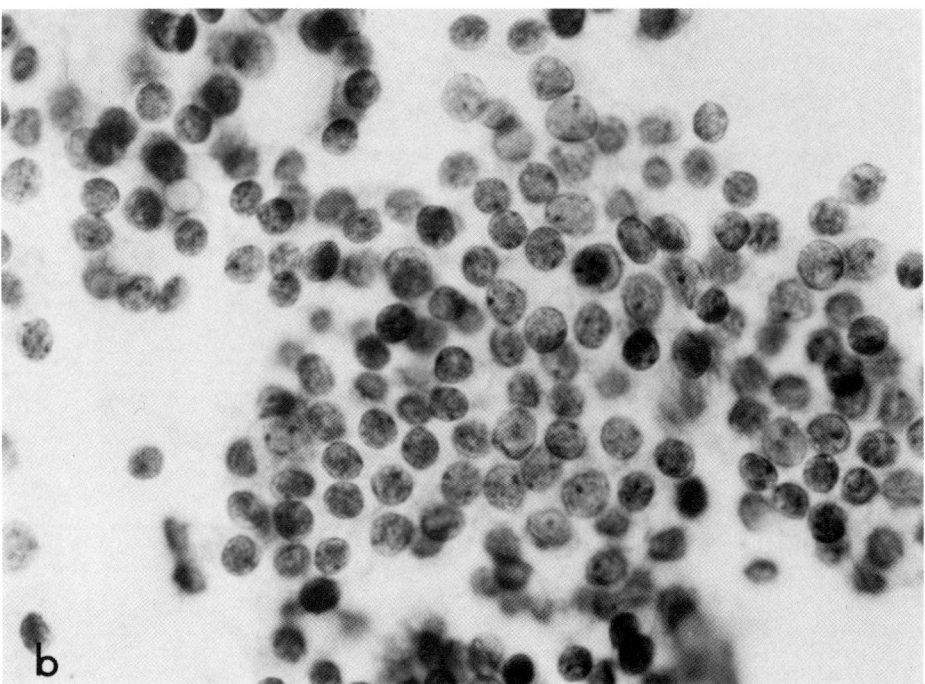

Fig. 6.9. A. Cellular adenoma. Several syncytial-type tissue fragments with marked crowding and overlapping of uniformly, but mildly, enlarged nuclei. There is no colloid in the
background. Papanicolaou preparation. × 160. B. Higher magnification of A showing
follicular pattern of tissue fragments. Note uniformly enlarged nuclei. Papanicolaou
preparation. × 630.

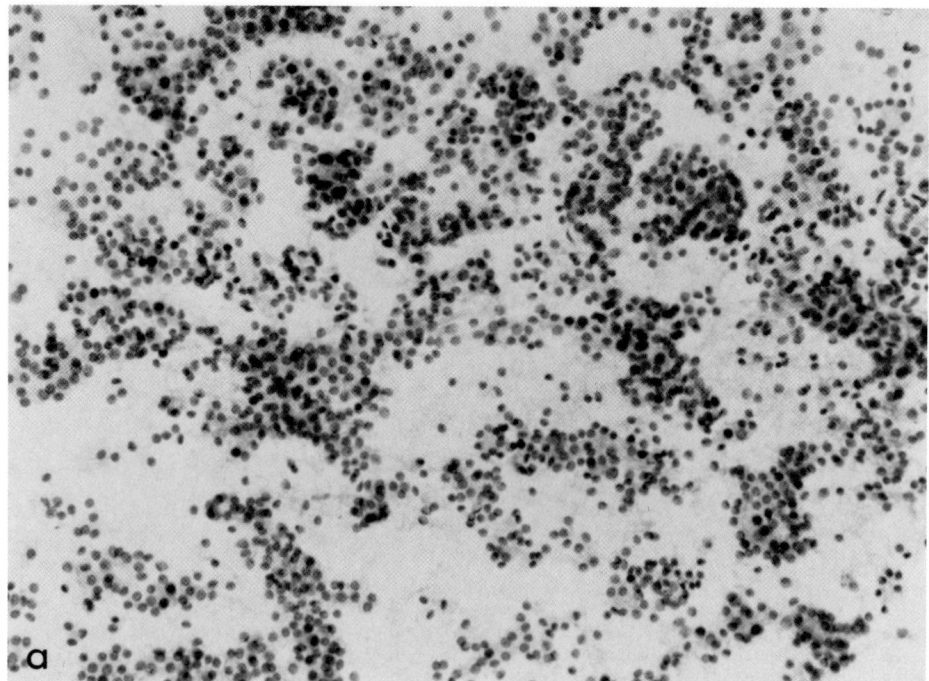

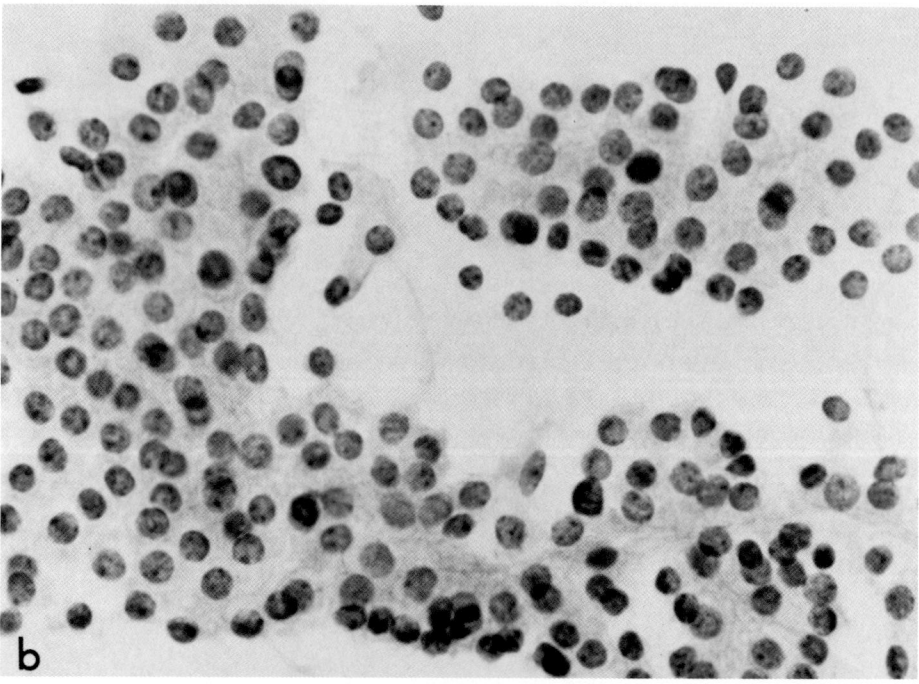

Fig. 6.10. A. Cellular adenoma. This cellular aspirate shows several tissue fragments of follicular epithelium with no colloid in the background. Papanicolaou preparation. × 160. **B.** Higher magnification of A showing syncytial arrangement, with slightly enlarged nuclei. Papanicolaou preparation. × 630.

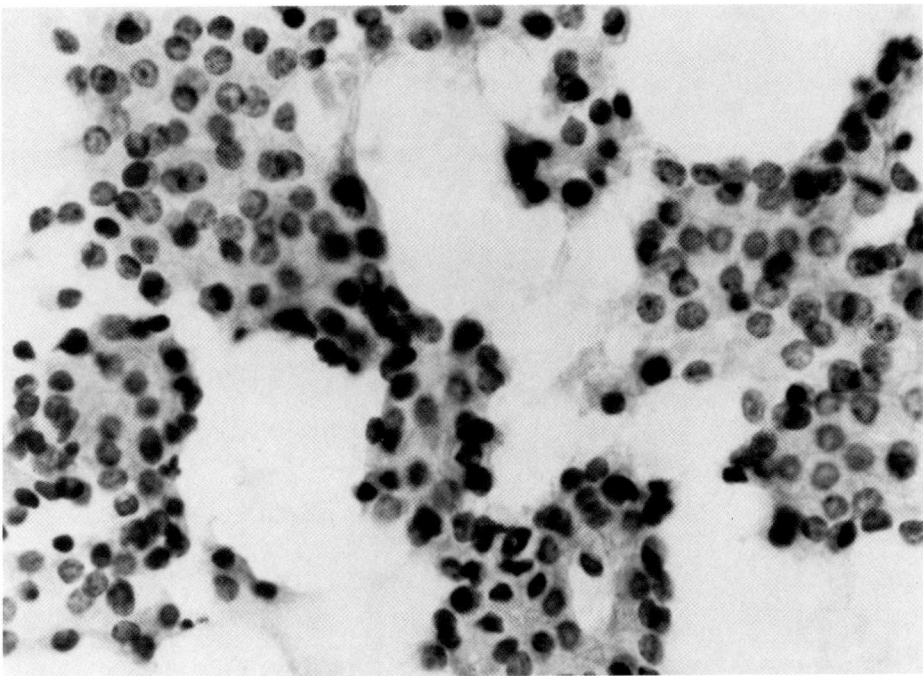

Fig. 6.11. Cellular adenoma showing syncytial-type tissue fragments with and without follicular pattern. The nuclei are uniformly enlarged. Papanicolaou preparation. × 630.

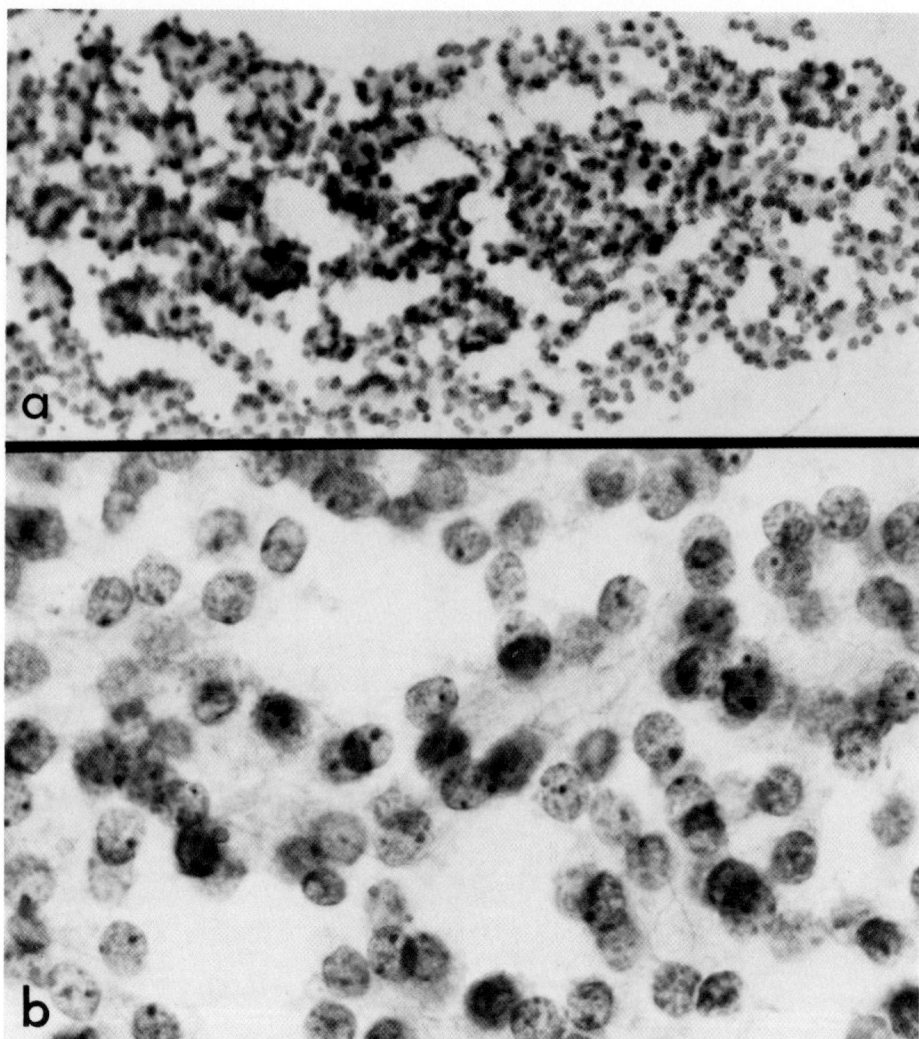

Fig. 6.12. A. Extremely cellular aspirate of cellular adenoma. The syncytial nature of the tissue fragments with follicular pattern and the absence of colloid is diagnostic. Papanicolaou preparation. × 63. **B.** Higher magnification of **A** showing large nuclei with nucleoli. This pattern may be interpreted as follicular carcinoma. Papanicolaou preparation. × 630.

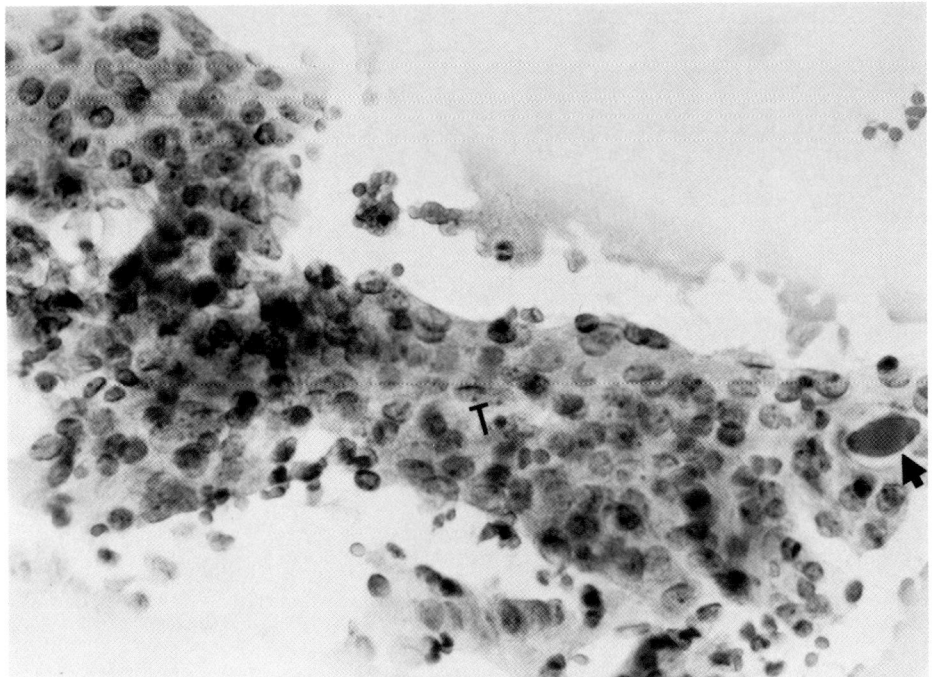

Fig. 6.13. Cellular adenoma with syncytial-type tissue fragments exhibiting a follicular *(arrow)* as well as trabecular *(T)* pattern. The enlarged nuclei have nucleoli. Papanicolaou preparation. × 400.

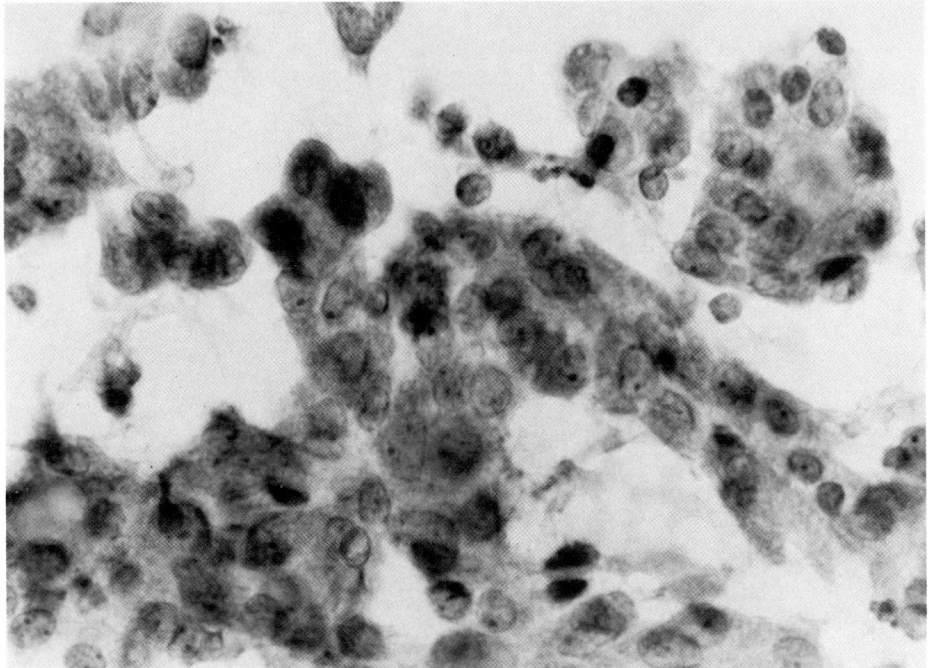

Fig. 6.14. Another field from same case as in Fig. 6.13 showing considerably enlarged, crowded, and overlapped nuclei containing nucleoli. This pattern is more consistent with a follicular carcinoma than with an adenoma. Papanicolaou preparation. × 630.

FOLLICULAR CARCINOMA

Follicular carcinomas are reported to represent 13–17% of thyroid carcinomas. Reported incidences vary depending on whether or not Hürthle cell carcinoma was included as part of the group. Follicular carcinomas are several times more common in women, but the age distribution differs from that of papillary carcinoma, being more frequent in middle and older age groups. A high incidence is reported in geographic areas with endemic goiters.[26] Follicular carcinomas can be distinguished from papillary carcinomas in several ways. They are well encapsulated, solitary, and rarely metastasize to cervical lymph nodes. They spread via the bloodstream to distant organs such as lungs and bone. The prognosis of the carcinoma is generally good, depending on the invasive characteristics of the tumor, but less favorable than for papillary carcinoma.[5,20,23,24,27]

Pathology

Like adenomas, follicular carcinoma grossly are well circumscribed and sharply demarcated from adjacent parenchyma (Fig. 6.15). Their invasive nature is not always evident to the naked eye. The cut surface shows a varied pattern ie, a bulging cut surface, fleshy areas, hemorrhage necrosis, calcification, etc. The microscopic pattern is as varied as that of the adenomas, ranging from well-developed follicles to a solid pattern with no evidence of differentiation (Fig. 6.16). The solid pattern may show trabeculae, alveoli, or large nests of carcinoma cells. Different growth patterns may be seen in the same tumor. The epithelial cells have larger nuclei with coarsely granular chromatin, often separated by clear areas. Nucleoli are frequent. The neoplastic cells can be functionally active, and thyroglobulin can be demonstrated by immunoperoxidase technique.

Classification of follicular carcinomas may be based on differentiation, eg, poorly or well-differentiated, or on extent of invasion such as capsular or blood vessel invasion, regardless of cytomorphology [9–14,17–22,9,11,15,16,19,21,22,25,27] (Figs. 6.17–6.19). We prefer to include atypical adenomas among the noninvasive carcinomas because histologically and in cytologic specimens the cytomorphology of neoplastic cells is very atypical (Table 6.2). Considerable confusion, controversy, and debate exist over what constitutes a capsular invasion and how much invasion is significant. Thus, the interpetation becomes subjective, and the diagnosis of encapsulated follicular lesions varies greatly.

TABLE 6.2. Classification of Follicular Carcinomas

1. Based on differentiation
     Well differentiated
     Poorly differentiated
2. Based on invasive characteristics
     a. Noninvasive (carcinoma in situ), malignant adenoma, atypical adenoma,
          carcinoma in adenoma, encapsulated carcinoma
          Well encapsulated with obvious malignant cytologic changes, but no evidence
               of invasive growth
     b. Minimally invasive (angioinvasive, encapsulated carcinoma)
          Minimal capsular or blood vessel invasion
     c. Moderate to markedly invasive
          Marked invasion of blood vessels or adjacent thyroid parenchyma

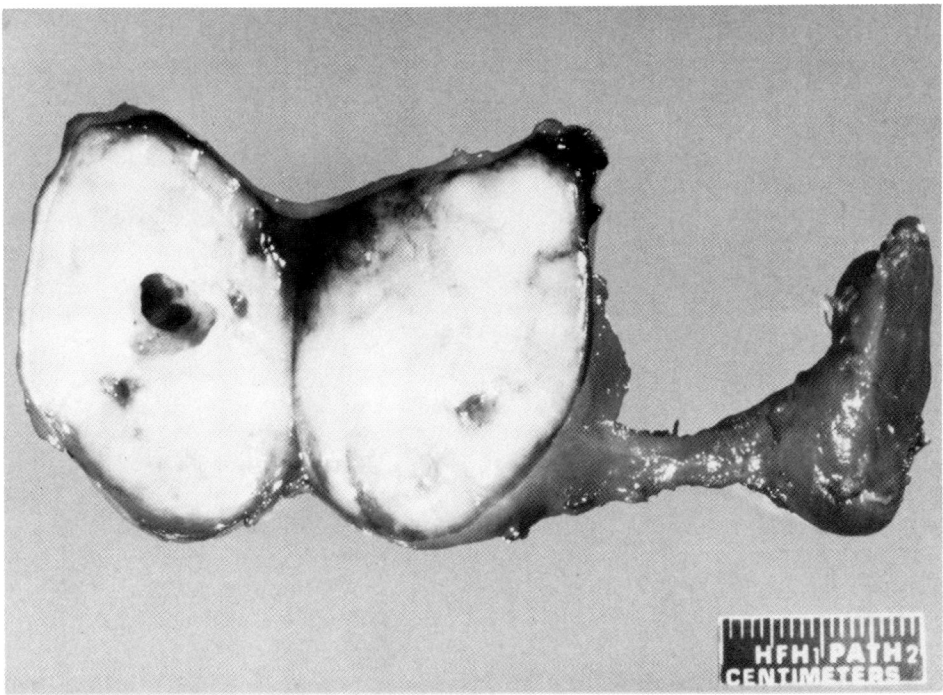

Fig. 6.15. Follicular carcinoma. A fleshy tumor replaces most of the right lobe.

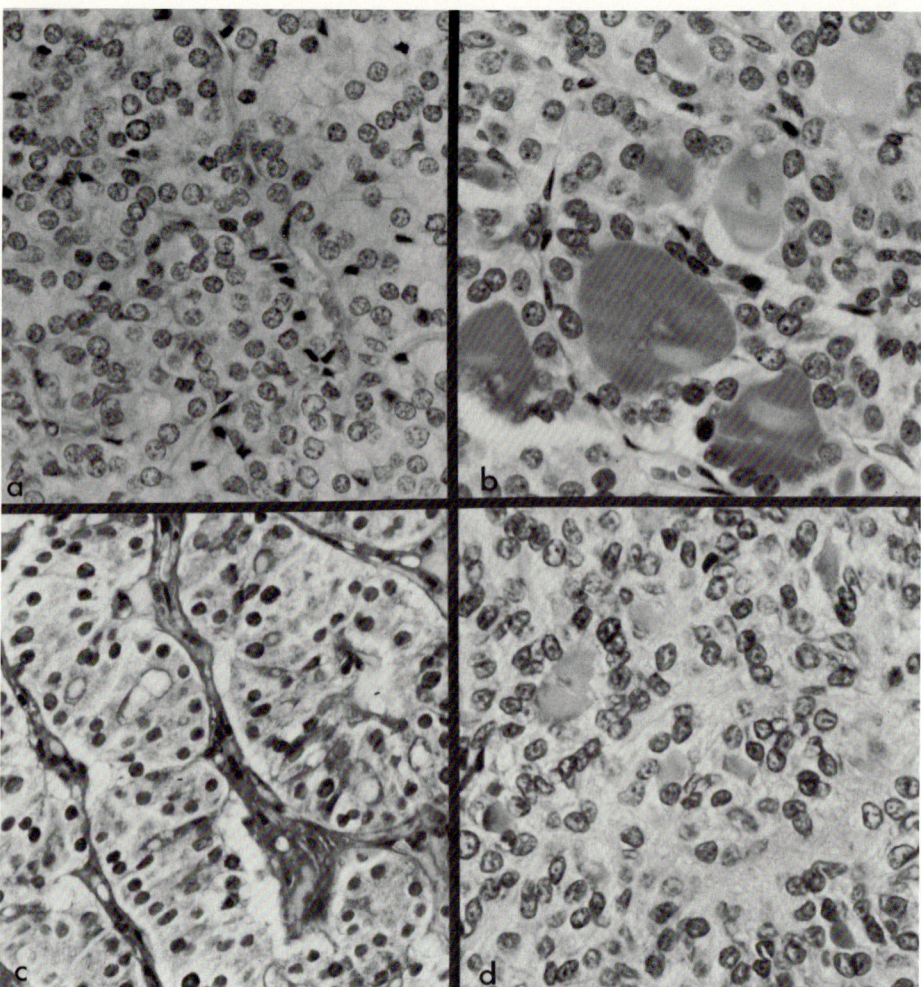

Fig. 6.16. Various histologic patterns of follicular carcinoma. **A.** Well-differentiated carcinoma with a microfollicular pattern, overlapping with that of microfollicular adenoma. Hematoxylin and eosin preparation. × 400. **B.** A well- differentiated microfollicular pattern, but with considerable nuclear atypia. Hematoxylin and eosin preparation. × 400. **C.** Trabecular pattern with no follicular differentiation. Note nuclear atypia. Hematoxylin and eosin preparation. × 400. **D.** Poorly differentiated carcinoma with solid pattern and marked nuclear atypia. Hematoxylin and eosin preparation. × 400.

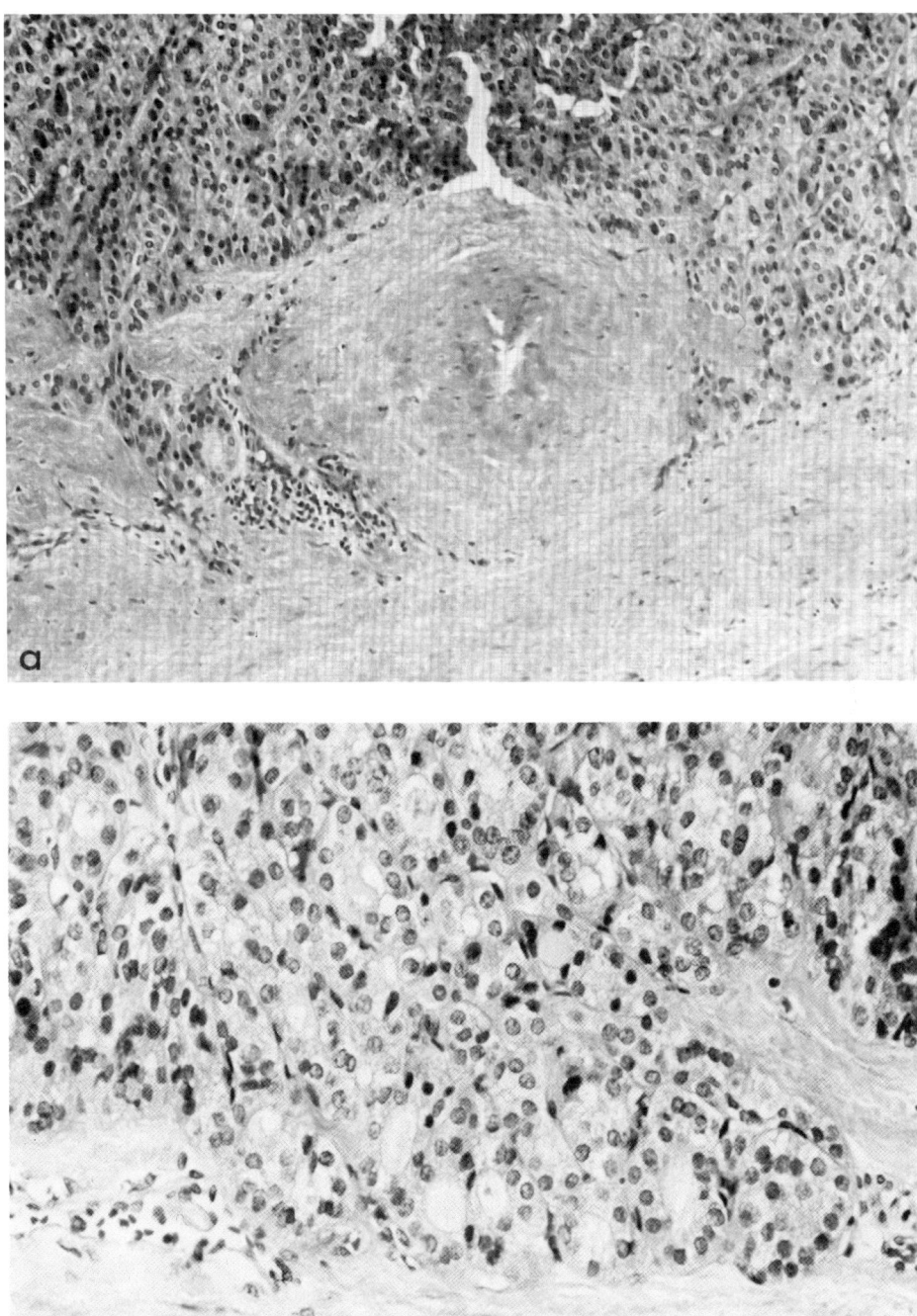

Fig. 6.17. **A.** Minimally invasive follicular carcinoma. Note small tongues of neoplastic epithelium in the capsule. Hematoxylin and eosin preparation. × 160. **B.** Higher magnification of another field from the same case as in **A**, showing a microfollicular pattern. This capsular involvement may not be considered sufficient by some for diagnosis of follicular carcinoma. Hematoxylin and eosin preparation. × 250.

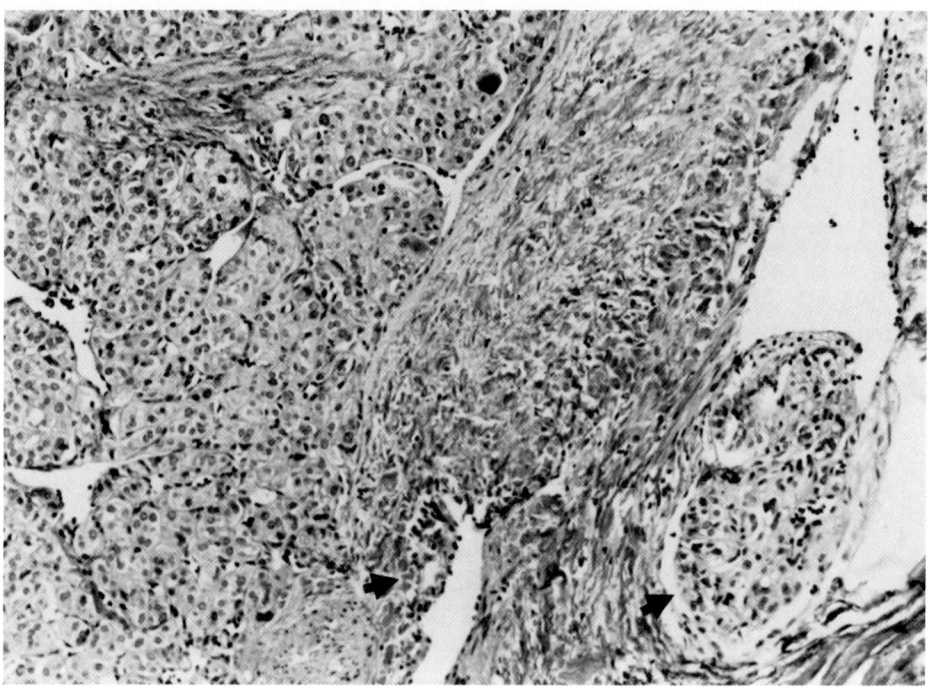

Fig. 6.18. Minimally invasive follicular carcinoma with vascular invasion *(arrow)*. Hematoxylin and eosin preparation. × 16.

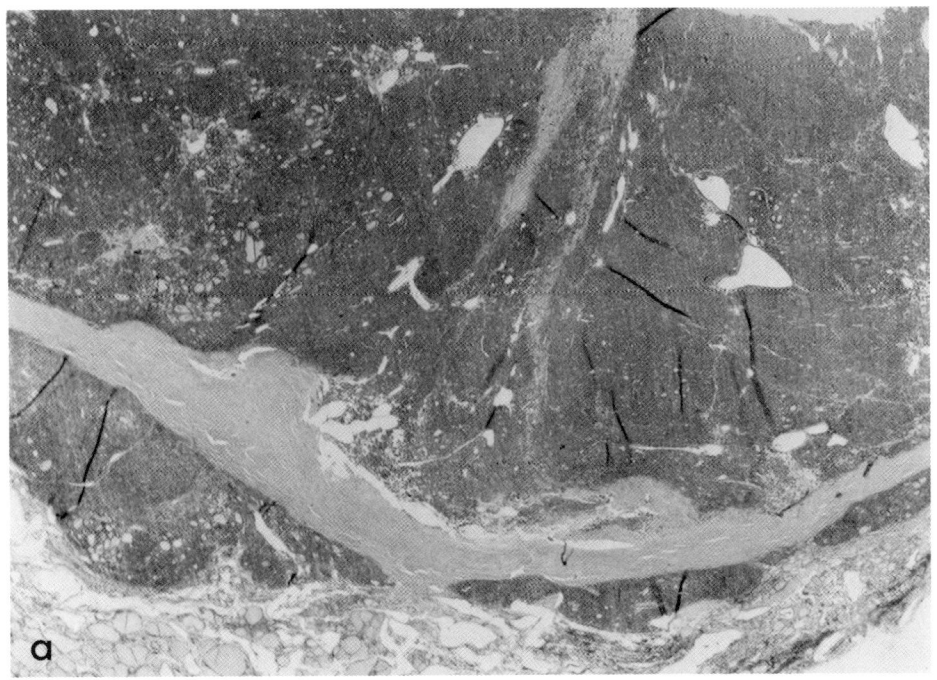

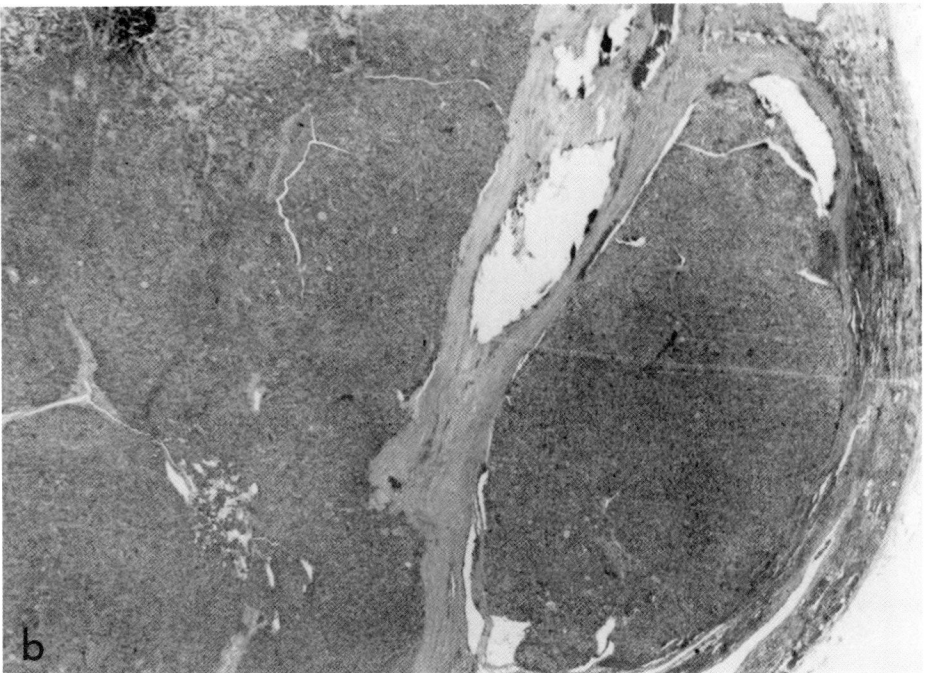

Fig. 6.19. A., B. Follicular carcinoma with moderate invasion of the surrounding parenchynma and blood vessels. Hematoxylin and eosin preparation. × 16.

Cytopathology

The aspirates of follicular carcinoma present a spectrum ranging from a pattern indistinguishable from that of cellular adenoma to one that is clearly recognizable

TABLE 6.3. Cytopathologic Features of Follicular Carcinoma

Pattern
   Syncytial-type tissue fragments with and without follicular pattern; follicles
      may be very irregular
   Marked crowding and overlapping of nuclei
Nuclei
   Round to oval, considerably enlarged in size
   Pleomorphism in size seen in less-differentiated neoplasms
   Very coarse chromatin granules with parachromatin clearing in some
   Single or multiple micronucleoli and/or macronucleoli always present
Cytoplasm
   Variable
   Colorless, pale to dense
Colloid
   Scanty, usually absent in background, but may be seen in follicular lumina

(Table 6.3). The patterns of well-differentiated to least-differentiated carcinomas gradually and imperceptibly merge (Figs. 6.20–6.26).

Aspirates are generally cellular and composed of syncytial-type tissue fragments of follicular epithelium, with or without a follicular pattern. Nuclei are very crowded and overlapped, and their density is much greater than that of follicular adenomas. The architecture of the follicles can be strikingly irregular. The nuclei are increased in size, round to oval, and either uniform or pleomorphic. The chromatin is coarsely granular in contrast with the dusty chromatin of papillary carcinoma cells. Parachromatin clearing is often seen. Micro- or macronucleoli are always present and intranuclear inclusions are rare, although Glant et al[6] reported one case in which they were present. The cells of follicular carcinoma tend to have more cytoplasm than those of adenoma. Colloid is very rarely seen in the background, but it may be present within the follicular lumina. The cytologic pattern suggestive or diagnostic of follicular carcinoma is seen in some follicular neoplasms that do not demonstrate invasive characteristics; these are referred to as atypical adenomas (Fig. 6.27).

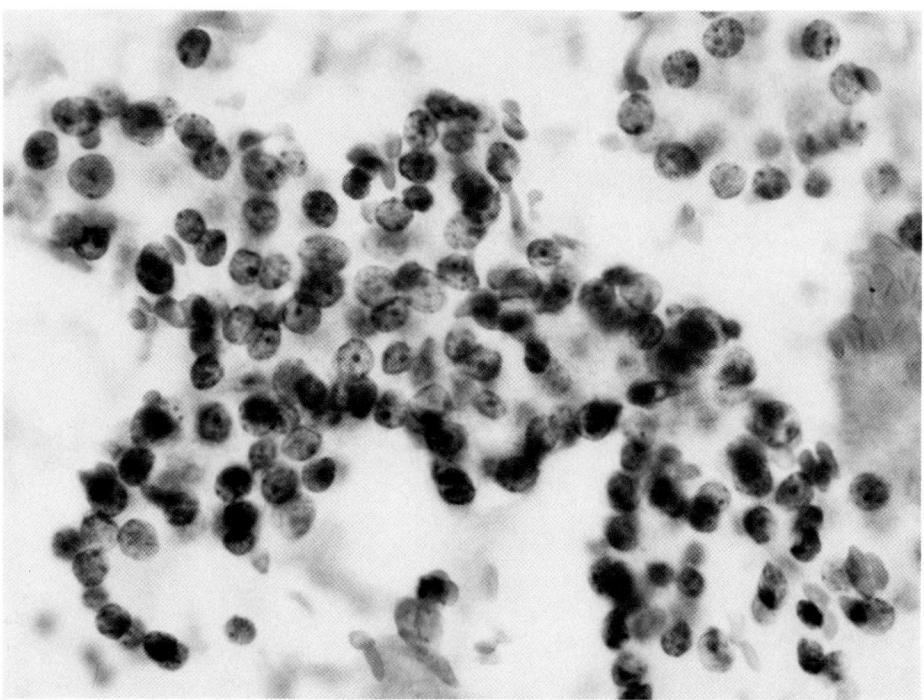

Fig. 6.20. Well-differentiated follicular carcinoma. The aspirate is cellular, with syncytial-type tissue fragments showing a follicular pattern. The nuclei are crowded, overlapped, and have nucleoli. Note the similarity to Fig. 6.12B. Papanicolaou preparation. × 630.

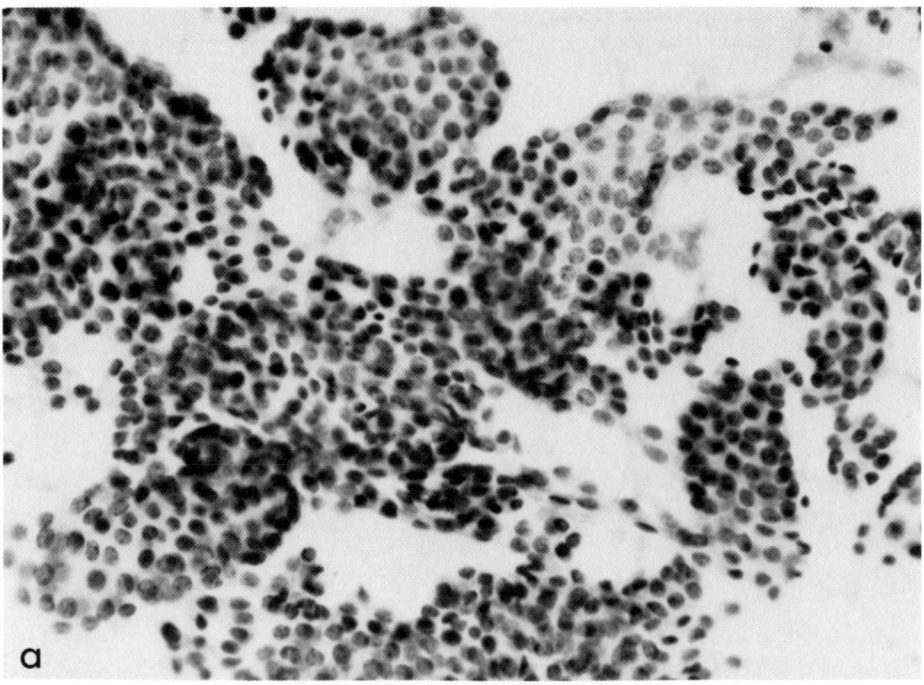

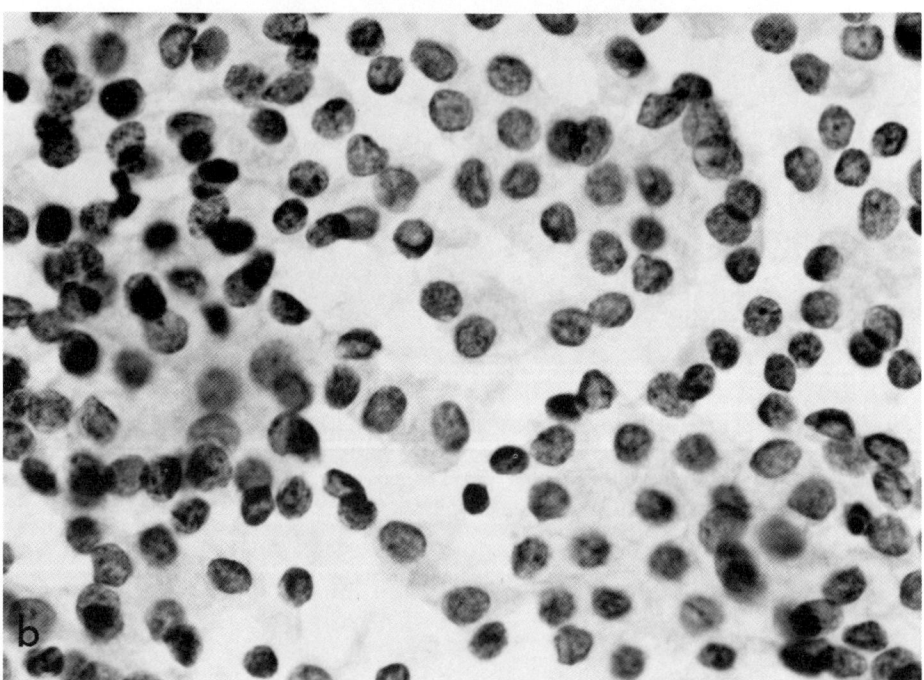

Fig. 6.21. Well-differentiated follicular carcinoma. **A.** The syncytial-type tissue fragments show marked crowding of enlarged nuclei. Papanicolaou preparation. × 400. **B.** Higher magnification showing a pattern very similar to the cellular adenomas shown in Figs. 6.10 and 6.11, except for nuclear size. Papanicolaou preparation. × 630.

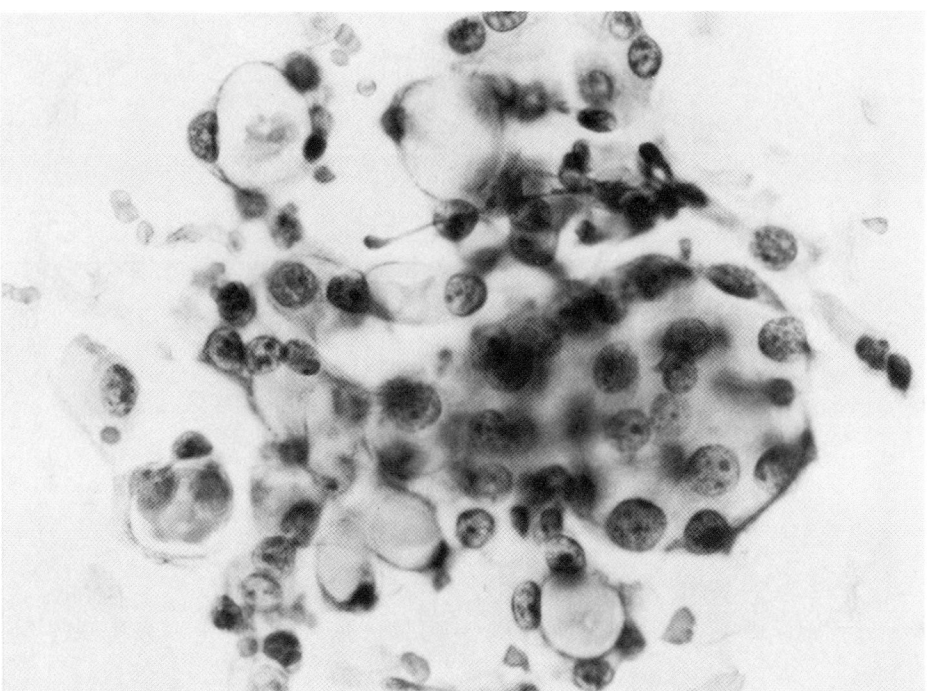

Fig. 6.22. Follicular carcinoma with markedly irregular follicles. The nuclei are pleomorphic and contain nucleoli. Papanicolaou preparation. × 630.

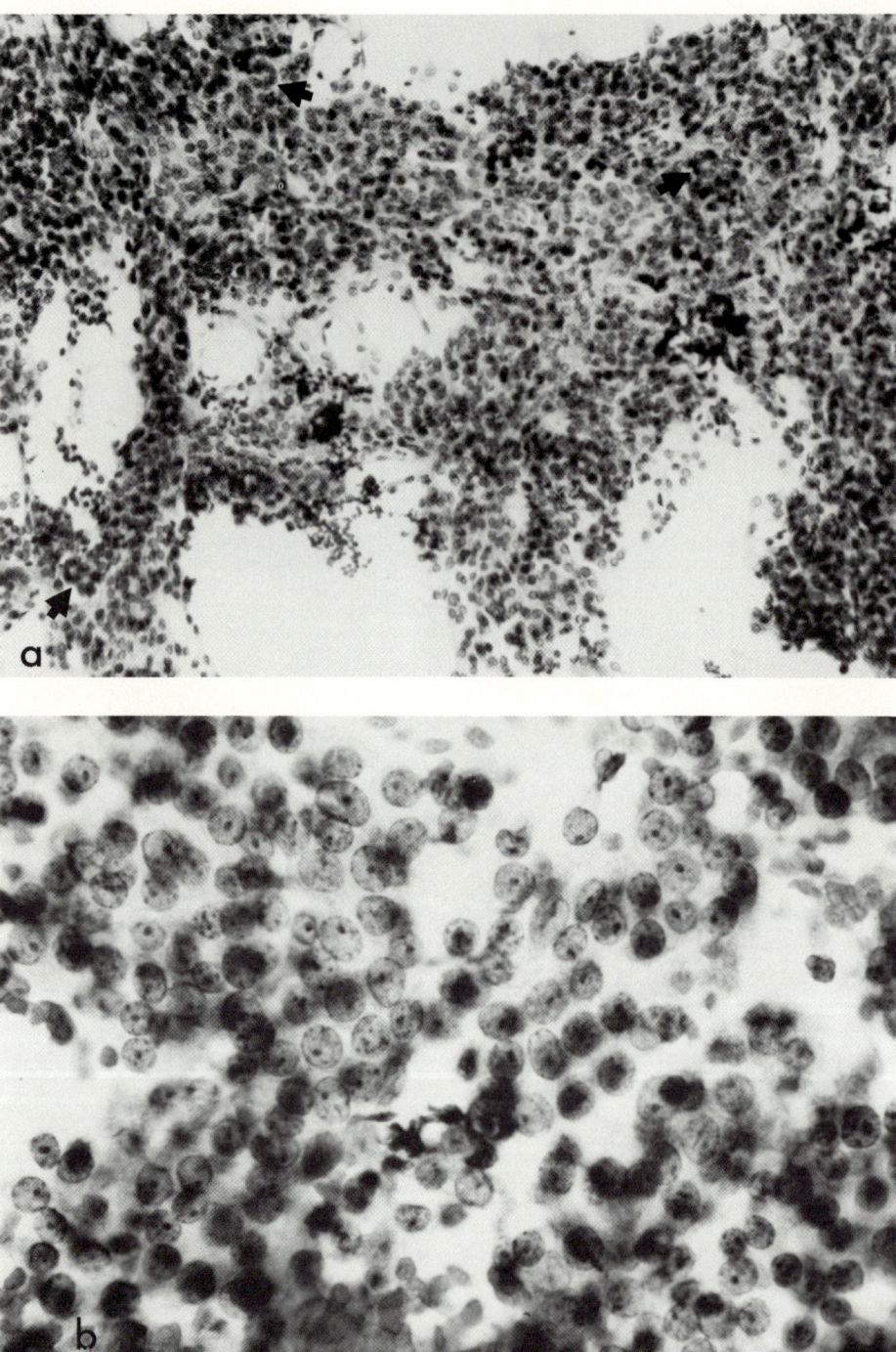

Fig. 6.23. Follicular carcinoma. **A.** The cellularity of the aspirate and marked density formed by extreme crowding of nuclei suggest the diagnosis of follicular carcinoma. Note the follicular pattern *(arrow)*. Papanicolaou preparation. × 160. **B.** Higher magnification of **A** showing large nuclei with nucleoli. Papanicolaou preparation. × 630.

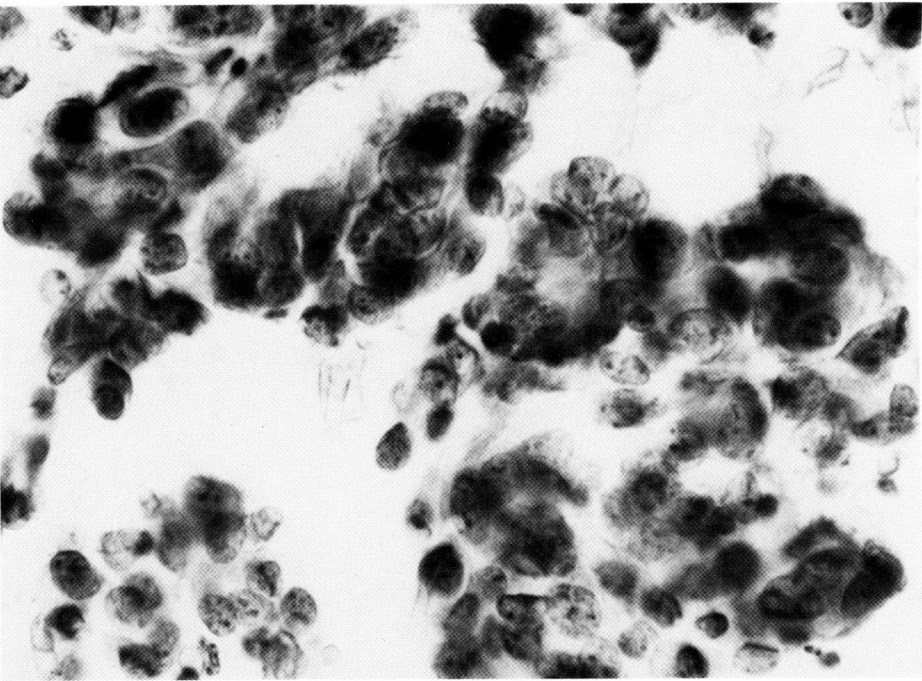

Fig. 6.24. Poorly differentiated follicular carcinoma. The architectural pattern and nuclear morphology allow an accurate diagnosis of follicular carcinoma. Papanicolaou preparation. × 630.

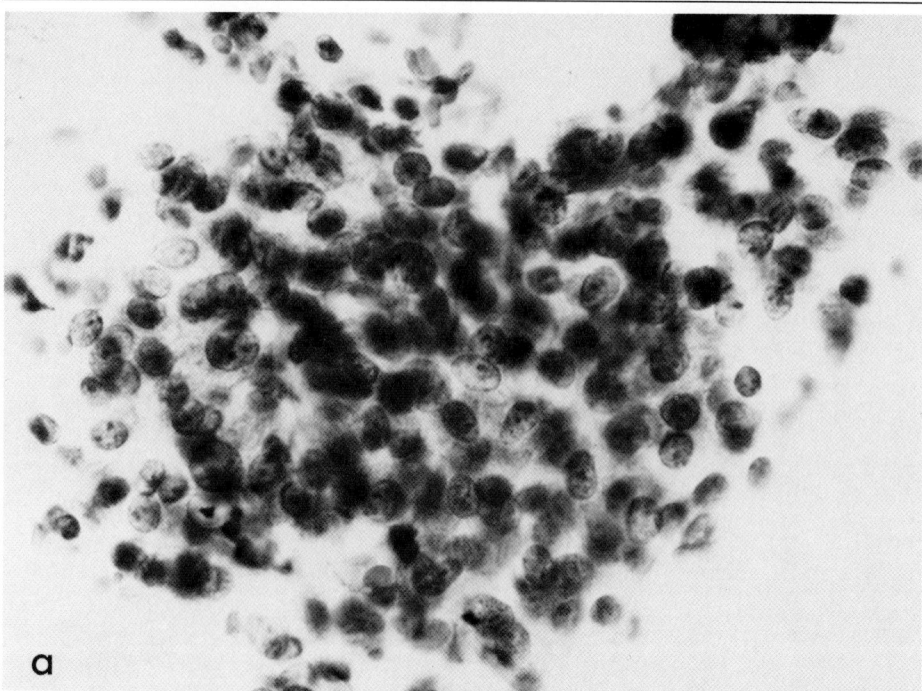

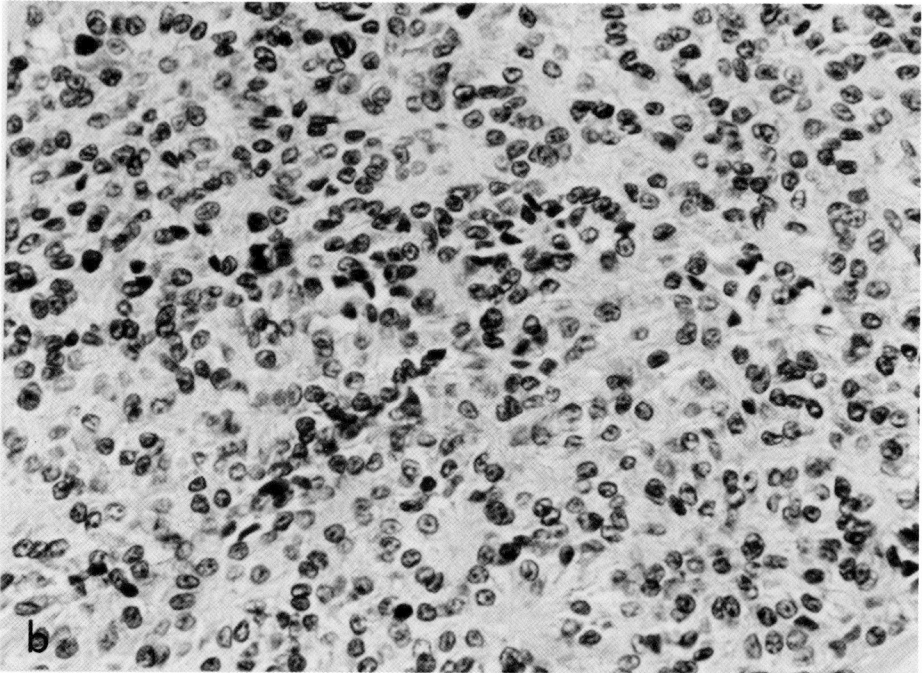

Fig. 6.25. A. Poorly differentiated follicular carcinoma with syncytial-type tissue fragments. Follicular pattern is not evident. Papanicolaou preparation. × 630. **B.** Histologic section showing a solid pattern. Hematoxylin and eosin preparation. × 250.

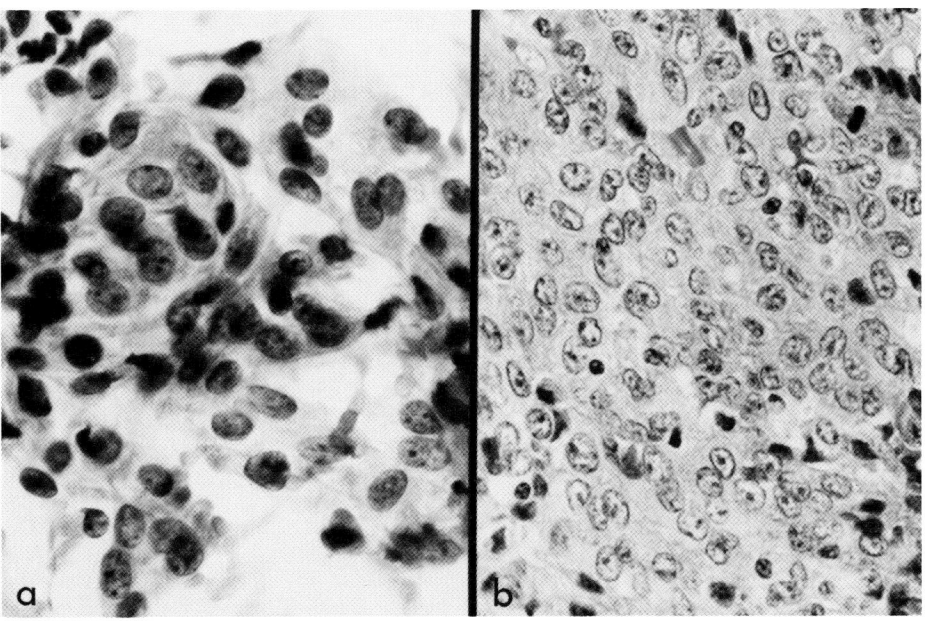

Fig. 6.26. A. Poorly differentiated follicular carcinoma. Papanicolaou preparation. × 630.
B. Histologic section showing a solid pattern. Hematoxylin and eosin preparation. × 400.

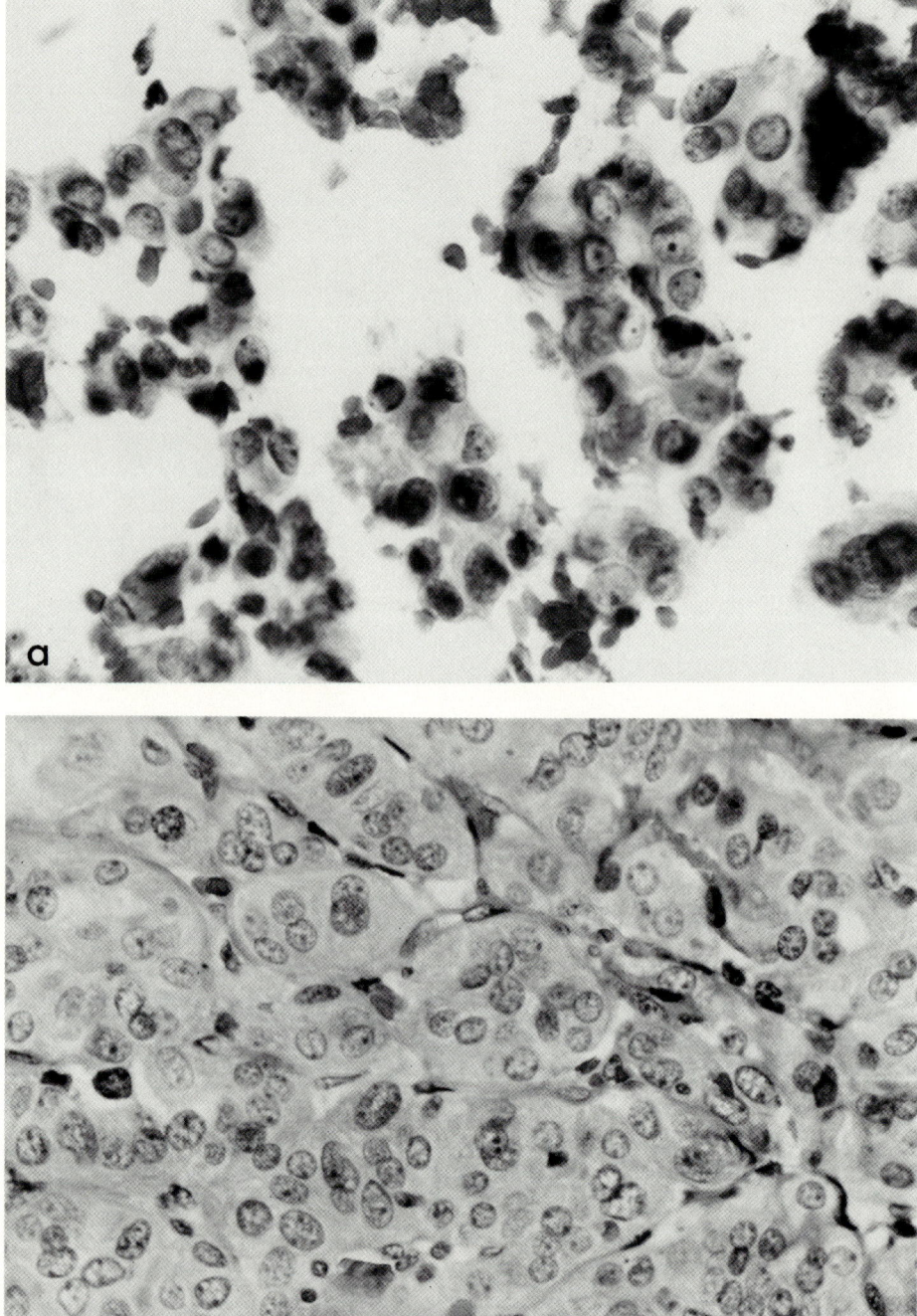

Fig. 6.27. Atypical adenoma. **A.** Cytologic pattern consistent with follicular carcinoma. Papanicolaou preparation. × 630. **B.** Histologically, this tumor failed to demonstrate invasive characteristics. Note the atypical cytomorphology. Hematoxylin and eosin preparation. × 630.

Diagnostic Accuracy

The diagnostic accuracy of follicular neoplasms is difficult to evaluate because of the overlapping patterns and because of the controversy and confusion over the histologic criteria for malignancy. Acceptable criteria include the presence of capsular and/or vascular invasion of an encapsulated follicular neoplasm. Nibbling of the capsule, even in multifocal areas, is not considered satisfactory evidence by some; others interpret the presence of neoplastic epithelium within a capsule as entrapment, and sometimes even displacement, due to an earlier needle biopsy procedure. For some, capsular transgression is required; for others, vascular invasion is the only acceptable criterion. Incomplete encapsulation or intralesional vascular involvement is also considered indicative of malignancy.

This confusion revolves around what constitutes true invasion, regardless of the cytomorphology. Neoplasms with obvious malignant cytologic changes are called atypical adenomas[8,20] if no invasive features are present, as they are known to follow a benign clinical course. Although an atypical adenoma is often interpreted cytologically as follicular carcinoma, in terms of cytohistologic correlation, this is considered a benign lesion, or a false-positive diagnosis. Likewise, a well-differentiated follicular carcinoma shares morphologic similarities with cellular adenoma, except for the invasive characteristics. However, cytologically it may be diagnosed as cellular adenoma and, therefore, will be considered a false-negative diagnosis. To avoid such disparities in cytohistologic correlation, Scandinavian authors[17,18] have combined all aspirates containing abundant follicular cells into one group called follicular neoplasms, indicating that cytologic differentiation between benign and malignant follicular neoplasms is not possible. As a result, many cold nodules that are not malignant or neoplastic are being surgically removed.

The purpose of the needle biopsy is defeated if no attempt is made to differentiate non-neoplastic from neoplastic, and benign from malignant, follicular lesions. Because of bias stemming from the practice of surgical pathology based on diagnostic criteria for follicular carcinoma using the Scandinavian reporting method, aspirates containing abundant follicular cells are being lumped together as follicular neoplasms. Rosai and Carcangiu[22] have expressed a somewhat different sentiment, as judged by their comments, "The importance of blood vessel invasion as the determining criterion for malignancy has been vastly exaggerated" and "it is not generally recognized that one of the classic papers[8] on encapsulated angioinvasive carcinoma stated that microscopic atypia are also nearly always present in these tumors." These atypical features in cytologic samples are represented by alterations in structural patterns of the tissue fragments of follicular epithelium and nuclear enlargement. Using these criteria, at least 70–75% of the follicular carcinomas may be identified accurately[15] (Table 6.4). These figures may be substantially lower if differentiation of follicular neoplasms is not attempted (Fig. 6.5). To support this view, the data presented in Tables 6.5 and 6.7 are divided into two time periods. In the earlier period, all cellular lesions were interpreted as follicular neoplasms, with recommendations of surgical removal for all. In the second period, cytologic differentiation was attempted. Table 6.6 gives cytohistologic correlation of all the follicular lesions and the incidence of follicular carcinoma with cytologic diagnosis of follicular adenoma. This incidence was lower when cytologic differentiation between adenoma and carcinoma was attempted: 14% versus 23% (Table 6.7).

TABLE 6.4. Cytologic Diagnosis of 52 Follicular Carcinomas

Follicular carcinoma	25	70%
Suspected follicular carcinoma	11	
Cellular follicular adenoma	14	
Nodular goiter	2	
Total	52	

TABLE 6.5. Histologic Diagnosis of 37 Cases Cytologically Interpreted as Follicular Carcinoma: Comparison of Two Time Periods

Histologic Diagnosis	First 3 yrs	Second 4 yrs
Follicular carcinoma	7 (53%)	18 (75%)
Atypical adenoma	1	3
Nodular Goiter	1	0
Follicular adenoma	3	3
Hashimoto's thyroiditis	1	—
Totals	13	24

TABLE 6.6. Cytohistologic Correlation of Follicular Lesions of Thyroid (Excluding Hürthle Cell Lesions)

Cytologic Diagnosis	No. of Cases	Histologic Diagnosis							
		FCA	FVPC	PCA	MCT	AA	FAD	NG	HASH
Nodular goiter	107	2	1	3	—	4	45	52	—
Follicular adenoma	158	14	4	9	2	5	83	37	4
Suspected FCA	46	11	—	—	—	5	18	10	2
FCA	37	25	—	—	—	4	6	1	1
Suspected FVPC	7	—	4	—	—	—	2	1	—
FVPC	24	—	24	—	—	—	—	—	—
Totals	379	52	33	12	2	18	154	101	7

AA, atypical ademona; FAD, follicular adenoma; FCA, follicular carcinoma; FVPC, follicular variant of papillary carcinoma; HASH, Hashimoto's thyroiditis; MCT, medullary carcinoma of the thyroid; NG, nodular goiter; PCA, papillary carcinoma.

TABLE 6.7. Histologic Diagnosis of 158 Thyroid Nodules Cytologically Interpreted as Cellular Adenoma: Comparison of First 3 and Second 4 Years

Histologic Diagnosis	First 3 yrs (Oct. 1976–1979)		Second 4 yrs (1980–1983)		Total
Papillary carcinoma	7		2		9
Follicular variant of papillary carcinoma	4		0		4
Follicular carcinoma	6		8		14
Medullary carcinoma	1		1		2
Atypical adenoma	1		5		6
Follicular adenoma	31		44		75
Nodular goiter	28	45%	14	19%	42
Hashimoto's thyroiditis	6		—		6
Totals	84		74		158
Percent carcinoma	21		14		18

The diagnostic errors in follicular neoplasms, thus, can be grouped into two main categories:

1. Non-neoplastic follicular lesions, eg, nodular goiter or follicular nodules in Hashimoto's thyroiditis versus follicular neoplasms

2. Benign follicular neoplasms (adenomas) versus malignant follicular neoplasms, eg., follicular carcinoma and follicular variant of papillary carcinoma

When non-neoplastic diseases are overcalled as neoplastic, the false-positive results do not generally cause concern, as most cold nodules would have been removed in prebiopsy era. The real concern is for false-negative diagnoses. Is it possible to undercall a follicular carcinoma? In our opinion, a follicular carcinoma may be undercalled as follicular adenoma, but the chances of it being diagnosed as nodular goiter or thyroiditis are very remote. The general tendency is to overcall. The diagnosis of carcinoma may be missed only if the specimen is poorly fixed or inadequate. With adequate cellularity, the diagnosis of follicular neoplasm is not apt to be missed.

It is important to avoid errors in the first category, non-neoplastic follicular lesions, to prevent unnecessary surgery. Errors in the second category, benign versus malignant follicular neoplasms, are not as consequential because surgery is recommended for both. The differentiation between adenoma and carcinoma is justified is the clinician prefers conservative management for adenomas in medically high-risk patients. The differentiating features are discussed in the next section, with the exception of follicular nodule in Hashimoto's thyroiditis, which is discussed in Chapter 11, Thyroiditis.

DIFFERENTIAL DIAGNOSIS OF FOLLICULAR LESIONS OF THYROID

Follicular lesions of thyroid include those that histologically present a follicular architecture[15,17] (Table 6.8; Fig. 6.28). If the lesions are cellular with scant or absent

TABLE 6.8. Cellular Follicular Lesions of Thyroid

1. Hyperplastic goiter
2. Cellular follicular adenoma
3. Follicular carcinoma
4. Follicular variant of papillary carcinoma

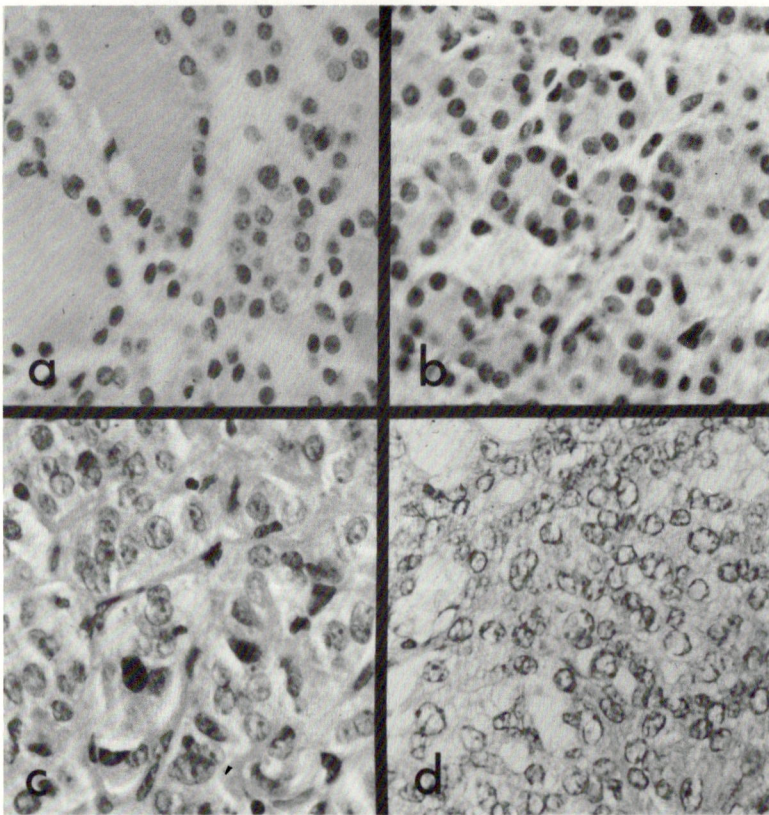

Fig. 6.28. Follicular lesions of thyroid. **A.** Hyperplastic goiter. Hematoxylin and eosin preparation. × 400. **B.** Cellular adenoma. Hematoxylin and eosin preparation. × 400. **C.** Follicular carcinoma. Hematoxylin and eosin preparation. × 400. **D.** Follicular variant of papillary carcinoma. Hematoxylin and eosin preparation. × 400.

colloid, the aspirates will show a large population of follicular cells isolated and in tissue fragments. The cytologic differentiation depends on the architectural pattern of the tissue fragments of the follicular epithelium, as well as on the cytomorphology (Plate 6.1).

The spectrum of histologic patterns in nodular goiters ranging from hyperinvoluted to hyperplastic overlap those of follicular adenomas ranging from macrofollicular to the cellular type. The follicular adenomas, in turn, overlap those of follicular carcinoma. Likewise, the cytologic samples from these lesions show similar overlap, with the patterns merging imperceptibly from one type to the other. This overlapping naturally creates some difficulty in diagnosis.

Nevertheless, certain features are noticeable (Fig. 6.29):

1. The amount of colloid decreases from macrofollicular adenoma to cellular adenoma and follicular carcinoma.

2. The architecture of tissue fragments of follicular epithelium is different in non-neoplastic and neoplastic lesions (sheets versus syncytia).

3. Follicular cell nuclei gradually increase in size.

4. The compact chromatin pattern of the follicular cell nuclei in nodular goiter changes to granular in cellular adenoma, and to coarsely granular with nucleoli and parachromatin clearing in follicular carcinoma.

Modified from Cervino , J.M.: et al - La Exploracion Citologica De La Glandula Tirodes Y Sus Correlaciones Anatomoclinicas. Anales De La Facultad de Medicina. 47:128-143, 1962

TABLE 6.9. Differential Diagnosis of Follicular Lesions of Thyroid (Excluding Hürthle Cell Lesions)

	Hyperplastic Nodular Goiter	Follicular Adenoma, Cellular Type	Follicular Carcinoma	Follicular Variant of Papillary Carcinoma
Cellularity	Usually cellular	Usually cellular	Usually cellular	Usually cellular
Colloid	Scant to absent	Scant to absent	Scant to absent	Scant to absent
Configuration of tissue fragments	Sheets of cells with honeycomb pattern; follicles uniform; nuclei well spaced, maintaining their polarity	Syncytial-type tissue fragments with and without follicular pattern; follicles irregular; crowding and overlapping of nuclei	Syncytial-type tissue fragments with and without follicular pattern; follicles very irregular; marked crowding and overlapping of nuclei	Syncytial-type tissue fragments with and without follicular pattern; follicles irregular with marked crowding and overlapping of nuclei
Nuclear size	Normal to slightly enlarged and uniform	Enlarged but uniform, no pleomorphism	Considerably enlarged, pleomorphic in size	Enlarged; pleomorphism may or may not be present
Chromatin	Finely granular, uniformly dispersed, sometimes compact	Fine to coarsely granular	Coarsely granular; hyperchromatin with parachromatin clearing frequent	Fine powdery chromatin, occasionally coarsely granular, chromatin ridge
Nucleolus	Generally absent	Infrequent	Micro- and macronucleoli	One or more micronucleoli
Intranuclear cytoplasmic inclusions	Not present	Not present	On extreme occasions	Usually present; may be diagnostic clue
Cytoplasm	Clear to pale; variable	Usually scant and pale	Variable; scant to pale, sometimes dense	Usually scanty
Helpful features	Cytologic changes of nodular goiter in same or in other slides			Cytologic features of papillary carcinoma in same or other slides

A cellular sample consisting of follicular cells—isolated or in tissue fragments, with or without follicular pattern—in a clear background containing little or no colloid will represent one of four entitites: hyperplastic goiter, cellular follicular adenoma, follicular carcinoma, or a follicular variant of papillary carcinoma (Table 6.8; Plate 6.1) If the architectural pattern is disregarded and emphasis is placed on cellularity alone, differentiation of follicular lesions is not possible. Hypercellularity is not synonymous with neoplasia. Many cold nodules are indeed hyperplastic goiter and will be removed surgically, if an attempt is not made to differentiate them from follicular neoplasms. If all cellular follicular neoplasms are removed surgically, the differentiation between an adenoma and a follicular carcinoma becomes an intellectual exercise that is of academic interest only. The differentiating features of various cellular follicular lesions are listed in Table 6.9 and illustrated in Plates 6.1–6.8.

It must be noted that the majority of cellular follicular adenomas (75–80%) are benign. The incidence of a follicular carcinoma in the group cytologically diagnosed as adenoma is 14–23% (Table 6.7). The latter figures are similar to those Vickery[25] projected for cellular follicular lesions diagnosed by core-needle biopsy. We have tried to differentiate cytologically those follicular adenomas that have a low probability for demonstrating invasive characteristics, realizing that there are limitations. Differentiation of cellular adenoma from a follicular carcinoma is based on nuclear characteristics, especially size, which is a good indicator of the possibility of malignancy. It has been well documented in studies of Boon et al,[2] who made a morphometric analysis of nuclear sizes of various follicular lesions (Table 6.10), and in the work of Cervino et al[3] more than 20 years ago, who measured the nuclear diameter of follicular cells in various thyroid lesions. Lang et al[14] have also confirmed this observation.

Differentiation of cellular adenoma or follicular carcinoma from a follicular variant of papillary carcinoma is based strictly on nuclear morphology,[4] as the tissue fragments present similar architectural patterns (Fig. 6.30) (see Chapter 8, Papillary Carcinoma). Because of the typical nuclear morphology, the diagnostic accuracy of the follicular variant of papillary carcinoma is very high (Table 6.6).

Rarely, medullary carcinoma may be typed as follicular neoplasm.[12] Differentiating features are discussed in Chapter 10, Medullary Carcinoma.

TABLE 6.10. Nuclear Area of Follicular Cells in Follicular Lesions

	Mean (μm^2)	SD (μm^2)
1. Nontoxic goiter	25	3
2. Follicular adenoma	74	23
3. Follicular carcinoma	131	23

SD, standard deviation.

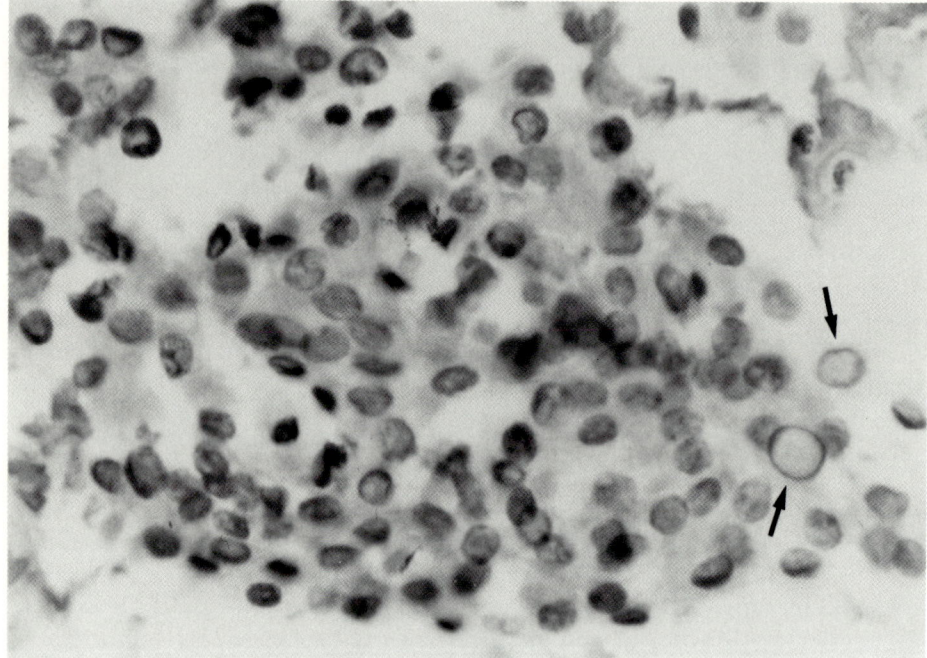

Fig. 6.30. Follicular variant of papillary carcinoma. The tissue fragments are syncytial type. The nuclei have powdery chromatin and cytoplasmic inclusions *(arrows)*. Papanicolaou preparation. × 630.

Summary of Overlapping Patterns of Follicular Lesions

I. Nodular goiter versus follicular adenoma and carcinoma

    A. Nodular goiter, ⟷ Follicular adenoma (macrofollicular
       hyperinvoluted type, colloid nodule)

Both show abundant colloid, sparse epithelial component with small follicles, and pyknotic nuclei. These two cannot be differentiated on cytologic bases, and they are diagnosed only on histologic criteria—encapsulated versus nonencapsulated. However, these are not likely to be interpreted as follicular carcinoma.

    B. Nodular goiter Follicular adenoma, simple type
       (admixture of involuted ⟷ (follicles generally of regular size, may
       and hyperplastic areas) be mixed with cellular areas)

Both show admixture of colloid and benign follicular epithelium. Architectural

pattern of tissue fragment depends on type of follicle. Cytologic pattern depends on areas sampled. Not likely to be overcalled as follicular carcinoma (see Plate 6.2).

                   common
    C. Nodular goiter, ⟶ Follicular adenoma (cellular
       hyperplastic ⟵ type)
                 unlikely

Features common to both are scant or absent colloid and increased cellularity. Architectural pattern of the tissue fragments—regular follicles and honeycomb sheets versus syncytial-type fragments with crowding and overlapping of nuclei and irregular follicles—is an important criterion that distinguishes the two entities (see Plate 6.3).

    D. Nodular goiter, hyperplastic ⤬ Follicular carcinoma

Although both show increased cellularity and scant or absent colloid, architectural pattern of tissue fragments of follicular epithelium and nuclear size are distinctly different. Cytologic pattern of follicular carcinoma is not likely to be interpreted as nodular goiter, or vice versa (see Plate 6.4).

II. Follicular adenoma versus follicular carcinoma

    A. Follicular adenoma, ⤬ Follicular carcinoma
       macrofollicular type (colloid
       nodule)

The cytopathologic patterns of these two entities are so different that it is very unlikely that one would be misinterpreted as the other (see Plate 6.5).

                  rare
    B. Follicular adenoma, ⟶ Follicular carcinoma
       simple type ⟵
                 rare

If the sampled area of the carcinoma adenoma is a cellular one, then the distinction between the two may be difficult on a cytologic basis.

often

C. Follicular adenoma, micro-   ──────────▶   Follicular carcinoma
    follicular and trabecular types ◀──────────
    (cellular adenoma)

often

Both show increased cellularity and scant or absent colloid. Both show syncytial-type tissue fragments of follicular epithelium containing crowded, overlapped nuclei with altered polarity. When the nuclear size of both follicular neoplasms are approximately the same, adenoma is difficult to differentiate from carcinoma. Increased density of nuclei within tissue fragments and presence of nucleoli favor malignancy. Despite features suggesting malignancy, invasive characteristics may not be demonstrated (see Plates 6.6 and 6.7).

D. Follicular adenoma, atypical   ◀──────────▶   Follicular carcinoma

Essentially the same cytologic pattern. If atypical adenoma is accepted as carcinoma in situ or noninvasive follicular carcinoma, the distinction is superfluous. Nuclei of ayptical adenoma may be much larger and atypical than those seen in follicular carcinoma (see Plate 6.8).

REFERENCES

1. Abele JS, Miller TR: Fine needle aspiration of the thyroid nodule: clinical applications. In Clark OH: *Endocrine Surgery of the Thyroid and Parathyroid Glands.* St. Louis, Mosby, 1985, pp. 293–335.

2. Boon ME, Löwhagen T, Williams JS: Planimetric studies on fine needle aspirates from follicular adenoma and follicular carcinoma of the thyroid. *Acta Cytol* 24:145–148, 1980.

3. Cervino JM, Paseyro P, Grosso O, Maggioto S: La exploracion citologic de la glandula tirodes y sus correlaciones anatomoclinicas. *An Facultad Med* 47:128–143, 1962.

4. Chen KTK, Rosai J: Follicular variant of thyroid papillary carcinoma: A clinicopathological study of six cases. *Am J Surg Pathol* 1:123–130, 1977.

5. Franssila D: Is the differentiation between papillary and follicular thyroid carcinoma valid? *Cancer* 32:853–864, 1973.

6. Glant MD, Berger EK, Davey DD: Intranuclear cytoplasmic inclusions in aspirates of follicular neoplasms of the thyroid. *Acta Cytol* 28:576–579, 1984.

7. Hazard JB, Kenyon R: Atypical adenoma of the thyroid. *Arch Pathol* 58:554–563, 1954.

8. Hazard JB, Kenyon R: Encapsulated angioinvasive carcinoma (angioinvasive adenoma of the thyroid gland. *Am J Clin Pathol* 24:755–766, 1954.

9. Heddinger CHR, Sobin LH: Histologic typing of thyroid tumors. In: *International Histologic Classification of Tumors*, NR 11, Geneva, WHO, 1974.

10. Iida F: Surgical significance of capsule invasion of adenoma of the thyroid. *Surg Gynecol Obstet* 144:710–712, 1977.

11. Kahn NF, Perzin KH: Follicular carcinoma of the thyroid: an evaluation of the histologic criteria used for diagnosis. *Pathol Annu* 18(part 1):221–253, 1983.

12. Kini SR, Miller JM, Hamburger JI, Purslow MJ: Cytopathology of follicular lesions of the thyroid gland. *Diagn Cytopathol* 1:123–132, 1985.

13. Kini SR, Miller JM, Hamburger JI, Smith MJ: Cytopathologic features of medullary carcinoma of the thyroid. *Arch Pathol Lab Med* 108:156–159, 1984.

14. Lang W, Atay Z, Georgi A: The cytologic classification of follicular tumors in the thyroid gland. *Virch Arch {A}* 378:199–211, 1978.

15. Lang W, Georgi A, Staveh G, Kienzle E: The differentiation of atypical adenomas and encapsulated follicular carcinomas in the thyroid gland. *Virch Arch {A}* 385:125–141, 1980.

16. LiVolsi VA, Merino MJ: Histopathologic differential diagnosis of the thyroid. *Pathol Annu* 16(part 2):357–406, 1981.

17. Löwhagen T: Thyroid. In Zajicek J: *Aspiration Biopsy Cytology. Part I. Cytology of Supradiaphragmatic Organs.* New York, Karger, 1974, pp. 67–69.

18. Löwhagen T, Spencer E: Cytologic presentation of thyroid tumors in aspiration biopsy smear. *Acta Cytol* 18:192–197, 1974.

19. Meissner WA: Follicular carcinoma of the thyroid. *Am J Surg Pathol* 1:171–173, 1977.

20. Meissner WA, Warren S: *Tumors of the Thyroid Gland.* Fascicle 4, Second Series, *Atlas of Tumor Pathology.* Washington, DC, Armed Forces Institute of Pathology, 1969.

21. Rosai J: *Ackerman's Surgical Pathology,* 6th ed. St. Louis, Mosby, 1981, pp. 357–360.

22. Rosai J, Carcangiu ML: Pathology of thyroid tumors, some recent and old questions. *Human Pathol* 15:1008–1012, 1984.

23. Sakamoto A, Kasai N, Sugoano H: Poorly differentiated carcinoma of the thyroid. A clinicopathologic entity for a high-risk group of papillary and follicular carcinomas. *Cancer* 52:1849–1855, 1983.

24. Selzer G, Kahn LB, Albertyn L: Primary malignant tumors of the thyroid gland: a clinicopathologic study of 254 cases. *Cancer* 40:1501–1510, 1977.

25. Vickery AL Jr: Needle biopsy pathology. In Williams ED: *Clinics in Endocrinology and Metabolism,* vol 10. Philadelphia, Saunders, 1981, pp. 275–292.

26. Williams ED, Doniach I, Bjarnason O, Michie W: Thyroid cancer in an iodide rich area. *Cancer* 39:215–222, 1977.

27. Woolner LB: Thyroid carcinomas: pathologic classification with data on prognosis. *Semin Nucl Med* 1:481–502, 1971.

7

Hürthle Cell Lesions

Hürthle cells—also called oncocytes, Askanazy cells, or oxyphils—are altered follicular cells. Although the cells described originally by Hürthle were probably parafollicular cells, the term "Hürthle cell" has become established in the medical literature. They are large polygonal cells (Fig. 7.1) with abundant granular cytoplasm, the granularity being the result of abundant mitochondria.[10] Hürthle cells generally do not synthesize thyroglobulin or concentrate radioactive iodine.

The Hürthle cell metaplasia of follicular cells probably reflects a functional state labeled by Friedman[6] as a "cellular involution." It is seen in several conditions affecting the thyroid, such as Hashimoto's thyroiditis, adenomatous goiter, Grave's disease, and others (Table 7.1). This change can be extensive, resulting in formation of clinically palpable nodules that cannot be differentiated from neoplasms and are often removed surgically. This chapter deals with the cytopathology of Hürthle cell neoplasms and non-neoplastic Hürthle cell nodules, which together constitute Hürthle cell lesions of the thyroid (Table 7.2).

HÜRTHLE CELL NEOPLASMS

Hürthle cell neoplasms have generated considerable interest over the decades.[4,5,11] Most authors regard these neoplasms as morphologic variants of follicular neoplasms and, depending on the invasive characteristics, use the terms "follicular adenoma" or "carcinoma, oxyphil type."[2,3,8,9,14,17,18,21,22] Proponents of this view believe that there is no justification for isolating Hürthle cell adenomas or carcinomas because their behavior parallels that of follicular adenoma or carcinoma, respectively. In sharp variance with this viewpoint is the study of Thompson et al.[19] These authors reviewed 25 Hürthle cell neoplasms and found that their biological behavior is unpredictable and that the distinction between an adenoma and carcinoma is not easily made by conventional criteria used for follicular neoplasms. According to Thompson et al,[19] Hürthle cell tumors follow an aggressive course with a frequent recurrence rate, distant metastasis, and a high incidence of fatal outcome, regardless of invasive

97

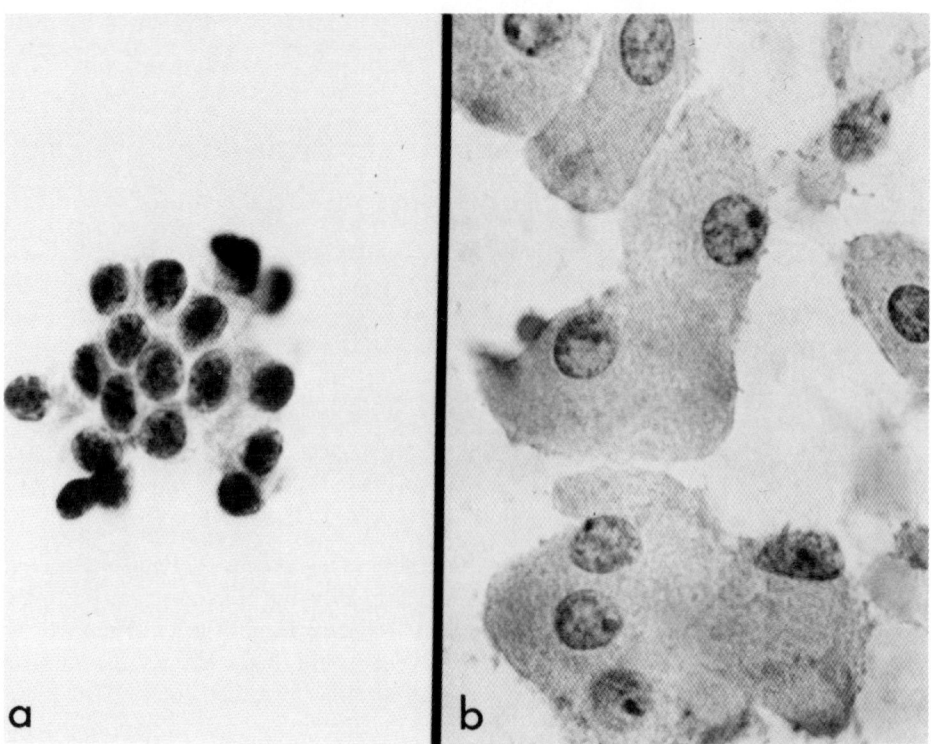

Fig. 7.1. Comparison of normal follicular cells with Hürthle cells. **A.** Follicular cells are small cuboidal, with scanty cytoplasm. The nuclei are round, with compact chromatin devoid of nucleoli. Papanicolaou preparation. × 1,000. **B.** Hürthle cells are large, polygonal with abundant, granular cytoplasm and slightly eccentric nuclei with prominent macronucleoli. Papanicolaou preparation. × 1,000.

TABLE 7.1. Conditions Associated with Hürthle
            Cell (Oxyphilic) Change

Hashimoto's thyroiditis
Adenomatous goiter
Grave's disease
Radiation
Myxedema
Partial thyroidectomy

TABLE 7.2. Differential Diagnosis of Hürthle Cell Lesions

Hürthle cell neoplasms
Hürthle cell nodules (involutional or non-neoplastic)
Hashimoto's thyroiditis
Adenomatous goiter
Graves' disease

characteristics. This observation was reconfirmed by Gundry et al.[7] Therefore, they assigned the term "Hürthle cell tumors" to all neoplasms comprising Hürthle cells and recommended total thyroidectomy. Since this study was published, it has been disputed and refuted by many who have proved otherwise. However, Tollefsen et al,[20] Rosai and Carcangiu,[15] and many others believe that although Hürthle cell adenomas behave in a benign fashion, Hürthle cell carcinomas represent an entity distinct from follicular carcinomas.

As Hürthle cell adenomas are included in the same category as follicular adenomas, their incidence is not reported separately. Hürthle cell carcinoma comprises 3–7% of thyroid malignancies.[20,22] They are common in women, with a peak incidence in the fifth through sixth decades. These carcinomas frequently involve lymph nodes (unlike follicular carcinomas), recur often, metastasize to distant organs, and do not concentrate radioactive iodine like follicular carcinomas. The patient's survival is short as well.

PATHOLOGY

Grossly, Hürthle cell tumors are well demarcated with a bulging cut surface that is tan-brown (Fig. 7.2). Areas of necrosis and hemorrhage are very common. Hürthle cell carcinomas tend to be large,[18] frequently exceeding 4 cm at the largest dimension, and bilaterality occurs frequently. Multicentricity is common in carcinomas, as is coexistence with other diseases.[22]

Microscopically, the Hürthle cell neoplasm is composed of large oval to polygonal cells arranged in follicles, cords, alveoli, or solid masses (Fig. 7.3), occasionally with a papillary pattern. The cells vary in size and contain deep eosinophilic granular cytoplasm. The nuclei are eccentric with frequent nucleoli. Pleomorphic, deep-staining nuclei are common in adenomas. Hürthle cell carcinomas are identified by demonstrating capsular or vascular invasion.[9,14,16,21]

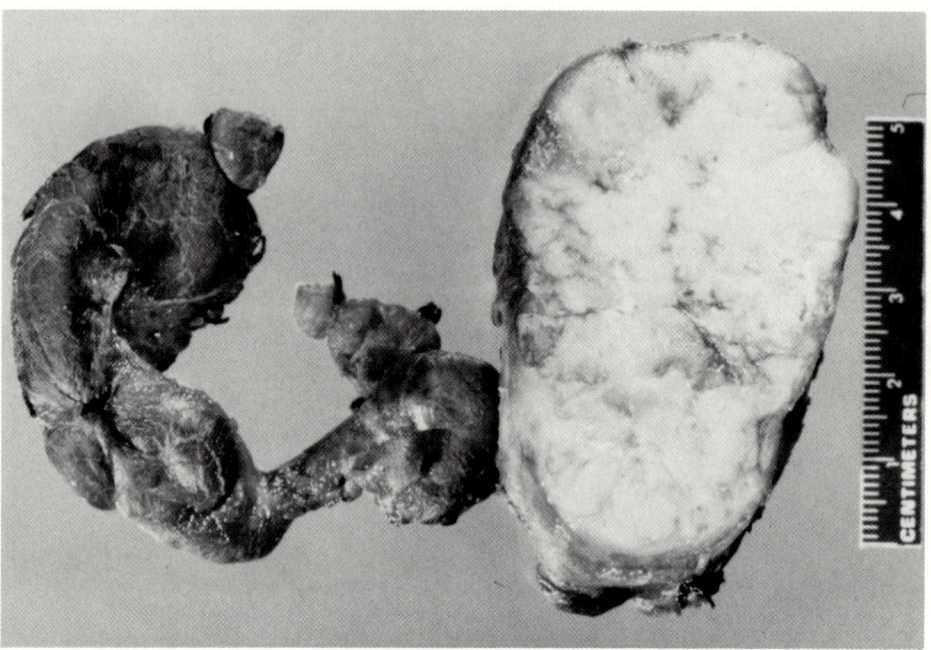

Fig. 7.2. Hürthle cell carcinoma involving the entire left lobe.

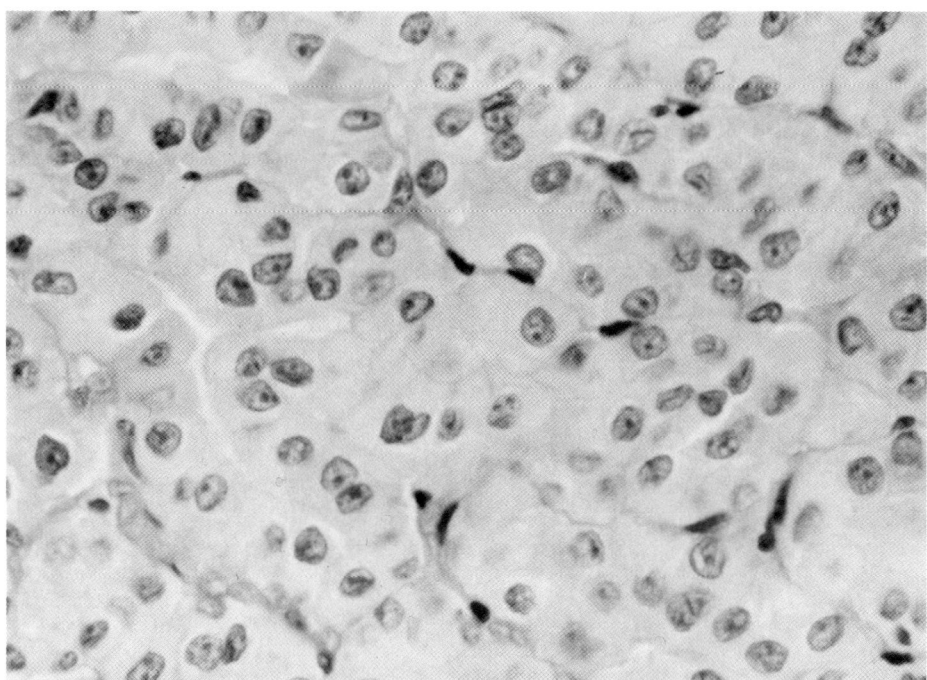

Fig. 7.3. Hürthle cell tumor with a trabecular pattern formed by large polygonal cells with abundant granular cytoplasm and uniform nuclei. Hematoxylin and eosin preparation. × 400.

CYTOPATHOLOGY

In general, the aspirates of Hürthle cell tumors are very cellular and present a strikingly monomorphic cell population (Table 7.3). Hürthle cells tend to present isolated or in loose cohesive groups, and infrequently in sheets or follicles. They are large, polygonal to oval, with well-defined cell borders. The cytoplasm is abundant and granular, and occasionally vacuolated. (Figs. 7.4 and 7.5) In Papanicolaou-stained preparations, the cytoplasm of Hürthle cells stains oxyphilic, cyanophilic, or amphophilic (Plate 7.1) in contrast with the consistent deep eosinophilia seen in formalin-fixed sections stained by hematoxylin and eosin. This variability in staining is particularly evident in spray-fixed smears (Plate 7.1).

Hürthle cell nuclei are often binucleated. The nuclei are slightly eccentrically located, small, uniform, round to oval and contain finely granular chromatin. The most characteristic feature is the presence of a single cherry-red macronucleolus. This feature is not prominently displayed in alcohol-fixed specimens (Plate 7.2). Aspirates of Hürthle cell tumors rarely show colloid in the background.

Cytologic features commonly seen in Hürthle cell tumors that are benign and do not demonstrate invasive characteristics are described in Table 7.3. Most Hürthle cell carcinomas exhibit subtle features that help differentiate them from their benign counterparts (Table 7.4).

TABLE 7.3. Cytopathologic Features of Hürthle Cell Tumor

Pattern	Monomorphic cell population
	Cells mostly isolated, loosely cohesive, in sheets or follicles
Cells	Large oval to polygonal; size variable, but uniform in a given tumor
Cytoplasm	Cell borders well defined; abundant granular cytoplasm with variable staining reaction
Nucleus	Binucleation common, slight eccentric location; small and round, with finely granular chromatin and single prominent cherry-red macronucleolus
Background	Colloid absent or scanty

The malignant behavior of the Hürthle cell tumors is suggested by the following:

1. Round to oval Hürthle cells, smaller in size, with relatively larger nuclei (Figs. 7.6 and 7.7), altering the nuclear/cytoplasmic ratio

2. Syncytial-type tissue fragments without any architectural pattern, with crowded and overlapped nuclei (Figs. 7.8 and 7.9)

3. Pleomorphism in nuclear size with one or more macronucleoli (Fig. 7.8)

4. Presence of intranuclear cytoplasmic inclusions. (Fig. 7.10)

Bondeson et al,[1] in their morphometric study of 26 oxyphilic thyroid tumors (13 benign and 13 malignant), found no difference between the nuclei of benign and malignant cells. Although mean nuclear size was larger in malignant neoplasms compared with that in the benign group, there was considerable overlap. Our experience with 29 Hürthle cell carcinomas suggests that although the nuclei do not show much enlargement, the nuclearcytoplasmic ratio is altered in favor of the nucleus in carcinomas. This is because the Hürthle cells in carcinomas are often considerably smaller in size, an observation also made by Horn.[11]

Hürthle cell carcinomas may present in the following unusual ways:

1. A papillary growth pattern is seen, but it may lack ground-glass nuclei (Fig. 7.11).

2. Psammoma bodies are seen occasionally (Fig. 7.12). They were identified in 5 of 29 cases of Hürthle cell carcinoma. The presence of a psammoma body does not warrant a diagnosis of papillary carcinoma. In general, the biological behavior of Hürthle cell carcinoma is more aggressive than that of papillary carcinoma.

TABLE 7.4. Cytopathologic Differentiation Between Hürthle Cell Adenoma and Hürthle Cell Carcinoma

	Adenoma	Carcinoma
Pattern	Isolated, loosely cohesive groups; sheets or, rarely, follicle formation	Isolated or in syncytial-type tissue fragments
Cell	Large ploygonal to oval; cytoplasm abundant, granular with low nuclear/cytoplasmic ratio	Much smaller, round to oval; abundant cytoplasm, more than in follicular cell but less than in adenoma; increased nuclear/cytoplasmic ratio
Nucleus	Round, uniform in size, with prominent single cherry-red macronucleolus	Nuclei variable in size, one or more prominent cherry-red macronucleoli, may be irregular
Intranuclear cytoplasmic inclusions	Not present	Occasionally present
Psammoma body	Not present	Occasionally present
Colloid	Variable	Absent

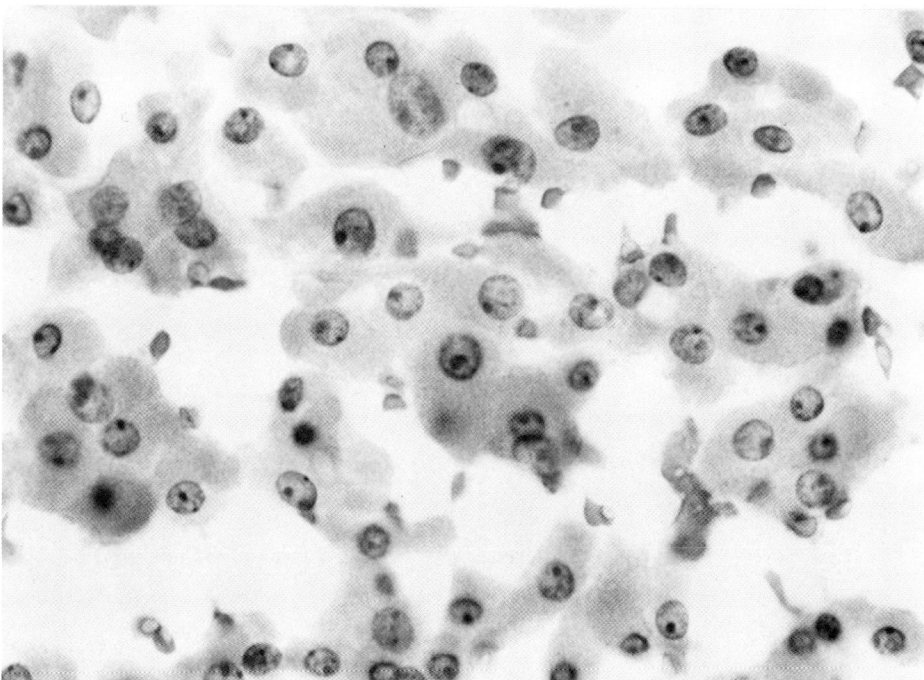

Fig. 7.4. Hürthle cell tumor showing large, polygonal cells with well-defined cell borders, abundant granular cytoplasm, eccentric nuclei, and prominent single macronucleolus. Papanicolaou preparation. × 630.

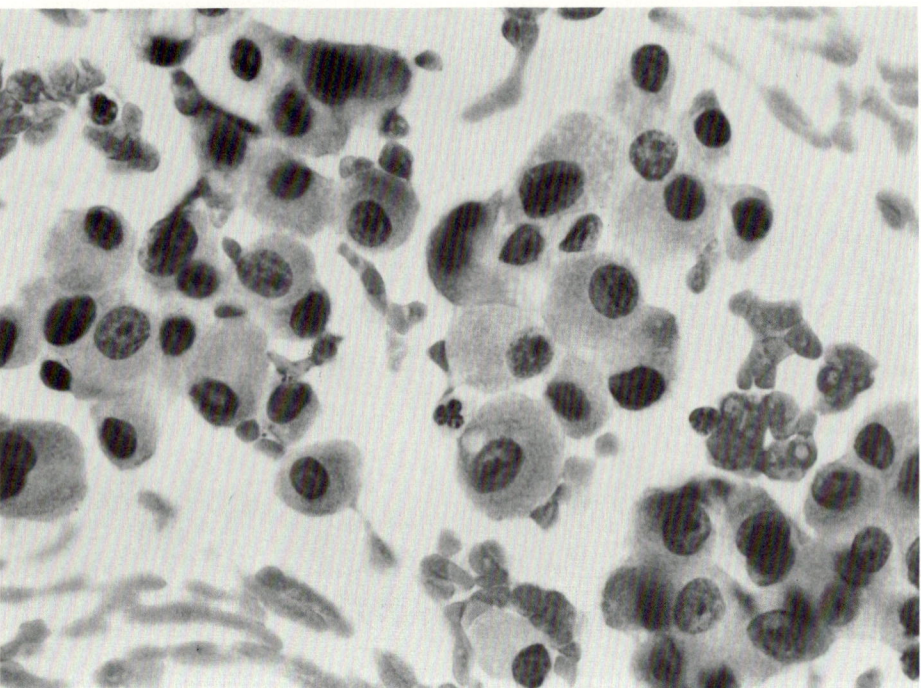

Fig. 7.5. Hürthle cell tumor showing discrete, round to oval cells with abundant granular cytoplasm and eccentric nuclei with prominent single macronucleolus. Papanicolaou preparation. × 630.

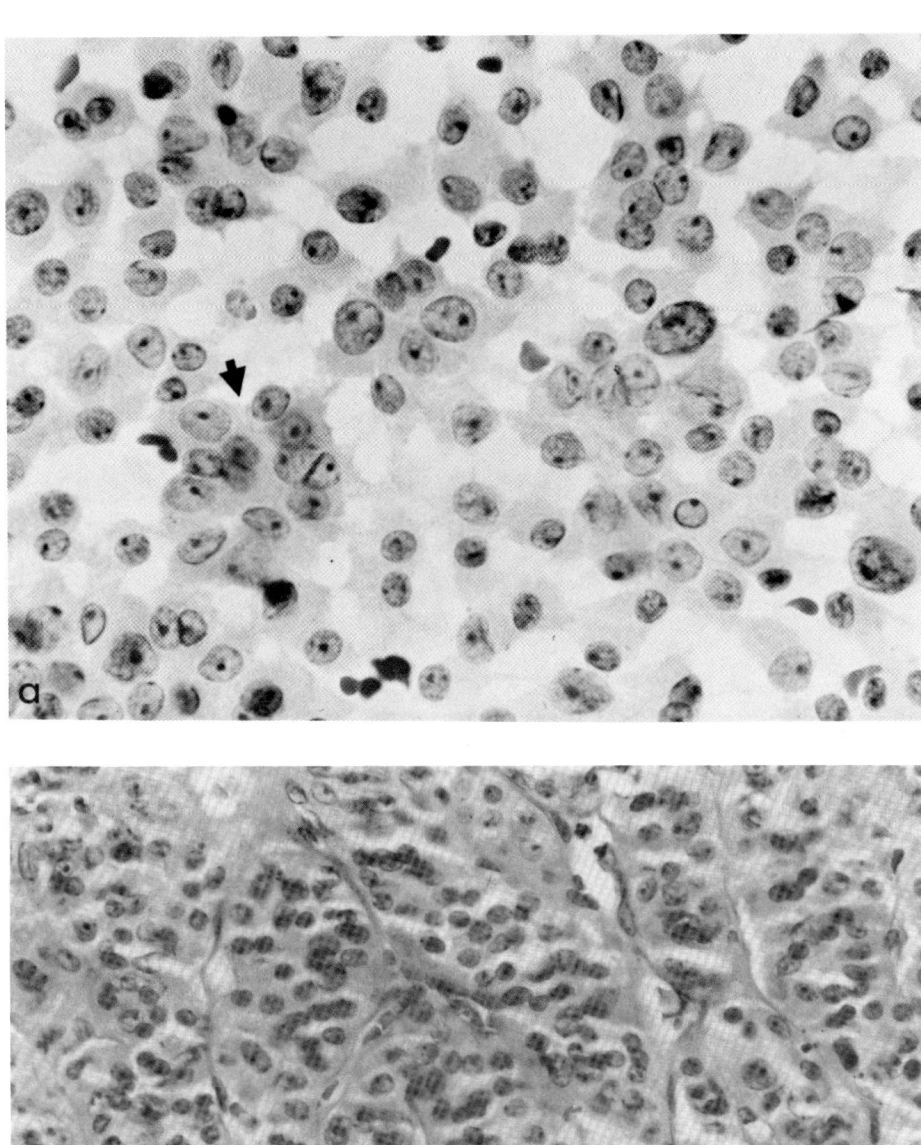

Fig. 7.6. A. Hürthle cell carcinoma. Note the small cells with relatively large nuclei, and mild pleomorphism in nuclear size. An occasional syncytial-type tissue fragment is present *(arrow)*. Papanicolaou preparation. × 630. **B.** This solid alveolar pattern with small cells is more often seen in Hürthle cell carcinoma than in adenoma. Hematoxylin and eosin preparation. × 400.

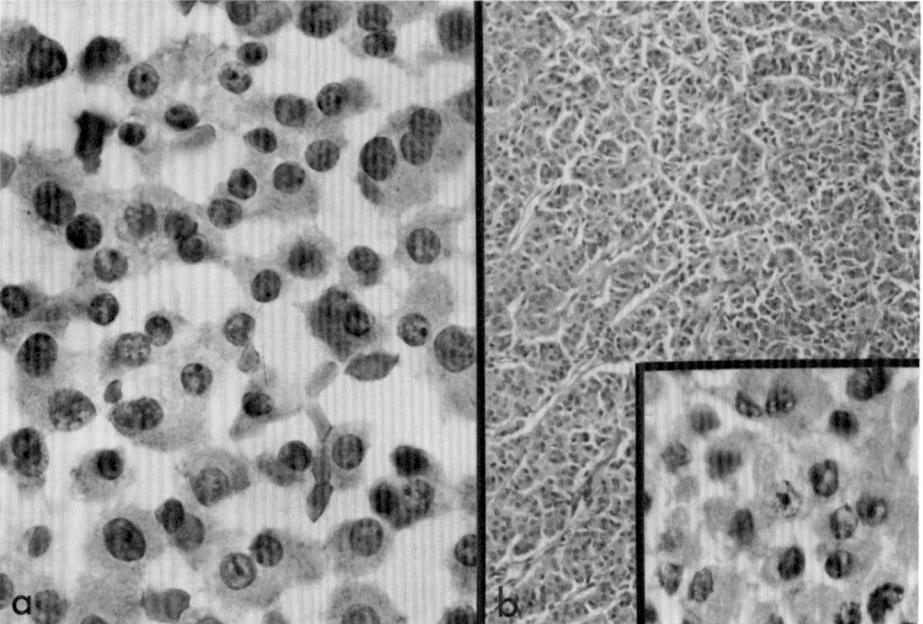

Fig. 7.7. Hürthle cell carcinoma. **A.** Aspiration biopsy specimen. Small cell size, considerably less but granular cytoplasm, slight nuclear pleomorphism, and high nuclear/cytoplasmic ratio suggest malignancy. Papanicolaou preparation. × 630. **B.** Histologic section showing pattern similar to that in Fig. 7.6 **B.** Hematoxylin and eosin preparation. × 100. *Inset:* Higher magnification of **B.** Hematoxylin and eosin preparation. × 400.

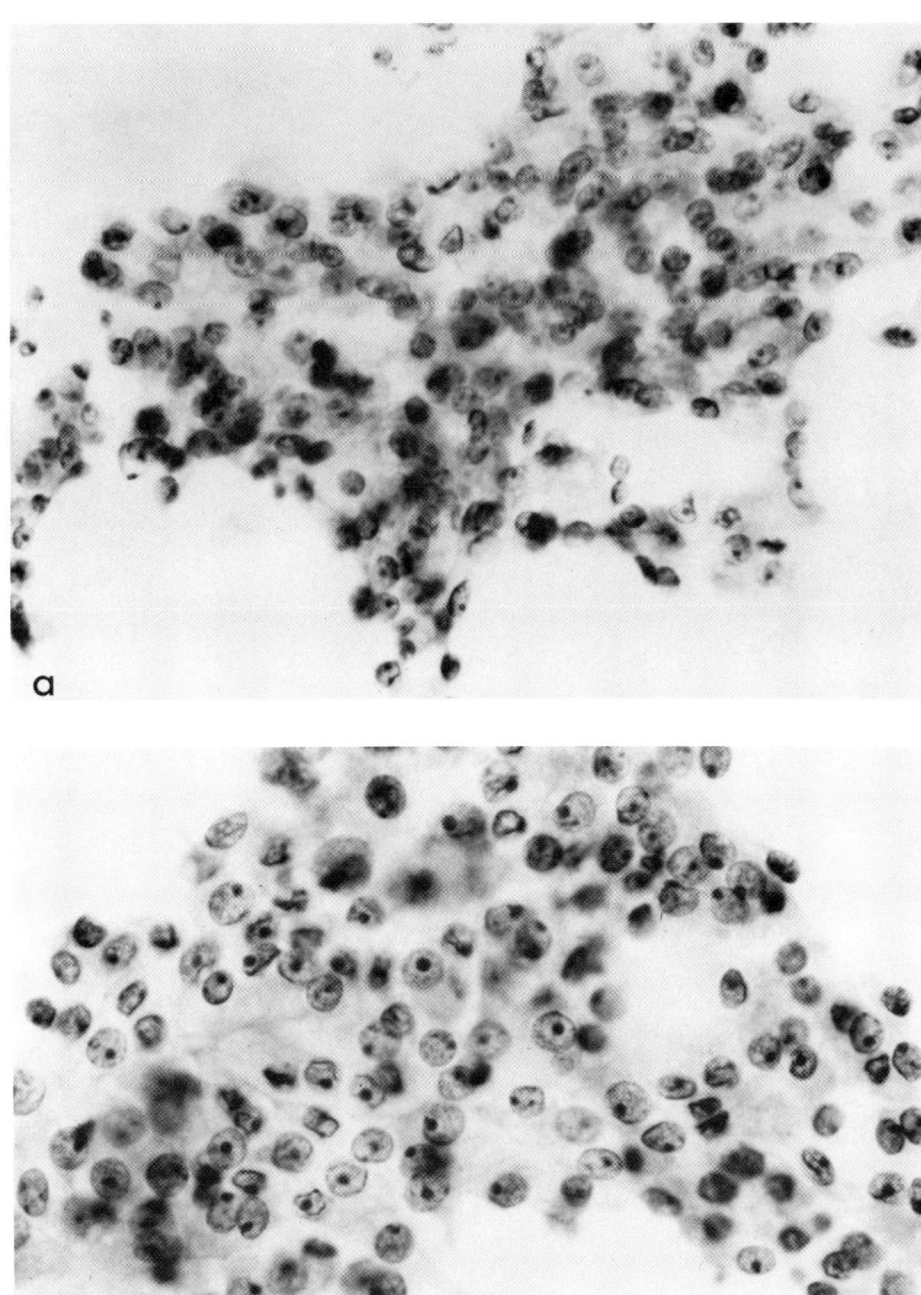

Fig. 7.8. A. Hürthle cell carcinoma, with syncytial-type tissue fragment of Hürthle cells. Monomorphic nuclear pattern is still retained. Papanicolaou preparation. × 400. B. Hürthle cells in syncytial-type tissue fragments, with crowding and overlapping of nuclei. The prominent single macronucleolus is characteristic, and the nuclear membranes are irregular. There is parachromatin clearing. This pattern is diagnostic of Hürthle cell carcinoma. Papanicolaou preparation. × 630.

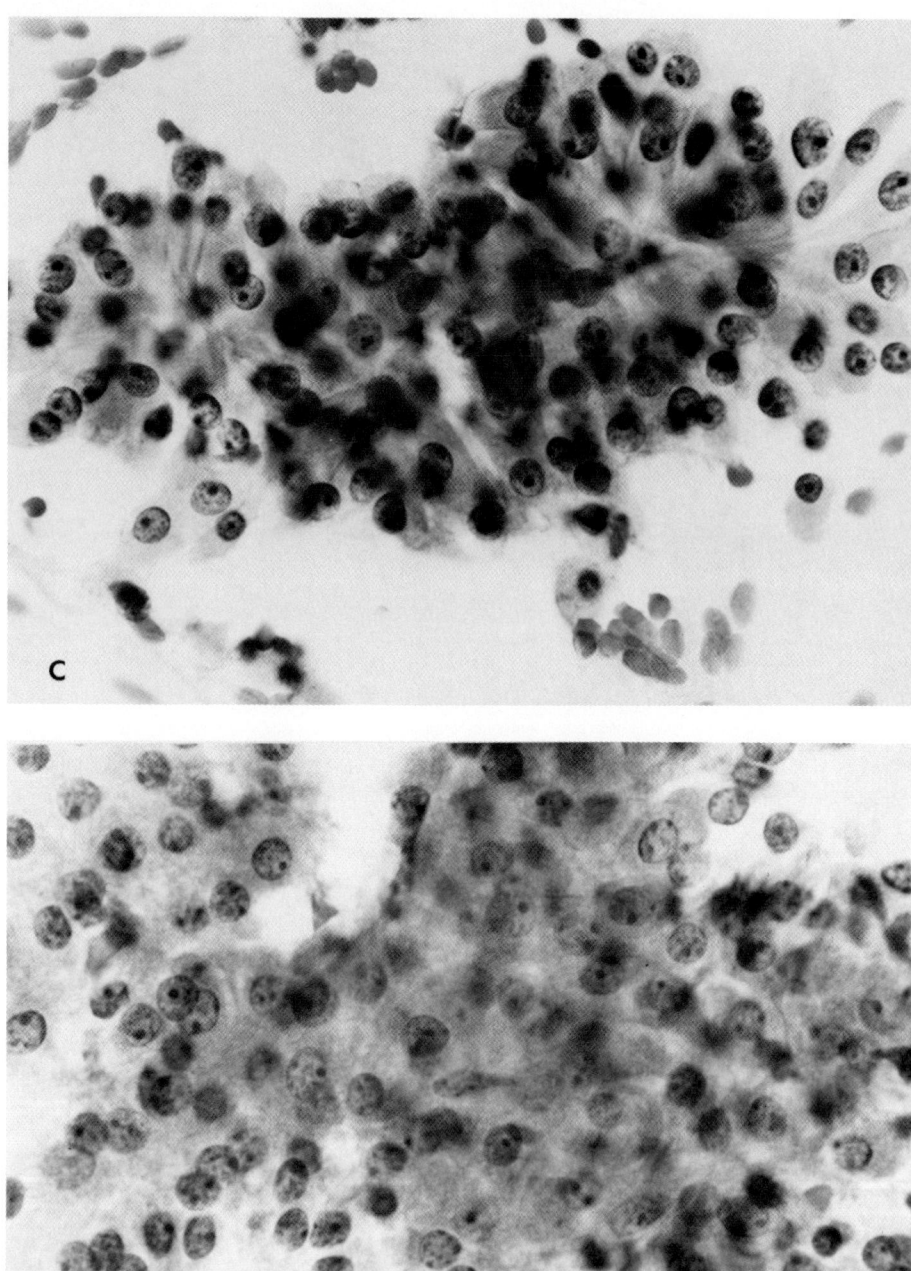

Fig. 7.8. **C.** Syncytial-type tissue fragment. Note that the Hürthle cells are elongated, oval to columnar, and still retain the characteristic nuclear morphology. Papanicolaou preparation. × 630. **D.** These syncytial-type arrangements of Hürthle cells with ill-defined cell borders, marked crowding, overlapping of nuclei, coarse chromatin, and multiple nucleoli suggest the diagnosis of Hürthle cell carcinoma. Invasive process was not demonstrated in surgically excised specimen. Papanicolaou preparation. × 630.

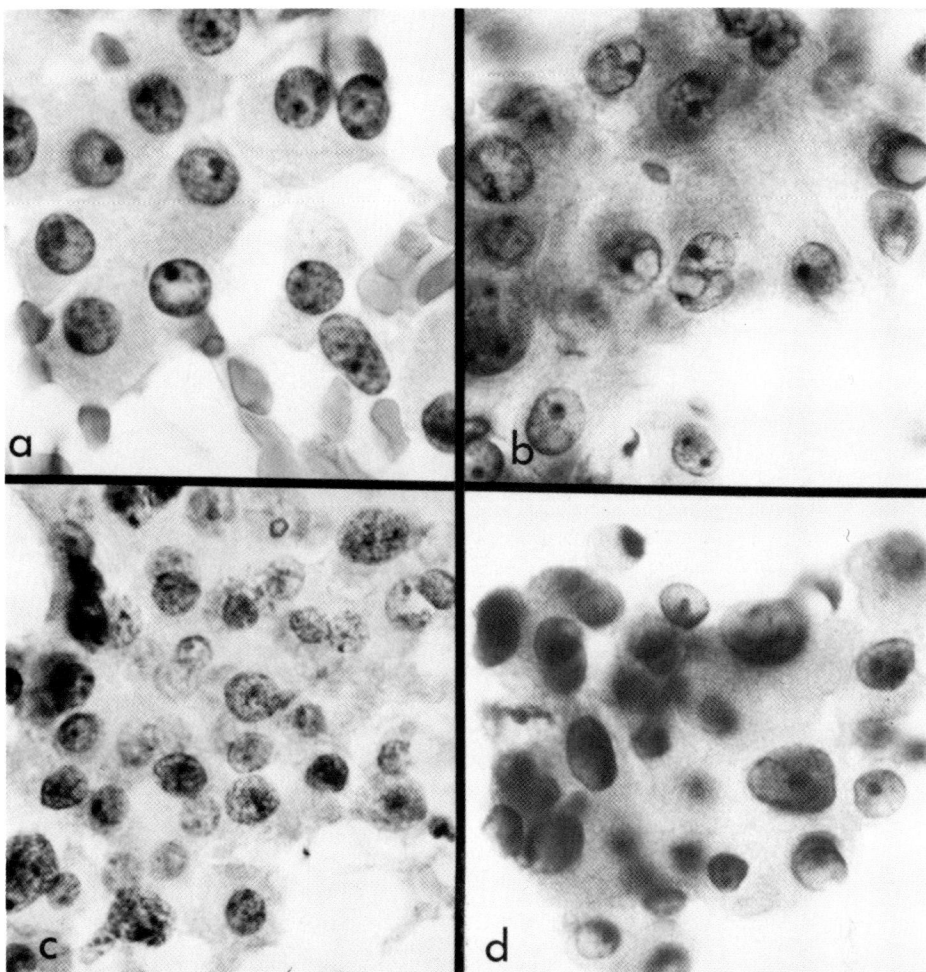

Fig. 7.9. Hürthle cell carcinoma. **A., B.** The carcinoma cells are small, with high nuclear/cytoplasmic ratios. Note the prominent nucleoli and the crisp nuclear details. Spray fixed. Papanicolaou preparation. × 630. **C., D.** These carcinoma cells show smudged nuclei. Nucleoli are not evident in all the cells. Alcohol fixed. Papanicolaou preparation. × 630.

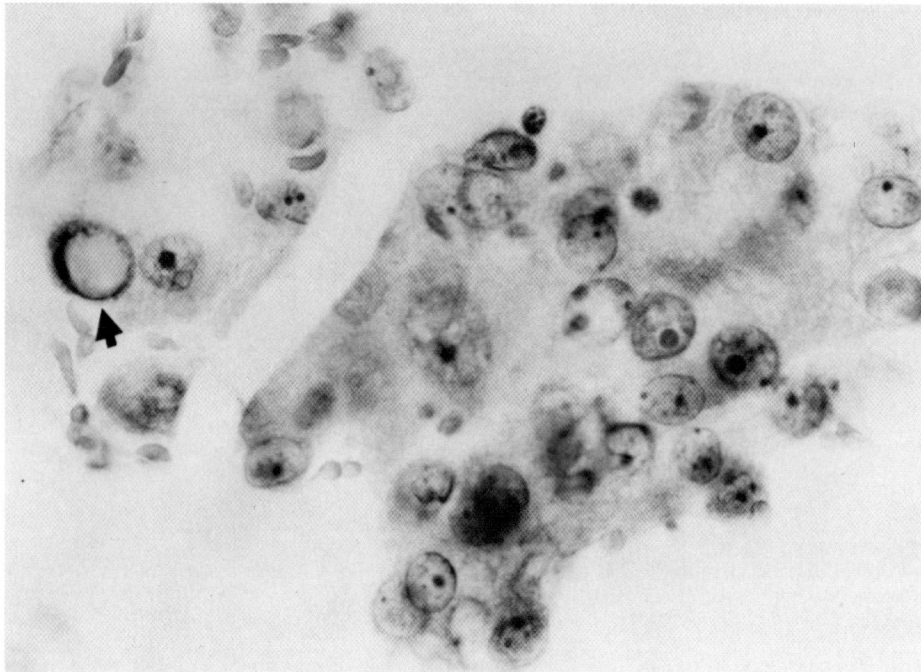

Fig. 7.10. Aspiration biopsy specimen of Hürthle cell carcinoma, metastatic to the spine. Note the syncytial-type tissue fragment with pleomorphic nuclei, multiple micro- and macronucleoli, and intranuclear cytoplasmic inclusions *(arrow)*. Papanicolaou preparation. × 630.

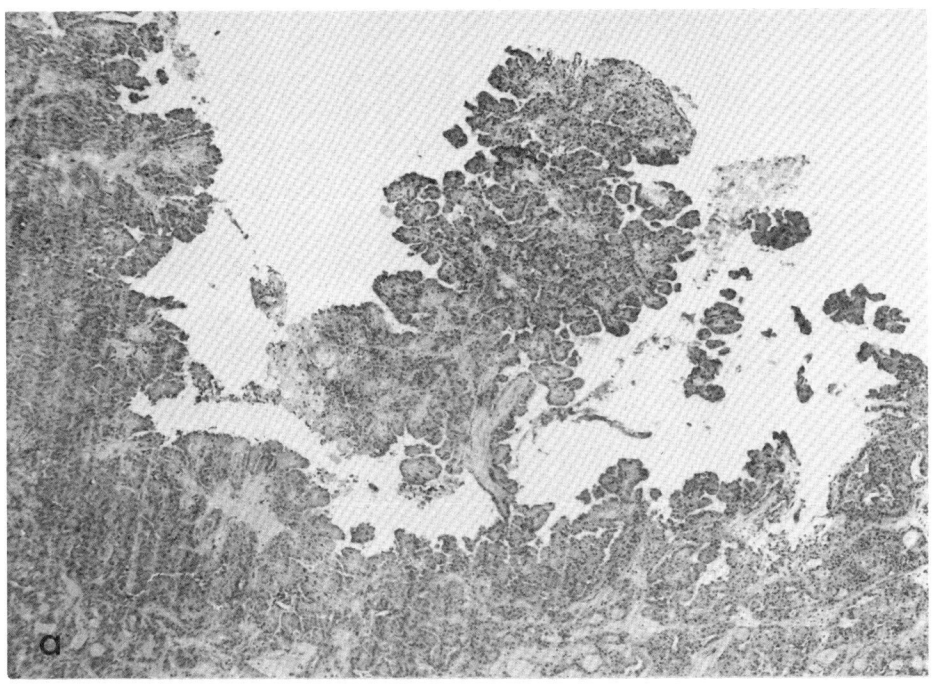

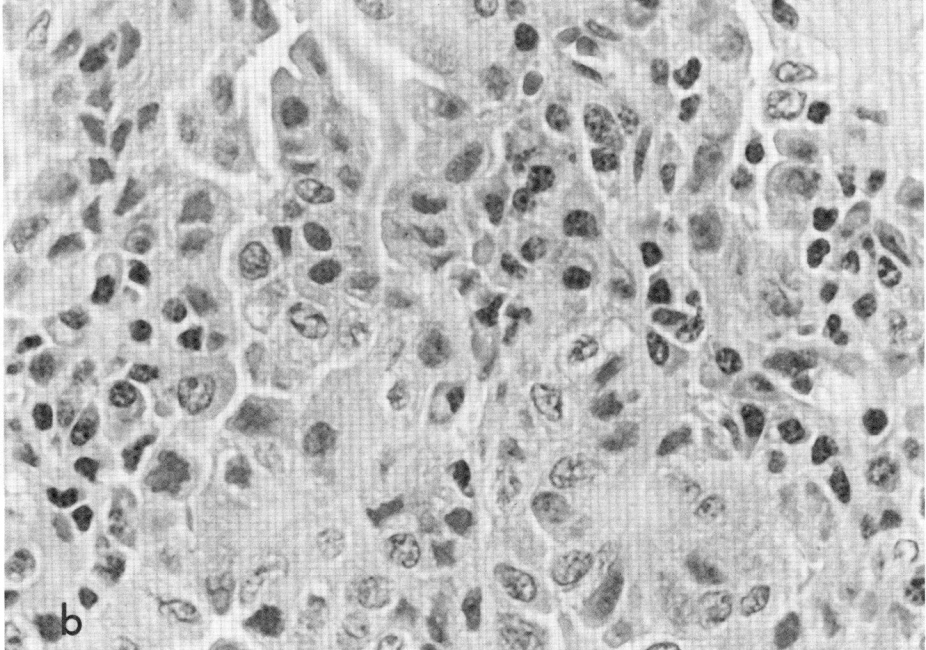

Fig. 7.11. A. Hürthle cell carcinoma. Papillary pattern. Hemotoxylin and eosin preparation. × 13. **B.** Higher magnification of **A** showing large Hürthle cells with abundant granular cytoplasm. Hematoxylin and eosin preparation. × 400.

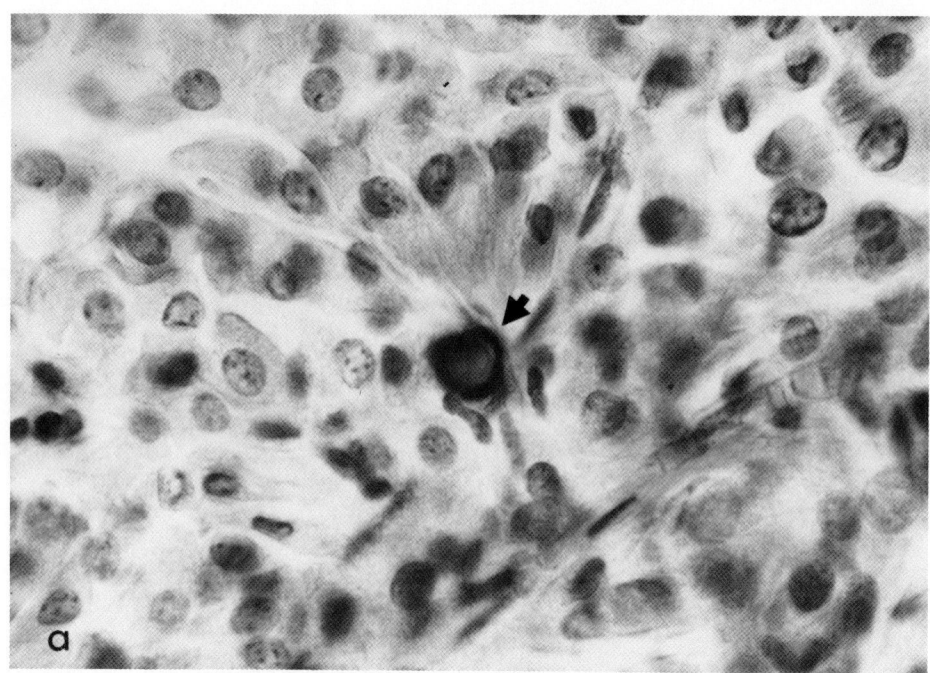

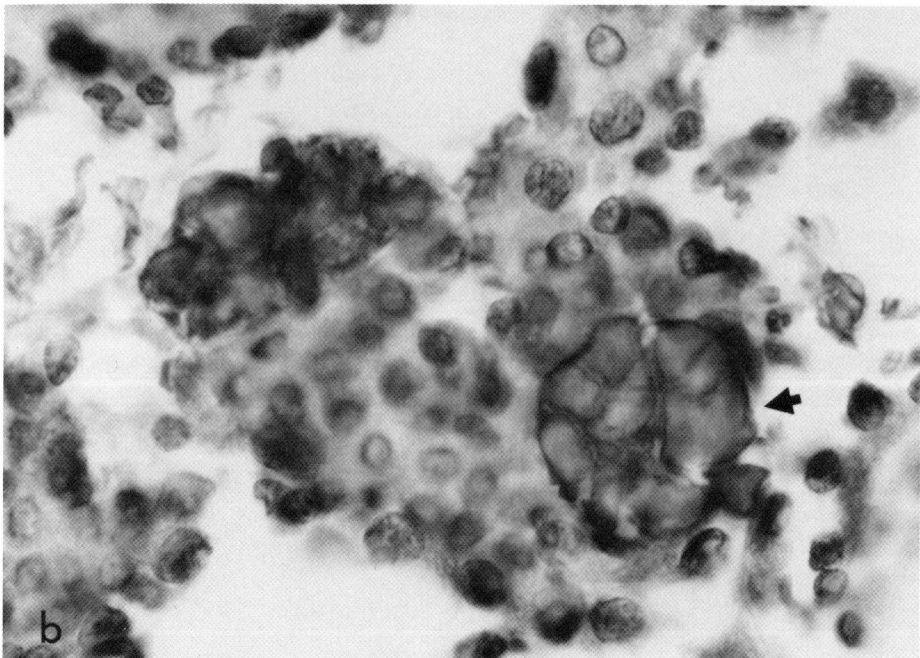

Fig. 7.12. A., B. Psammoma bodies *(arrow)* in aspirates of Hürthle cell carcinoma. Papanicolaou preparation. × 630.

DIAGNOSTIC ACCURACY

Because of their characteristic cytomorphology, high diagnostic accuracy can be expected for Hürthle cell neoplasms. However, in actual practice, it does not seem to be so due to continual controversy over the nomenclature and diagnostic criteria.

Usual diagnostic errors include false-positive or false-negative results as well as mistyping the neoplasm.

False-positive diagnoses involve misinterpretation of non-neoplastic or involutional nodules frequently seen in nodular goiter or Hashimoto's thyroiditis as Hürthle cell neoplasms.

False-negative diagnoses may occur if a Hürthle cell carcinoma is typed as an adenoma, or if a diagnosis of Hürthle cell adenoma or carcinoma is missed and the specimen is instead interpreted as nodular goiter or thyroiditis. A true false-negative diagnosis is possible only if the specimen is inadequate, as Hürthle cells are easily recognized and the general tendency is to overdiagnose.

If all the neoplasms composed of Hürthle cells are diagnosed as Hürthle cell tumors and treated in the same fashion, an attempt to separate Hürthle cell adenoma from a carcinoma becomes a futile exercise. The diagnostic accuracy of Hürthle cell neoplasms on the whole should be in the range of 85–90% (Table 7.5). On the other hand, if surgical treatment is different for Hürthle cell carcinoma than for adenoma, such a distinction must be attempted on a cytologic basis. In our series, Hürthle cell carcinomas tended to be overdiagnosed cytologically, with an accuracy in the range of 60% (Table 7.5). The actual accuracy may differ due to inconsistencies among pathologists regarding the diagnostic criteria for Hürthle cell carcinoma.

Our attempt to differentiate Hürthle cell adenoma from carcinoma on a cytologic basis began strictly as an academic exercise after 3 years of biopsy experience. Of six cases of Hürthle cell carcinoma diagnosed cytologically as Hürthle cell tumor from a group of 73 Hürthle cell tumors, four occurred during the first 3 years of our experience. The other two cases presented cytomorphology indistinguishable from those that followed a benign course or showed a lack of invasive features. One case was diagnosed by an outside consultant as carcinoma strictly on the basis of the large tumor size (more than 4 cm). The other case demonstrated vascular invasion (Fig. 7.13).

DIFFERENTIAL DIAGNOSIS OF HÜRTHLE CELL LESIONS

Hürthle Cell Tumors Versus Hürthle Cell Nodules

Large, clinically palpable nodules formed entirely of Hürthle cells are seen in nodular goiter as well as in Hashimoto's thyroiditis and sometimes in post-Graves' disease. Clinically and on imaging, they cannot be differentiated from a neoplasm. Cyto-pathologic distinction is not always easy.[13] Some difficulties are encountered even

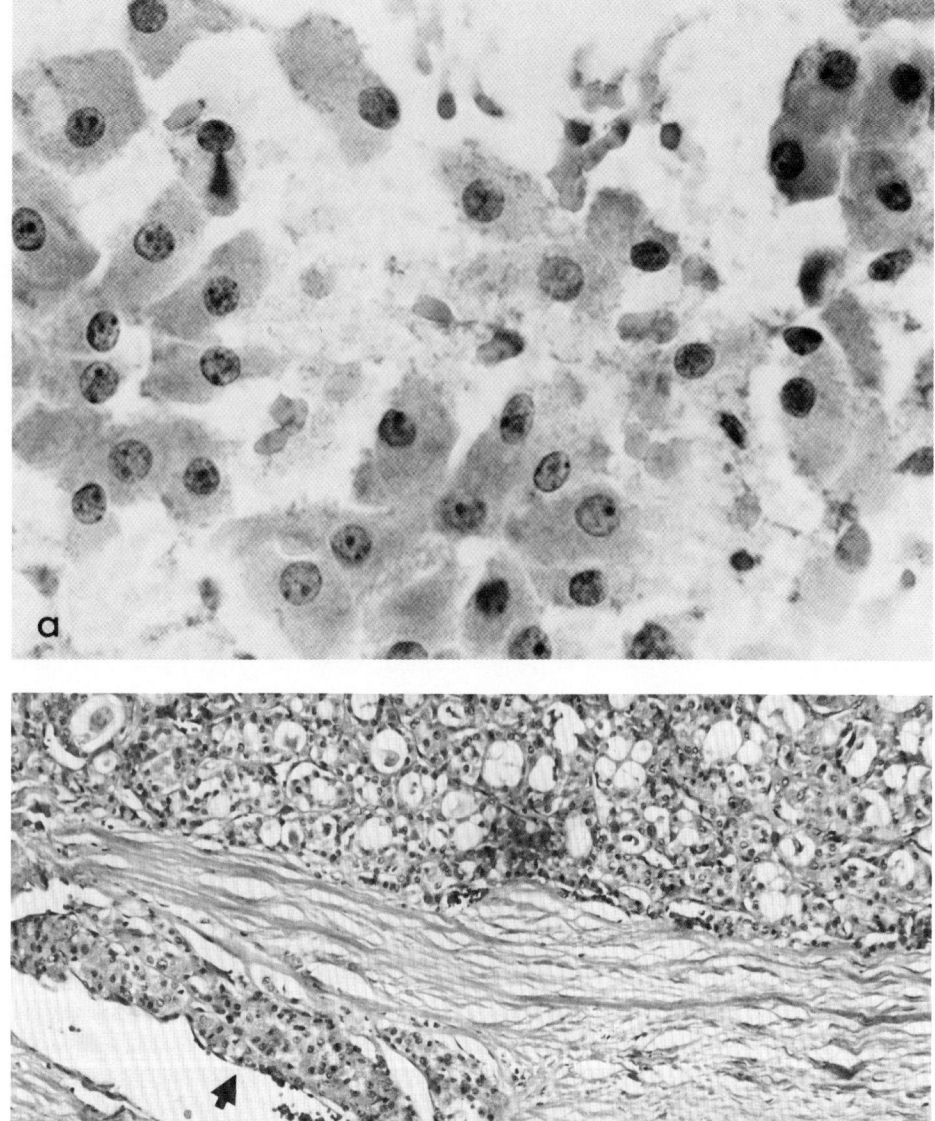

Fig. 7.13. A. Hürthle cell carcinoma. These neoplastic Hürthle cells are discrete, large, and monomorphic, a pattern generally consistent with benign behavior, yet they showed vascular invasion. Papanicolaou preparation. × 630. **B.** Histologic section of the tumor in **A** showing vascular invasion *(arrow)*. Hematoxylin and eosin preparation. × 160.

TABLE 7.5. Cytohistologic Correlation of Hürthle Cell Tumors

Cytologic Diagnosis	Histologic Diagnosis			
		Hürthle Cell Adenoma	Hürthle Cell Carcinoma	Nodular Goiter	Hashimoto's Thyroiditis
Hürthle cell tumors	73	53	6	10	4
Suspected Hürthle cell carcinoma	17	14	3	0	0
Hürthle cell carcinoma	35	14	20	0	1*
Totals	125	81	29	10	5
		88%		12%	

*Final diagnosis was Hashimoto's thyroiditis with atypical Hürthle cell nodule.

when the entire thyroid is available for examination.[11,19] The cytologic criteria for differentiating Hürthle cell neoplasms from Hürthle cell nodules are listed in Table 7.6. These criteria are subtle and recognizing them requires experience. Our error rate of 12% (Table 7.5) reflects inexperience during the early years.

Hürthle Cell Tumor Versus Hürthle Cell Metaplasia in Nodular Goiter

A few scattered Hürthle cells along with benign follicular cells are often present in aspirates from nodular goiter (Fig. 7.14; Plate 7.3). Hürthle cells aspirated from non-neoplastic Hürthle cell nodules tend to be cohesive and present as sheets of epithelium with well-defined cell borders and abundant cytoplasm that is either dense or granular and contains centrally placed (Figs. 7.14 and 7.15) nuclei. A follicular pattern is not uncommon. Transitional forms from regular follicular cells to large polygonal cells are usually present. The nuclei may be uniform, but do not show macronucleoli as a consistent feature. Colloid is present in the background, but variable and can be abundant. The nuclear chromatin is coarsely granular. Pyknotic forms are very frequent in Hürthle cell nodules. This entire picture differs from that of Hürthle cell neoplasm, which is characterized by disassociated monomorphic cells with nuclei containing macronucleoli. Although nuclear pleomorphism is a feature of non-neoplastic Hürthle cell nodules, the nuclei lack the malignant criteria seen in Hürthle cell carcinomas, ie, crowded and overlapping of nuclei with altered nuclearcytoplasmic ratio, chromatin coarsely granular but sharply defined from the parachromatin, and one or more macronucleoli.

Hürthle Cell Tumor Versus Hürthle Cell Nodules in Hashimoto's Thyroiditis

Hürthle cell metaplasia with nodule formation is a routine histologic feature of Hashimoto's disease. An aspirate of a cold nodule in the background of a diffusely

TABLE 7.6. Cytopathologic Differentiation Between Hürthle Cell Tumors and
Hürthle Cell Nodules, Non-Neoplastic

	Hürthle Cell Tumor	*Hürthle Cell Nodules, Adenomatous Goiter*	*Hürthle Cell Nodules, Hashimoto's Thyroiditis*
Pattern	Isolated, or loosely cohesive cells with a monomorphic pattern; syncytial-tissue fragments in Hürthle cell carcinoma	Hürthle cells isolated or in sheets	Predominantly tight cohesive groups
Cells	Uniform large oval to polygonal, with well-defined cell borders, granular abundant cytoplasm	Large isolated cells, very pleomorphic in size, mixed with normal follicular cells; sheets of Hürthle cells with honeycomb pattern; transitional forms from follicular cells to Hürthle cells	Pleomorphic in size
Nucleus	Generally uniform in size, single or multiple, round to oval, finely granular chromatin with prominent cherry-red macronucleolus	Variable in size; small, similar to follicular cell nucleus, to large; dense staining; cherry-red macronucleolus rare	Pleomorphic in size with compact chromatin
Background	Inflammatory cells, if present, are neutrophilic type, suggesting necrosis	Not present	Lymphocytes and plasma cells
Colloid	Absent	May be abundant	Absent

enlarged goiter showing many or predominantly Hürthle cells with a few lympho-cytes and plasma cells can be identified as a non-neoplastic Hürthle cell lesion. Experience helps in recognizing such lesions. To the uninitiated eye, a predominant Hürthle cell component in an aspirate will suggest a diagnosis of a neoplasm[12] (Fig. 7.16; Plate 7.3). This is discussed in detail in Chapter 11, Thyroiditis.

Hürthle Cell Carcinoma Versus Other Tumors

Hürthle cell carcinomas share morphologic similarities with medullary carcinoma and are often typed as such. The differentiating features are discussed in Chapter 10, Medullary Carcinoma.

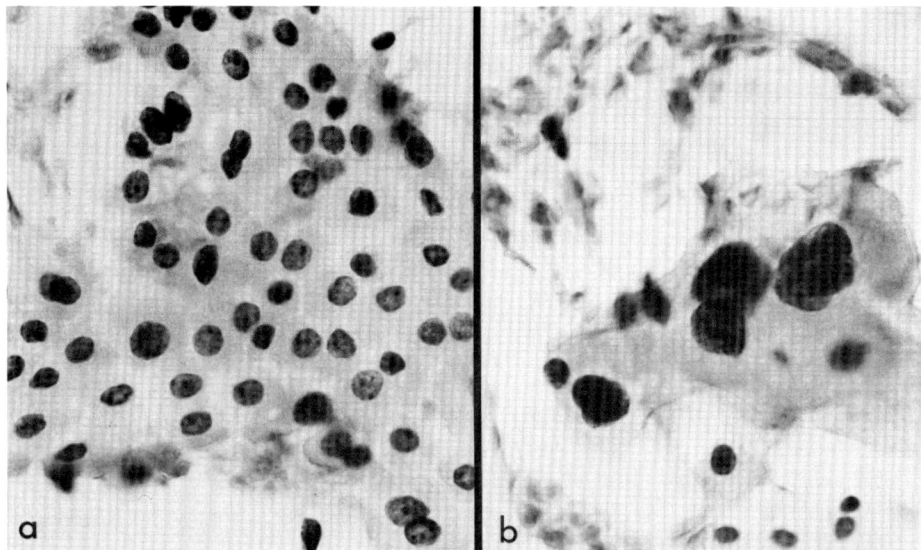

Fig. 7.14. Hürthle cell metaplasia in nodular goiter. **A.** Metaplastic Hürthle cells often occur in sheets with a honeycomb pattern. The nuclei are similar to those of follicular cells, regular type. The only change is abundant cytoplasm. Macronucleoli are rare. Papanicolaou preparation. × 630. **B.** Pyknosis and multinucleation is frequent in metaplastic Hürthle cells. Papanicolaou preparation. × 630.

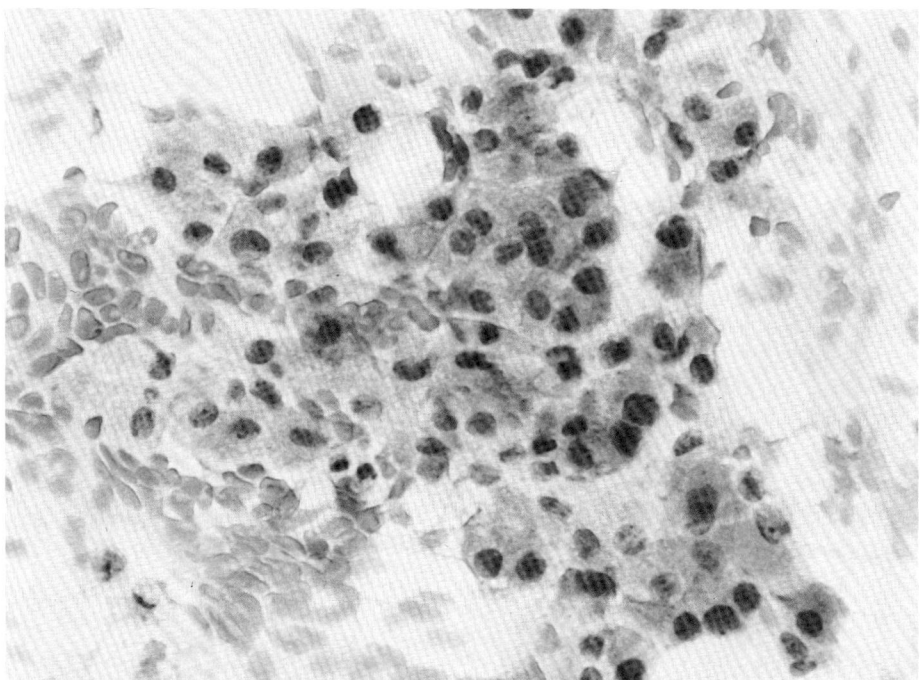

Fig. 7.15. Hürthle cell metaplasia in nodular goiter. Sheet of Hürthle cells with abundant cytoplasm. Cohesive pattern and lack of nucleoli suggest metaplasia, rather than neoplasia. Papanicolaou preparation. × 630.

117

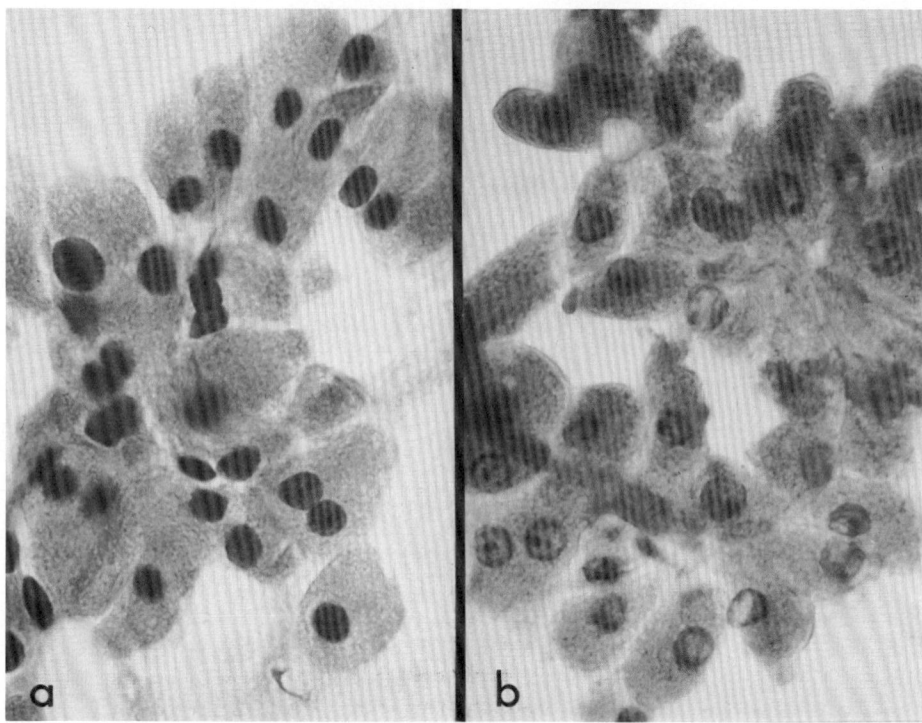

Fig. 7.16. A. Involutional nodule in Hashimoto's thyroiditis. The Hürthle cells have dense nuclei and are lacking macronucleoli. Papanicolaou preparation. × 630. **B.** Typical morphology of neoplastic Hürthle cells with monomorphic pattern. Nuclei have finely granular chromatin and a single macronucleolus. Papanicolaou preparation. × 630.

SUMMARY

Hürthle cell tumors with benign behavior often show large, loosely cohesive cells with well-defined cell borders, abundant granular cytoplasm with variable staining characteristics, and eccentric nuclei with prominent cherry-red macronucleoli and present a monomorphic pattern. Hürthle cell tumors with malignant behavior can be recognized by small cell size, syncytial-type tissue fragments, and high nuclearcytoplasmic ratio. Unusual features include intranuclear cytoplasmic inclusions and psammoma bodies. Hürthle cell carcinoma may be mistyped as medullary thyroid carcinoma. Diagnostic pitfalls include involutional nodules from nodular goiter or Hashimoto's thyroiditis.

REFERENCES

1. Bondeson L, Bondeson AG, Ljungberg K, Ljungberg O, Tibblin S: Morphometric studies on nuclei in smears of fine needle aspirates from oxyphilic tumors of the thyroid. *Acta Cytol* 27:437–440, 1983.

2. Bondeson L, Bondeson AG, Ljungberg O, Tibblin S: Oxyphil tumors of the thyroid. *Am Surg* 196:677–680, 1981.

3. Caplan RH, Abellera M, Kisken W: Hürthle cell tumors of the thyroid gland; a clinicopathologic review and long-term follow up. *JAMA* 251:3114–3177, 1984.

4. Chesky VE, Droese WC, Hellwig CA: Hürthle cell tumors of the thyroid gland: a report on 25 cases. *J Clin Endocrinol* 11:1535–1548, 1951.

5. Frazell EI, Duffy BJ: Hürthle cell cancer of the thyroid, a review of forty cases. *Cancer* 4:952–956, 1951,

6. Friedman NB: Cellular involution in the thyroid gland: significance of Hürthle cells in myxedema, exhaustion atrophy. Hashimoto's disease and the 'reactions to radiation,' thiouracil therapy and subtotal resection. *J Clin Endocrinol* 9:874–882, 1949.

7. Gundry SR, Burney RE, Thompson NW, Lloyd R: Total thyroidectomy for Hürthle cell neoplasm of the thyroid. *Arch Surg* 118:529–532, 1983.

8. Gusain AK, Clark OH: Hürthle cell neoplasms malignant potential. *Arch Surg* 119:515–519, 1984.

9. Heddinger CR, Sobin LH: Histologic typing of thyroid tumors. In: *International Histological Classification of Tumors*, NR 11, Geneva, 1974.

10. Heiman P, Ljungren JH, Löwhagen T, Hjern B: Oxyphilic adenoma of the human thyroid, a morphological and biochemical study. *Cancer* 31:246–254, 1973.

11. Horn RC: Hürthle cell tumors of the thyroid. *Cancer* 7:234–244, 1954.

12. Kini SR, Miller JM, Hamburger JI: Problems in the cytologic diagnosis of the 'cold' thyroid nodule in patients with lymphocytic thyroiditis. *Acta Cytol* 25:506–512, 1981.

13. Kini SR, Miller JM, Hamburger JI: Cytopathology of Hürthle cell lesions of the thyroid gland by fine needle aspiration. *Acta Cytol* 25:647–652, 1981.

14. Meissner WA, Warren S: Tumors of the Thyroid Gland. Fascicle 4, Second Series, *Atlas of Tumor Pathology*. Washington, DC, Armed Forces Institute of Pathology, 1969, pp. 135.

15. Rosai J, Carcangiu ML: Pathology of thyroid tumors, some recent and old questions. *Hum Pathol* 15:1008–1012, 1984.

16. Rosai J: Thyroid gland. In Ackerman (ed): *Surgical Pathology*, ch. 8, vol 1, 6th ed. St. Louis, Mosby 1981, pp. 352–356.

17. Saull SC, Kimmelman CP: Hürthle cell tumors of the thyroid gland. *Otolaryngol Head Neck Surg* 93:58–62, 1985.

18. Savino D, Silbey RK, Summer H: Significance of Hürthle cells in thyroid neoplasms, recommendations of an old but persistent problem. *Lab Invest (Abst)* 44–59A, 1981.

19. Thompson NW, Dunn EL, Batsakis JG, Nishiyama RH: Hürthle cell lesions of the thyroid gland. *Surg Gynecol Obstet* 139:555–560, 1974.

20. Tollefsen RH, Shah PJ, Juvos AG: Hürthle cell carcinoma of the thyroid; *Am J Surg* 130:390–394, 1974.

21. Vickery AL Jr: Needle biopsy pathology. In Williams ED: *Clinics in Endocrinology and Metabolism*, vol 10. Philadelphia, Saunders, 1981, pp. 283–292.

22. Watson RG, Brennan MD, Goellner JR, et al: Invasive Hürthle cell carcinoma of the thyroid, natural history and management. *Mayo Clin Proc* 59:851–855, 1984.

8

Papillary Carcinoma

Papillary carcinoma, the most common malignant neoplasm of thyroid, comprises about 60% of all thyroid carcinomas in the United States. It occurs more frequently in women, with a female to male ratio of 3:1. Papillary carcinomas are seen in all age groups, with a peak in the third decade. They have a tendency for intraglandular spread and cervical lymph node metastasis, but demonstrate less predilection for hematogenous spread than do follicular carcinomas. These tumors are slow-growing and follow an indolent course. The prognosis for papillary thyroid carcinoma is generally considered favorable; however, it depends on the patient's age; the extension stage, eg, occult, intrathyroidal, or extrathyroidal; and the histologic differentiation.[4,10,29,30,33,34,37]

PATHOLOGY

The gross appearance of papillary carcinoma varies with size. Large tumors are typically fleshy, velvety, fragile, and may extend to the capsule (Fig. 8.1). They are nonencapsulated, but have a tendency for fibrosis that results in partial encapsulation.[5] Cystic changes due to degeneration are very common, as is calcification (Fig. 8.2). Small papillary carcinomas (less than 1.5 cm), called occult,[16] are quite often sclerotic, resembling minute scars (Fig. 8.3).

Microscopically, papillary carcinomas present varied patterns[5,14] (Figs. 8.4–8.8). A typical papillary carcinoma is characterized by neoplastic epithelium arranged on fibrovascular stalks. The papillary fronds may be well developed, with a complex branching pattern, or they may be rudimentary without discernable fibrovascular stalks. Generally, the covering epithelium is single layered, although it may be multilayered. The neoplastic cells can be cuboidal, columnar, or squamoid, with variable cytoplasm surrounding a central ovoid nucleus. These nuclei have pale chromatin, with peripheral condensation that gives a ground-glass or watery appearance[5,13] that is typical of papillary carcinoma. Mitoses are extreme rare.

121

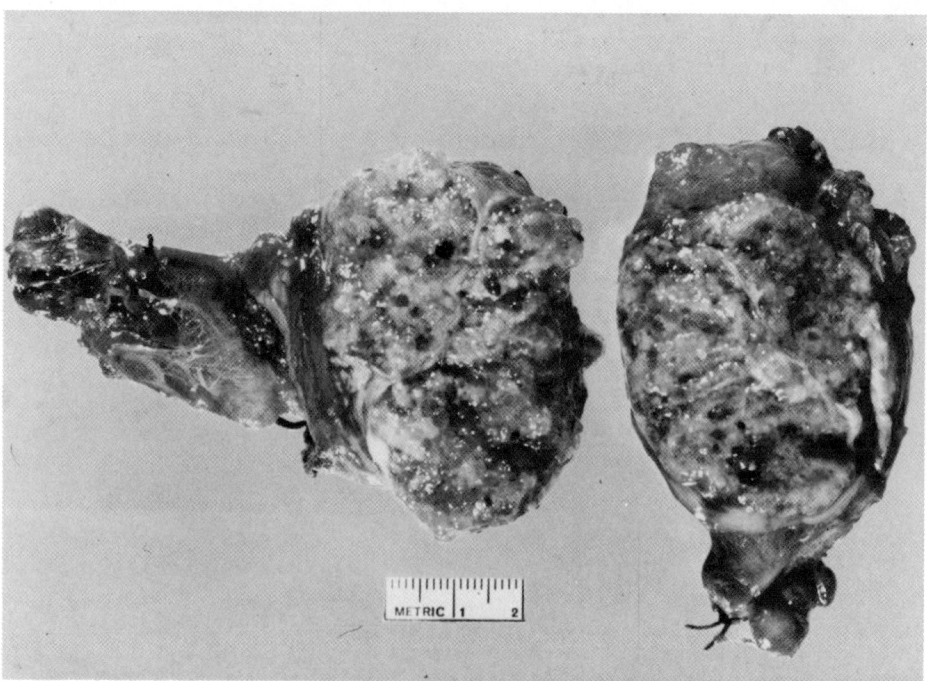

Fig. 8.1. Papillary carcinoma of the thyroid. The tumor is fleshy, with bulging variegated cut surface mottled by small cystic cavities and fibrosis.

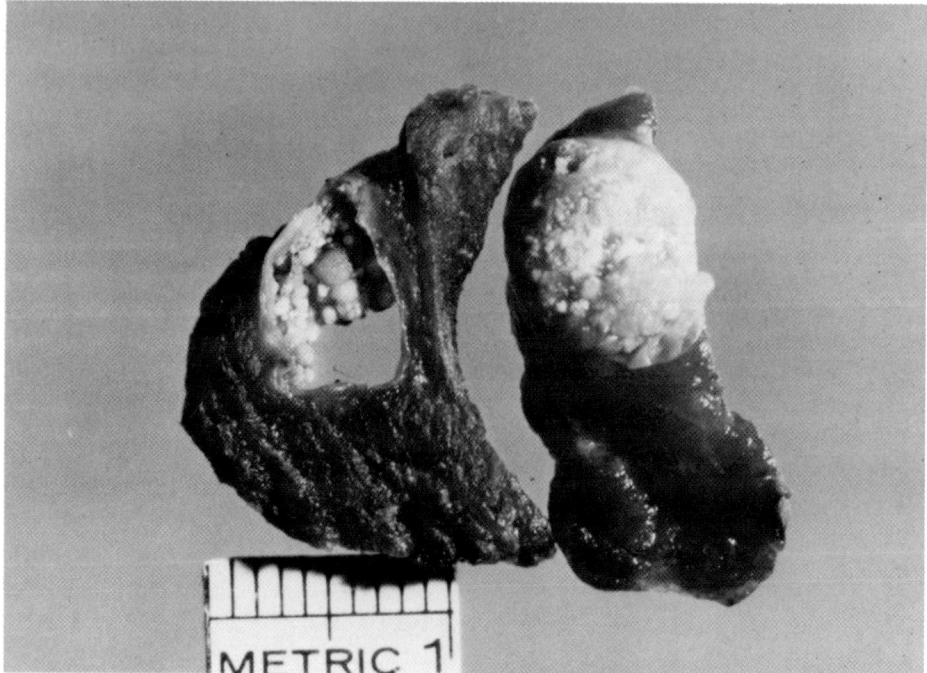

Fig. 8.2. Cystic papillary carcinoma.

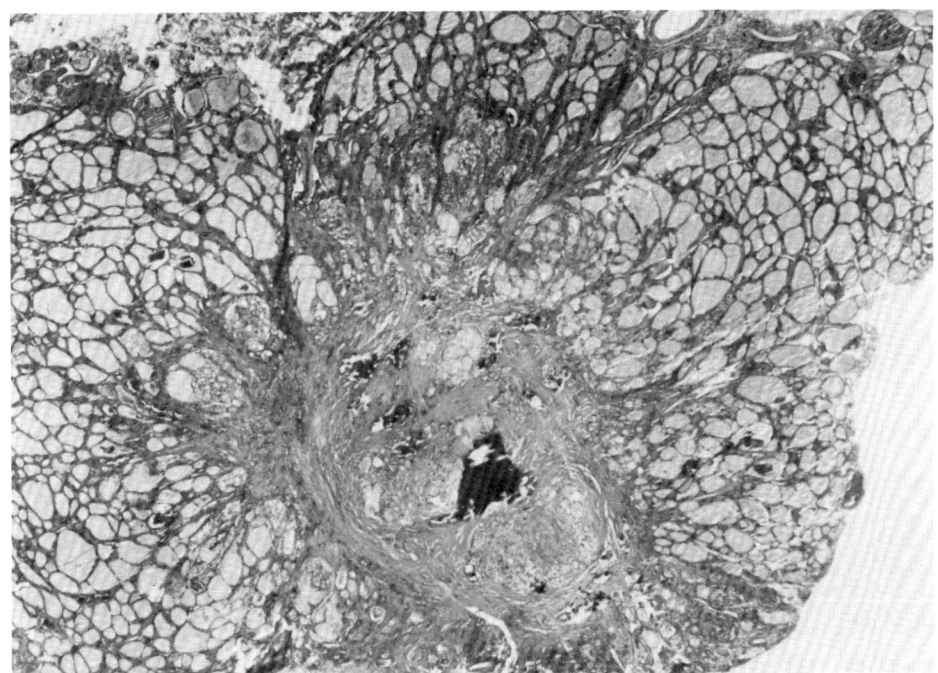

Fig. 8.3. Occult papillary carcinoma of thyroid resembling a scar due to marked desmoplasia. Hematoxylin and eosin preparation. × 40.

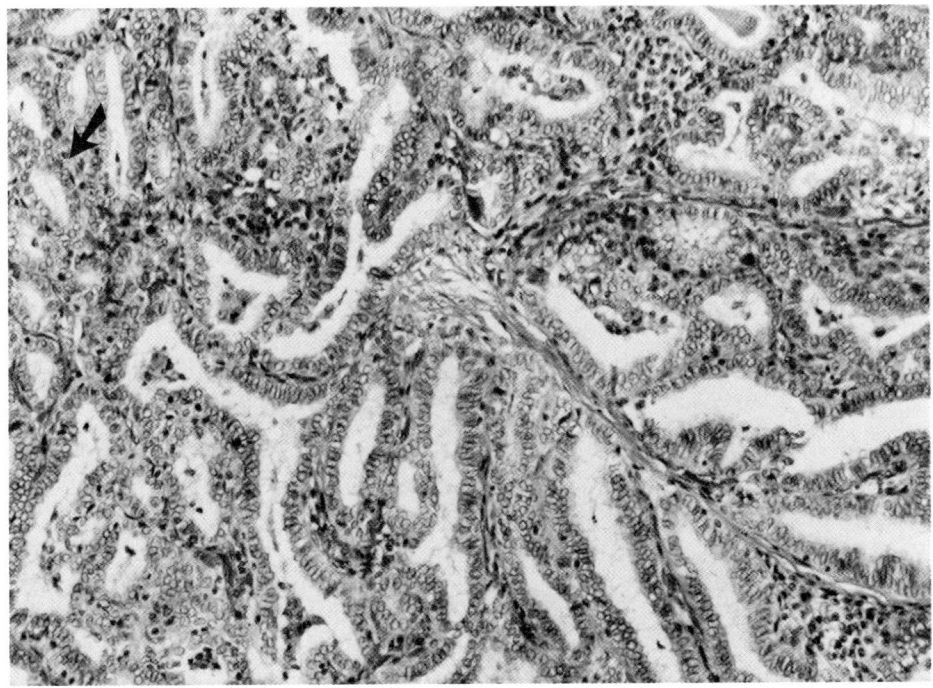

Fig. 8.4. Papillary carcinoma with branching papillary fronds. Note the glandular component (arrow). The lining epithelium is single-layered with ground-glass nuclei. Hematoxylin and eosin preparation. × 160.

123

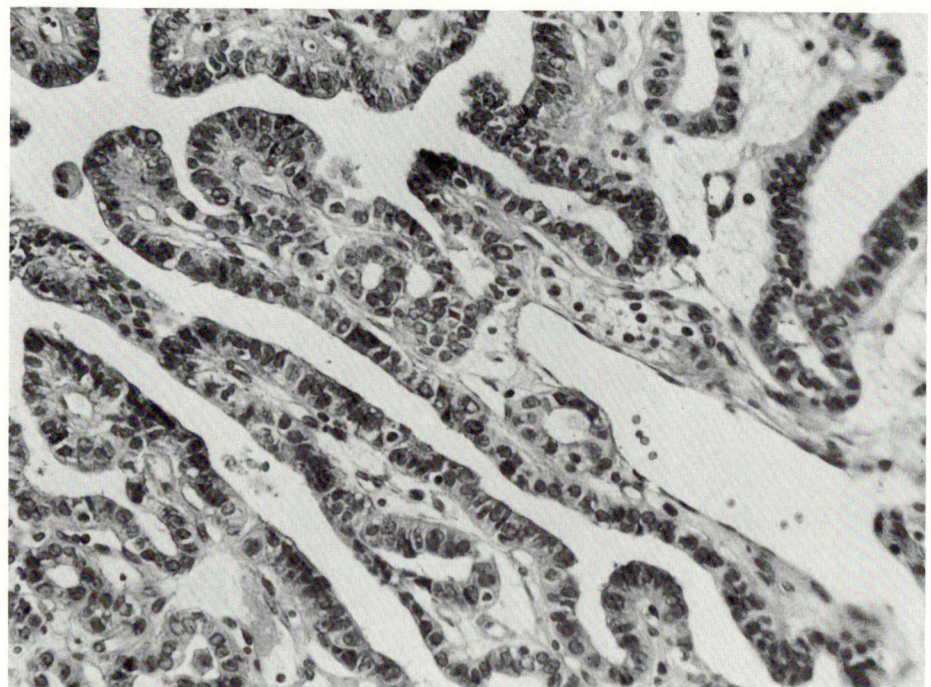

Fig. 8.5. Papillary carcinoma with papillary fronds containing central core of fibrovascular stroma. Hematoxylin and eosin preparation. × 160.

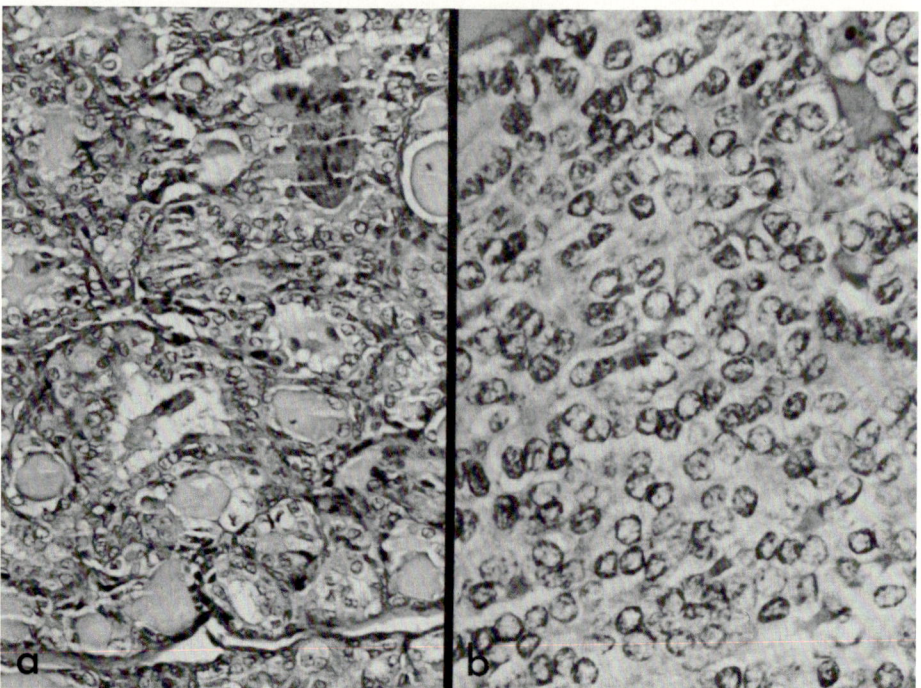

Fig. 8.6. A. Follicular variant of papillary carcinoma. Hematoxylin and eosin preparation. × 400. **B.** Solid component of papillary carcinoma. Hematoxylin and eosin preparation. × 400. The nuclei in both **A** and **B** are clear or ground glass.

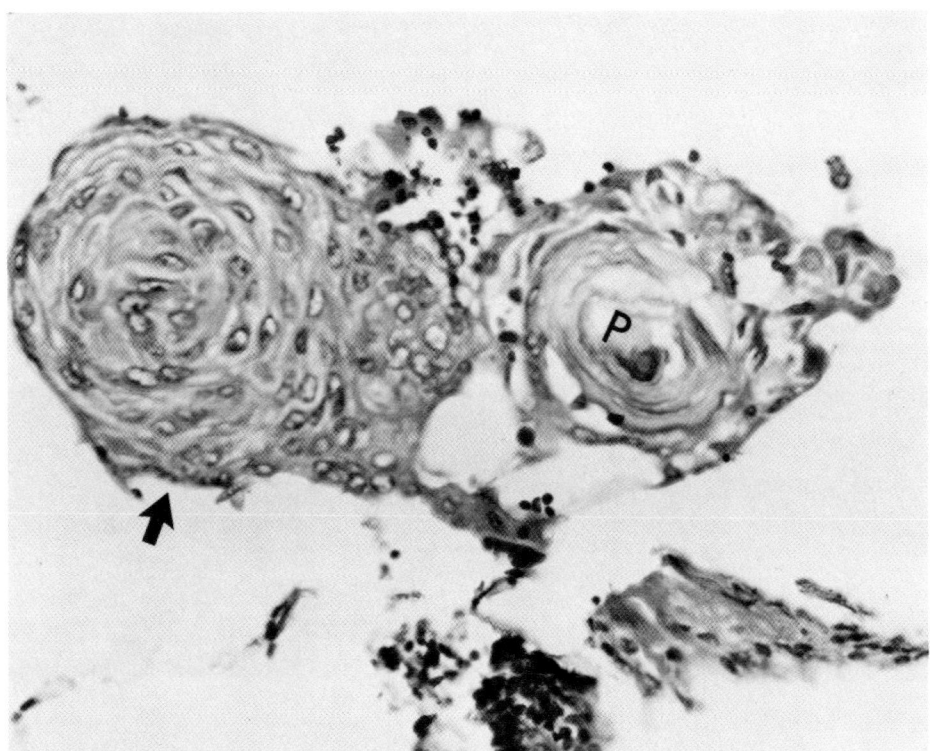

Fig. 8.7. Papillary carcinoma with squamous metaplasia *(arrow)* and a psammoma body (P). Hematoxylin and eosin preparation. × 400.

Papillary carcinomas are often mixed, with a follicular pattern in variable proportions. At times, this pattern is present to the exclusion of the papillary component; the common denominator is the watery nuclei. Such tumors are referred to as a follicular variant of papillary carcinoma.[5,6,21,29] They behave in the same way as ordinary papillary carcinomas.

Papillary carcinomas also show a solid pattern, squamous metaplasia, and oxyphilia.[14] Roughly 40–60% have lamellated calcific spherules called psammoma bodies, microliths, or calcospherites.[5,10,25,30] These are basophilic, nonbirefringent 5–100 μm in size, and seem to arise between epithelial cells. They are also found within hyalinized stroma at the tip of a papilla. "Naked" psammoma bodies may be found in thyroid tissue adjacent to or even distant from the cancer. The colloid in papillary carcinoma is dense staining.[29] Multinucleated giant cells are commonly seen.

Cystic degeneration is very common. Carcangiu et al,[5] in their series of 241 papillary carcinomas, reported an incidence of 52.5%, with marked cystic changes in 9.1%. Cystic changes also develop in nodal metastasis; 19.7% of papillary carcinomas may clinically present with nodal metastasis.[4]

Lymphocytic infiltrate is frequent. Franssila[10] reported this feature in 31% of his cases, and Carcangiu et al[5] reported it in 26.7%. Whether this infiltrate represents Hashimoto's thyroiditis or a reaction to the neoplasm is not certain. Desmoplasia is variable and could be extensive.[5]

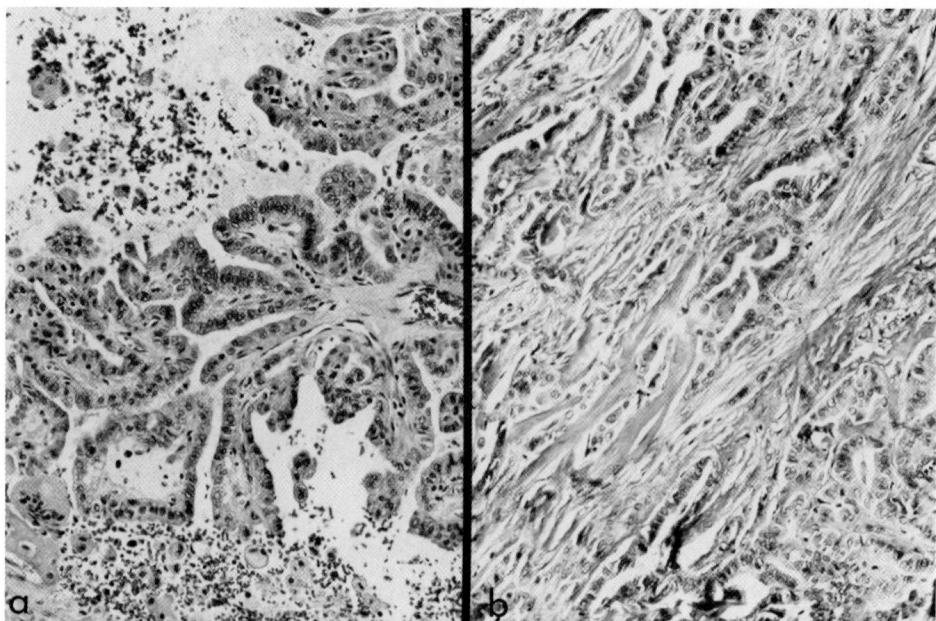

Fig. 8.8. A. Papillary carcinoma with degeneration. Note inflammatory cells including histiocytes in the background. Hematoxylin and eosin preparation. × 160. **B.** Papillary carcinoma with marked desmoplasia. Hematoxylin and eosin preparation. × 160.

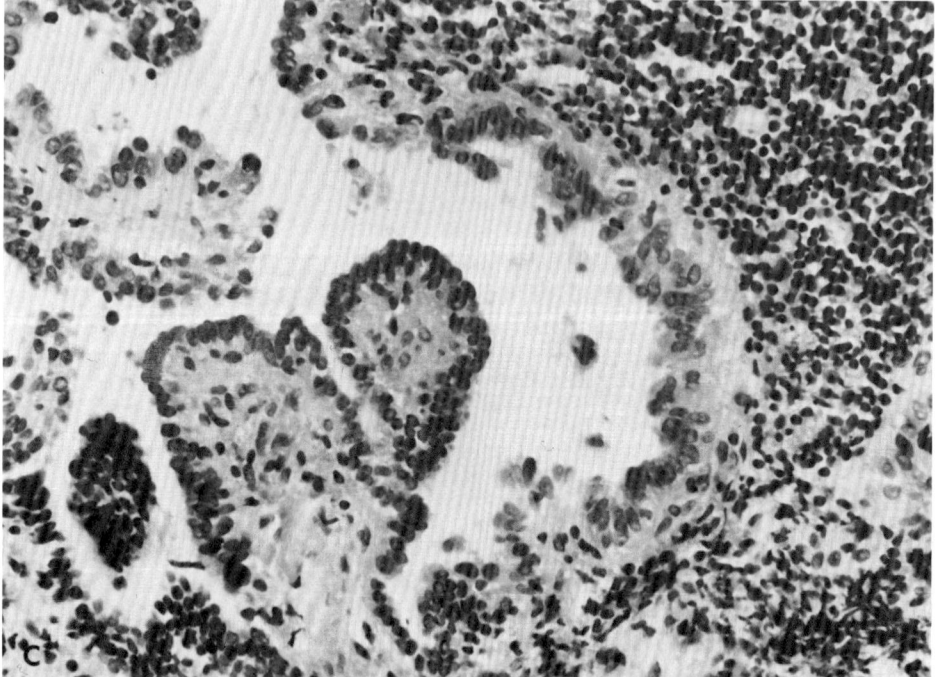

Fig. 8.8. C. Papillary carcinoma with lymphocytic infiltrate. Hematoxylin and eosin preparation. × 400.

TABLE 8.1. Cytopathologic Features of Papillary Carcinoma

Pattern	Malignant cells, isolated and in tissue fragments (latter more common) Tissue fragment: papillary with branching fronds, monolayered, or syncytial with and without follicular pattern
Cells	Cuboidal, columnar, oval, polygonal, Hürthloid, or squamoid, spindle shaped
Nucleus	Approximately 18–50 μm or larger, round to oval; finely granular, powdery dusty chromatin, slightly eccentric location, with linear chromatin ridge; pale or watery appearance Multiple micro- or macronucleoli Intranuclear cytoplasmic inclusions
Cytoplasm	Variable in quality and quantity, pale, foamy, vacuolated, or dense
Adjunct feature	Psammoma bodies
Background	Multinucleated foreign- body-type giant cells (in the absence of degeneration) Sticky colloid in the background, in strands or blobs, dense staining Degenerative changes—histiocytes with or without hemosiderin Lymphocytic infiltrate

CYTOPATHOLOGIC FEATURES OF PAPILLARY CARCINOMA

Because of the diversity of the morphologic patterns, cytopathologic criteria, as reflected in cytologic samples, are numerous and complex (Table 8.1). The diagnosis of papillary carcinoma cannot be made based on just one criterion because any one feature listed in the Table 8.1 can be seen in benign diseases. It is important, therefore, to be familiar with the typical cytopathologic features in order to appreciate the variations and diagnostic pitfalls. For this reason, the usual and typical cytopathologic features are first individually described in detail, and then discussed as to their significance.

Because papillary carcinomas are generally soft, fragile, and with minimal stroma, they yield very cellular aspirates. The cellularity is often overwhelming. Characteristic structural patterns of tissue fragments are mixed with a large population of pleomorphic, isolated neoplastic cells that provide a correct diagnosis when viewed under a low-power objective (Fig. 8.9).

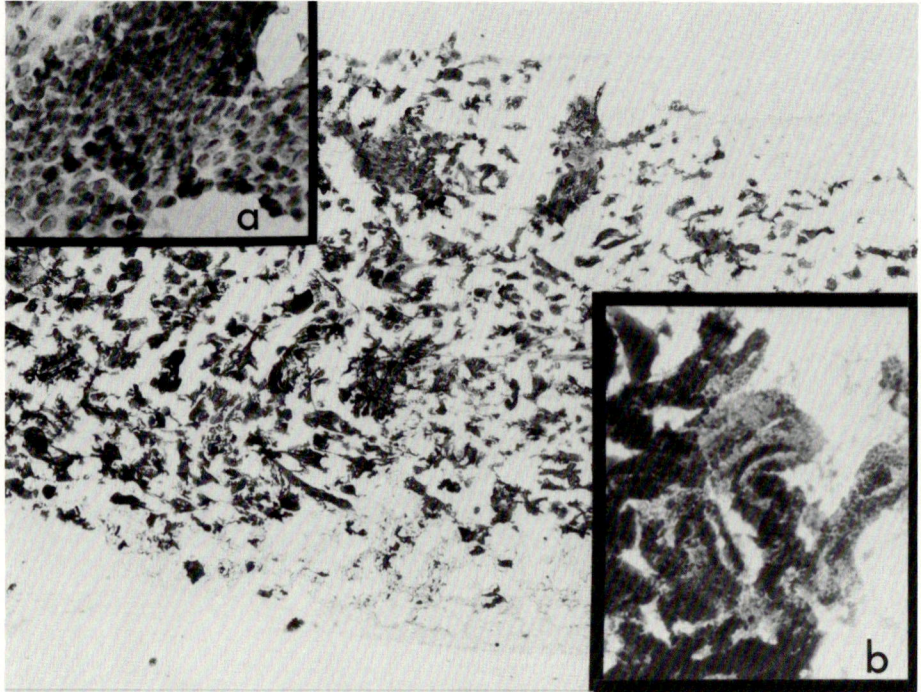

Fig. 8.9. Overwhelmingly cellular aspirate with myriads of tissue fragments exhibiting a complex branching pattern, some monolayered. Papanicolaou preparation. × 40. *Inset a:* Monolayered tissue fragment. Papanicolaou preparation. × 630. *Inset b:* Papillary tissue fragments. Papanicolaou preparation. × 160.

Cells of Papillary Carcinoma

Cells of papillary carcinoma (Figs. 8.10–8.13) are so varied that practically any shape and size may be encountered. They may be cuboidal, columnar, ovoid, polygonal, squamoid, and even spindle shaped. The cell borders in single cells are well defined. The scant to abundant cytoplasm may be pale, foamy, vacuolated, or dense. The carcinoma cells with abundant, dense cytoplasm appear Hürthloid. Nuclei are generally slightly eccentric in position, round to oval, and vary in size. In well-differentiated papillary fronds, they appear small because they are closely packed together. In monolayered tissue fragments, they are considerably larger. The nuclear membranes are sharp. The chromatin is so finely granular, dusty to powdery, that the nuclei appear clear, pale, or watery. Single or multiple micro- and or macronucleoli are always seen. A nonspecific feature is the presence of a chromatin ridge along the long axis of the nucleus. This is probably due to irregular infolding of the nuclear membrane, as seen in electromicrographs.[5] Another characteristic feature is the presence of intranuclear cytoplasmic inclusions (see below).

   The nuclear characteristics of papillary carcinomas are diagnostic. In cytologic material, the tetrad of pale enlarged nuclei with dusty chromatin, nucleoli, chromatin ridge, and intranuclear cytoplasmic inclusions are virtually pathognomonic of papillary carcinoma.

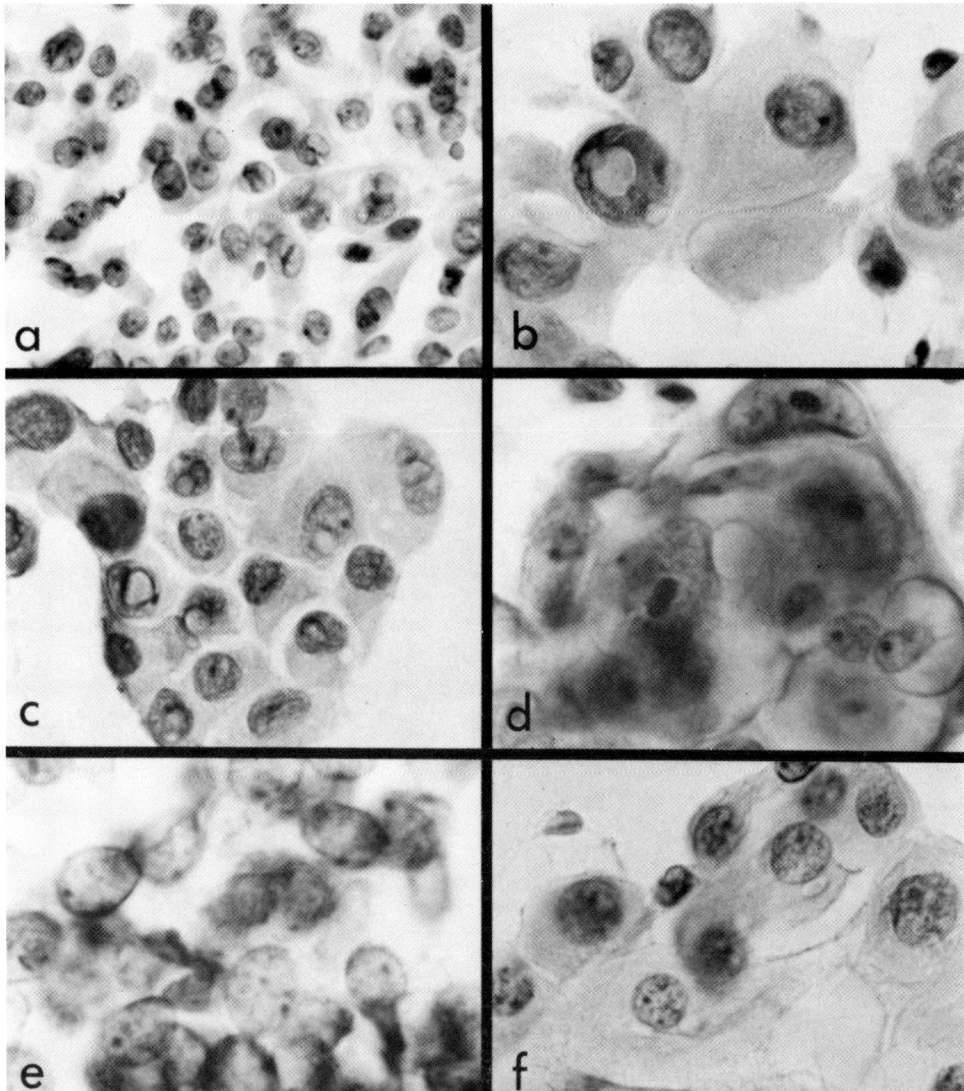

Fig. 8.10. Cells of papillary carcinoma. **A.** Small oval and columnar-shaped cells. Papanicolaou preparation. × 630. **B.** Large cells with dense cytoplasm resembling Hürthle cells. Papanicolaou preparation. × 630. **C.** Large cuboidal cells with well-defined cell borders. Papanicolaou preparation. × 630. **D.** Tissue fragment with very pleomorphic nuclei and vacuolated cytoplasm. Papanicolaou preparation. × 630. **E.** Scanty cytoplasm but large watery nuclei. Papanicolaou preparation. × 630. **F.** Squamoid cells. Papanicolaou preparation. × 630.

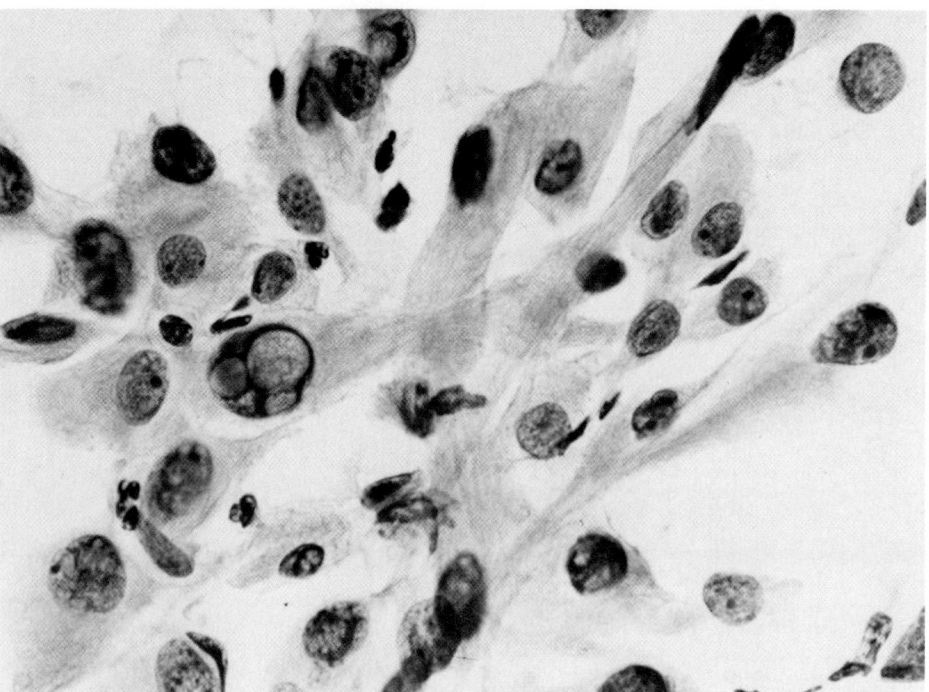

Fig. 8.11. Cells of papillary carcinoma. Note cellular pleomorphism with spindle cell pattern. The nuclei exhibit typical morphology of papillary carcinoma. Papanicolaou preparation. × 630.

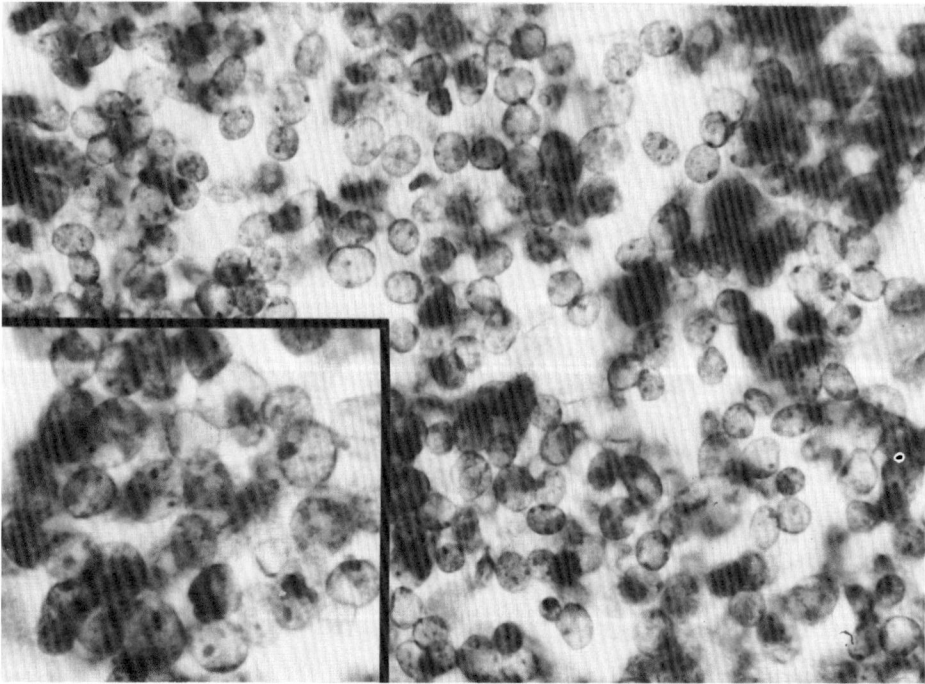

Fig. 8.12. Papillary carcinoma cells with characteristic nuclear morphology. The nuclei are large, appear empty due to peripheral condensation of the chromatin, and contain micronucleoli, giving the typical "Orphan Annie" appearance. Papanicolaou preparation. × 400. *Inset:* Higher magnification. Papanicolaou preparation. × 630.

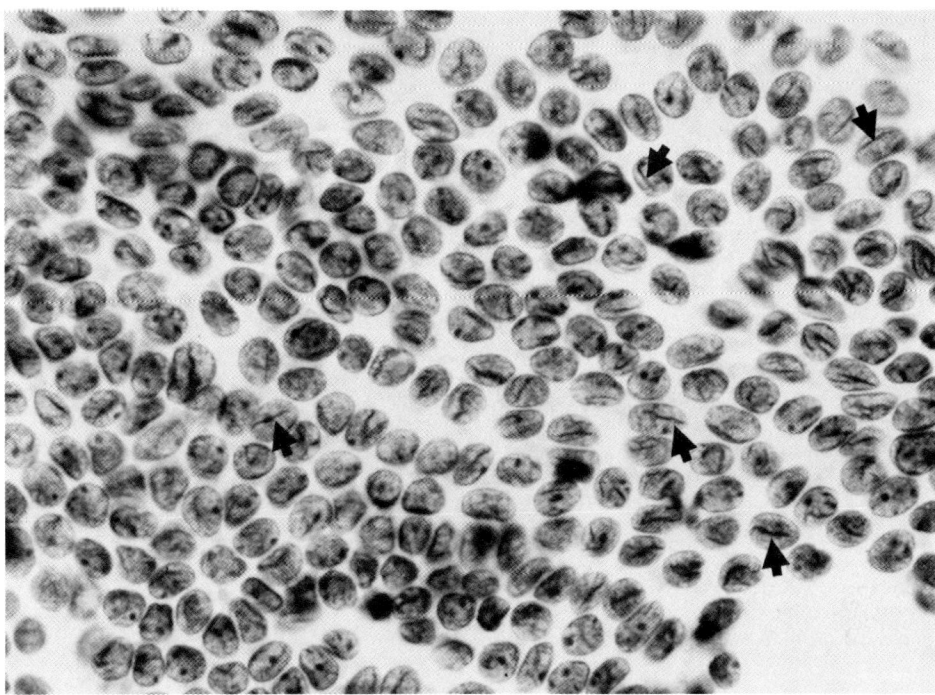

Fig. 8.13. Cells of papillary carcinoma with characteristic nuclear ridges *(arrows)*. Papanicolaou preparation. × 630.

Syncytial-Type Tissue Fragments With and Without Follicular Patterns

Cancer cells grow irregularly. They have ill-defined cell borders and altered nuclear polarity with crowded, overlapped nuclei that form syncytial-type tissue fragments (Figs. 8.14 and 8.15). Such a structural pattern is seen in any type of carcinoma, and papillary carcinoma is no exception. Some tissue fragments may show a follicular pattern, indicating a follicular component of the carcinoma. Their cells generally exhibit typical nuclear morphology of papillary carcinoma.

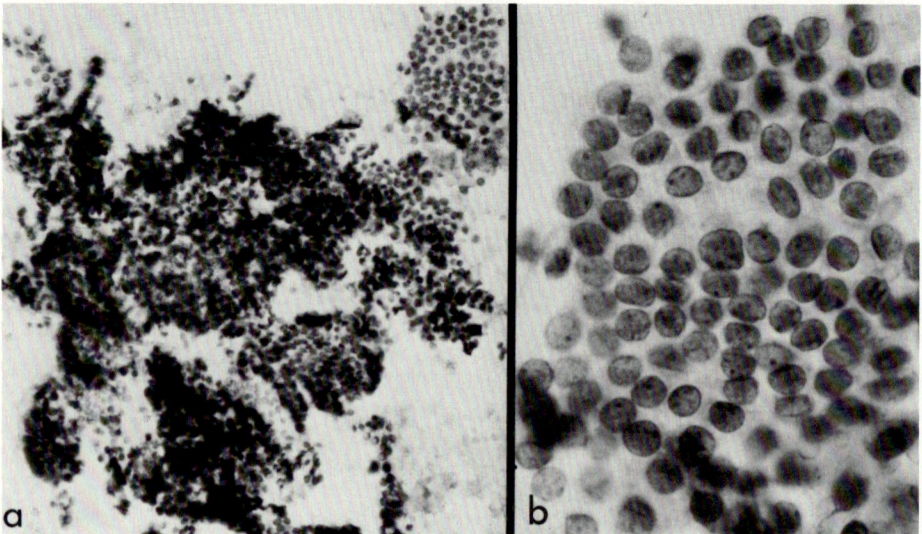

Fig. 8.14. A. Syncytial-type tissue fragments of papillary carcinoma. Papanicolaou preparation. × 160. **B.** Higher magnification of **A** showing a monolayered pattern with typical nuclear morphology. Papanicolaou preparation. × 630.

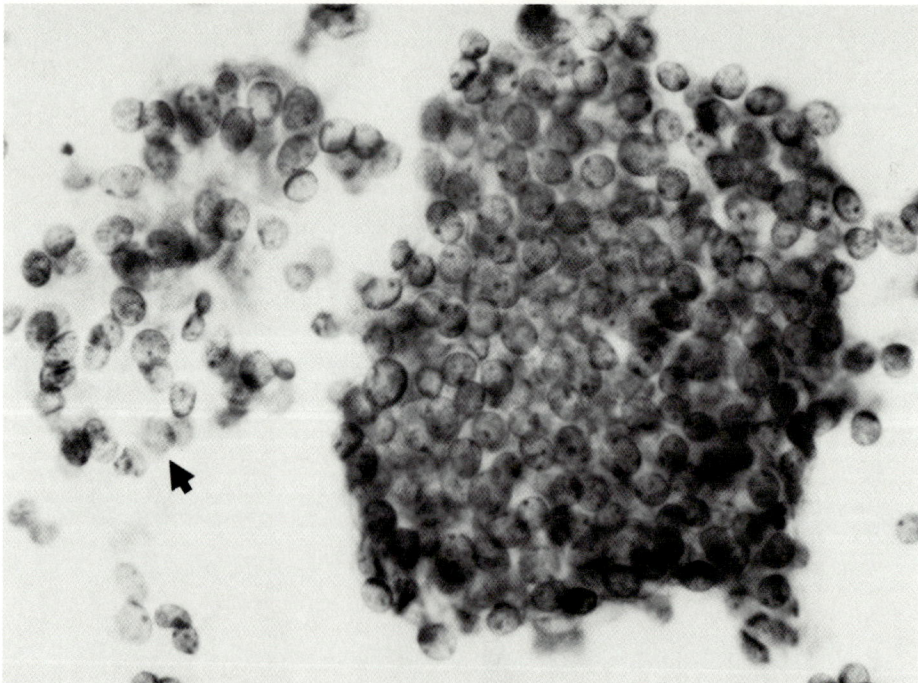

Fig. 8.15. Syncytial-type tissue fragments with *(arrow)* and without follicular pattern. The nuclei have fine, powdery chromatin with periphral condensation, thus appearing pale or clear. Papanicolaou preparation. × 630.

Papillary Tissue Fragments

Papillary tissue fragments (Figs. 8.16–8.19; Plate 4.6) are syncytial and have a simple or complex branching pattern characterized by a smooth, external contour and peripheral palisading of the nuclei. The component cells are closely packed, have poorly defined cell borders, and their cytoplasm is hardly visible. The nuclei are crowded and overlapped, and exhibit characteristic morphology. The tips of the papillary fronds may be seen as three-dimensional clusters, with smooth external boundaries.

In well-fixed, well-stained preparations, the papillary tissue fragments demonstrate central fibrovascular stroma containing capillary loops (Plate 8.1). Neoplastic cells arising from such a stromal core are either low, cuboidal, or columnar, and give a feathery pattern to the papillary fragment.

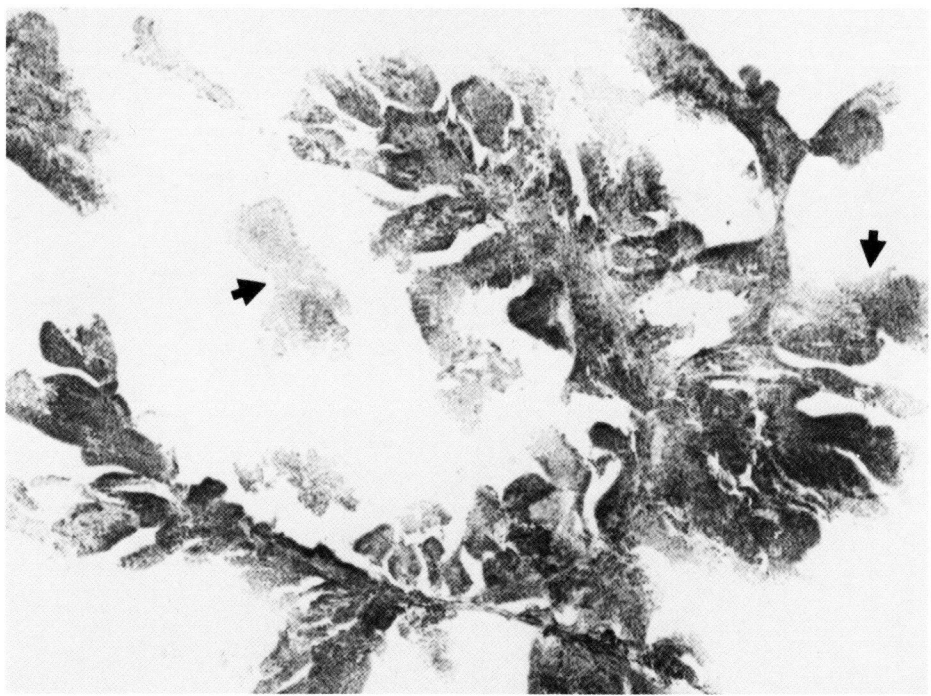

Fig. 8.16. Tissue fragments with complex branching pattern. Some appear monolayered (*arrow*), a characteristic pattern that allows a diagnosis when viewed with a low-power objective. Papanicolaou preparation. × 63.

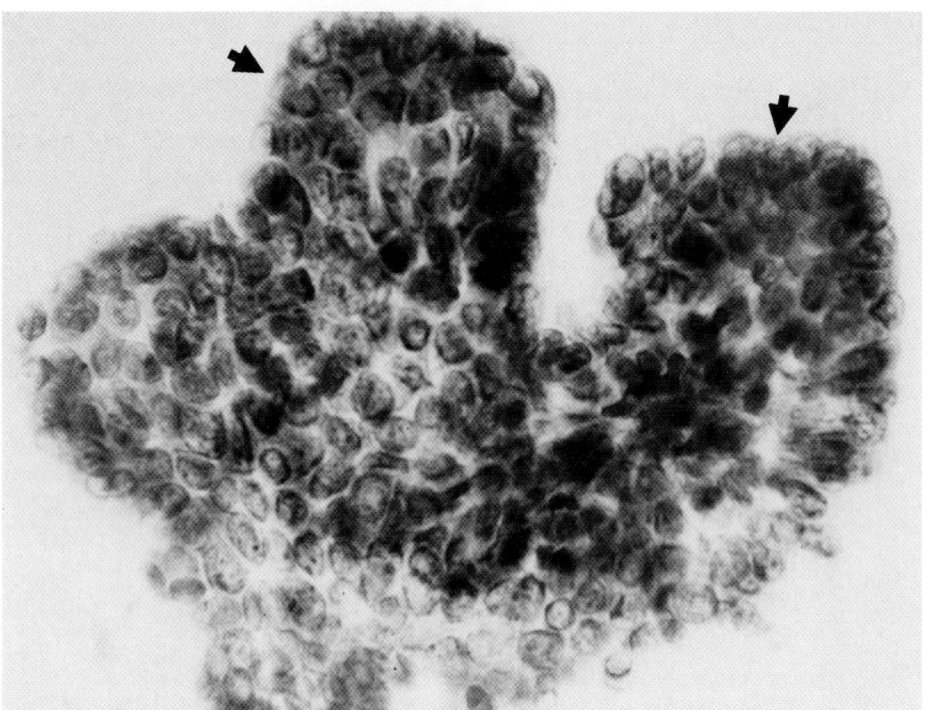

Fig. 8.17. Higher magnification of branching papillary tissue fragment with syncytial pattern. Note smooth external contour and peripheral palisading of nuclei *(arrows)*. Papanicolaou preparation. × 630.

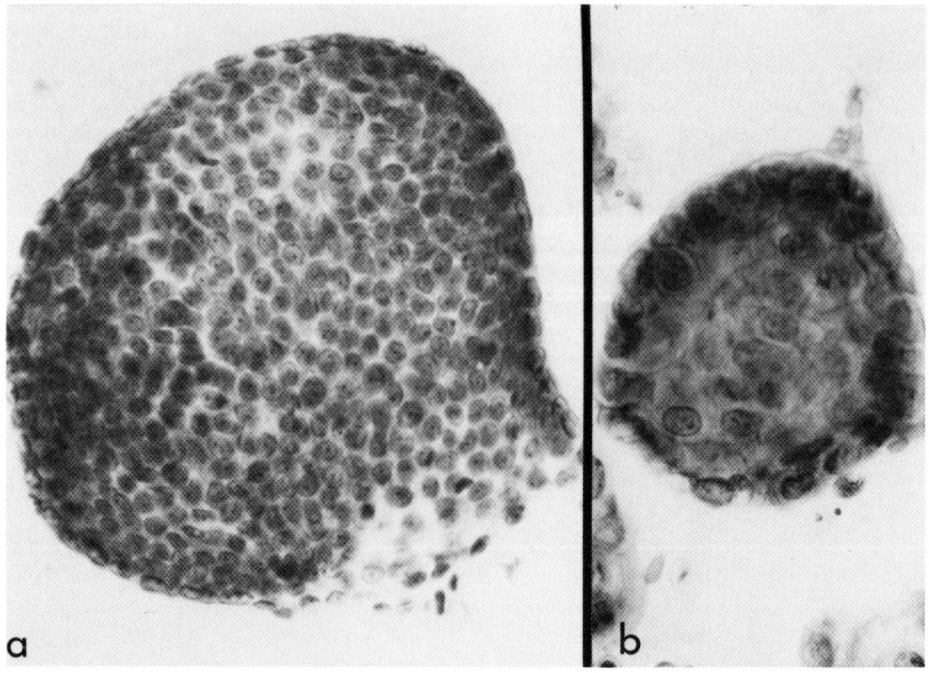

Fig. 8.18. A. Single papillary tissue fragment with smooth external contour and peripheral palisading of nuclei. Papanicolaou preparation. × 400. B. Cluster of carcinoma cells, probably representing tip of the papilla. Note smooth external border and three-dimensional configuration. Papanicolaou preparation. × 630.

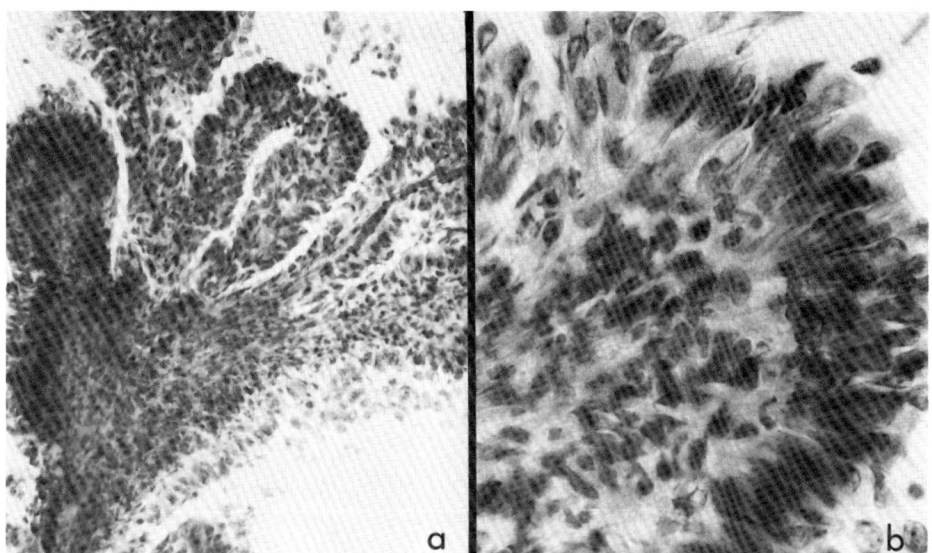

Fig. 8.19. **A.** Branching papillary tissue fragment with central fibrovascular core. Papanicolaou preparation. × 160. **B.** Higher magnification of **A** showing columnar cells lining the outer surface, with overlapped nuclei. Papanicolaou preparation. × 630.

Monolayerd Tissue Fragments

The presence of monolayered tissue fragments (Figs. 8.20–8.24) is characteristic of papillary carcinoma. They probably represent the papillary fronds seen en face (see Chapter 4, Concepts Basic to Thyroid Cytopathology). This impression is supported by the fact that many fragments are large, with branching, sweeping curves. The tissue fragments are commonly referred to as monolayered sheets because they often show a two-dimensional pattern, ie, cells are in one plane of focus. The component cells usually have poorly defined cell borders, with a syncytial pattern. Nuclei are generally large and pleomorphic in size with altered polarity, and the nuclear chromatin is finely granular and powdery. Micro- and macronucleoli are frequently present. The nuclei show morphology characteristic of papillary carcinoma. Intranuclear cytoplasmic inclusions are conspicuous. The cytoplasm is variable, generally abundant, pale, foamy to dense, giving a Hürthloid appearance. This dense cytoplasm is considered a diagnostic feature by Abele and Miller.[1]

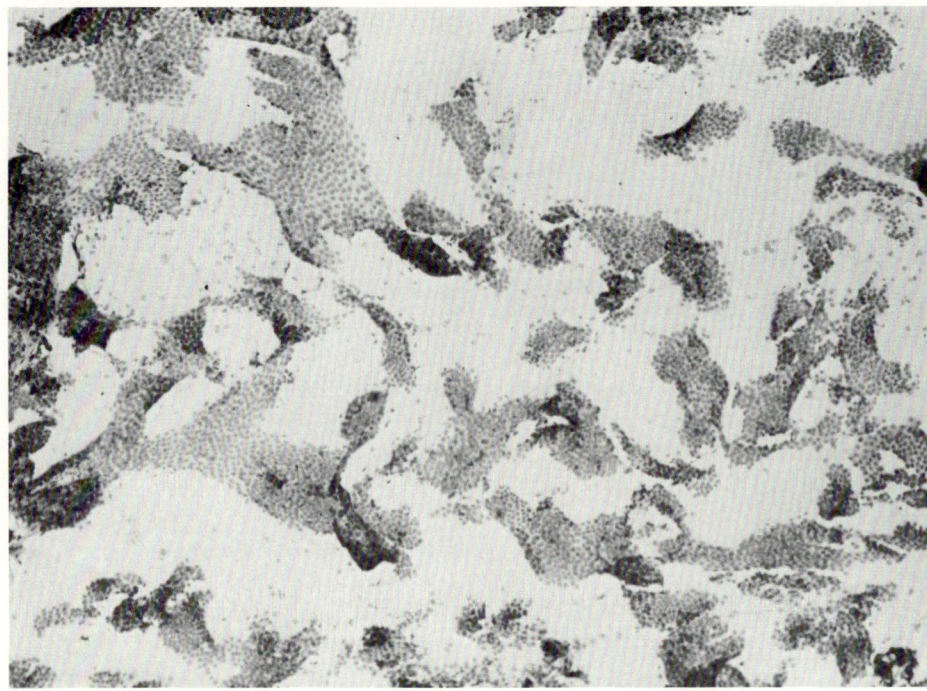

Fig. 8.20. Papillary carcinoma showing monolayered tissue fragments with branching, sweeping curves. Papanicolaou preparation. × 63.

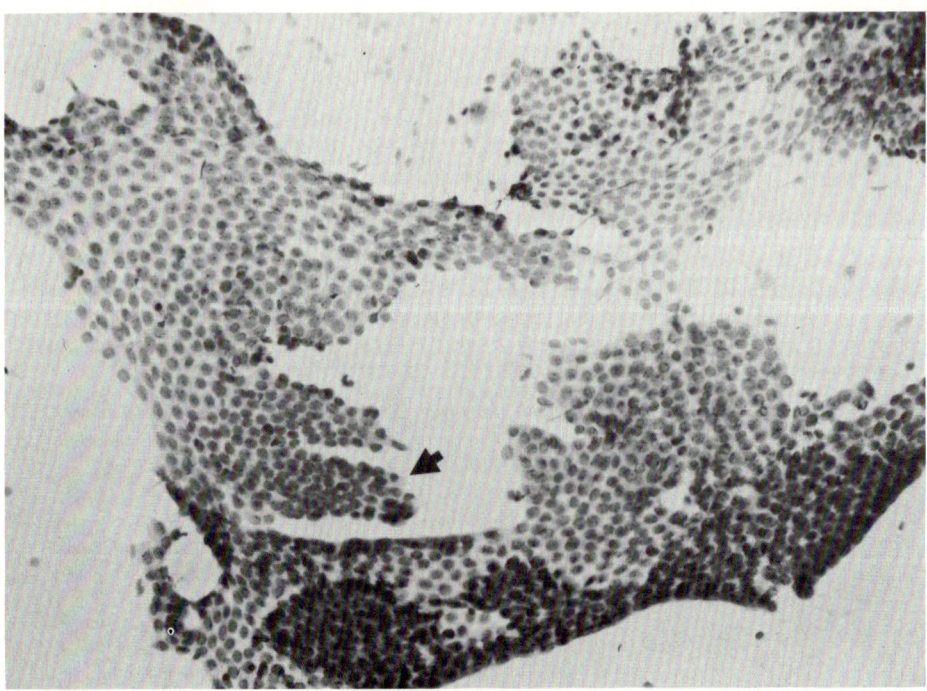

Fig. 8.21. Monolayered tissue fragments of papillary carcinoma, with suggestion of branching pattern *(arrow)*. Papanicolaou preparation. × 160.

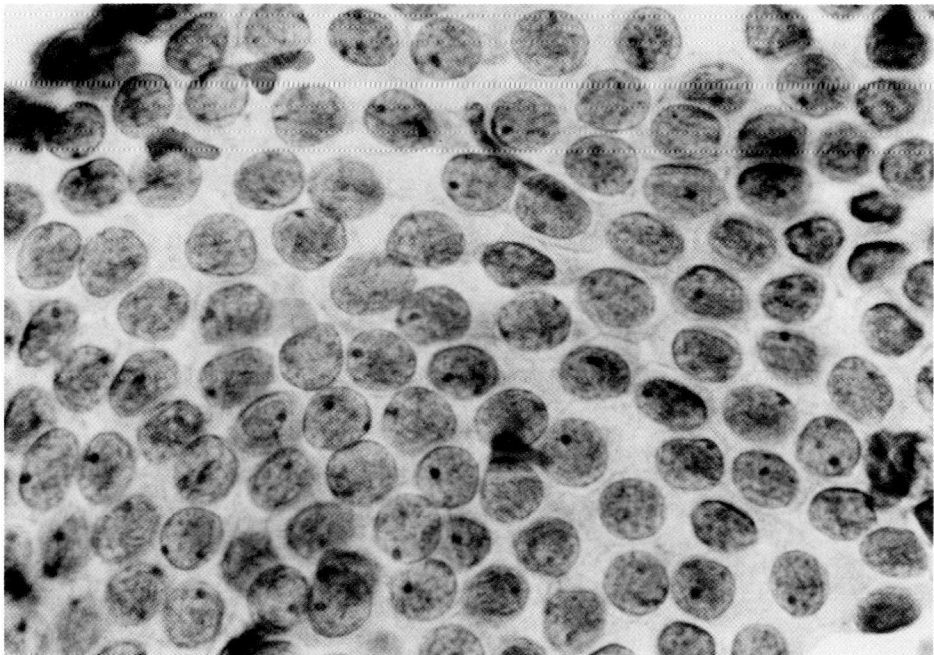

Fig. 8.22. Monolayered tissue fragment of papillary carcinoma. The nuclei are considerably enlarged with fine, dusty chromatin and multiple micronucleoli. Papanicolaou preparation. × 1000.

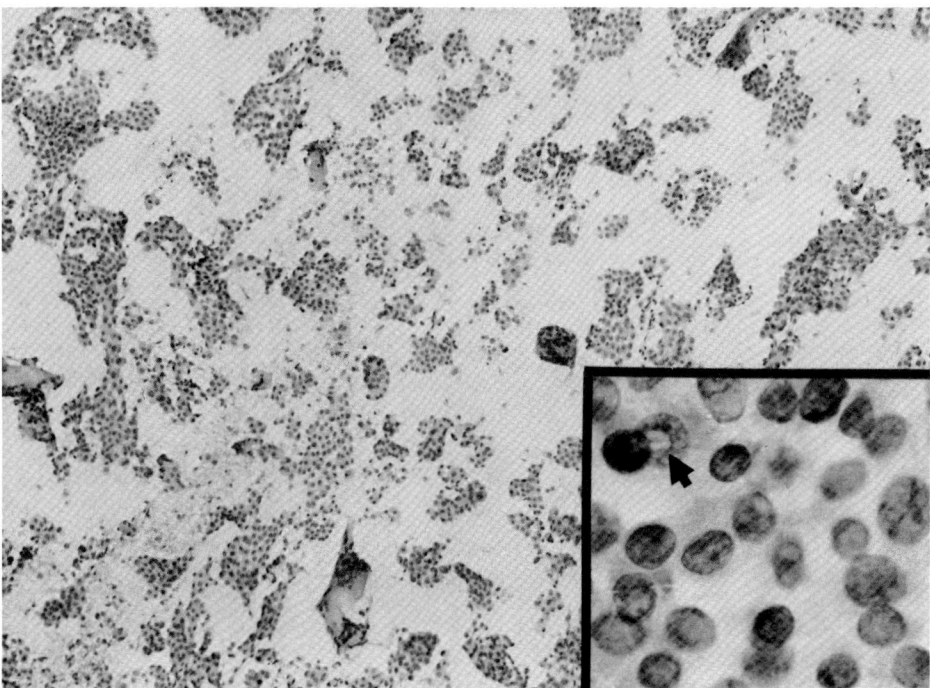

Fig. 8.23. Monolayered tissue fragments of papillary carcinoma. Papanicolaou preparation. × 63. *Inset:* Note enlarged nuclei with altered polarity, fine powdery chromatin, nucleoli, chromatin ridge, and intranuclear cytoplasmic inclusion *(arrow).* Papanicolaou preparation. × 630.

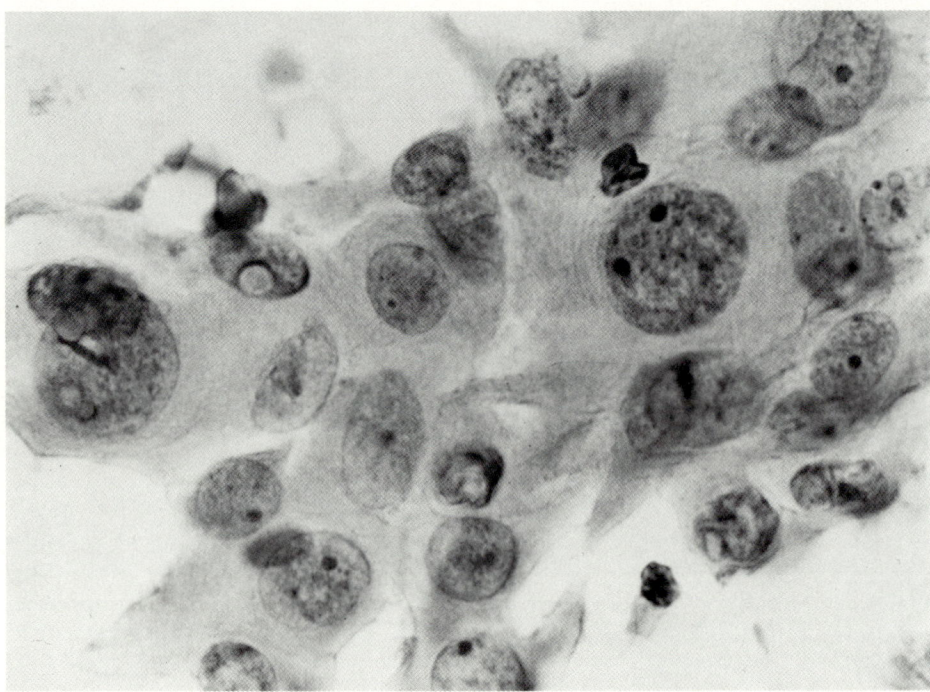

Fig. 8.24. Monolayered tissue fragment of papillary carcinoma composed of large polygonal cells with abundant dense cytoplasm. The pleomorphic nuclei exhibit a typical morphology of papillary carcinoma. Papanicolaou preparation. × 1000.

Intranuclear Cytoplasmic Inclusions

Intranuclear cytoplasmic inclusions (Fig. 8.25) are a consistent feature in aspirates of papillary carcinoma.[7] They occur as sharply defined, clear, round inclusions bordered by condensed chromatin. They may be large and single, occupying the entire nucleus, or small and multiple. According to Abele and Miller[1] an intranuclear inclusion should take up at least 10% of the total nuclear surface area to distinguish it from nonspecific vacuoles, which are often seen in air-dried preparations. Also, the sharp border is the differentiating feature from vacuoles seen in some degenerating nuclei, where the vacuoles merge with the chromatin.

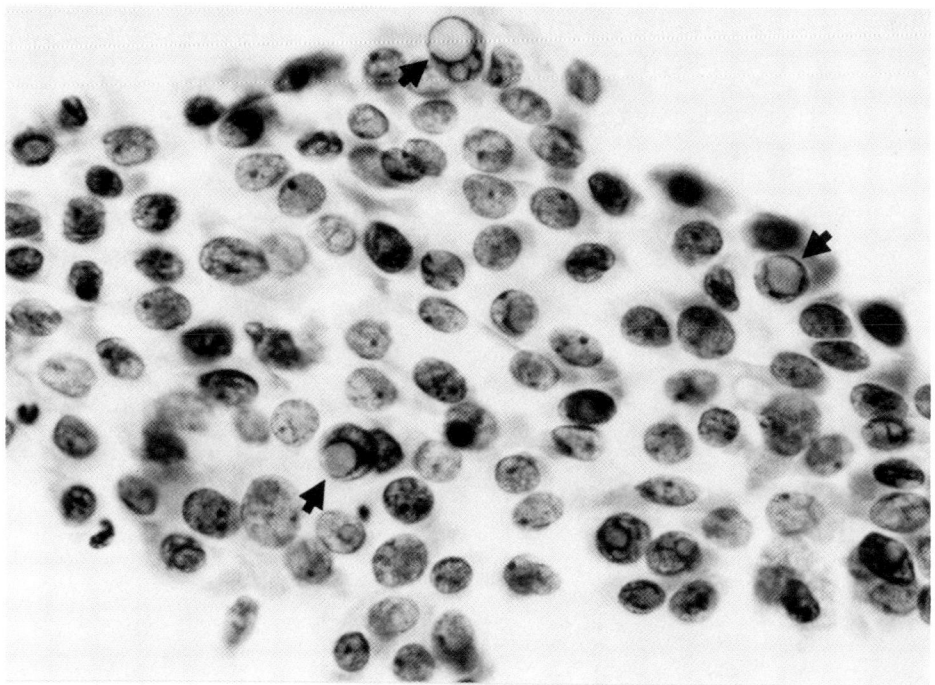

Fig. 8.25. Monolayered tissue fragment. The nuclei are large, pleomorphic in size, with powdery chromatin. Intranuclear cytoplasmic inclusions are seen in several of the nuclei *(arrow)*. Note the sharply condensed chromatin bordering the inclusions. Papanicolaou preparation. × 630.

Psammoma Bodies

Psammoma bodies (Fig. 8.26; Plates 8.2 and 8.5) are a diagnostic feature of papillary carcinoma.[35] They are easily recognized by basophilic concentric lamellation, generally incorporated within a tissue fragment of follicular cells. In Papanicolaou-stained preparations, psammoma bodies not only stain basophilic, but also stain lavender, golden-brown, or amphophilic. The architecture may also be different. In addition to concentric lamellation, they may have a starburst and refractile appearance, or may resemble a Maltese cross. The nuclei of the cells forming the tissue fragments that incorporate the psammoma body show typical morphology of papillary carcinoma.

Multinucleated Foreign-Body–Type Giant Cells

Although giant cells are not generally described in the literature on the histopathology of papillary carcinoma, their presence appears to be ubiquitous in

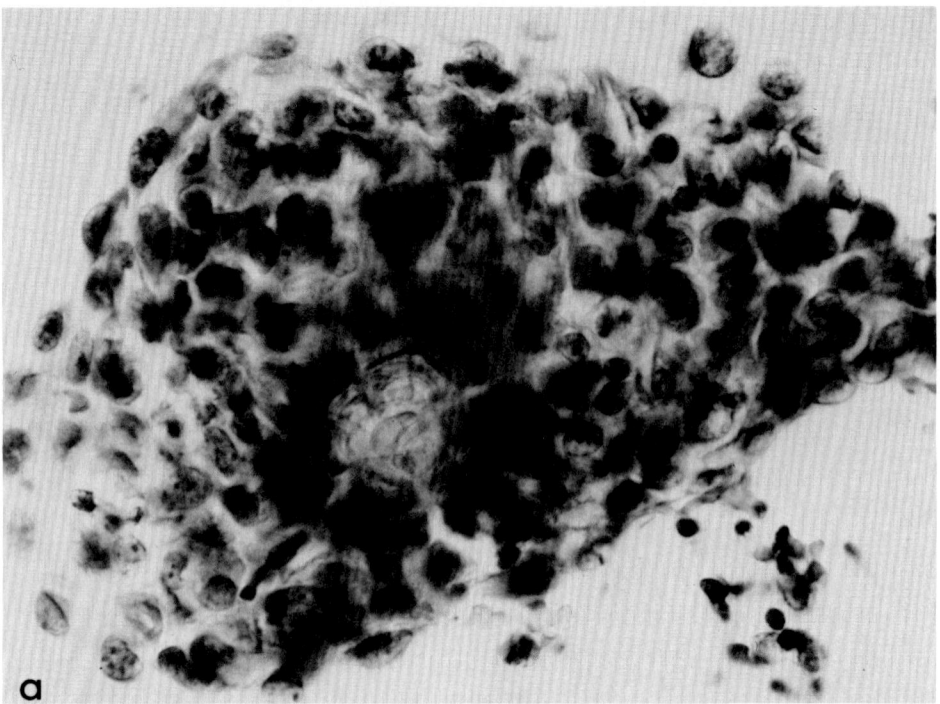

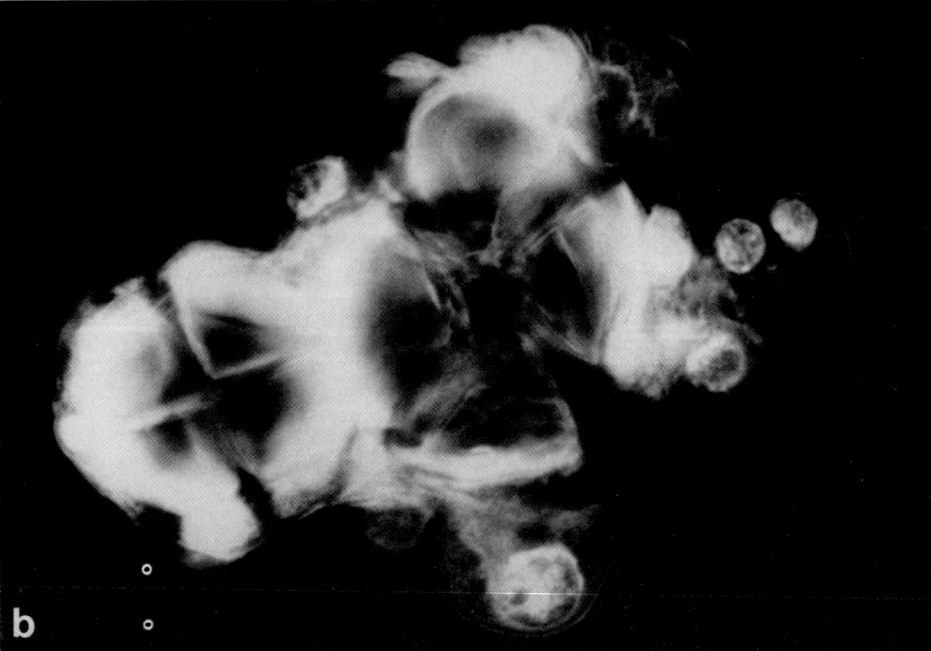

Fig. 8.26. **A.** Psammoma body with concentric lamellation, incorporated in a syncytial-type tissue fragment. The nuclei show typical morphology of papillary carcinoma. Papanicolaou preparation. × 630. **B.** Negative print showing a Maltese cross appearance of psammoma body. Papanicolaou preparation. × 630.

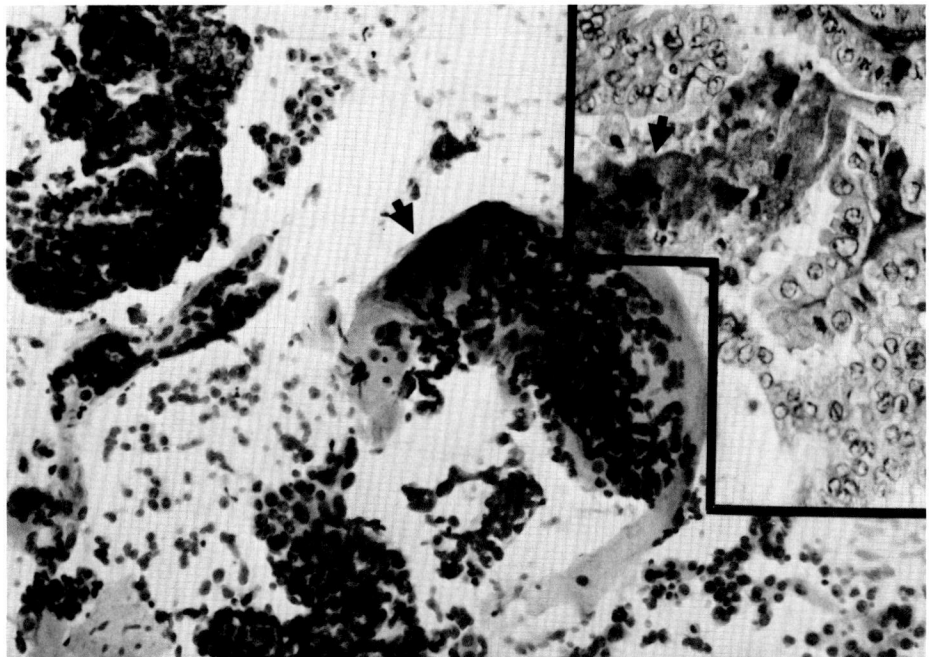

Fig. 8.27. Multinucleated foreign-body–type giant cells in an aspirate of papillary carcinoma. These can be enormous *(arrow)*. Papanicolaou preparation. × 160. *Inset:* Histologic section showing similar cells *(arrow)*. Hematoxylin and eosin preparation. × 400.

cytologic and histologic material (Fig. 8.27). They are seen in the absence of degeneration, and do not seem to be phagocytic or histiocytic in origin. These giant cells vary in size from small to enormous, and may fill an entire high-power field. Their cytoplasm is dense and not dirty granular or vacuolated, like that of the histiocytic-type giant cells. Abele and Miller[1] aptly described the cytoplasm they observed as "abundant, wavy, resembling wind-blown stratus cloud." The nuclei vary in number, and often resemble those of carcinoma cells. Giant cells are always intimately associated with papillary or monolayered fragments, a feature appreciated in histologic material as well. Hidvegi et al[15] suggested that the giant cells are perhaps derived from cancer cells.

Colloid Strands

As described by Löwhagen et al,[23] ropy strands of colloid (Fig. 8.28) are often seen in aspirates from papillary carcinoma. The colloid may also be dense staining and is frequently observed in blobs or follicular luminal casts (Plate 8.3).

Degeneration

Degenerative changes with cyst formation (Fig. 8.29) are frequently observed in papillary carcinomas. They are manifested in the aspirate by the presence of histiocytes with or without hemosiderin.

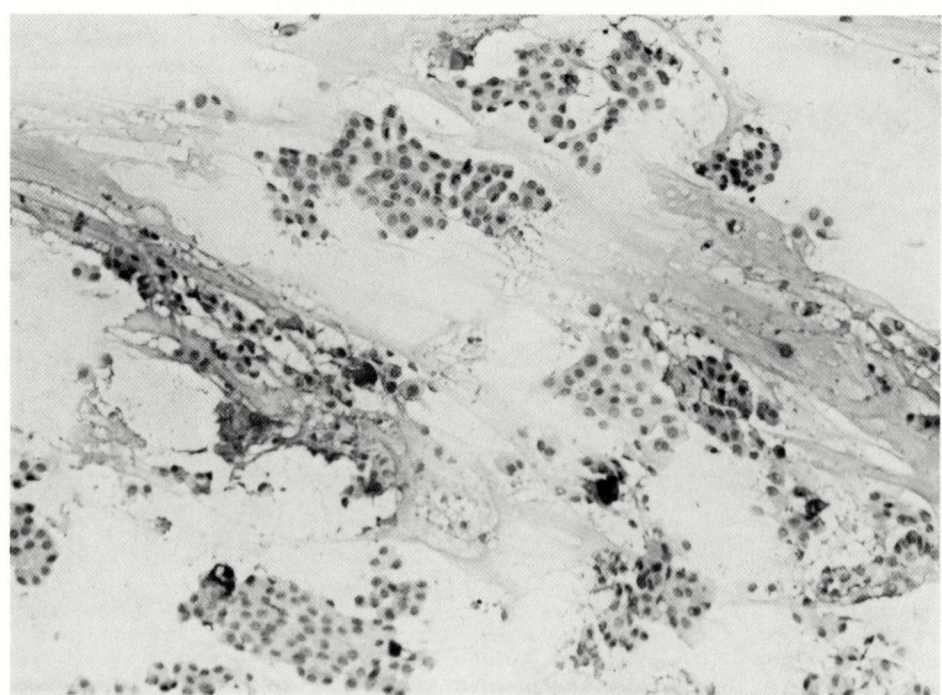

Fig. 8.28. Strands of dense, sticky colloid, a frequent but nonspecific feature of papillary carcinoma. Papanicolaou preparation. × 160.

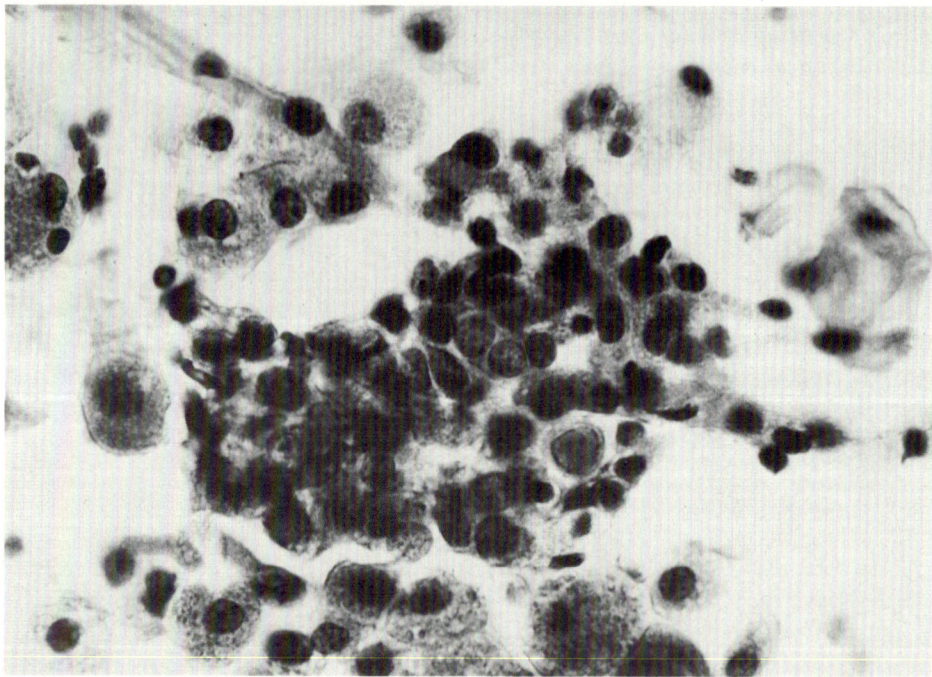

Fig. 8.29. Papillary carcinoma cells surrounded and obscured by hemosiderin-containing histiocytes, indicating degeneration and hemorrhage. Such an aspirate may offer diagnostic difficulties. Papanicolaou preparation. × 630.

142

TABLE 8.2. Difficulties in Cytologic Diagnosis of
Papillary Carcinoma

1. Follicular variant of papillary carcinoma
2. Papillary carcinoma with cystic changes
3. Single cell pattern
4. Inadequate sample

Lymphocytic Infiltrate

The presence of lymphocytes indicates underlying or coexisting Hashimoto's thyroiditis, features of which may be seen along with the cytologic features of papillary carcinoma (see Chapter 11, Thyroiditis). According to some, papillary carcinomas elicit a host reaction characterized by a lymphocytic infiltrate,[22] although Carcangiu et al[5] have disputed that concept.

DIAGNOSTIC DIFFICULTIES

Most papillary carcinomas are easily identified from fine-needle aspirates because they have several diagnostic features. However, certain types and certain presentations pose diagnostic difficulties (Table 8.2). These include the follicular variant of papillary carcinoma and papillary carcinoma with cystic changes. An aspirate with a single cell pattern or a sample that is poorly cellular are equally challenging.

Follicular Variant

First described by Lindsay,[21] the follicular variant of papillary carcinoma (Figs. 8.30–8.33; Plate 8.3) is characterized by an exclusively or predominantly follicular pattern with abortive papillae. Despite the follicular architecture, the nuclei share morphologic similarities with those of papillary carcinoma—they are clear with a ground-glass appearance. These carcinomas behave in the same fashion as ordinary papillary carcinoma.[29] The aspirates show syncytial-type tissue fragments with or without a follicular pattern, very similar to those seen in follicular neoplasms (see Chapter 6, Follicular Adenoma and Carcinoma). The nuclei are enlarged, crowded, and overlapped. The nuclear chromatin is generally fine and powdery, with one or several micronucleoli. Intranuclear cytoplasmic inclusions are frequently seen.

As follicular variants may have an abortive papillary pattern, the aspirates usually show only a few cytologic features of papillary carcinoma, such as an occasional papillary fragment or a monolayered sheet of cancer cells. Psammoma bodies are only infrequently observed, and giant cells are seldom seen. The colloid is rather sticky and dense. With a follicular presentation in the cytologic material, the fine powdery chromatin and intranuclear cytoplasmic inclusions serve as a clue to a correct diagnosis. The ground-glass pattern of the nuclei in papillary carcinomas is not always generalized, but can be focal. Because of sampling, in such cases aspirated neoplastic cells may not show the typical nuclear cytomorphology. Instead, the nuclei have coarse chromatin similar to those of follicular carcinoma, and the tumor is apt to be interpreted as a follicular neoplasm.

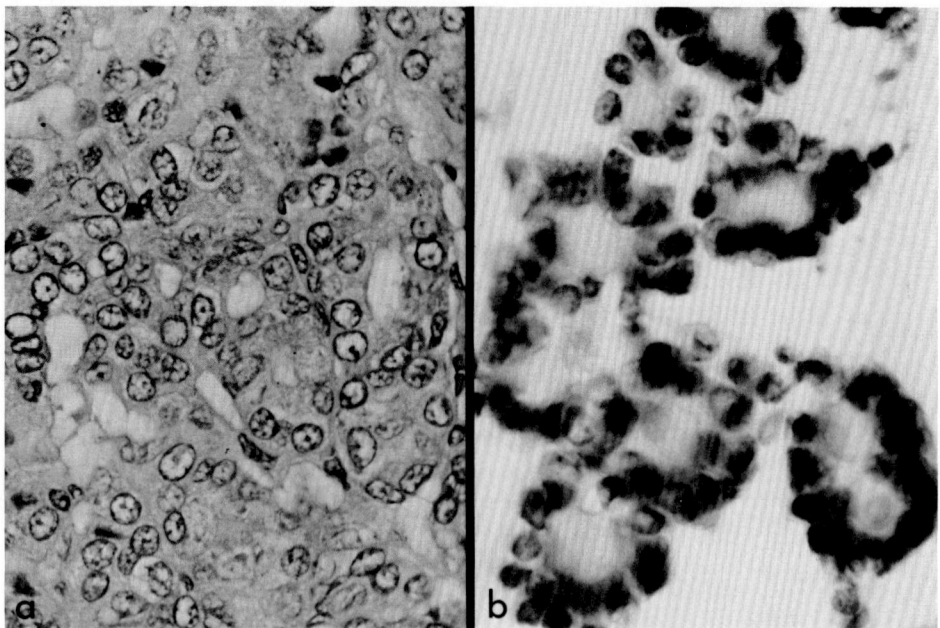

Fig. 8.30. A. Follicular variant of papillary carcinoma. Hematoxylin and eosin preparation. × 400. **B.** Aspirate with follicular pattern. The nuclei show typical morphology of papillary carcinoma. Papanicolaou preparation. × 630.

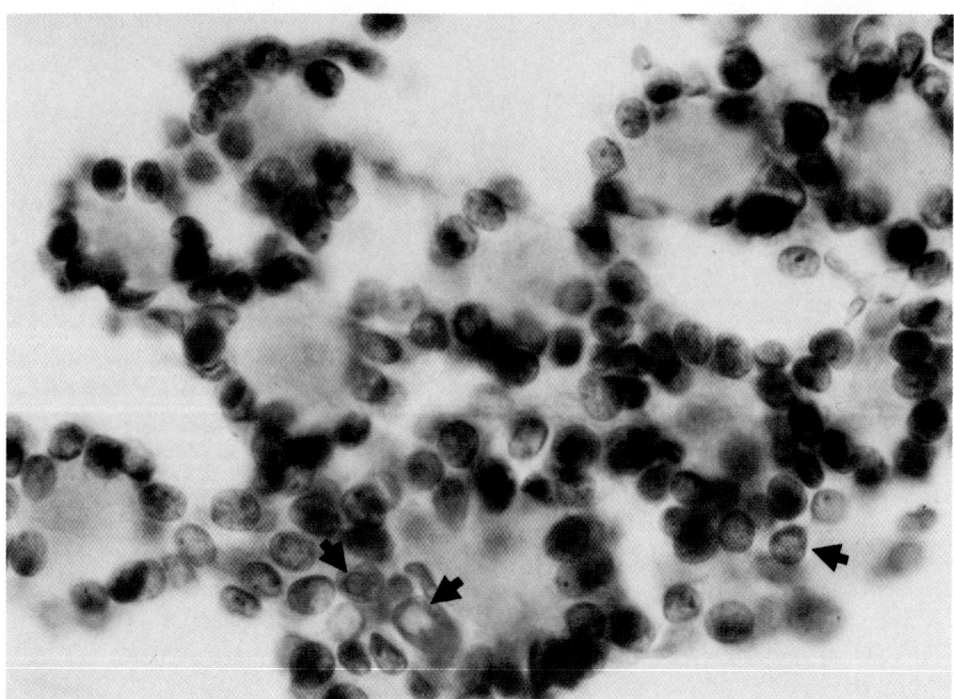

Fig. 8.31. A striking example of follicular variant of papillary carcinoma. The nuclei have powdery chromatin and cytoplasmic inclusions *(arrows)*. The colloid within the follicles is quite dense. Papanicolaou preparation. × 630.

144

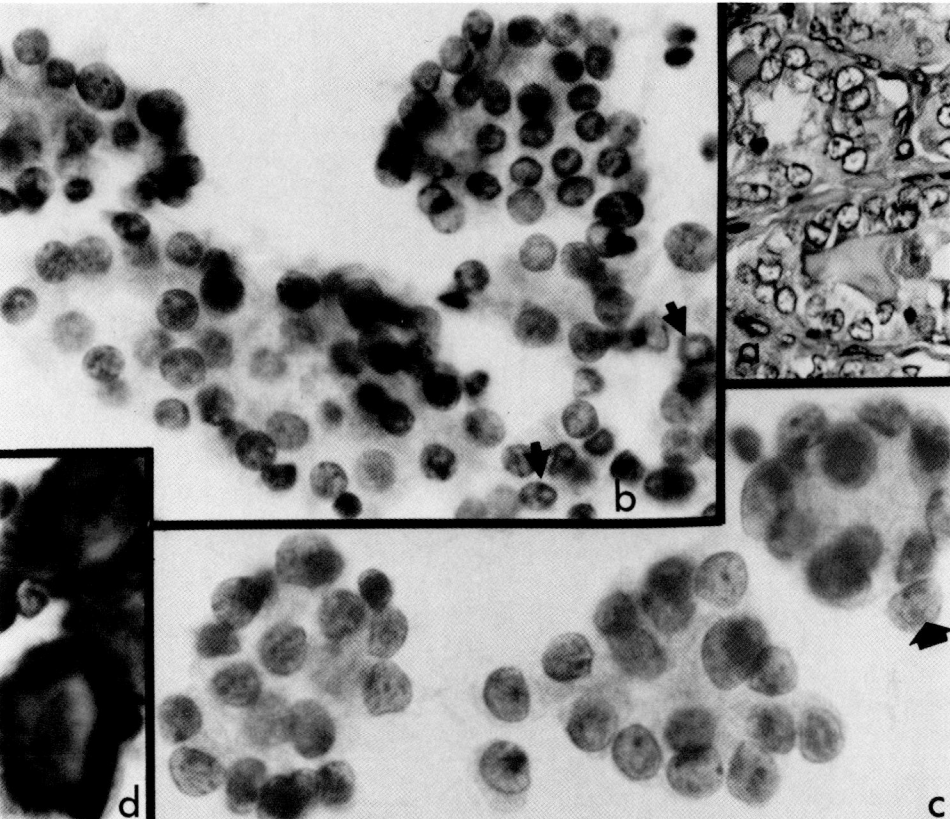

Fig. 8.32. A. Follicular variant of papillary carcinoma. Hematoxylin and eosin preparation. × 400. **B., C.** Syncytial-type tissue fragments with follicular pattern. The nuclei have powdery chromatin and cytoplasmic inclusions *(arrows)*. Papanicolaou preparation. × 630. **D.** Presence of psammoma bodies is not essential for a diagnosis of papillary carcinoma, but is helpful. Papanicolaou preparation. × 630.

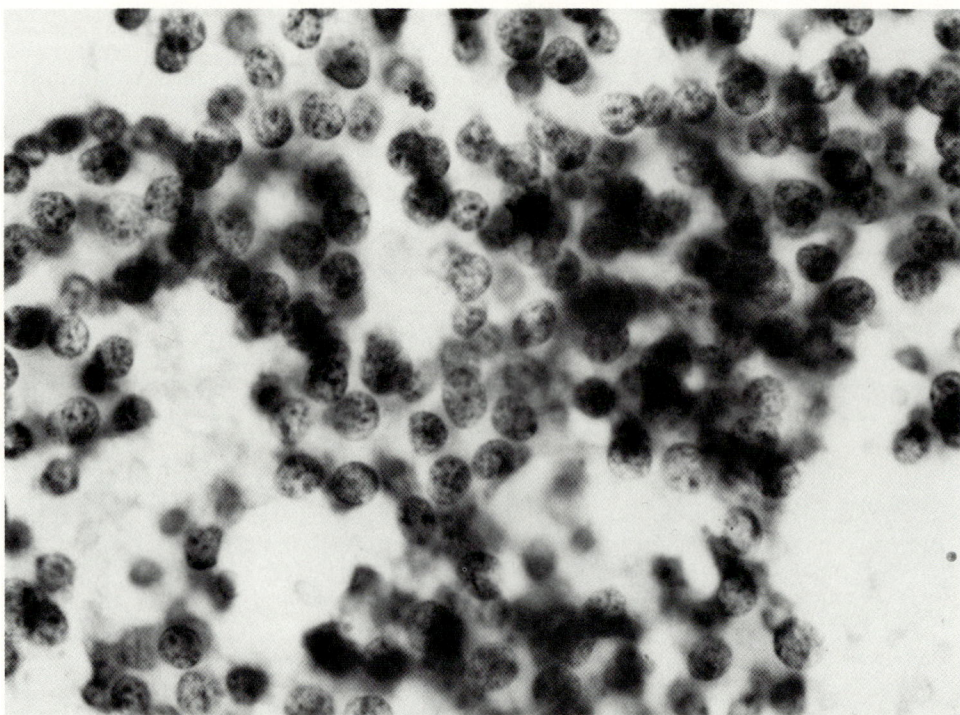

Fig. 8.33. Follicular variant of papillary carcinoma. Note syncytial-type tissue fragments with follicular pattern. The nuclei have coarse chromatin. This pattern is likely to be typed as follicular carcinoma. Papanicolaou preparation. × 630.

Cystic Papillary Carcinoma

The aspirates from cystic papillary carcinomas (Figs. 8.34–8.38; Plate 8.4) are often difficult to interpret for several reasons:

1. The specimens are frequently poorly cellular and, thus, are inadequate for interpretation. The low cellularity may be the result of failure of the needle to penetrate the thick, fibrous, and often calcified capsule that is found in cystic carcinomas. The long-standing cystic carcinomas may not contain much cellular material in the cystic cavity, and the aspirated fluid may be thin, watery, and low in cellularity. If these specimens are not properly processed to salvage the scanty cellular material, the diagnosis may be missed, and the incidence of false-negative diagnoses could be high.[26,36]

2. The cellular and inflammatory debris resulting from hemorrhage and necrosis obscure the cytomorphology of neoplastic cells. Interpretation of scanty cellular material in the background of extensive cellular debris can be very challenging.

3. Retrogressive changes initiated in the fluid medium can mask the diagnostic criteria of cancer cells (see Chapter 14, Cysts of Thyroid). If the scanty cellular material shows follicular epithelium with atypical changes suggestive of papillary carcinoma, repeat aspiration biopsy is needed to confirm the diagnosis.

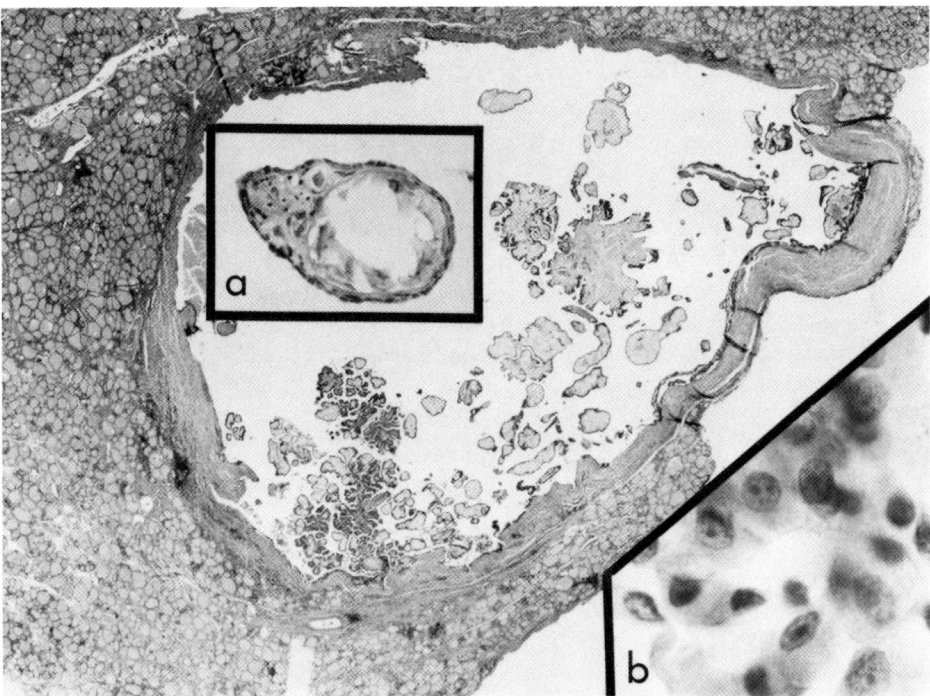

Fig. 8.34. Cystic papillary carcinoma with a thick, fibrous capsule. The cavity is only partially filled with detached papillary fronds having edematous stroma covered by flattened epithelium. Hematoxylin and eosin preparation. × 40. *Inset a:* Detached papillary frond. Hematoxylin and eosin preparation. × 160. *Inset b:* Exfoliated carcinoma cells with foamy cytoplasm display insufficient criteria for a diagnosis of papillary carcinoma. Papanicolaou preparation. × 630.

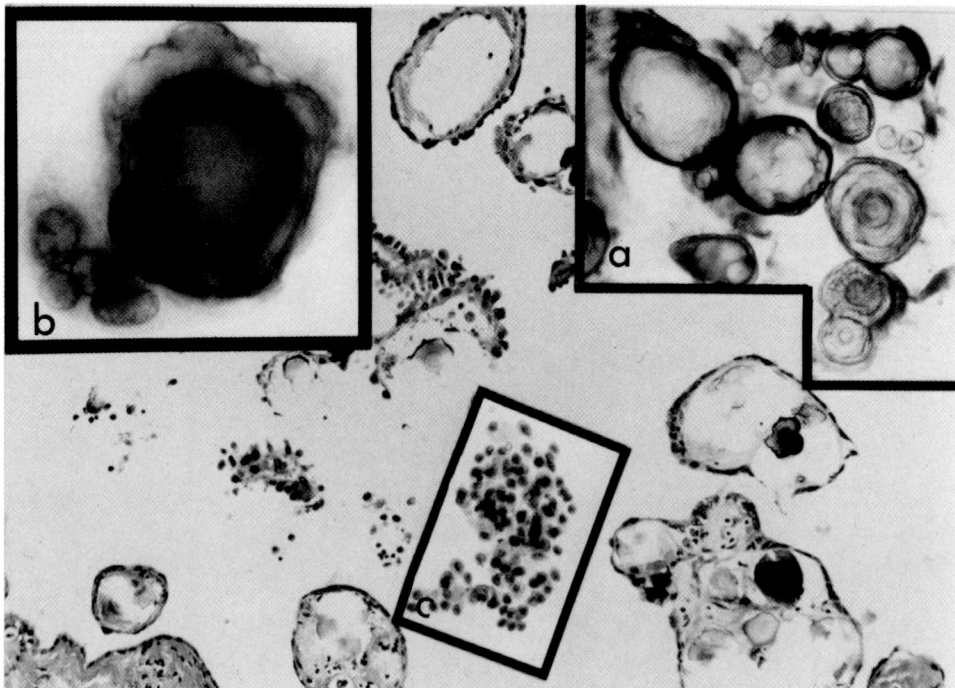

Fig. 8.35. Contents of a cystic papillary carcinoma may be scanty, with very few papillary tissue fragments and insufficient diagnostic criteria. *Inset a:* "Naked" psammoma bodies. Papanicolaou preparation. × 630. *Inset b:* Psammoma body surrounded by very few cells. The nuclear morphology suggests papillary carcinoma. Papanicolaou preparation. × 630. *Inset c:* Papillary carcinoma cells in a cystic environment are often degenerated. Papanicolaou preparation. × 160.

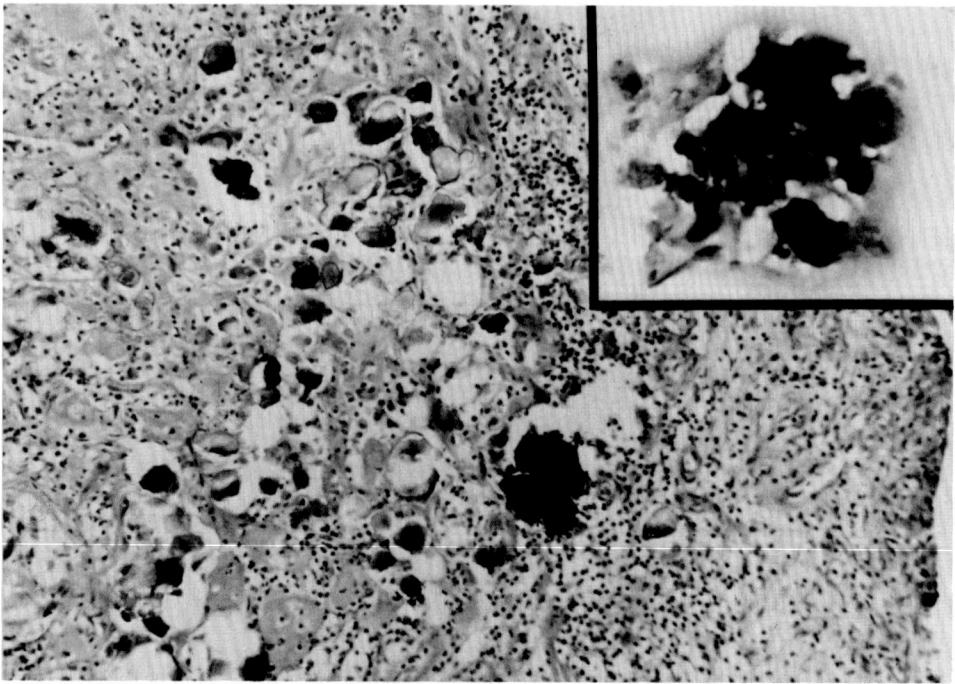

Fig. 8.36. Contents of cystic papillary carcinoma may be hemorrhagic with inflammatory, cellular, and calcific debris, as well as psammoma bodies. Hematoxylin and eosin preparation. × 160. *Inset:* "Naked" psammoma bodies aspirated from such a lesion are difficult to interpret. Papanicolaou preparation. × 630.

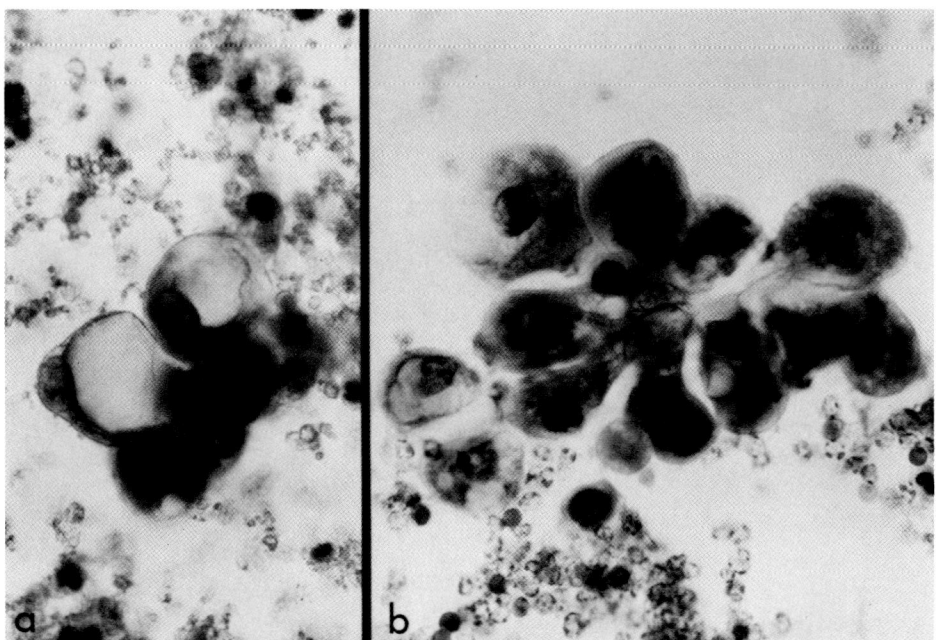

Fig. 8.37. A., B. Cystic papillary carcinoma. These carcinoma cells in the background of cellular debris show cytoplasmic vacuoles. The nuclei are obscured and difficult to evaluate. Papanicolaou preparation. × 630.

Papillary Carcinoma With Single Cell Pattern in Aspirates

A cytologic diagnosis of papillary carcinoma is easily and accurately made because of the architectural pattern of tissue fragments and the typical cytomorphology of component cells (Fig. 8.39). Indeed, most papillary carcinomas yield tissue fragments on needle biopsy. On rare occasions, perhaps due to less differentiation of the carcinoma, the aspirate may show a large population of discrete cells, either monomorphic or pleomorphic, without other diagnostic features of papillary carcinoma. Such an aspirate may be typed as medullary carcinoma because of the morphologic similarity of its cells, eg, cuboidal, short columnar, or oval cells; eccentric nuclei; and intranuclear cytoplasmic inclusions. An occasional syncytial-type tissue fragment does not help in typing the lesion, and other diagnostic modalities are necessary to confirm the diagnosis (see Chapter 10, Medullary Carcinoma).

Inadequate Specimen

An inadequate specimen (Fig. 8.40) with insufficient cytologic criteria is always a diagnostic problem. There are many reasons for obtaining an inadequate needle-biopsy specimen (see Chapter 3, Table 3.1). Experience is the only guide for suspecting papillary carcinoma on marginal cellularity. Repeat biopsy is recommended to confirm the diagnosis.

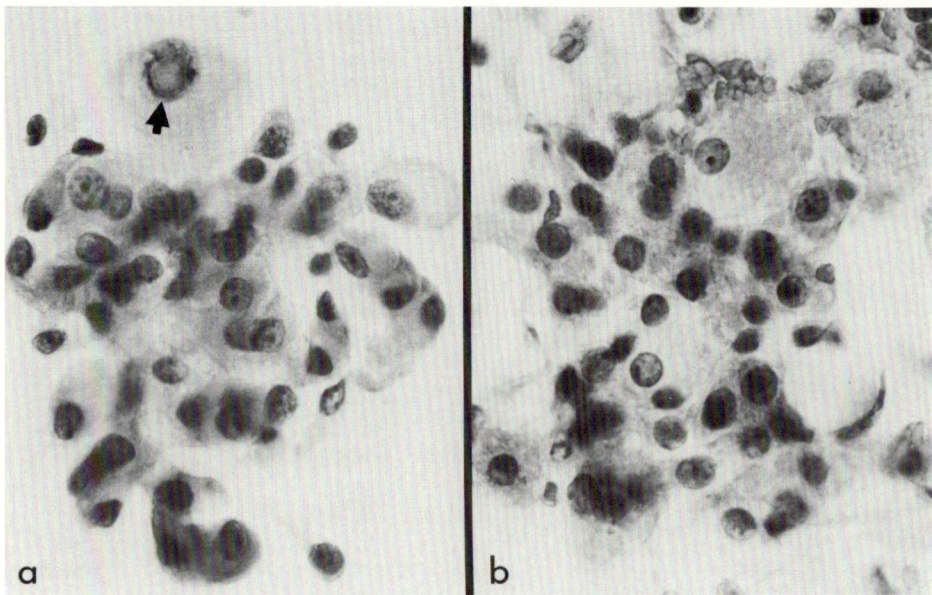

Fig. 8.38. A. Carcinoma cells from cystic papillary carcinoma. The nuclear details are poor. Except for an intranuclear inclusion *(arrow)*, these cells resemble degenerating follicular cells in nodular goiter. Papanicolaou preparation. × 630. **B.** Degenerating follicular cells in nodular goiter. Papanicolaou preparation. × 630.

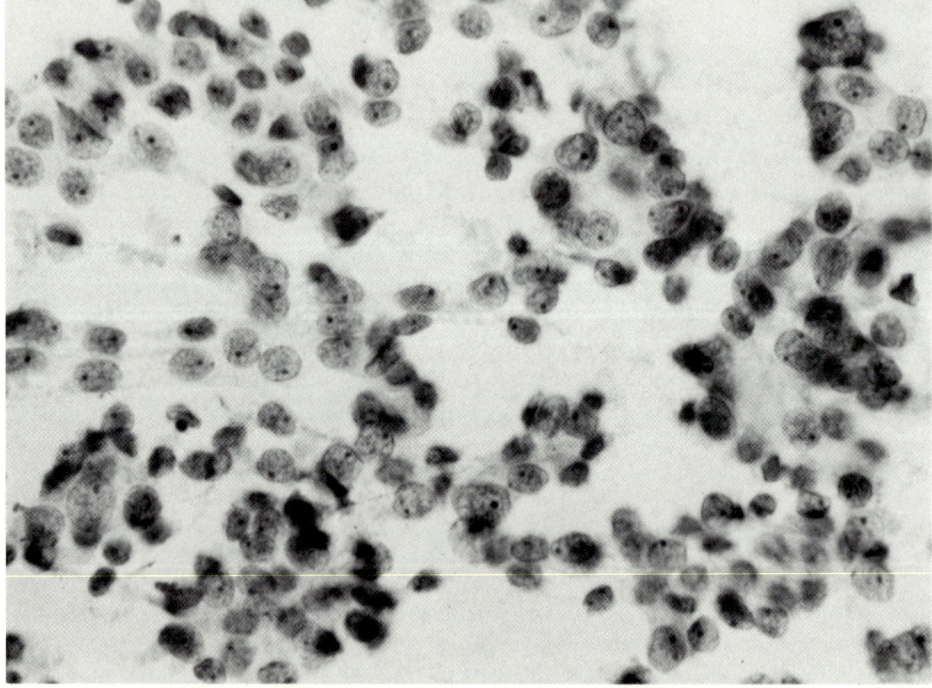

Fig. 8.39. Papillary carcinoma with single cell pattern. The nuclear chromatin is finely granular. This pattern may be mistaken for medullary thyroid carcinoma. Papanicolaou preparation. × 630.

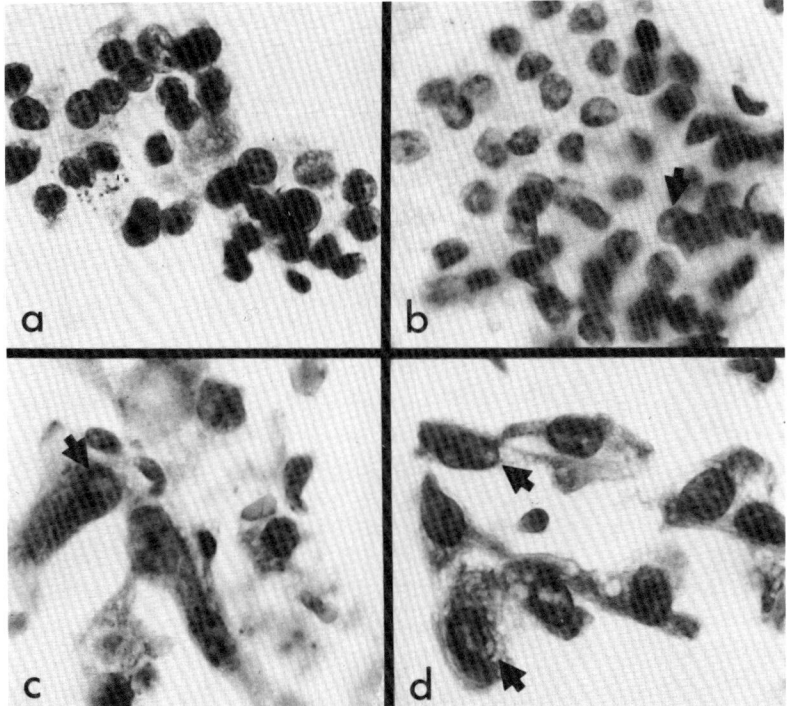

Fig. 8.40. The only cellular material aspirated from four papillary carcinomas. Experience is necessary to appreciate the minimal atypia presented by these cells. **A.** Note syncytial-type tissue fragments with enlarged nuclei and nucleoli. **B.** Powdery chromatin and intranuclear inclusions *(arrow)*. **C., D.** Intranuclear inclusions *(arrow)*. A diagnosis of papillary carcinoma is only suggested. Papanicolaou preparation. × 630.

DIAGNOSTIC ACCURACY

The diagnostic accuracy of papillary carcinoma should approach 90–94% (Table 8.3), provided the aspirate obtained by fine-needle biopsy is adequate for cytologic interpretation.

TABLE 8.3. Cytologic Diagnosis of 349 Papillary Carcinomas

Papillary carcinoma including follicular variant	303*
Suspected papillary carcinoma	18
Medullary carcinoma	2
Cellular adenoma	13
Benign	4[†]
Unsatisfactory (acellular, bloody)	9
Total	349

*Two cases were initially benign (lymphocytic thyroiditis). However, on repeat biopsy, papillary carcinoma was the diagnosis. Sampling error was the reason for the discrepancy.

[†]Four cases of nodular goiter (see Table 8.4).

Errors in cytologic diagnosis of papillary carcinoma can be grouped into three categories: (1) false-negative results; (2) false-positive results; and (3) typing errors (Figs. 8.41–8.51).

False-Negative Results

The cytologic diagnosis of papillary carcinoma may be missed only if the specimen is acellular; poorly cellular, demonstrating insufficient diagnostic criteria; or if there is a sampling error (Tables 8.3 and 8.4).

Acellular aspirates or a poor cellular yield on a fine-needle biopsy are inevitable in some instances, eg, large cystic papillary carcinoma, marked desmoplasia, or a thick fibrous, calcified capsule.

Three false-negative cases of papillary carcinoma in our series reflect a combination of poorly cellular specimens and inexperience in recognizing the minimal cytologic atypia as possibly indicative of papillary carcinoma. In one case of papillary carcinoma in which repeated attempts at fine-needle biopsy were made—including one on a "residual" palpable mass—only histiocytes were found. A large-needle biopsy on the residual mass confirmed the diagnosis. Of 349 papillary carcinomas, 9 were acellular on fine-needle biopsy (2.5%). If fine-needle biopsies on large nodules are unsuccessful and there are strong clinical suggestions of carcinoma, a cutting-needle biopsy is recommended.

A false-negative diagnosis may also occur as a result of sampling error. Two of our cases were initially and correctly diagnosed as lymphocytic thyroiditis. One year later, repeat biopsy on both cases showed all the criteria of papillary carcinoma coexistent with lymphocytic thyroiditis. The initial biopsies had sampled the parenchyma adjacent to the carcinoma. For this reason, a few unremarkable follicular cells aspirated from a thyroid containing a large nodule should not be considered adequate and benign.

False-Positive Results

False-positive diagnoses (Table 8.5) involve misinterpretation of aspirates from benign non-neoplastic diseases of the thyroid as malignant neoplasms when they superficially mimic some cytologic criteria of papillary carcinoma. The same problem is faced with cellular aspirates from a follicular adenoma, especially with degeneration and pseudopapillary change. Most often, the errors are made if too much emphasis is placed on just one cytologic feature, especially when the aspirate is overwhelmingly cellular. Of 316 cytologic diagnoses of papillary carcinoma, 11 were false-positive diagnoses (Table 8.6 and 8.7).

A diagnosis of suspected papillary carcinoma is generally given when:

1. The aspirate is marginally cellular and exhibits atypical features suggestive, but not diagnostic, of papillary carcinoma.
2. The aspirate is adequately cellular, with features of a benign disease (nodular goiter, Hashimoto's thyroiditis, follicular adenoma); but, in addition, shows a few follicular cells with atypia (Table 8.5). The features that may be mistaken for papillary carcinoma are: (a) tissue fragments of spindle cells forming a whorled pattern, with atypical nuclei; (b) an occasional monolayered tissue fragment of follicular cells, with abundant dense cytoplasm, and large irregular nuclei with

TABLE 8.4. Analysis of 13 False-Negative Diagnoses of Papillary Carcinoma

Patient No.	Cytologic Findings	Comments
1	Cyst fluid; cellular debris, histiocytes, calcospherites	No well-preserved follicular epithelium present; calcospherites, some surrounded by cells obscured by cellular and hemorrhagic debris
2	Few groups of follicular cells	Partially air-dried and scanty specimen; intranuclear inclusions overlooked; *inadequate for diagnosis, but suspicious*
3	Rare group of follicular cells	*Inadequate for diagnosis*; only one group of follicular cells, syncytial arrangement, large nuclei not appreciated due to inexperience
4	Bilateral nodules, aspirated; similar pattern, features of nodular goiter with few tissue fragments showing pale nuclei	Few groups of atypical follicular cells in the background of nodular goiter, generally of no significance; possible reason for negative diagnosis: sampling error
5	Cyst fluid hemorrhagic, only histiocytes	True false-negative diagnosis
6–13	Acellular	True false-negative diagnosis

TABLE 8.5. Circumstances Resulting in a Possible False-Positive Diagnosis of Papillary Carcinoma

1. Scanty specimen with insufficient criteria
2. Cystic nodular goiter
3. Follicular cell atypia in background of nodular goiter
4. Hyperplastic nodular goiter with papillary and monolayered tissue fragments
5. Occasional psammoma body in background of nodular goiter
6. Inspissated colloid simulating psammoma body
7. Papillary hyperplasia in Hashimoto's thyroiditis
8. Follicular hyperplasia with intranuclear cytoplasmic inclusions in Hashimoto's thyroiditis
9. Simple follicular adenoma

TABLE 8.6. Histologic Diagnosis of 316 Cases with Cytologic Diagnosis of Papillary Carcinoma

Papillary carcinoma	303
Medullary carcinoma	2
Follicular adenoma	4
Nodular goiter	4
Hashimoto's thyroiditis	3
Total	316

powdery chromatin and nucleoli; (c) an occasional follicular cell showing intranuclear cytoplasmic inclusions; (d) a rare papillary tissue fragment with crowded nuclei; or (e) a rare psammoma body.

These isolated findings by themselves may be extremely worrisome, but when present in the background of a benign disease, they should be judged with extreme caution.

Of 42 cases of suspected papillary carcinoma, 36 underwent surgery (Table 8.8). Eighteen cases were confirmed. Two were follicular carcinomas and two follicular adenomas, indicating a typing error. Thirteen were benign non-neoplastic diseases of thyroid. Surgery was not recommended for six patients because the cytologic features on repeat biopsy were diagnostic of benign disease. As the diagnostic accuracy of papillary carcinoma is very high with an adequate aspirate, it is advisable to have a definitive diagnosis before surgery. The decision to recommend surgical excision after a cytologic diagnosis of suspicious papillary carcinoma depends on such factors as age and sex of the patient, size of the nodule, lymphadenopathy, history of radiation to head and neck, and unsatisfactory attempts at repeat fine-needle biopsy.

Typing Errors

Typing errors are not as consequential as false-positive results because surgery is recommended for most thyroid neoplasms. Tumors that may be confused with papillary carcinomas are follicular neoplasms—both cellular follicular adenoma and follicular carcinoma—as well as medullary carcinoma. Similarities and differentiating features are discussed in other chapters. The cases where the atypical cytologic features lead us in the interpretative traps are listed in Tables 8.7 and 8.9 and illustrated in Figs. 8.41–8.51.

TABLE 8.7 Analysis of 11 False-Positive Diagnoses of Papillary Carcinoma

Patient No.	Cytologic Findings	Surgery	Comments
1	Single psammoma body; papillary tissue fragments; background features of nodular goiter; repeat fine-needle biopsy: nodular goiter	Total thyroidectomy; nodular goiter with papillary hyperplasia	Diagnosis of papillary carcinoma based on single psammoma body, architectural pattern (papillary) of the tissue fragment; cells lacked typical cytomorphology of papillary carcinoma
2	Single psammoma body; rare group of atypical follicular cells; several monolayered tissue fragments of follicular epithelium with honeycomb pattern (Fig. 8.41)	Total thyroidectomy; multiple follicular adenomas	Tissue fragment containing psammoma body lacked typical cytomorphology of papillary carcinoma; other features of papillary carcinoma not present; tissue fragments of follicular epithelium suggested diagnosis of nodular goiter
3	Cyst fluid; hemorrhagic, large papillary tissue fragments; psammoma bodies	Total thyroidectomy; Hürthle cell adenoma with cystic degeneration	Cytomorphology altered by the hemorrhage; psammoma bodies were atypical, perhaps colloid
4	Multiple psammoma bodies	Total thyroidectomy; multiple follicular adenomas	Inspissated colloid within follicles simulated psammoma bodies
5	Hypercellular aspirate, large numbers of monolayered sheets of follicular epithelium	Right lobectomy; simple adenoma	Emphasis on cellularity and architectural pattern of tissue fragments without cytomorphology of papillary carcinoma
6	Hypercellular aspirate, papillary tissue fragments	Total thyroidectomy; diffuse hyperplasia	Emphasis on cellularity and architectural pattern; cytomorphology of papillary carcinoma lacking
7	Extremely cellular aspirate; branching papillary tissue fragments; crowded nuclei with nucleoli	Total thyroidectomy; follicular adenoma with atypical papillary change	Papillary fragments; crowded nuclei with nucleoli, chromatin not powdery; intranuclear inclusions and chromatin ridge

TABLE 8.7. Continued

Patient No.	Cytologic Findings	Surgery	Comments
			Absent; other features of papillary carcinoma not present; specimens from other areas of nodule showed features of nodular goiter
8	Papillary tissue fragments with powdery chromatin (Fig. 8.43)	Total thyroidectomy: nodular goiter with papillary hyperplasia, one focus of atypical hyperplasia	Marginal cellularity, partial air-drying with suboptimal cytomorphology; insufficient criteria for diagnosis of papillary carcinoma
9	Syncytial-type tissue fragments; enlarged crowded nuclei with nucleoli; chromatin finely granular; features of lymphocytic thyroiditis; history of lobectomy for papillary carcinoma (Fig. 8.51)	Lobectomy: Hashimoto's thyroditis	Insufficient criteria for diagnosis of papillary carcinoma; history of carcinoma influenced the diagnosis
10	Features of lymphocytic thyroiditis; occasional papillary fragment of follicular epithelium (Fig. 8.66)	Total thyroidectomy: Hashimoto's thyroiditis with papillary hyperplasia	Typical nuclear cytomorphology absent
11	Features of lymphocytic thyroiditis; occasional papillary fragment of follicular epithelium	Total thyroidectomy: Hashimoto's thyroiditis with papillary hyperplasia	Typical nuclear cytomorphology absent

TABLE 8.8. Histologic Diagnosis of 36 Cases Cytologically
Suspected of Papillary Carcinoma

Papillary carcinoma	18
Follicular carcinoma	2
Follicular adenoma	3
Nodular goiter	11
Hashimoto's thyroiditis	2
Total	36

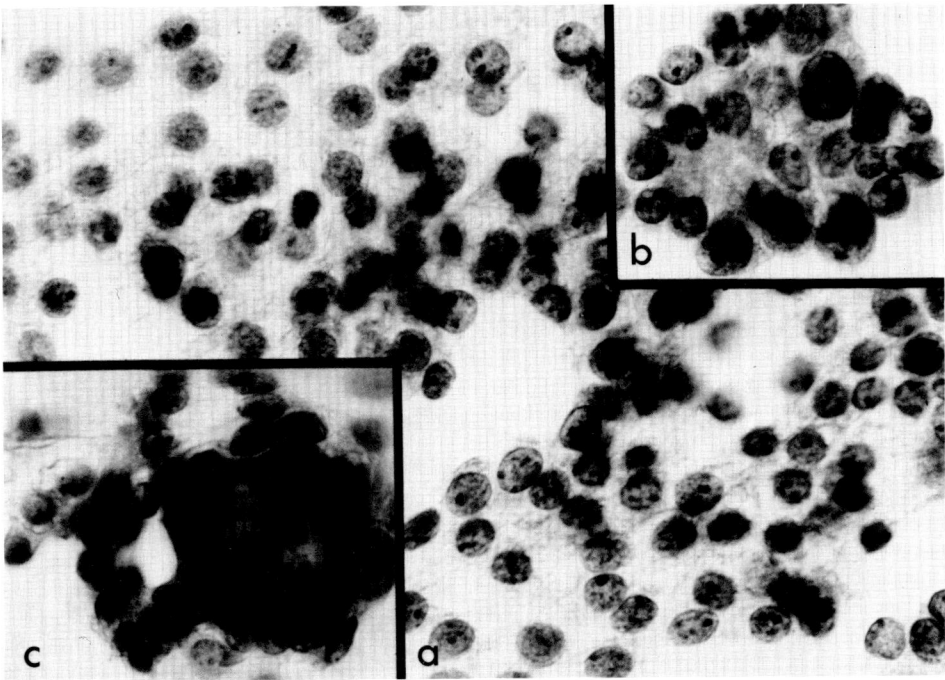

Fig. 8.41. This aspirate was diagnosed cytologically as papillary carcinoma (see Table 8.7, case 2). **A.**, **B.** Moderately enlarged nuclei, with finely granular chromatin and nucleoli. Papanicolaou preparation. × 630. **C.** Even a psammoma body is present. Papanicolaou preparation. × 630. Thyroidectomy showed nodular goiter with psammoma bodies.

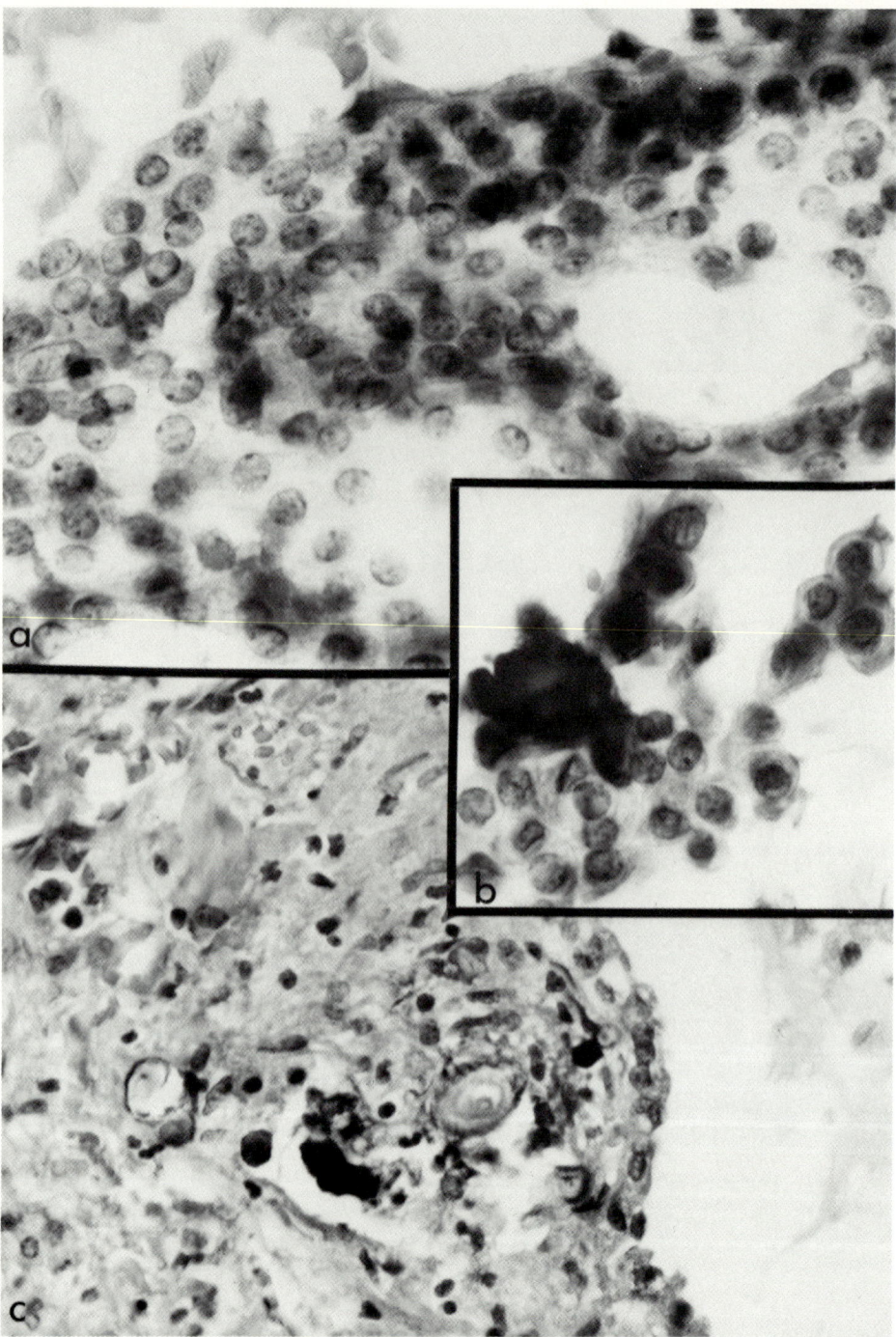

Fig. 8.42. This aspirate was interpreted as suspicious for papillary carcinoma. **A.** Mono-layered tissue fragment. Because of folding, it appears to be syncytial. The nuclei show only modest enlargement, with finely granular chromatin. Nucleoli are present. Papanicolaou preparation. × 630. **B.** Single psammoma body. The cytomorphology of surrounding cells is suggestive of papillary carcinoma, but not diagnostic. Papanicolaou preparation. × 630. **C.** Thyroidectomy showed a follicular adenoma with psammoma bodies in the stroma (see Table 8.9, case 11). Hematoxylin and eosin preparation. × 400.

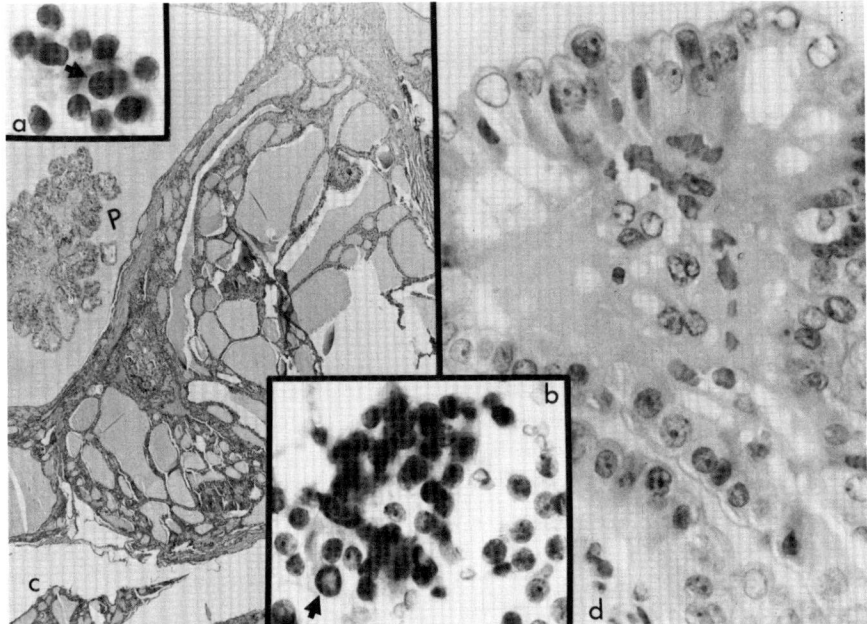

Fig. 8.43. Marginally cellular aspirate interpreted as papillary carcinoma (see Table 8.7, case 8) because of features shown in **A** and **B**. **A.** Finely granular chromatin. Papanicolaou preparation. × 630. **B.** Possible intraranuclear cytoplasmic inclusions *(arrow)*. Papanicolaou preparation. × 630. Thyroidectomy showed a nodular goiter with papillary hyperplasia. **C.** Note a branching papillary tissue fragment *(p)* floating in a dilated follicle. Hematoxylin and eosin preparation. × 63. **D.** Higher magnification showing very atypical nuclei, some with clear chromatin pattern of papillary carcinoma. Hematoxylin and eosin preparation. × 630.

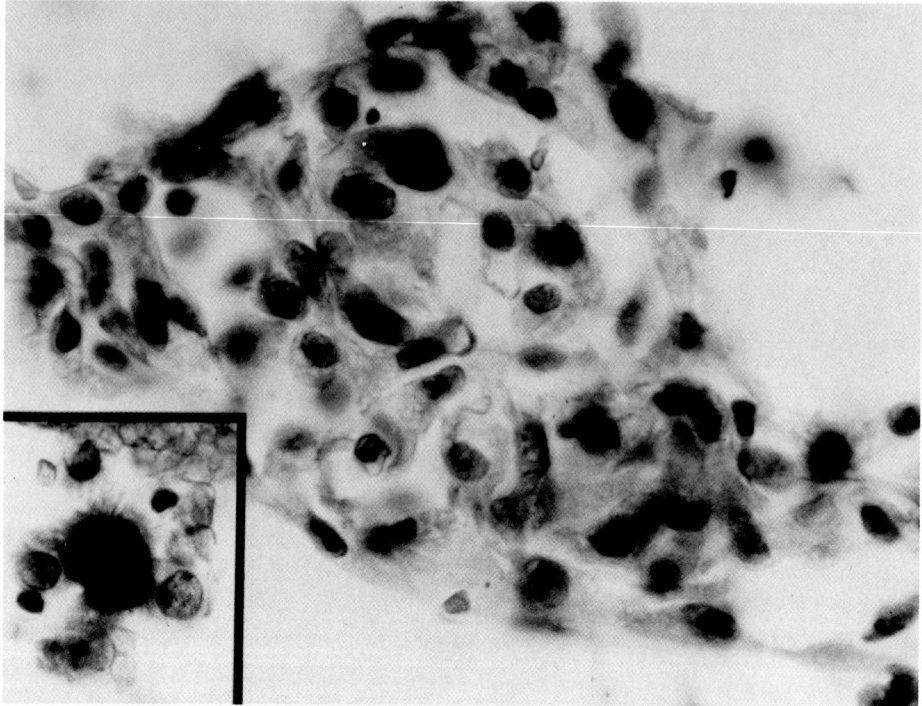

Fig. 8.44. Group of atypical follicular cells. Papanicolaou preparation. × 630. *Inset:* Psammoma body. The nuclei do not have typical morphology of papillary carcinoma. Papanicolaou preparation. × 630. The background features were consistent with nodular goiter. Thyroidectomy did not confirm papillary carcinoma (see Table 8.9, case 9).

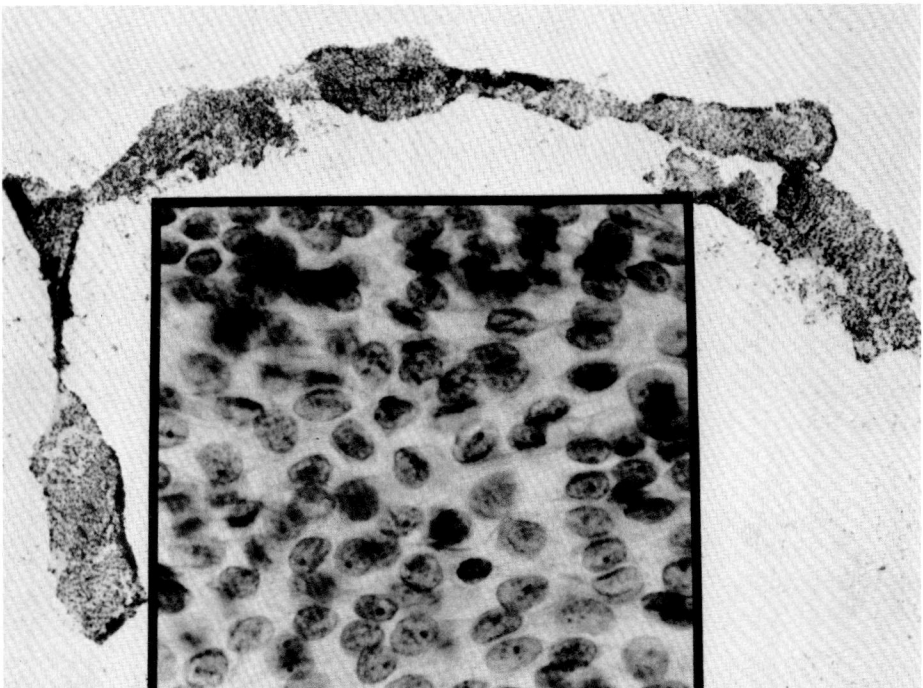

Fig. 8.45. This aspirate was cytologically suspected of papillary carcinoma. Most of the aspirated material was diagnostic of nodular goiter, except for a large syncytial-type tissue fragment. Papanicolaou preparation. × 160. *Inset:* Nuclei with powdery chromatin and nucleoli. Papanicolaou preparation. × 630.

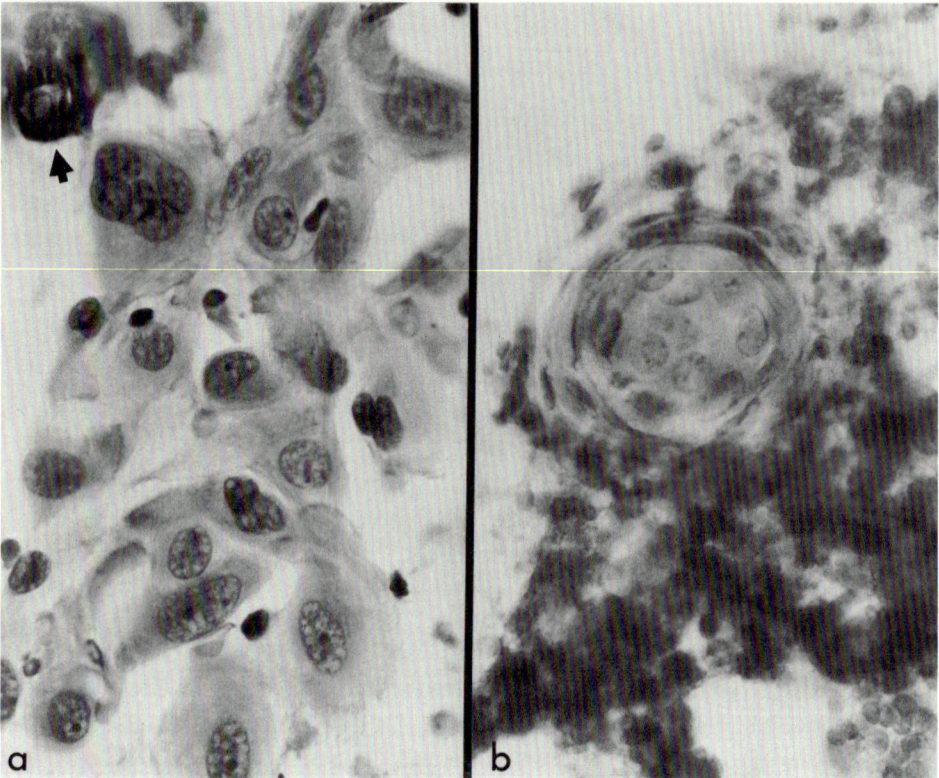

Fig. 8.46. A. From the aspirate shown in Fig. 8.45, a group of large cells with pleomorphic nuclei, dense cytoplasm, and possible psammoma body *(arrow)*. Papanicolaou preparation. × 630. **B.** From the aspirate shown in Fig. 8.45, squamous metaplasia. Papanicolaou preparation. × 630. Thyroidectomy showed papillary hyperplasia in an adenoma (see Table 8.9, case 4).

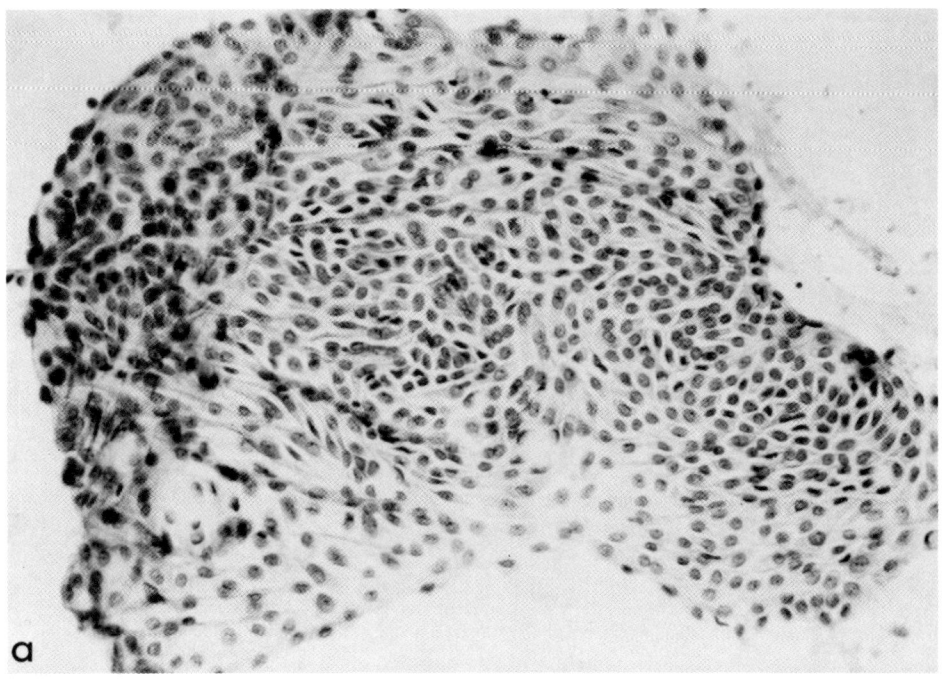

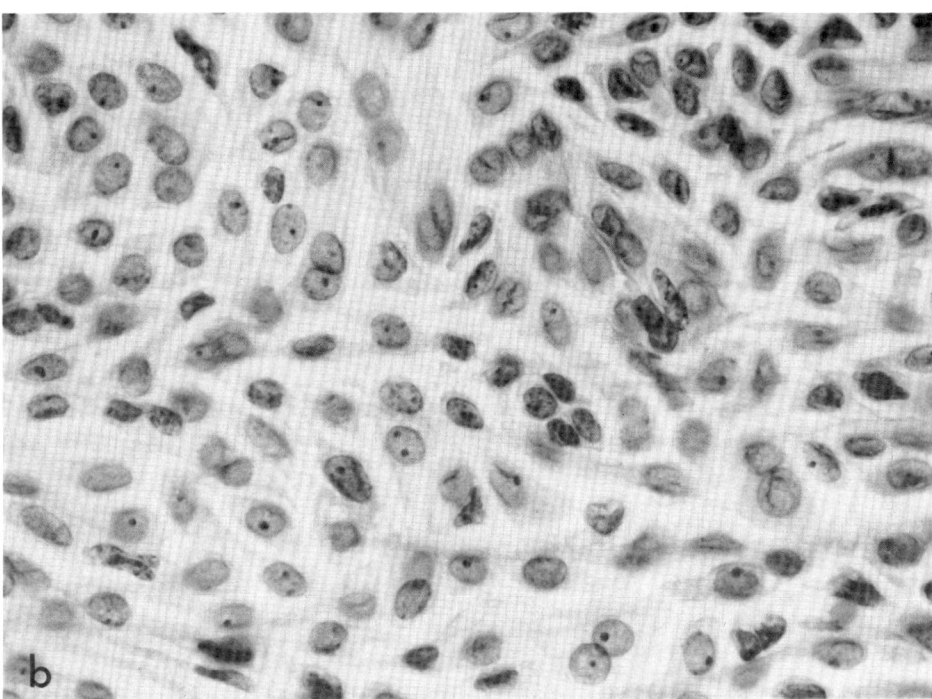

Fig. 8.47. **A.** A tissue fragment of spindle cells in the background of nodular goiter (not shown). Papanicolaou preparation. × 160. **B.** Higher magnification of **A** showing enlarged nuclei with powdery chromatin, nucleoli, and nuclear ridge. Papanicolaou preparation. × 630. The features are highly suggestive of papillary carcinoma. Thyroidectomy did not confirm the diagnosis of papillary carcinoma (see Table 8.9, case 8)

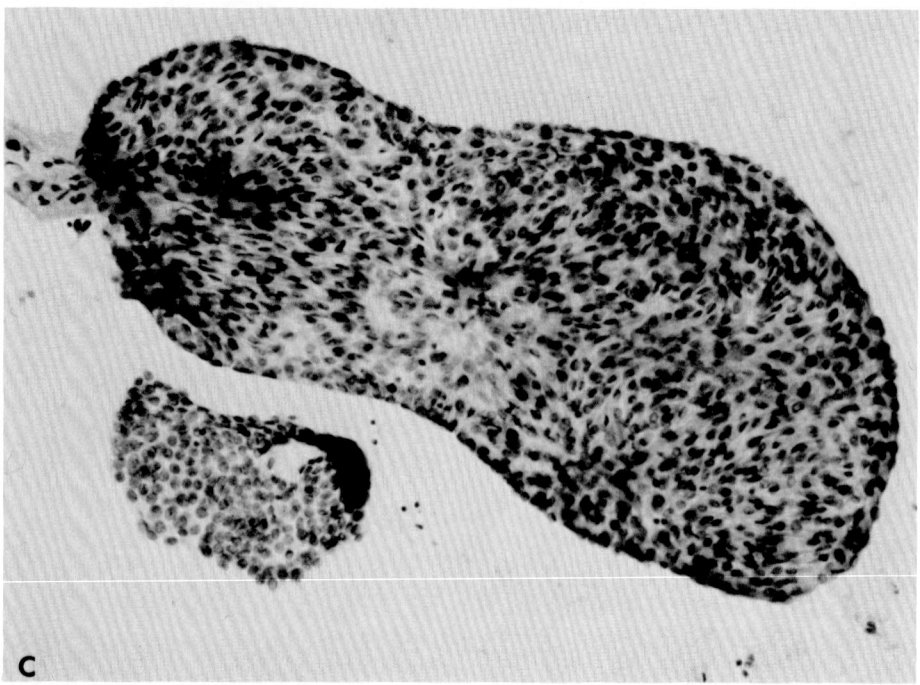

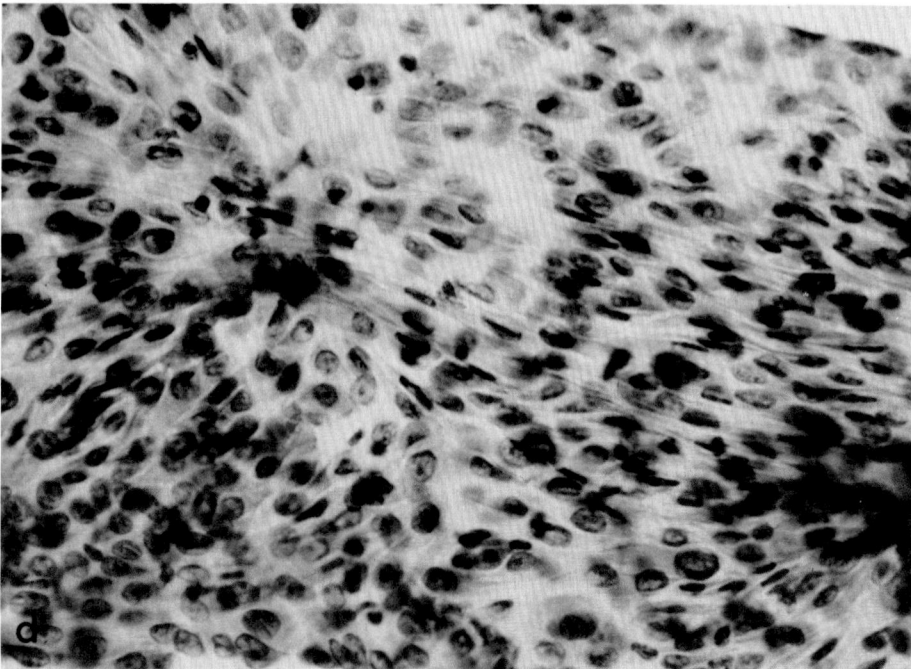

Fig. 8.47. C. Tissue fragment of spindle cells from papillary carcinoma. Papanicolaou preparation. × 160. D. Higher magnification of C showing cells with morphology indistinguishable from that seen in B. Papanicolaou preparation. × 630.

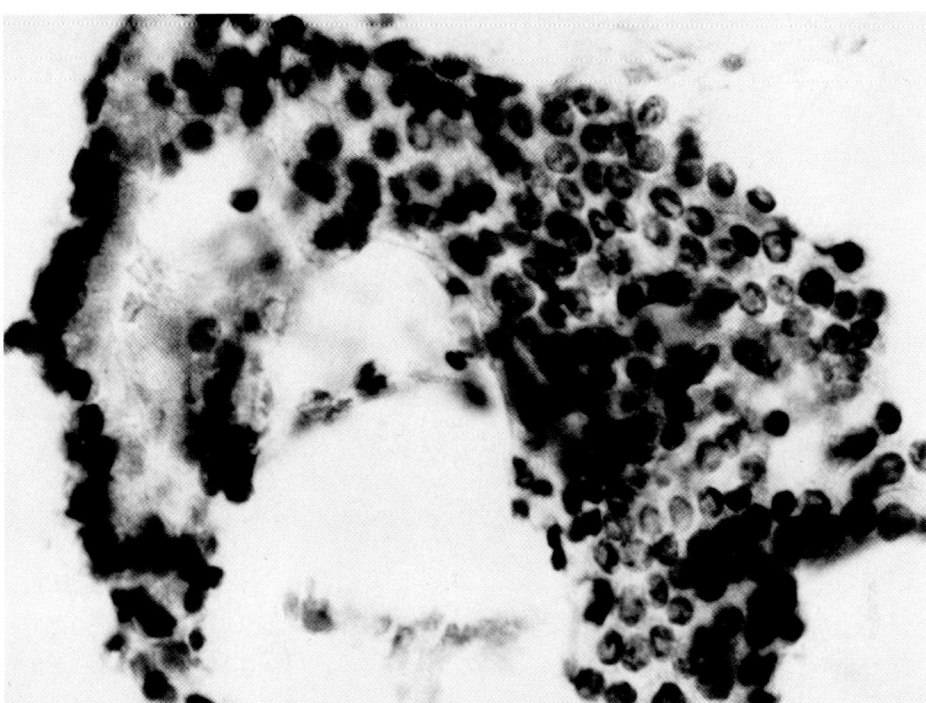

Fig. 8.48. This papillary tissue fragment in the background of lymphocytic thyroiditis suggested the possibility of papillary carcinoma. Note that typical nuclear morphology is not present (see Table 8.9, case 14). Papanicolaou preparation. × 630.

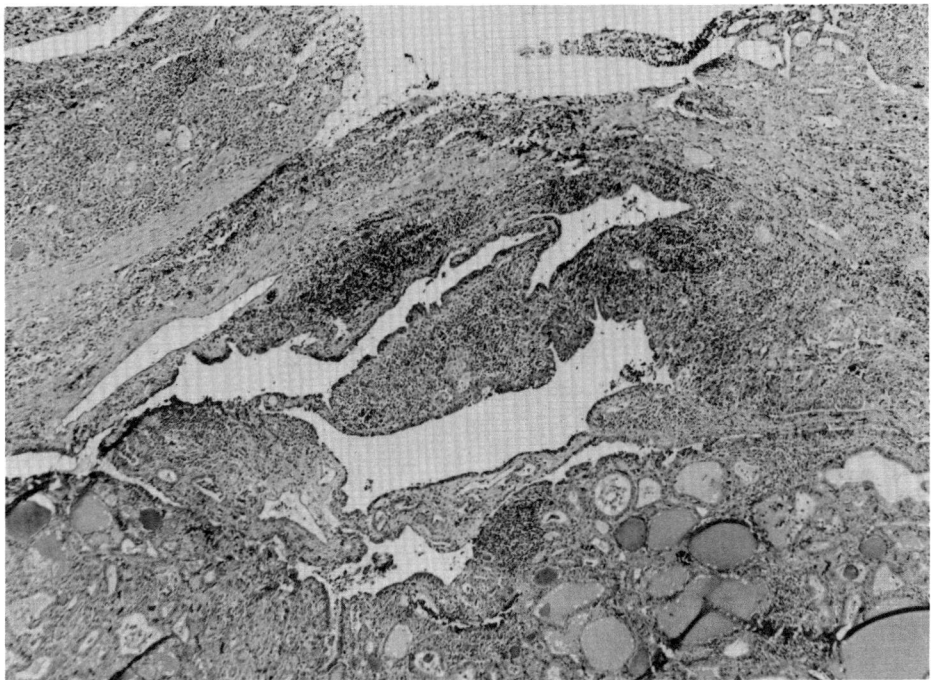

Fig. 8.49. Thyroidectomy showed Hashimoto's thyroiditis and papillary hyperplasia. Hematoxylin and eosin preparation. × 63.

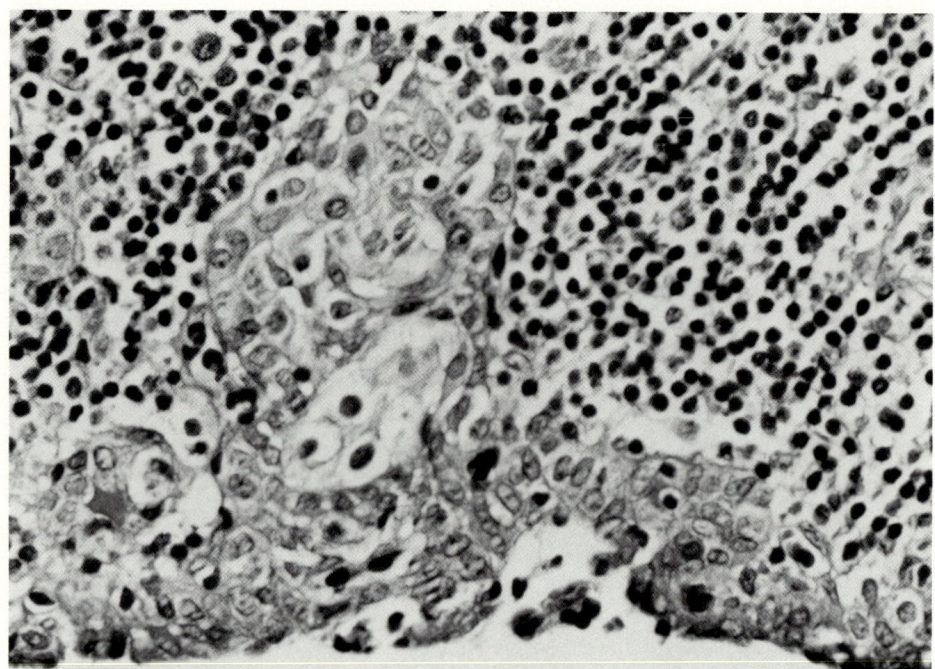

Fig. 8.50. Higher magnification of specimen shown in Fig. 8.49 showing papillary hyperplasia, explaining the cytologic presentation. Hematoxylin and eosin preparation. × 400.

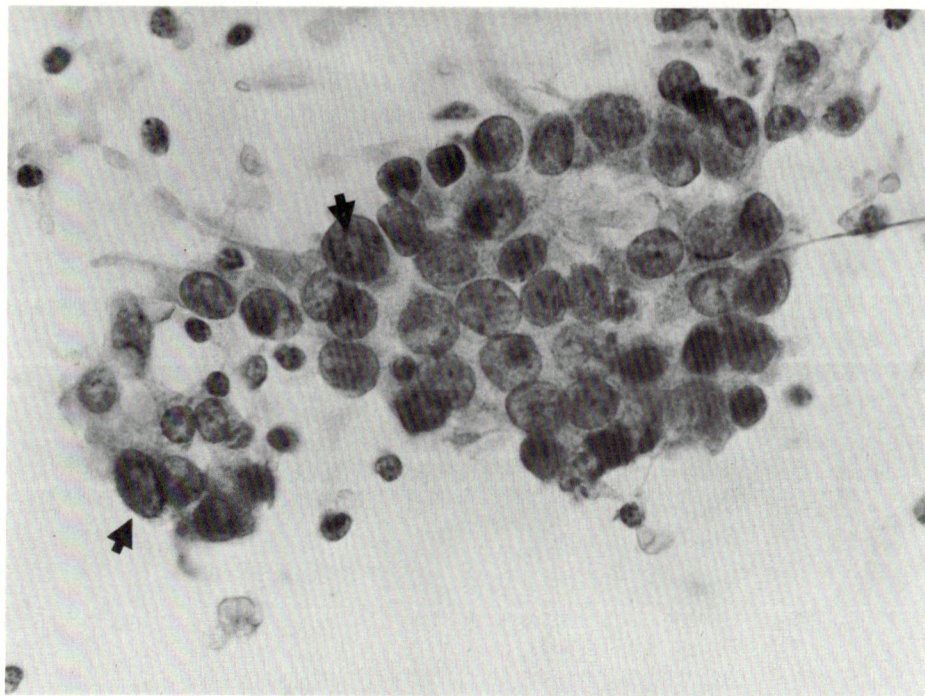

Fig. 8.51. This syncytial-type tissue fragment shows large nuclei with powdery chromatin and nucleoli. There is only a suggestion of intranuclear inclusion *(arrow)*. Lymphocytes are present in the background. A diagnosis of papillary carcinoma was not confirmed histologically in this patient, who had a history of papillary carcinoma (see Table 8.7, case 9). Papanicolaou preparation. × 630.

TABLE 8.9. Critical Analysis of 16 Cases Cytologically Suspected of Papillary Carcinoma with Histologic Diagnoses of Benign Disease Following Surgery

Patient No.	Cytologic Findings	Surgery	Comments
1	Hypercellular aspirate; large monolayered sheets of follicular epithelium; occasional papillary pattern; multiple micronucleoli	Nodular goiter with infarct	Emphasis on hypercellularity as well as architectural pattern; lacked typical cytomorphology of papillary carcinoma
2	Features of nodular goiter; few groups of atypical follicular cells with large nuclei and multiple nucleoli	Nodular goiter	Few groups of atypical cells in background of nodular goiter, generally of no significance; misinterpretation due to inexperience
3	Cyst fluid; histiocytes and tissue fragments of follicular epithelium with foamy cytoplasm, enlarged nuclei, and nucleoli	Nodular goiter with cyst	Degenerative changes in epithelium from cyst fluid mimicking neoplasia; important diagnostic pitfall
4	One group of pleomorphic cells with atypical nuclei; one psammoma body; one very large monolayered sheet of follicular epithelium; nucleoli present (Fig. 8.46)	Nodular goiter	Marginal cellularity; cytomorphology of papillary carcinoma not present
5	Hypercellular aspirate; large number of monolayered sheets of follicular epithelium	Simple adenoma	Emphasis on only one criterion, ie, monolayered sheets; typical nuclear morphology of papillary carcinoma absent
6	Hypercellular aspirate; large number of monolayered sheets of follicular epithelium	Simple adenoma	Emphasis on only one criterion, ie, monolayered sheets; typical nuclear morphology of papillary carcinoma absent
7	Occasional papillary tissue fragment(?)psammoma body	Simple adenoma	Pseudopsammoma body (inspissated colloid simulating psammoma body)
8	Few tissue fragments of atypical cells; spindle forms; nucleoli; swirling arrangement suggesting papillary configuraton; background of nodular goiter (Fig. 8.47)	Hyperplastic goiter	Adequate aspirate with features of nodular goiter; only few tissue fragments of atypical cytomorphology; nuclei did not show cytoplasmic inclusions; mostly coarse chromatin

TABLE 8.9. Continued

Patient No.	Cytologic Findings	Surgery	Comments
9	Few tissue fragments of atypical follicular epithelium; two psammoma bodies; many histiocytes and giant cells (Fig. 8.44)	Nodular goiter	Psammoma bodies not surrounded by cells that exhibit typical cytomorphology of papillary carcinoma; features of papillary carcinoma not present
10	Cystic hemorrhage with cellular debris; few fragments of follicular epithelium; vacuolated cytoplasm (Fig. 8.42)	Nodular goiter	Poorly cellular specimen; nuclear cytomorphology not seen; degenerated follicular cells with nuclear atypia
11	Psammoma bodies and features of nodular goiter	Hyperplastic goiter with single psammoma	True psammoma body, but lacked nuclear features of papillary carcinoma
12	Psammoma body; few groups of atypical cells; occasional monolayered tissue fragments	Nodular goiter	Marginal cellularity; typical cytomorphology of papillary carcinoma absent; emphasis only on psammoma body
13	Features of nodular goiter; calcific debris and multinucleated giant cells; rare psammoma body	Nodular goiter	Features of papillary carcinoma not present; emphasis only on calcospheries
14	Cytologic features of lymphocytic thyroiditis; occasional papillary tissue fragment with overlapping nuclei (Fig. 8.48)	Hashimoto's thyroiditis	Papillary tissue fragments; lacked typical cytomorphology
15	Features of lymphocytic thyroiditis; occasional tissue fragment with papillary configuration; discrete cells with intranuclear inclusions	Hashimoto's thyroiditis	Except for intranuclear inclusions, papillary tissue fragments lacked nuclear morphology of papillary carcinoma
16	Cellular debris and hemorrhage;(?)syncytial-type tissue fragments	Hyperplastic goiter	Only(?)syncytial-tissue fragments; typical nuclear cytomorphology not present

TABLE 8.10. Frequency of Occurrence of Various Cytologic Criteria in 329 Cases of Papillary Carcinoma

	No.	Percent
Syncytial-type tissue fragments	329	100
Papillary tissue fragments	283	86
Monolayered sheets	198	60
Syncytial-type tissue fragments with follicular pattern	174	50
Intranuclear cytoplasmic inclusions	308	93
Psammoma bodies	68	20
Foreign-body type, giant cells, multinucleated	200	60
Colloid strings	100	30
Powdery chromatin	329	100
Chromatin ridge	290	88
Micro- and/or macronucleoli	329	100

Minimal Criteria for Cytologic Diagnosis

Cytologic preparations of papillary carcinoma have several diagnostic features, but not all may be present in aspirates of every case. Some features are essential, whereas others are adjunct. Their frequency also depends on the histologic pattern of the tumor.

In a review and analysis of cytopathologic features of 329 cases of papillary carcinoma, all the features listed in Table 8.1 were present in only 27 cases. Table 8.10 indicates the frequency of occurrences of various cytologic features of papillary carcinoma. These figures differ somewhat from those reported in our earlier review of 87 cases of papillary carcinoma,[18] perhaps because of better cytologic preparation in subsequent years and more careful review. Usually one or two features predominated. The most consistent features were enlarged nuclei containing fine powdery, dusty chromatin that appeared pale or watery (100%), a linear chromatin ridge or groove (88%), single or multiple micro- and/or macronucleoli (100%), and intranuclear cytoplasmic inclusions (93%).

The minimal criteria for the diagnosis of papillary carcinoma thus include a *syncytial-type tissue fragment of follicular epithelium, that regardless of the architectural pattern, shows a typical nuclear morphology, ie, pale-appearing enlarged nuclei with fine dusty, powdery chromatin; chromatin bar or ridge; single or multiple micro- and/or macronucleoli; and intranuclear cytoplasmic inclusions* (Figs. 8.52–8.54; Table 8.11).

The results of an analysis of cytologic preparations of 65 papillary carcinomas with marginal cellularity (Table 8.12) were similar to those for the overall analysis of 329 cases, thus substantiating the minimal criteria of the cytologic diagnosis of papillary carcinoma (Figs. 8.53–8.55). Abele and Miller[1] have subclassified cytopathologic features in primary and secondary groups. Their primary features include intranuclear cytoplasmic inclusions (92%), cells with dense cytoplasm (89%), and papillary fronds

(92%). Their secondary features included septate cytoplasmic vacuoles (64%), huge multinucleated giant cells (50%), psammoma bodies (36%), monolayered sheets with atypical nuclei (36%), and "bubble gum" colloid (14%).

TABLE 8.11. Minimal Criteria for Cytologic Diagnosis of Papillary Carcinoma

1. Syncytial-type tissue fragments with or without any architectural pattern
2. Enlarged nuclei with very fine dusty or powdery chromatin
3. Multiple micro- and/or macronucleoli
4. Intranuclear cytoplasmic inclusions
5. Linear chromatin ridge

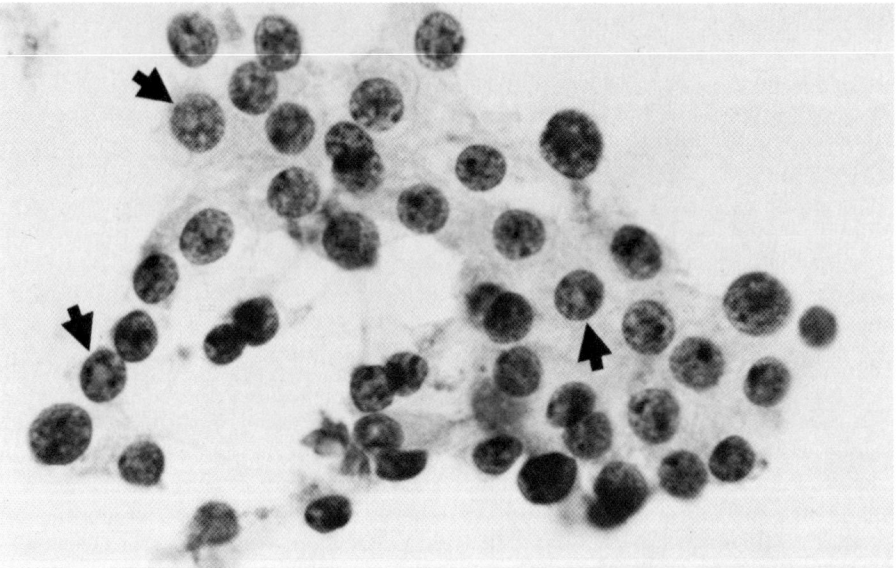

Fig. 8.52. This syncytial-type tissue fragment is suspicious of but not diagnostic of, papillary carcinoma. The nuclei are mildly pleomorphic in size, with powdery chromatin containing nuclei and only a suggestion of intranuclear inclusions *(arrow)*. A diagnosis of carcinoma cannot be given based only on this fragment. Papanicolaou preparation. × 630.

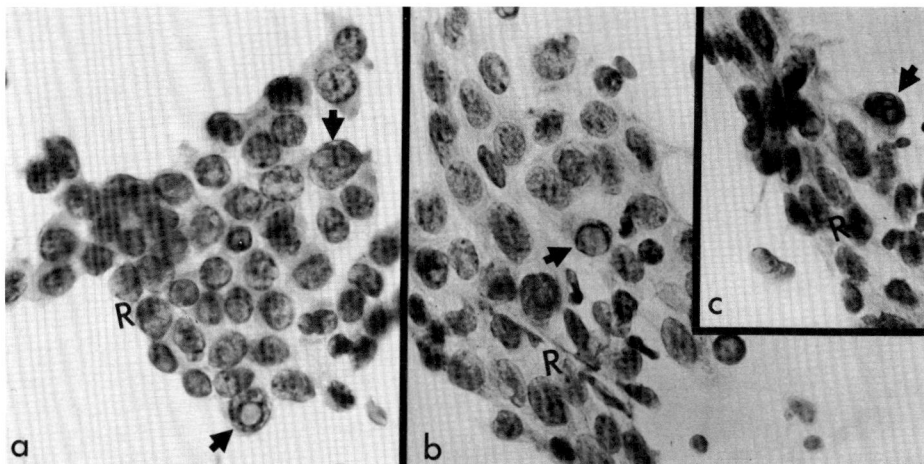

Fig. 8.53. A–C. These syncytial-type tissue fragments from three different, marginally cellular aspirates present minimal criteria for the diagnosis of papillary carcinoma. Note enlarged nuclei with altered polarity, powdery chromatin, single or multiple nucleoli, intranuclear cytoplasmic inclusions *(arrow)*, and chromatin ridge *(R)*. A definite diagnosis of papillary carcinoma may be justified in each case. Papanicolaou preparation. × 630.

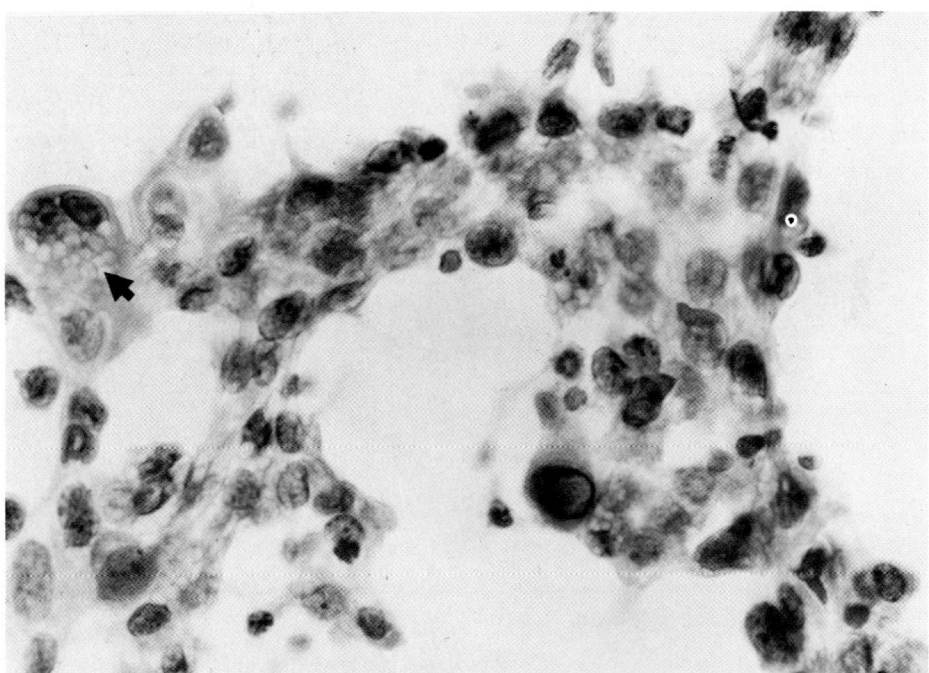

Fig. 8.54. This aspirate was almost acellular except for what is depicted here. Minimal criteria of papillary carcinoma are seen, thus justifying a diagnosis from the scanty specimen. Note the septate, vacuoles *(arrow)*, as described by Abele and Miller.[1] Papanicolaou preparation. × 630.

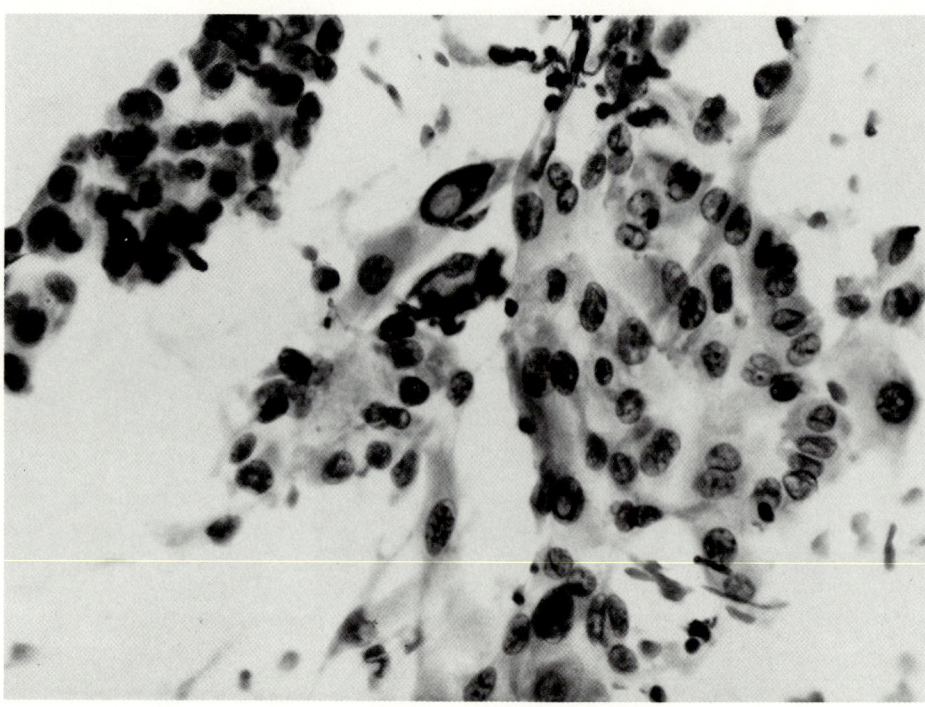

Fig. 8.55. This aspirate was almost acellular except for what is depicted here. Minimal criteria of papillary carcinoma are seen, thus justifying a diagnosis from the scanty specimen. Papanicolaou preparation. × 630.

TABLE 8.12. Frequency of Occurrences of Various Cytologic Criteria in 65 Cases of Papillary Carcinoma with Marginal Cellularity

	No.	Percent
Syncytial-type tissue fragments with or without follicular pattern	65	100
Papillary fragments	34	52
Monolayered sheets	13	20
Powdery chromatin	65	100
Intranuclear inclusions	55	84.5
Chromatin ridge	54	83
Psammoma bodies	15	23
Giant cells, multinucleated foreign-body type	19	29
Degeneration	14	21
Colloid strings	2	3

TABLE 8.13. Papillary Tissue Fragments in Cytologic Samples*

1. Papillary carcinoma
2. Papillary hyperplasia in nodular goiter
3. Papillary change in follicular adenoma
4. Hashimoto's thyroiditis

*Although papillary hyperplasia is seen in Graves' disease, it is not included here because no fine-needle aspiration biopsies were performed on functioning nodules.

TABLE 8.14. Cytologic Differentiation Between Papillary Hyperplasia and Papillary Carcinoma

	Papillary Hyperplasia	*Papillary Carcinoma*
Architecture of tissue fragments	Papillary	Papillary
Peripheral palisading of nuclei	Present	Present
Component cells	Honeycomb pattern with well-defined cell borders; uniform, small nuclei maintain their polarity	Syncytial-type pattern, with crowded and overlapped large nuclei; altered polarity
Nuclear chromatin	Granular, uniformly distributed	Dusty, fine powdery
Chromatin ridge	Absent	Present
Nucleoli	Micronucleoli may be present	Multiple micro- and/or macronucleoli
Intranuclear cytoplasmic inclusions	Absent	Present

No single cytopathologic feature is diagnostic of papillary carcinoma. A diagnosis based on one feature will often prove to be a false-positive result (Tables 8.7 and 8.9). Therefore, some of the criteria are discussed as to their significance.

Papillary Tissue Fragments

Papillary architecture can be seen in several conditions affecting the thyroid gland that present clinically as cold nodules[22] (Figs. 8.56–8.59; Table 8.13). Fine-needle aspirates of thyroid nodules of any of these diseases yield papillary tissue fragments of follicular epithelium. Their occurrence in lesions other than papillary carcinoma, however, is infrequent. The papillary tissue fragment is one of the most common features in cytologic material of papillary carcinoma. Of 329 papillary carcinomas, 283 aspirates showed either only papillary or predominantly papillary tissue fragments. Such a pattern was not appreciated in only 46 cases.

Despite its frequency, the diagnosis of papillary carcinoma based on papillary architecture alone is difficult both cytologically and histologically. This problem is covered in several articles that offer criteria helpful for differentiating between benign and malignant lesions on a histologic basis.[35] Carcangiu et al[5] stressed the cytologic criteria in the diagnosis of papillary carcinoma. The cytomorphology of the cells forming the papillary tissue fragment is critically important.

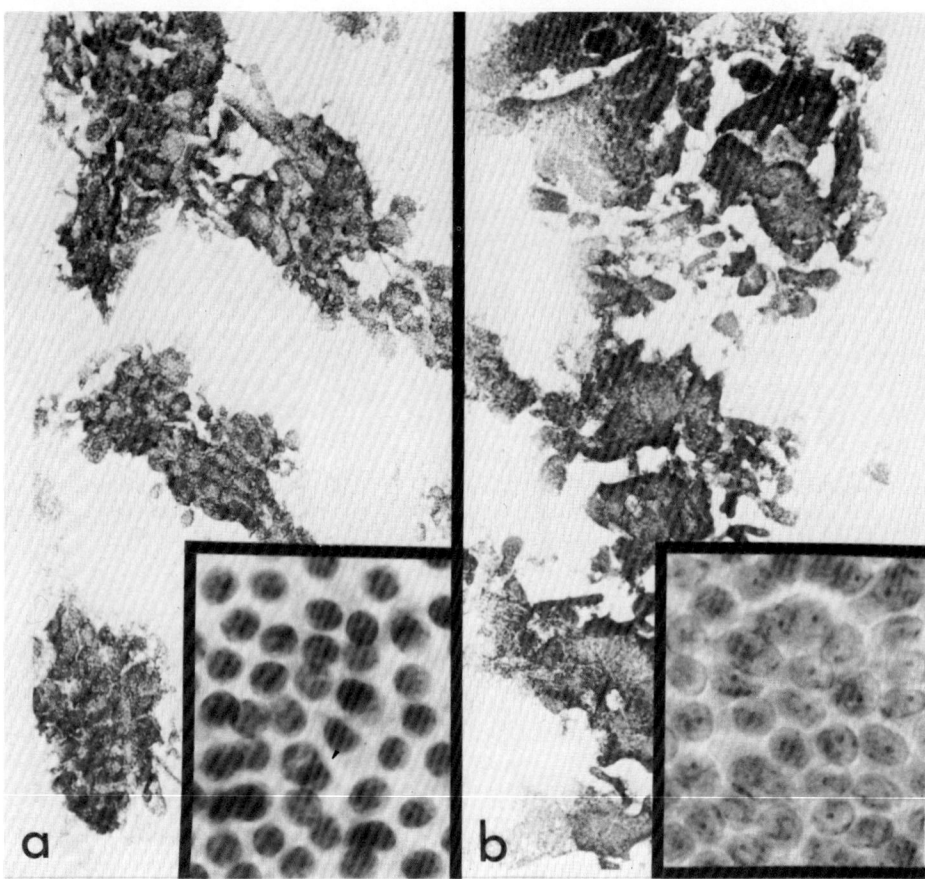

Fig. 8.56. Papillary hyperplasia and papillary carcinoma. **A.** Several branching papillary tissue fragments from nodular goiter are seen under low power, suggesting a diagnosis of carcinoma. Papanicolaou preparation. × 63. *Inset:* Higher magnification showing uniform, small nuclei, compact chromatin; and honeycomb pattern. Papanicolaou preparation. × 630. **B.** Under lower magnification, these papillary tissue fragments have an architectural pattern similar to that shown in **A.** Papanicolaou preparation. × 63. *Inset:* But they show syncytial arrangement and typical nuclear changes of papillary carcinoma. Papanicolaou preparation. × 630.

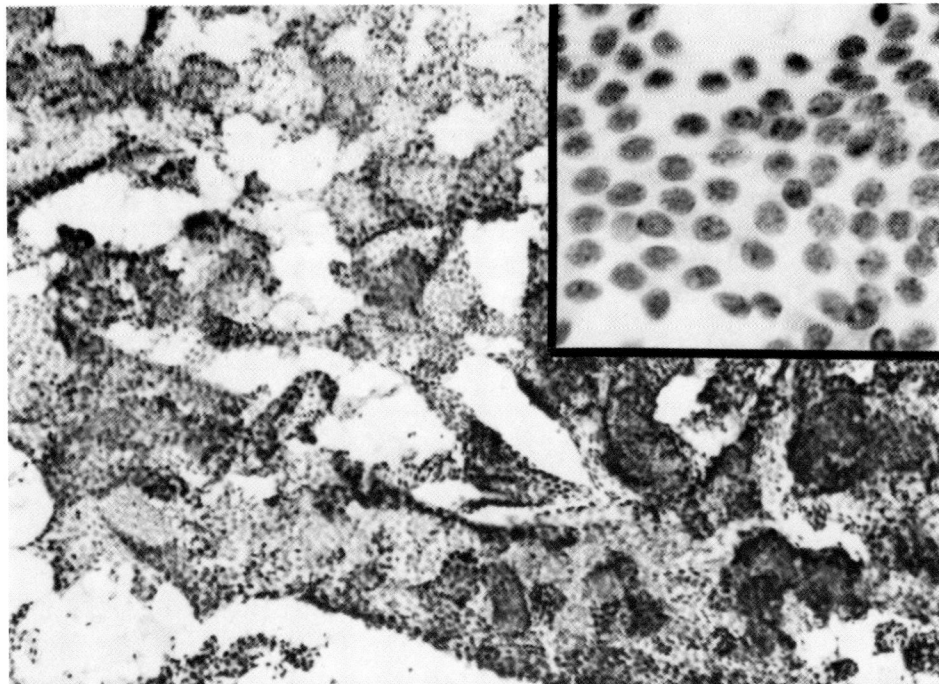

Fig. 8.57. Branching monolayered and papillary tissue fragments. A false-positive diagnosis of papillary carcinoma can easily be made if attention is not paid to component cells. Papanicolaou preparation. × 160. *Inset:* Component cells with uniform small nuclei and honeycomb pattern. Papanicolaou preparation. × 630.

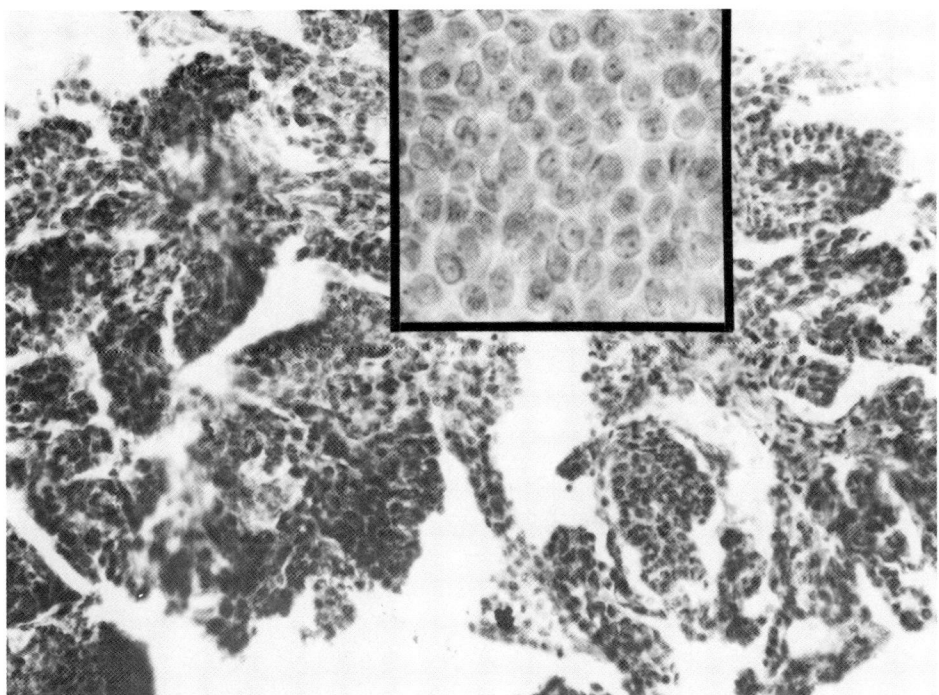

Fig. 8.58. Irregularly branching tissue fragments. Papanicolaou preparation. × 160. *Inset:* Papillary carcinoma cells with typical nuclear morphology. Papanicolaou preparation. × 630.

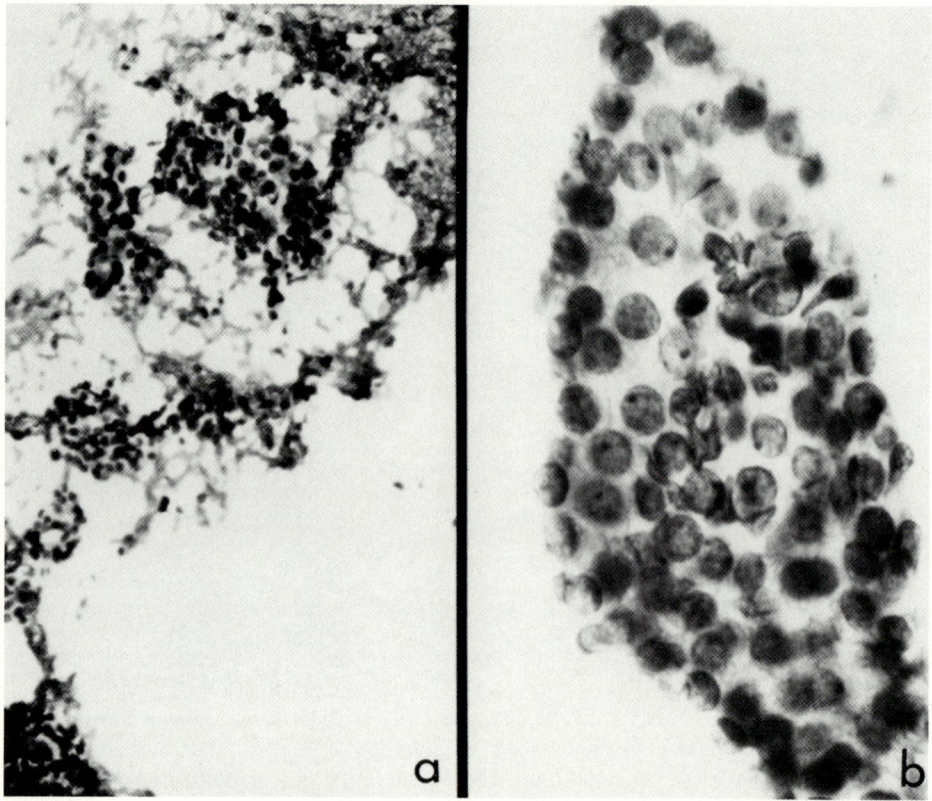

Fig. 8.59. Lymphocytic thyroiditis and papillary hyperplasia. **A.** This aspirate was suspected of being papillary carcinoma coexistent with lymphocytic thyroiditis because of the tissue fragments of follicular epithelium with papillary configuration. There are lymphocytes in the background. Papanicolaou preparation. × 160. **B.** Higher magnification of a papillary tissue fragment. Note that the typical nuclear morphology is lacking. Papanicolaou preparation. × 630. Thyroidectomy did not confirm papillary carcinoma (see Table 8.7, case 11).

The cytologic differentiation between benign and papillary fragments and papillary carcinoma is listed in Table 8.14.

Monolayered Tissue Fragments

Monolayered tissue fragments of carcinoma cells (Figs. 8.60–8.66) were seen in 60% of the aspirates of papillary carcinoma in our series. As described earlier, they probably represent papillary fronds seen en face. Being single layered, they exhibit a two-dimensional pattern and share a morphologic similarity with tissue fragments of nodular goiter. An overwhelmingly cellular aspirate of hyperplastic goiter or one with myriads of monolayered tissue fragments may be mistaken for papillary carcinoma, especially when viewed under a low-power objective. However, closer examination will reveal a different cytomorphology. The monolayered tissue fragments of nodular goiter have a honeycomb pattern, with well-defined cell borders; uniform, small nuclei with regular polarity; and compact chromatin. They show none of the features exhibited by monolayered tissue fragments of cancer cells (Table 8.15).

Monolayered tissue fragments may also be seen in simple follicular adenomas or Hashimoto's thyroiditis with papillary hyperplasia, but they lack the typical nuclear morphology of papillary carcinoma.

TABLE 8.15. Cytologic Differentiation Between Monolayered Tissue Fragments of Nodular Goiter and Papillary Carcinoma

	Nodular Goiter	Papillary Carcinoma
Architecture	Monolayered, honeycomb pattern	Monolayered, no honeycomb pattern
Cell borders	Well defined	May or may not be well defined
Nuclei	Uniform, small in size (7–9μm), polarity maintained	Pleomorphic with considerable variation in size, polarity altered; nuclear membrane may be irregular, some overlapping may be seen
Nuclear chromatin	Finely granular, even distribution, may appear compact	Fine powdery, dusty and pale
Chromatin ridge	Absent	Present
Nucleoli	Generally absent	Multiple micro- and/or macronucleoli
Intranuclear cytoplasmic inclusions	Absent	Present
Cytoplasm	Pale and variable	Variable; may be abundant and dense

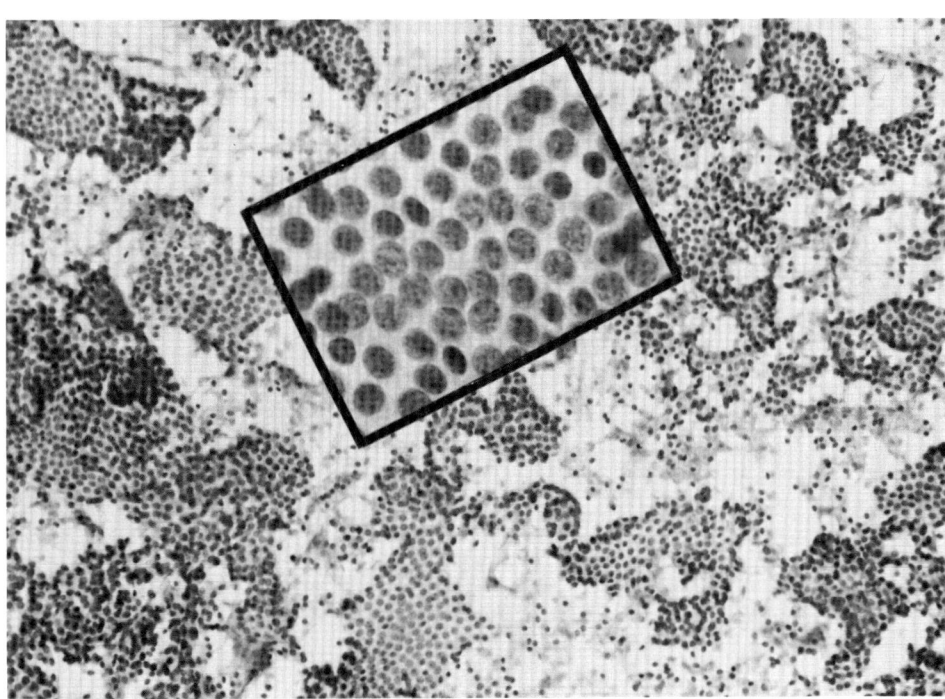

Fig. 8.60. Very cellular aspirate from hyperplastic nodular goiter. These large monolayered tissue fragments can easily be mistaken for papillary carcinoma. Papanicolaou preparation. × 160. *Inset:* Higher magnification gives a correct diagnosis of nodular goiter. The tissue fragment has a honeycomb pattern, with small nuclei. The nuclear chromatin is finely granular. Intranuclear inclusions are not present. Nucleoli are present, which may be seen in hyperplastic goiter. Papanicolaou preparation. × 630.

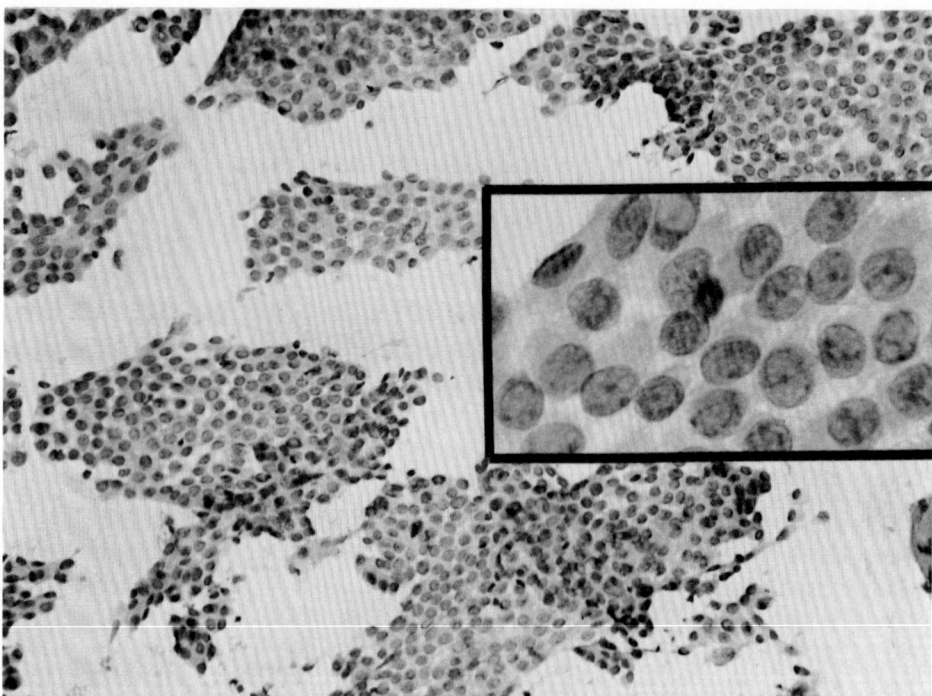

Fig. 8.61. In contrast to Fig. 8.60, these monolayered tissue fragments from papillary carcinoma exhibit typical nuclear morphology. Papanicolaou preparation. × 160. *Inset:* Higher magnification of same specimen. Papanicolaou preparation. × 630.

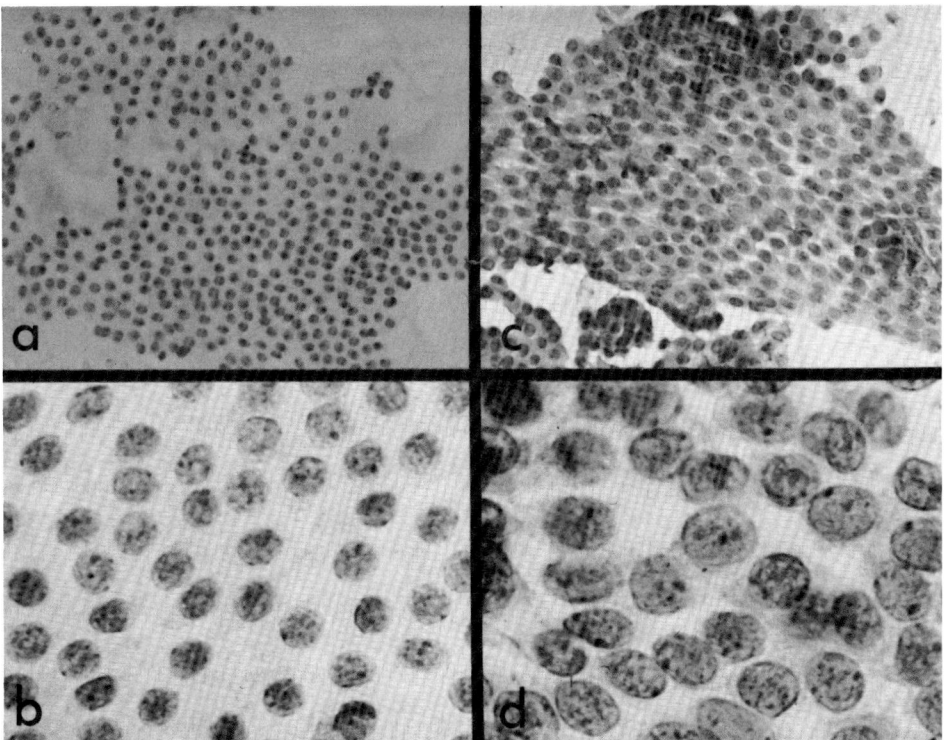

Fig. 8.62. Morphologic differences between monolayered tissue fragment in nodular goiter and monolayered fragment of papillary carcinoma. **A.** Nodular goiter. Papanicolaou preparation. × 160. **B.** Nodular goiter. Papanicolaou preparation. × 630. **C.** Papillary carcinoma. Papanicolaou preparation. × 160. **D.** Papillary carcinoma. Note the typical nuclear characteristics. Papanicolaou preparation. × 630.

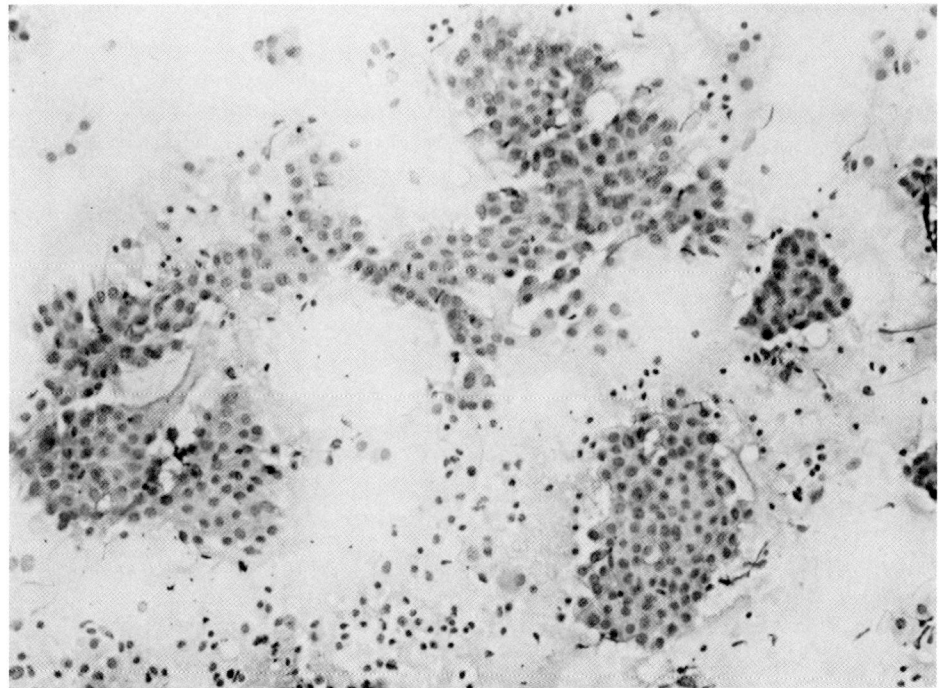

Fig. 8.63. A cellular aspirate showing several monolayered tissue fragments with lymphocytes in the background. Papanicolaou preparation. × 160.

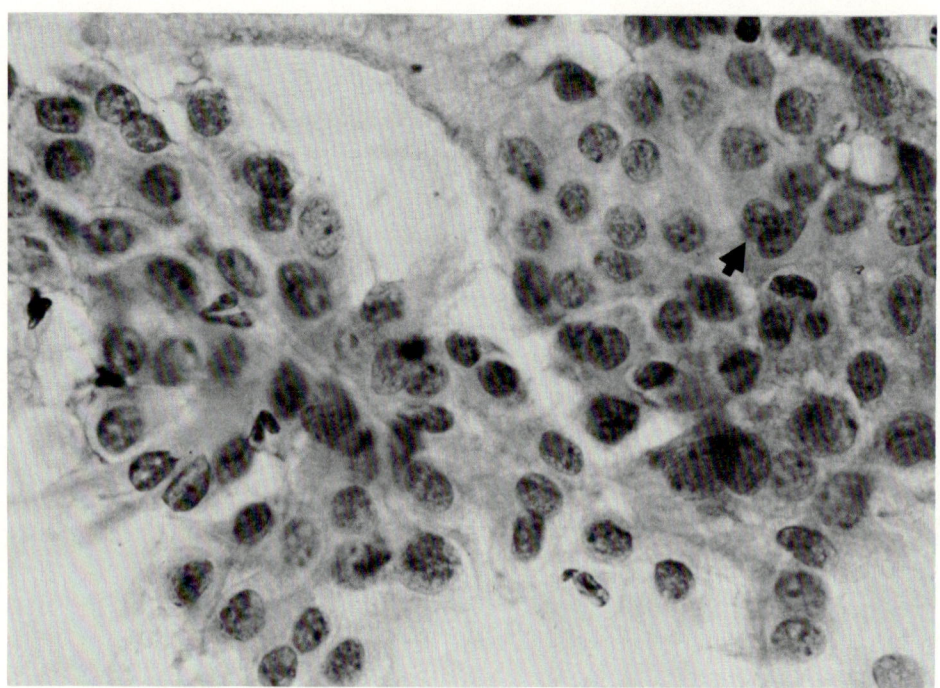

Fig. 8.64. Higher magnification of specimen shown in Fig. 8.63 showing enlarged nuclei with nucleoli and possible intranuclear inclusions *(arrow)*. A diagnosis of papillary carcinoma coexistent with Hashimoto's thyroiditis was made. Papanicolaou preparation. × 630.

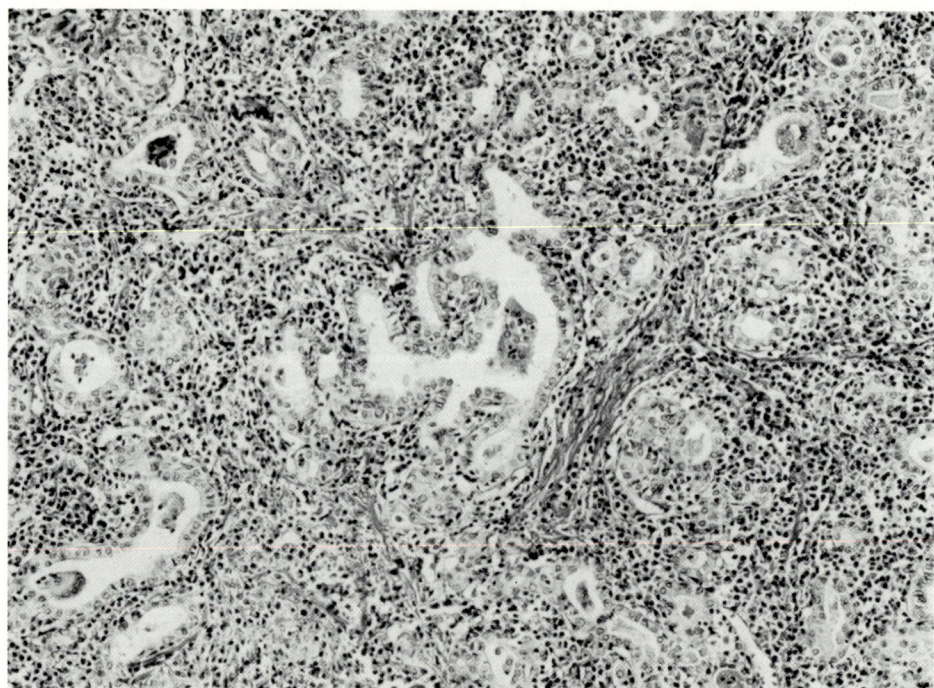

Fig. 8.65. Thyroidectomy in the case shown in Fig. 8.64 showed Hashimoto's thyroiditis and papillary hyperplasia. Hematoxylin and eosin preparation. × 160.

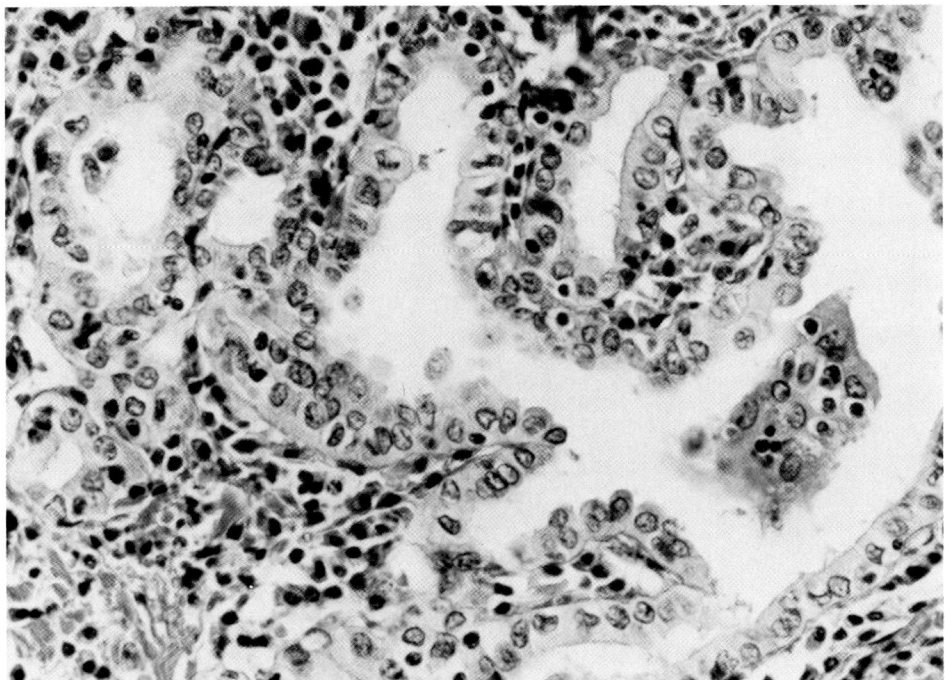

Fig. 8.66. Higher magnification of specimen shown in Fig. 8.65. Papillary carcinoma was not confirmed (see Table 8.7, case 10). Hematoxylin and eosin preparation. × 400.

Intranuclear Cytoplasmic Inclusions

Intranuclear cytoplasmic inclusions were first noted by Söderström[32] and Bjorklund[32] to be an important criterion of malignancy in fine-needle aspirate smears of papillary carcinoma of the thyroid. They were present in 308 of 329 cases (93%) of papillary carcinoma in our series. Löwhagen and Sprenger[24] found them in 5 of 10 (50%), Christ and Haja[7] in 20 of 22 (91%), and Frable[9] in 7 of 7 (100%). Intranuclear inclusions are often considered synonymous with the ground-glass or "Orphan Annie" appearance of the nuclei of papillary thyroid carcinoma. However, ground-glass or watery nuclei are a more or less generalized finding due to finely granular, powdery nuclei. Intranuclear inclusions are seen in both cytologic and histologic sections, but in a small proportion of cells. Ultrastructurally, they are seen as membrane bound, spheroidal masses of cytoplasm intruding into the nuclei[2,12,31] that contain cytoplasmic organelles.

Although a frequent feature of papillary carcinoma, intranuclear inclusions are also present in other thyroid malignancies. They are a remarkably consistent finding in medullary carcinoma[17,20] and are sometimes seen in Hürthle cell carcinomas,[27] as well as in anaplastic carcinoma. Glant et al[11] reported their presence in follicular neoplasms, both adenoma and carcinoma, and Droese[8] found them in benign non-neoplastic conditions. We have seen three aspirates from Hashimoto's thyroiditis with follicular cell nuclei containing cytoplasmic inclusions (Fig. 8.67). Intranuclear cytoplasmic inclusions are present not only in cells of thyroid neoplasms, but they are also observed in several different types of malignancies, eg, malignant melanoma,

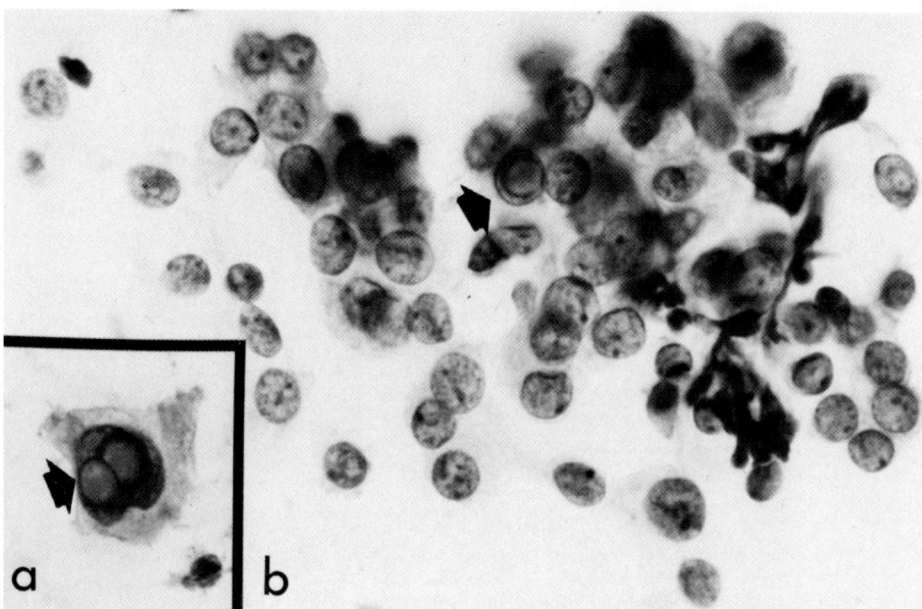

Fig. 8.67. A diagnosis of papillary carcinoma was suspected in two cases of Hashimoto's thyroiditis because of intranuclear cytoplasmic inclusions *(arrow)*. In the case shown in **A**, the nodule disappeared after suppression therapy; in the case shown in **B**, thyroidectomy failed to confirm the malignancy. Papanicolaou preparation. × 630.

liver cell carcinoma, adenocarcinoma of the lung, breast carcinomas, and soft tissue sarcomas.

   Intranuclear cytoplasmic inclusions are diagnostically important only when present in a proper setting. In thyroid aspirates, syncytial-type tissue fragments of any architectural pattern, with nuclei containing powdery chromatin and cytoplasmic inclusions, may be diagnostic of papillary carcinoma. On the other hand, aspirates showing only isolated cells with intranuclear inclusions may either be medullary carcinoma[17] of the thyroid or papillary carcinoma (see Chapter 10, Medullary Carcinoma). For this reason, diagnosis of papillary carcinoma should never be based on the presence of intranuclear cytoplasmic inclusions alone.

Psammoma Bodies

Psammoma bodies (Figs. 8.68 and 8.69; Plate 8.5) are considered a pathognomonic feature of papillary carcinoma.[35] The reported incidence in histologic material varies from 40–60%, but they are not seen with such frequency in cytologic material (Table 8.11). We found them in 20% of the aspirates from papillary carcinomas. Psammoma bodies are so rarely seen in benign disorders of the thyroid[3,19,28] that their presence in the otherwise normal-appearing thyroid gland or even in a cervical lymph node should be regarded as evidence for the presence of carcinoma until proved otherwise.[5] Because of such views, the presence of psammoma bodies in aspirates of thyroid nodules causes a diagnostic dilemma if other cytologic features of papillary carcinoma are not present. Can a diagnosis of papillary carcinoma be made

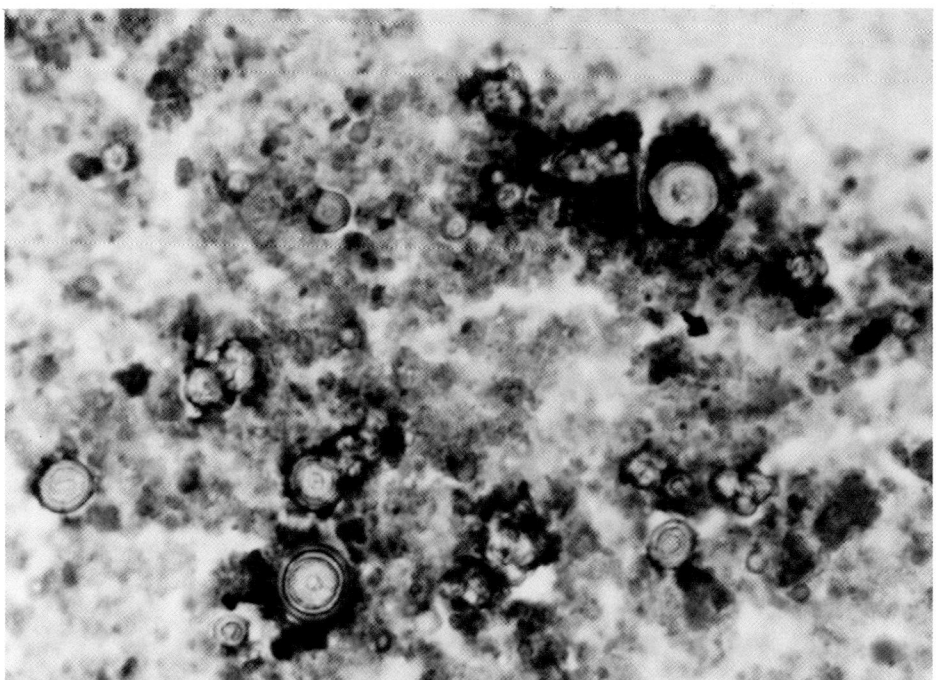

Fig. 8.68. Calcific debris with "naked" psammoma bodies. Although papillary carcinoma was not cytologically diagnosed, the mere presence of psammoma bodies influenced the clinician to recommend surgery. Thyroidectomy revealed only multinodular goiter. Papanicolaou preparation. × 400.

unequivocally in the above situations? Should a surgical procedure be recommended to confirm the diagnosis of papillary carcinoma? As indicated earlier, minimal criteria for the diagnosis of papillary carcinoma do not include a psammoma body. Initially, we placed considerable emphasis on psammoma bodies alone in making a diagnosis of papillary carcinoma, but later it was noted that they may not be of diagnostic importance in the absence of other features of papillary carcinoma. "Naked" psammoma bodies or a rare psammoma body incorporated in a tissue fragment without minimal criteria of papillary carcinoma must be interpreted with caution, as these may be seen in nodular goiter. Two of our false-positive cases fell in this category (Table 8.7). A diagnosis of suspected papillary carcinoma was given in nine cases, solely because of psammoma bodies. Five patients underwent surgery with a final diagnosis of adenomatous goiter. The other four cases had a diagnosis of nodular goiter based on results of a repeat fine-needle or large-needle biopsy. All nine cases had features of nodular goiter in the background, and the typical cytomorphology of papillary carcinoma was either lacking or insufficient. The cellular material exhibited insufficient criteria for the diagnosis of papillary carcinoma.

A psammoma body can be mimicked by dense inspissated colloid within a follicle, or because of its tendency to crack in a linear fashion.

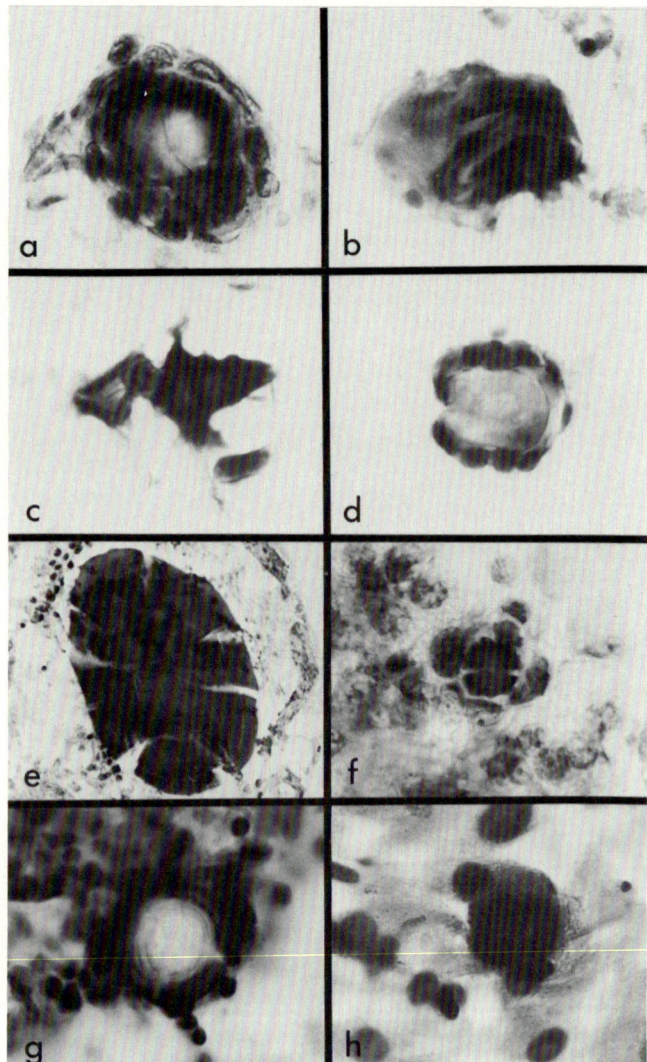

Fig. 8.69. Differential diagnosis of psammoma bodies. **A.** Typical psammoma body incorporated in a syncytial-type tissue fragment with nuclear features of papillary carcinoma. Papanicolaou preparation. × 630. **B., C.** These two psammoma bodies with degenerating follicular cells are difficult to interpret. Papanicolaou preparation. × 630. **D.** Inspissated colloid within a follicle simulating a psammoma body. Papanicolaou preparation. × 630. The surrounding cells have small nuclei with compact chromatin, not diagnostic of papillary carcinoma. Papanicolaou preparation. × 630. **E.** Large droplet of inspissated colloid with linear cracks simulating a psammoma body. Papanicolaou preparation. × 160. **F.** True psammoma body incorporated in a tissue fragment. Note morphologic similarity to that shown in **E.** Papanicolaou preparation. × 630. **G.** Psammoma body from nodular goiter. The component cells of the tissue fragment have small, uniform nuclei, Papanicolaou preparation. × 630. **H.** An isolated "naked" psammoma body from Hürthle cell carcinoma. Papanicolaou preparation. × 630.

SUMMARY

Papillary carcinoma of the thyroid is the most common of thyroid malignancies. It is also the least difficult to diagnose from cytologic samples, provided that the *aspirate is adequate*. It has a diagnostic accuracy of over 90%. Although there are several cytologic features, the minimal criteria include a syncytial-type tissue fragment that, irrespective of architectural pattern, shows typical nuclear morphology of pale, watery nuclei due to powdery, dusty chromatin; micro- and/or macronucleoli; chromatin ridge; and intranuclear cytoplasmic inclusions. False-positive diagnoses result from interpretations based on insufficient criteria.

REFERENCES

1. Abele JS, Miller TR: Fine needle aspiration of the thyroid nodule: clinical applications. In Clark OH: *Endocrine Surgery of the Thyroid and Parathyroid Glands.* St. Louis, Mosby, 1985, pp. 293–365.

2. Albores-Saavedra J, Altamirano-Dimas M, Alcurta-Anguizola B, Smith M: Fine structure of human papillary thyroid carcinoma. *Cancer* 28:763–744, 1971.

3. Batsakis JG, Nishiyama RH, Rich CR: Microlithiasis (calcospherites) and carcinoma of the thyroid gland. *AMA Arch Pathol* 69:493–498, 1960.

4. Carcangiu ML, Zampi G, Pupi A, Castagnuli A, Rosai J: Papillary carcinoma of the thyroid: a clinicopathologic study of 241 cases treated at the University of Florence, Italy. *Cancer* 55:805–828, 1985.

5. Carcangiu ML, Zampi G, Rosai J: Papillary thyroid carcinoma: a study of its many morphologic expressions and clinical correlates. In Sommers S, Rosen PD: *Pathology Annuals, Part I.* Norwalk CT. Appleton-Century-Crofts, 1985, pp. 1–44.

6. Chen KTK, Rosai J: Follicular variant of thyroid papillary carcinoma: a clinicopathologic study of six cases, *Am J Surg Pathol* 1:123–130, 1977.

7. Christ M, Haja J: Intranuclear cytoplasmic inclusions (invaginations) in thyroid aspriations, frequency and specificity, *Acta Cytol* 23:327–331, 1979.

8. Droese M: Cytological aspiration biopsy of the thyroid gland. Stuttgart, FF Schattauer Verlag, 1980, pp. 62–63.

9. Frable W: Thin needle aspriation biopsy. In Bennington JL: *Major Problems in Pathology*, vol 14. Philadelphia, Saunders, 1983, pp. 162, 170–171.

10. Franssila KO: Is the differentiation between papillary and follicular thyroid carcinoma valid? *Cancer* 32:853–864, 1973.

11. Glant MD, Berger EK, Davey DD: Intranuclear cytoplasmic inclusions in aspirates of follicular neoplasms of the thyroid. *Acta Cytol* 28:576–579, 1984.

12. Gray A, Doniach J: Morphology of the nuclei of papillary carcinoma of the thyroid. *Br J Cancer* 23:49–51, 1969.

13. Hapke M, Dehner L: The optically clear nucleus: a reliable sign of papillary carcinoma of the thyroid? *Am J Surg Pathol* 3:31–58, 1979.

14. Hawk WA, Hazard JB: The many appearances of papillary carcinoma of the thyroid. *Cleve Clin Quart* 43:207–216, 1976.

15. Hidvegi DF, Heltgren S, Gallagher L: Origin of giant cells from papillary carcinoma of the thyroid: immunologic, enzymatic and ultrastructural aspects of cytopreparations. *Acta Cytol* 25:742, 1981.

16. Hubert JP Jr, Kiernan PD, Bearhs OH, McConahey WM, Woolner LB: Occult papillary carcinoma of the thyroid. *Arch Surg* 115:394–398, 1980.

17. Kini SR, Miller JM, Hamburger JI: Cytopathological features of medullary carcinoma of the thyroid. *Arch Pathol Lab Med* 108:156–159, 1984.

18. Kini SR, Miller JM, Hamburger JI, Smith MJ: Cytopathology of papillary carcinoma of the thyroid. *Acta Cytol* 24:511–521, 1980.

19. Klinck GH, Winship T: Psammoma bodies and thyroid cancer. *Cancer* 12:656–662, 1959.

20. Lew W, Orell S, Henderson DW: Intranuclear vacuoles in nonpapillary carcinoma of the thyroid. *Acta Cytol* 28:581–586, 1984.

21. Lindsay S: *Carcinoma of the Thyroid Gland; A Clinical and Pathologic Study of 293 Patients at the University of California Hospital.* Springfield, IL, Charles C Thomas, 1960.

22. LiVolsi VA, Merino MJ: Histopathological differential diagnosis of the thyroid. *Pathol Annu* 16(part 2):357–406, 1981.

23. Löwhagen T, Giremberg PO, Lundell G: Aspiration biopsy cytology (ABC) in nodules of the thyroid gland suspected to be malignant. *Surg Clin N Am* 59:3–18, 1979.

24. Löwhagen T, Sprenger E: Cytologic presentation of thyroid tumors in aspiration biopsy smear: a review of 60 cases. *Acta Cytol* 18:192–197, 1974.

25. Meissner WA, Adler A: Papillary carcinoma of the thyroid: a study of the pathology of 226 cases. *Arch Pathol* 66:518–525, 1958.

26. Muller N, Cooperburg PL, Suen KCH, Thorsson SC: Needle aspiration in cystic papillary carcinoma of the thyroid. *Am J Radiol* 144:251–253, 1985.

27. O'Morchoe PJ, Lee DC: Intranuclear cytoplasmic inclusions in carcinoma of the thyroid gland (letter to the editor). *Acta Cytol* 28:621, 1984.

28. Patchefsky AS, Hoch WS: Psammoma bodies in diffuse toxic goiter. *Am J Clin Pathol* 57:551–556, 1972.

29. Rosai J, Zampi G, Carcangiu ML: Papillary carcinoma of the thyroid: a discussion of the several morphologic expressions with particular emphasis on the follicular variant. *Am J Surg Pathol* 7:809–817, 1983.

30. Selzer G, Kahn LB, Albertyn L: Primary malignant tumors of the thyroid gland: a clinicopathologic study of 254 cases. *Cancer* 40:1501–1510, 1977.

31. Sobel HJ, Schwarz R, Marquet E: Non-viral nuclear inclusions. *Arch Pathol* 87:179–192, 1969.

32. Söderström M, Bjorklund A: Intranuclear cytoplasmic inclusions in some types of thyroid cancer. *Acta Cytol* 17:191–197, 1973.

33. Strate SM, Lee EL, Childers JM: Occult papillary carcinoma of the thyroid with distant metastasis. *Cancer* 54:1093–1100, 1984.

34. Tscholl-Durommun J, Hedinger CE: Papillary thyroid carcinomas: morphology and prognosis, *Virchows Arch {A}* 396:19–39, 1982.

35. Vickery AL Jr: Thyroid papillary carcinoma: pathological and philosophical controversies. *Am J Surg Pathol* 7:797–807, 1983.

36. Walfish PG, Hazani E, Strawbridge HTH, Miskin M, Rosen IB: Combined ultrasound and needle aspiration cytology in the assessment and management of hypofunctioning nodule. *Ann Intern Med* 87:270–274, 1977.

37. Woolner LB: Thyroid carcinoma: pathologic classification with data on prognosis. *Semin Nucl Med* 1:481–502, 1971.

9
Anaplastic Carcinoma

Anaplastic carcinoma of thyroid comprises 5–15% of all thyroid carcinomas.[5,8,11,13] One of the most aggressive thyroid neoplasms, it is almost always fatal within a few months of detection. It is found in older individuals, and is rare in patients under 60 years of age. In a Mayo Clinic report,[11] the mean age was 66.6 years (range, 37–90 years), and only three patients were under 50 years of age. Anaplastic carcinomas are slightly more common in women. Some patients have a long history of goiter or a nodule. They present with a rapidly growing, painful goiter with pressure symptoms, such as dysphagia, dyspnea, and hoarseness of voice of short duration. The tumor is locally invasive and metastasizes widely at distant sites. It is rapidly fatal.

PATHOLOGY

Grossly, the tumor is bulky and fleshy, extensively infiltrating the thyroid (Fig. 9.1). It often extends beyond the capsule into surrounding tissues, and is often necrotic and even cystic. Microscopically (Figs. 9.2–9.5), two distinct types are recognized, spindle and giant cell, although Carcangiu et al[5] included squamous carcinoma in this group. Transitional and intermediate forms often occur. Generally, small cell carcinomas—considered a type of anaplastic carcinoma of the thyroid—are either malignant lymphomas, medullary thyroid carcinomas, or poorly differentiated carcinomas of the thyroid.[2–5,9,12,13,15]

The spindle cell type is present alone or in combination with giant cells. Its appearance is like that of a sarcoma, and in most areas it is indistinguishable from a true sarcoma. The nuclei are hyperchromatic, with numerous atypical mitoses. Spindle cell anaplastic carcinomas may either resemble fibrosarcomas because of collagenized stroma and a fascicular arrangement; or malignant fibrous histiocytomas because of scattered giant cells, a storiform pattern of growth, and inflammatory

189

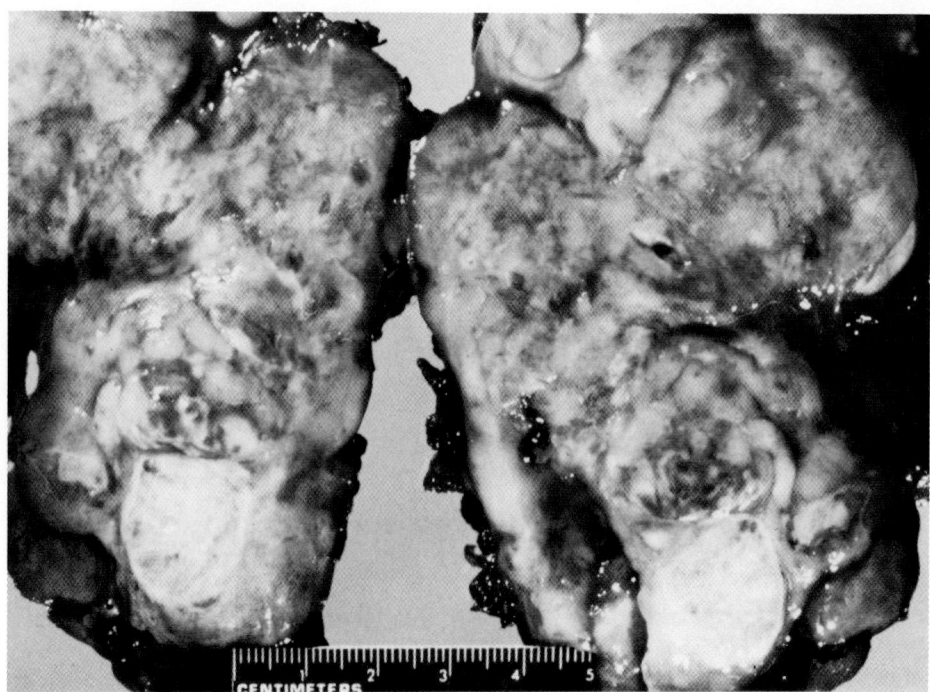

Fig. 9.1. Anaplastic carcinoma. Note bulky, fleshy tumor with necrotic areas.

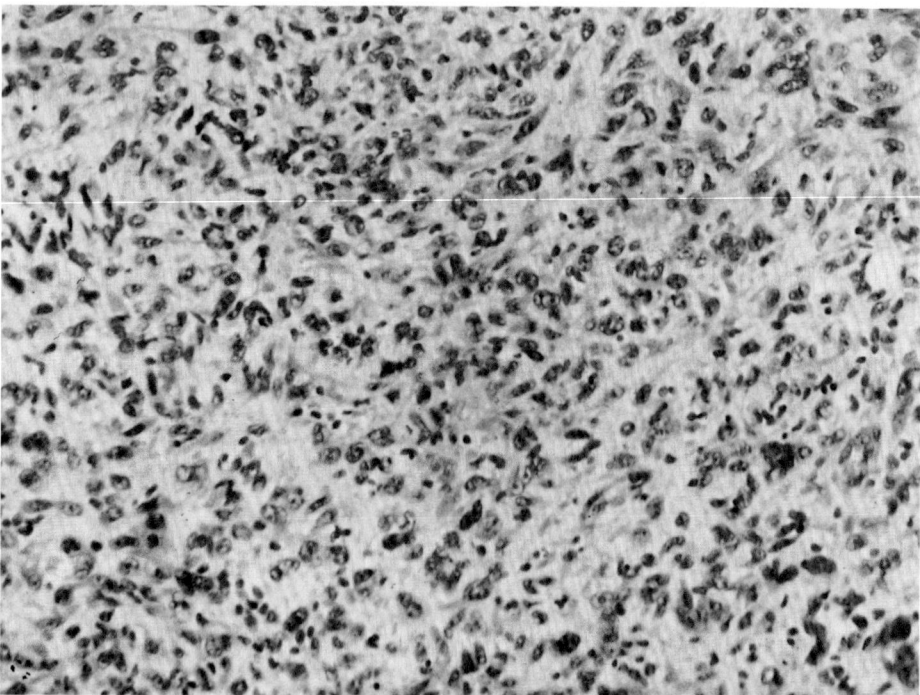

Fig. 9.2. Anaplastic carcinoma with spindle cell pattern. Hematoxylin and eosin preparation. × 160.

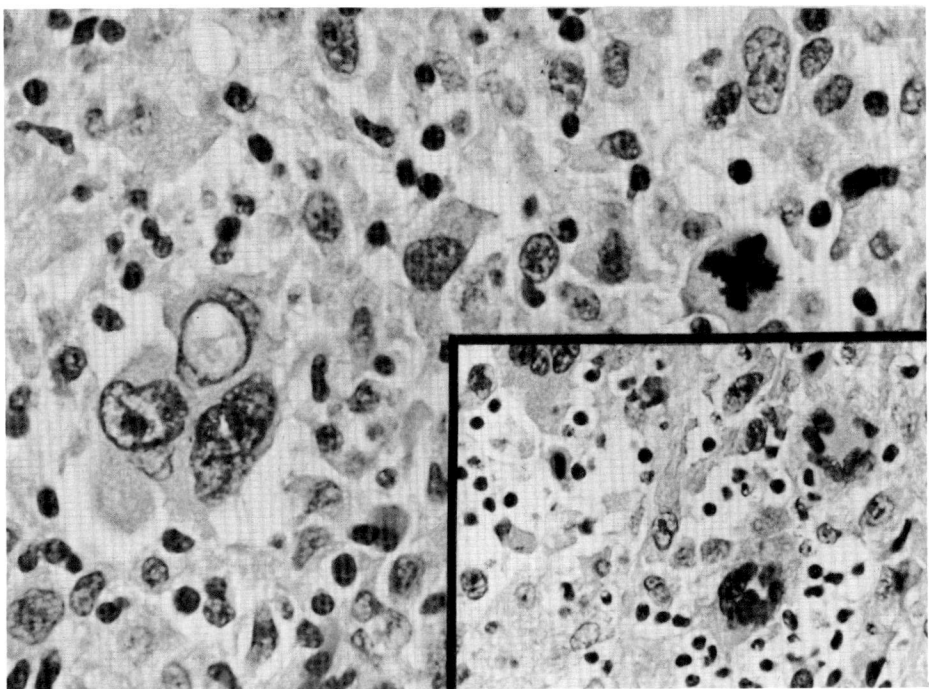

Fig. 9.3. Anaplastic carcinoma, giant cell type, with bizarre nuclei and quadripolar mitosis. Note inflammatory cells in the background due to necrosis. Hematoxylin and eosin preparation. × 630. *Inset:* Osteoclast-type giant cells. Hematoxylin and eosin preparation. × 630.

infiltrate. Permeation of the blood vessel[5] is a common phenomenon, and extensive desmoplasia is often seen.

The giant cell pattern is characterized by a striking degree of pleomorphism, exhibited by giant tumor cells containing bizarre single or multiple nuclei and abundant acidophilic cytoplasm. The giant cells may be interspersed among the smaller mononuclear tumor cells with similar cytoplasmic features. The pattern of growth is solid.

In either type, necrosis can be extensive with a heavy inflammatory component. Giant tumor cells may contain neutrophils. Multinucleated cells with an osteoclast-like appearance among the neoplastic cells have been reported.[6,7] In a number of cases, residual foci of papillary or follicular carcinoma are seen, indicating dedifferentiation of preexisting differentiated cancers.[5,8,13,14]

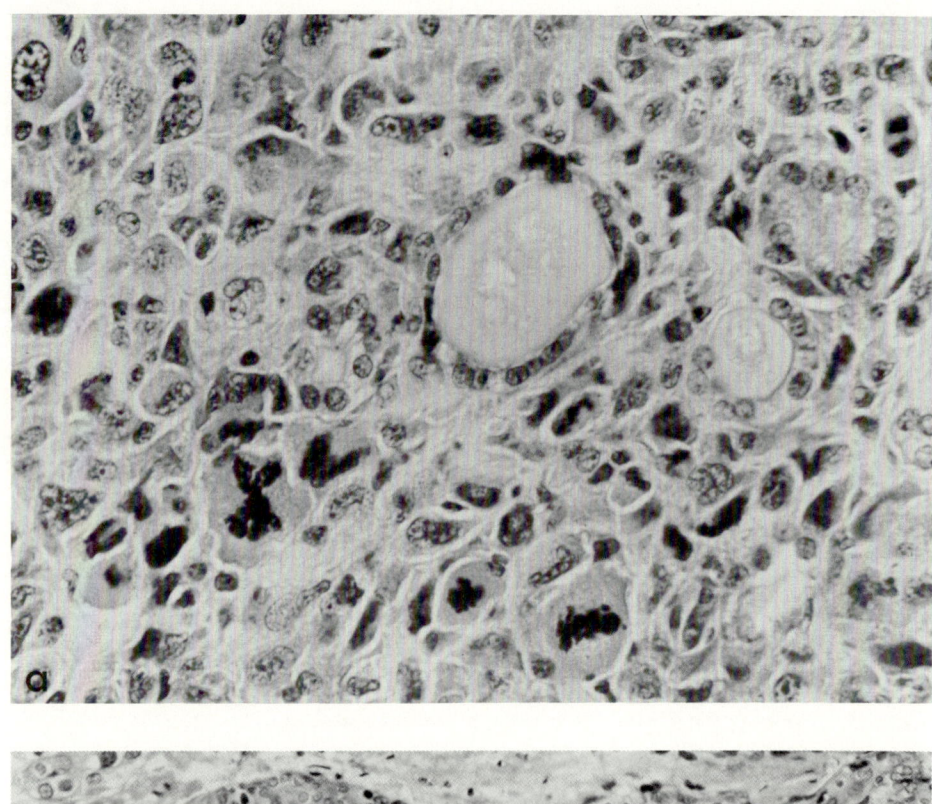

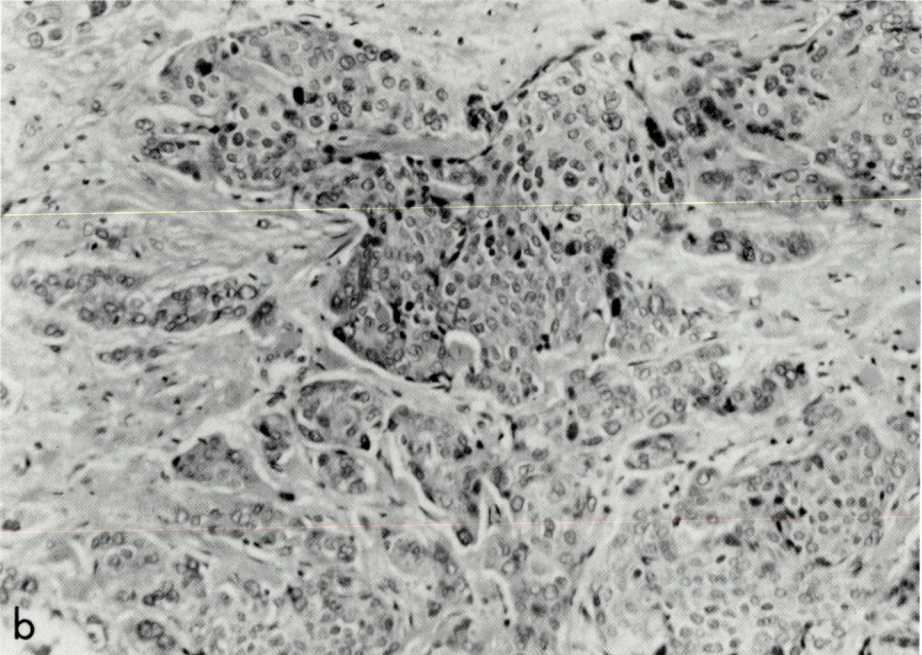

Fig. 9.4. A. Anaplastic carcinoma with bizarre nuclear pattern and frequent, atypical mitoses. Follicles containing colloid suggest origin from preexisting follicular carcinoma. Hematoxylin and eosin preparation. × 400. **B.** Anaplastic carcinoma with squamous cell component. Hematoxylin and eosin preparation. × 160.

CYTOPATHOLOGY

In aspirates of an anaplastic carcinoma of thyroid (Figs. 9.6–9.12), cellularity is inversely proportional to stromal component. Anaplastic carcinomas with a marked desmoplastic reaction, seen particularly with the spindle cell type, yield acellular or inadequate samples.

With adequate cellularity, the diagnosis is obvious even to a novice (Table 9.1). The malignant cells are seen usually isolated or in tissue fragments, with extreme pleomorphism in the size and shape. The cells of a giant cell carcinoma can be small to very large, with occasional multinucleation (Figs. 9.6–9.8). Nuclei are usually eccentric and bizarre, with irregular clumps of chromatin, separated by excessively clear parachromatin. The chromatinic membrane is often irregular and scalloping, and the nuclei have multiple and irregular nucleoli. Mitotic figures may be present. The nuclei may be multilobulated, and intranuclear cytoplasmic inclusions are also seen. The cytoplasm of the giant cell carcinoma cells is usually dense and abundant, with a strong resemblance to Hürthle cells. However, unlike Hürthle cells ultrastructurally, anaplastic carcinoma cells contain no, or very few, mitochondria.[5] With dense cytoplasm and sharp cell borders, anaplastic carcinoma cells also appear similar to keratinized squamous cells. Cytoplasmic vacuolization is frequent, and leukophagocytosis is not uncommon (Fig. 9.12). Osteoclast-like giant cells have been also reported in aspirates of anaplastic carcinoma.[17] Aspirates of spindle cell type anaplastic carcinoma contain isolated or groups of pleomorphic spindle cells (Fig. 9.9) with bizarre nuclei. The cytoplasm is pale, dense, and sometimes vacuolated.

Anaplastic carcinomas are frequently mixed with both giant and spindle cell patterns, and the aspirates from such cases show an admixture of both cell types (Figs. 9.10 and 9.11).

Necrosis and inflammation are frequent findings in anaplastic carcinoma, characterized by tumor diathesis with cellular and inflammatory debris in the background. With extensive necrosis, malignant cells are difficult to identify amid cellular debris.[16]

TABLE 9.1. Cytopathologic Features of Anaplastic Carcinoma of Thyroid

Pattern	Cells isolated and in tissue fragments
Cells	Extremely pleomorphic in size and shape; small to giant forms; round, oval, or spindle shapes
Nucleus	Large bizarre shapes; clumped chromatin with excessive parachromatin clearing; nucleoli large, multiple, and irregular; intranuclear cytoplasmic inclusions frequent; mitotic figures may be present
Cytoplasm	Abundant, pale, vacuolated or dense; resembles keratinized squamous or Hürthle cells; leukophagocytosis common
Background	Tumor diathesis; osteoclast-like cells may be present

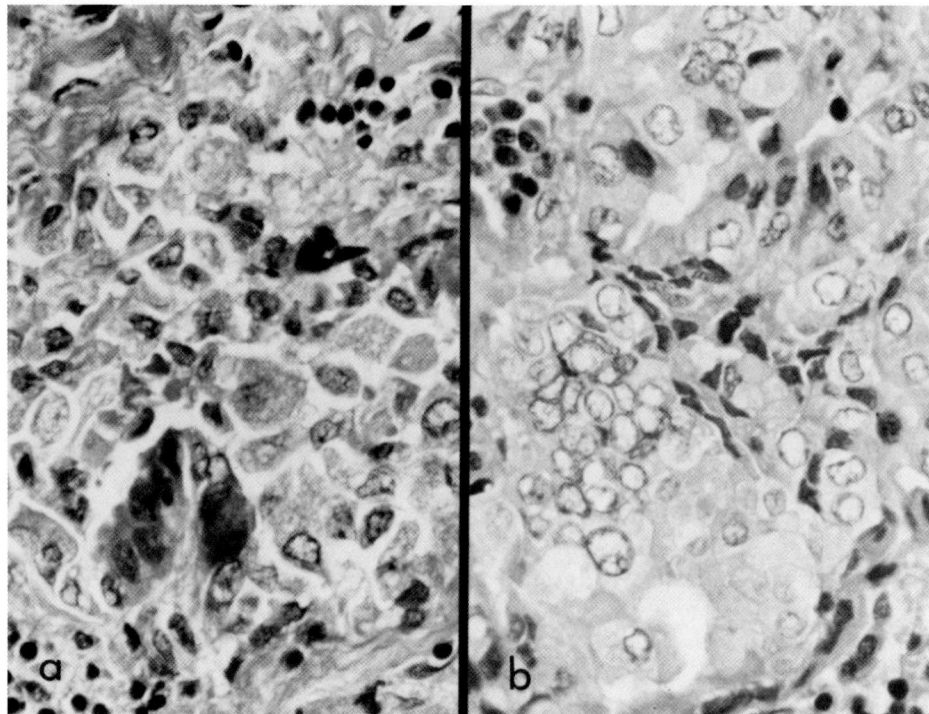

Fig. 9.5. Anaplastic carcinoma. **A.** Abortive papilla. Hematoxylin and eosin preparation. × 400. **B.** Area of tumor cells containing watery, clear nuclei. Hematoxylin and eosin preparation. × 400. These features suggest origin from a preexisting papillary carcinoma.

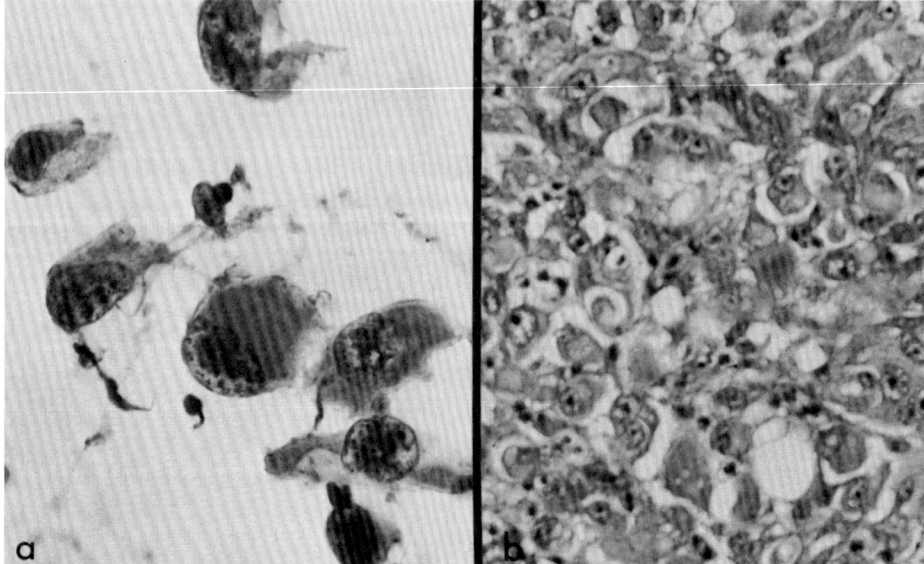

Fig. 9.6. Anaplastic carcinoma, giant cell type. **A.** Discrete, large cancer cells with bizarre nuclei and abundant dense cytoplasm. Papanicolaou preparation. × 630. **B.** Histologic section of the same case shown in **A.** Hematoxylin and eosin preparation. × 400.

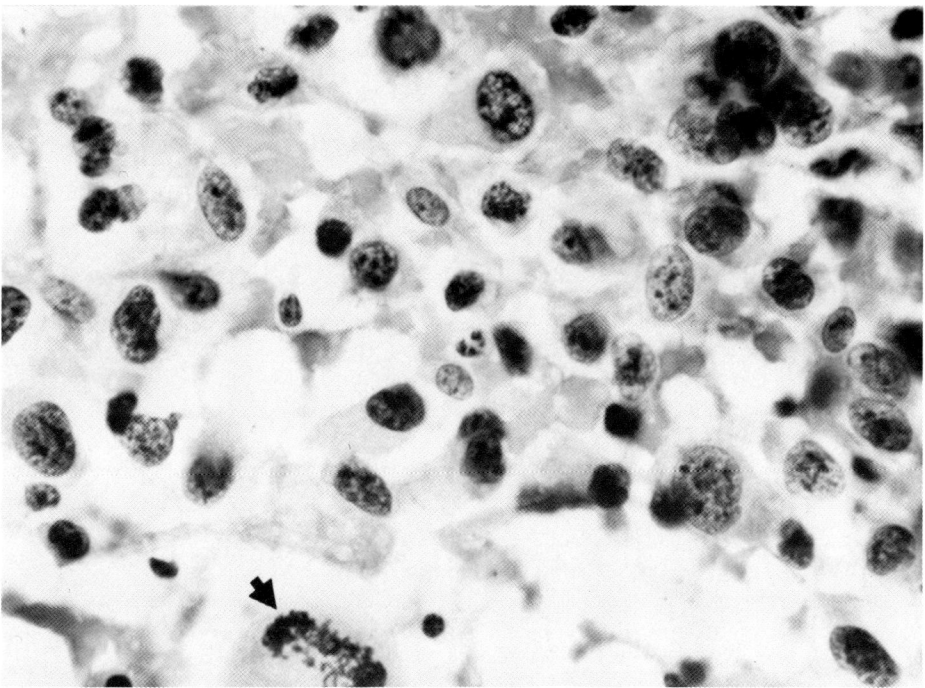

Fig. 9.7. Anaplastic giant cell carcinoma. Discrete pleomorphic carcinoma cells with bizarre nuclei and a mitotic figure *(arrow)*. Papanicolaou preparation. × 630.

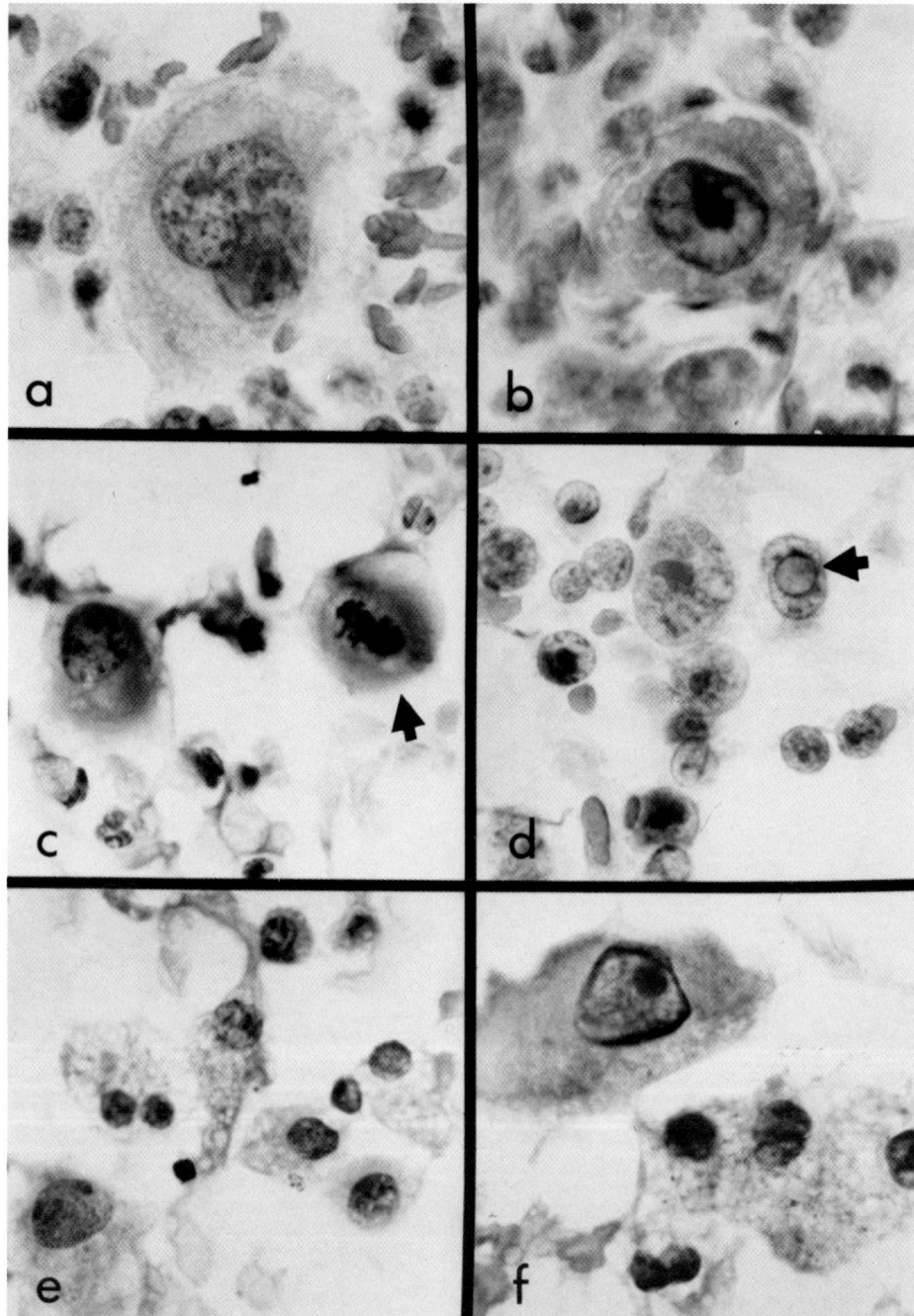

Fig. 9.8. Cells of anaplastic carcinoma, giant cell type. **A.** Giant carcinoma cells with lobulated nucleus. Papanicolaou preparation. × 630. **B.** Dense cytoplasm, well-defined cell borders, and central nucleus; morphology similar to squamous cell carcinoma. Papanicolaou preparation. × 630. **C.** Discrete carcinoma cells with mitotic figure *(arrow)*. Papanicolaou preparation. × 630. **D.** Small to large giant cells with intranuclear cytoplasmic inclusion *(arrow)*. Papanicolaou preparation. × 630. **E.** Foamy, vacuolated cytoplasm and cytoplasmic process. Papanicolaou preparation. × 630. **F.** Foamy, vacuolated cytoplasm due to degeneration. Papanicolaou preparation. × 630.

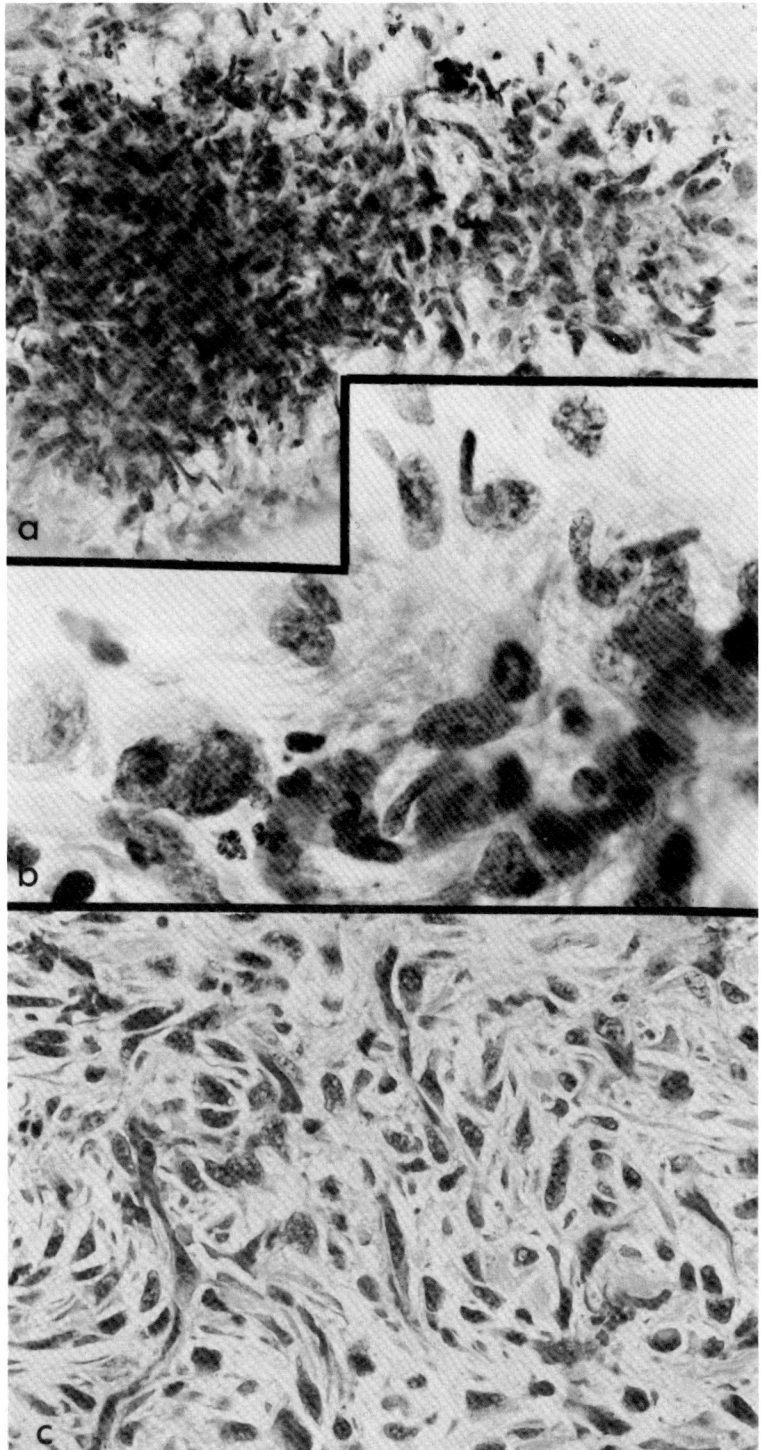

Fig. 9.9. Anaplastic carcinoma, spindle cell type. **A.** Group of pleomorphic spindle cells. Papanicolaou preparation. × 160. **B.** Spindle cells with bizarre nuclei. Papanicolaou preparation. × 630. **C.** Histologic section showing spindle cell carcinoma resembling fibrosarcoma. Hematoxylin and eosin preparation. × 400.

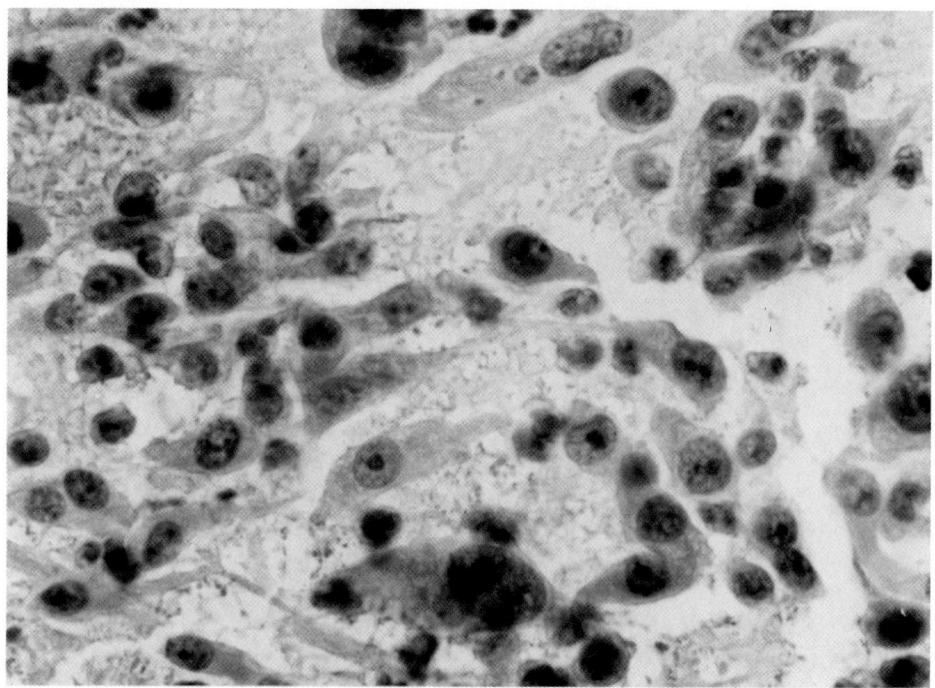

Fig. 9.10. Anaplastic carcinoma of thyroid. Group of very pleomorphic giant and spindle cells with bizarre nuclei. Note multinucleation. Papanicolaou preparation. × 630.

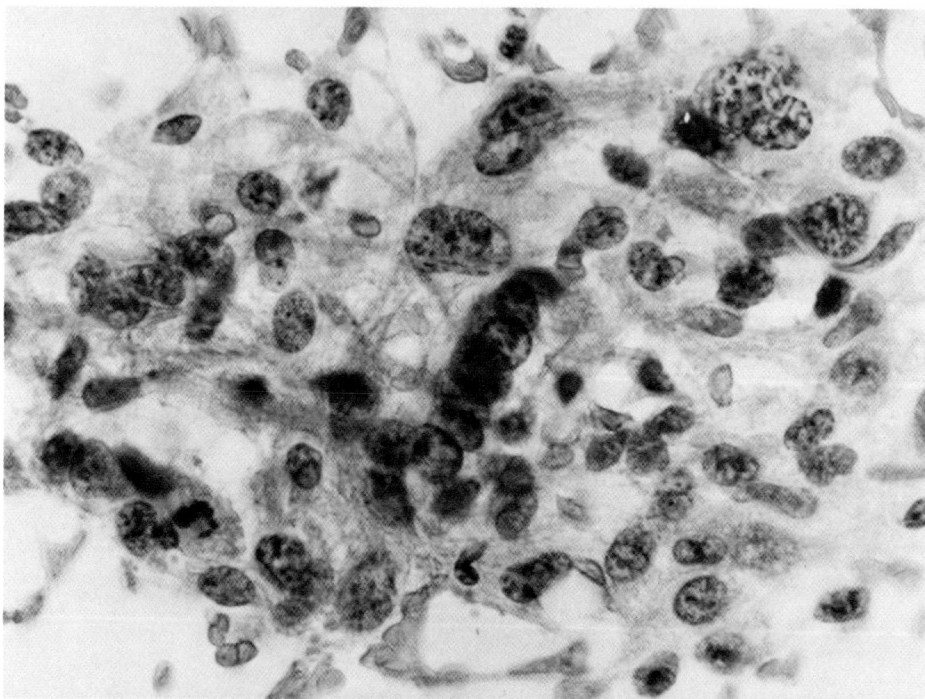

Fig. 9.11. Anaplastic carcinoma showing mixture of giant cells and spindle-shaped cells with pleomorphic nuclei and dense, abundant cytoplasm. Note amorphous debris in background. Papanicolaou preparation. × 630.

198

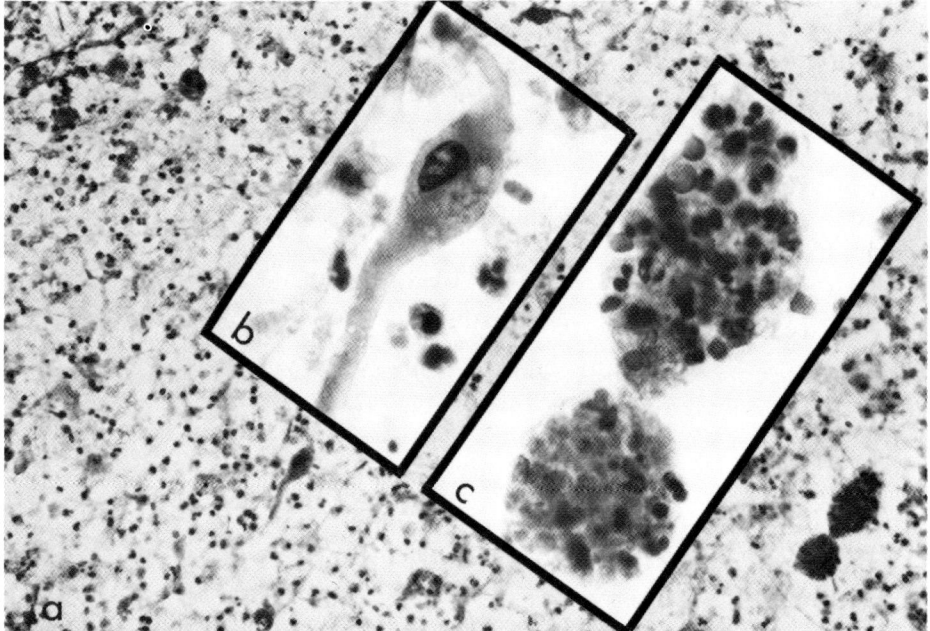

Fig. 9.12. A. Anaplastic carcinoma with extensive necrosis.Papanicolaou preparation. × 160. **B.** Bizarre carcinoma cells. Papanicolaou preparation. × 630. **C.** Carcinoma cells exhibiting leukophagocytosis. Papanicolaou preparation. × 630. Identification of cancer cells can be very difficult from such an aspirate.

DIFFERENTIAL DIAGNOSIS

The cytologic pattern of anaplastic carcinoma of the thyroid presents no diagnostic challenge. Because of its bizarre nuclear cytomorphology, anaplastic carcinoma is easy to diagnose accurately and cannot be confused with any other lesion. However, the converse is not true (Table 9.2).

Several types of benign cells may be misinterpreted as anaplastic carcinoma. Proliferating fibroblasts from granulation tissue or tissue fragments of stroma constitute a diagnostic pitfall. The nuclei of the fibroblasts have an alarming appearance because they are large and contain macronucleoli (Fig. 9.13). However, the nuclear chromatin is rather bland and extremely pleomorphic; nuclei characteristics of anaplastic carcinoma cells are lacking. Large tissue fragments of the connective tissue stroma are often aspirated and may present diagnostic difficulties (Figs. 9.14 and 9.15). The same may hold true for histiocytes (Fig. 9.16) or for follicular cells undergoing regressive changes (Figs. 9.17 and 9.18). This is especially true in patients who are undergoing therapy. Clinically, subacute thyroiditis with a painful, enlarged thyroid may simulate symptoms of anaplastic carcinoma. If stromal cells are aspirated, it is easy to interpret them as anaplastic carcinoma.

Neoplasms that may be misinterpreted as undifferentiated carcinoma are medullary carcinoma of the thyroid, and, on extremely rare occasions, a metastatic, poorly differentiated, malignant neoplasm to the thyroid, which masquerades as a primary thyroid cancer. Differentiation between metastatic anaplastic carcinoma and a primary anaplastic tumor may be very difficult on a cytologic basis. Because immunoperoxidase stains for thyroglobulin are weakly positive or negative in anaplastic carcinomas of the thyroid,[1] they may not be diagnostically rewarding.

TABLE 9.2. Differential Diagnosis of Anaplastic Carcinoma of Thyroid

I. Benign cells misinterpreted as anaplastic carcinoma

    Fibroblasts, eg, granulation tissue, stroma, granuloma
    Histiocytes
    Atypical follicular cells secondary to ^{131}I therapy
    Degenerating follicular cells

II. Malignant neoplasms misinterpreted as anaplastic carcinoma

    Medullary carcinoma
    Metastatic, poorly differentiated, malignant neoplasms to thyroid

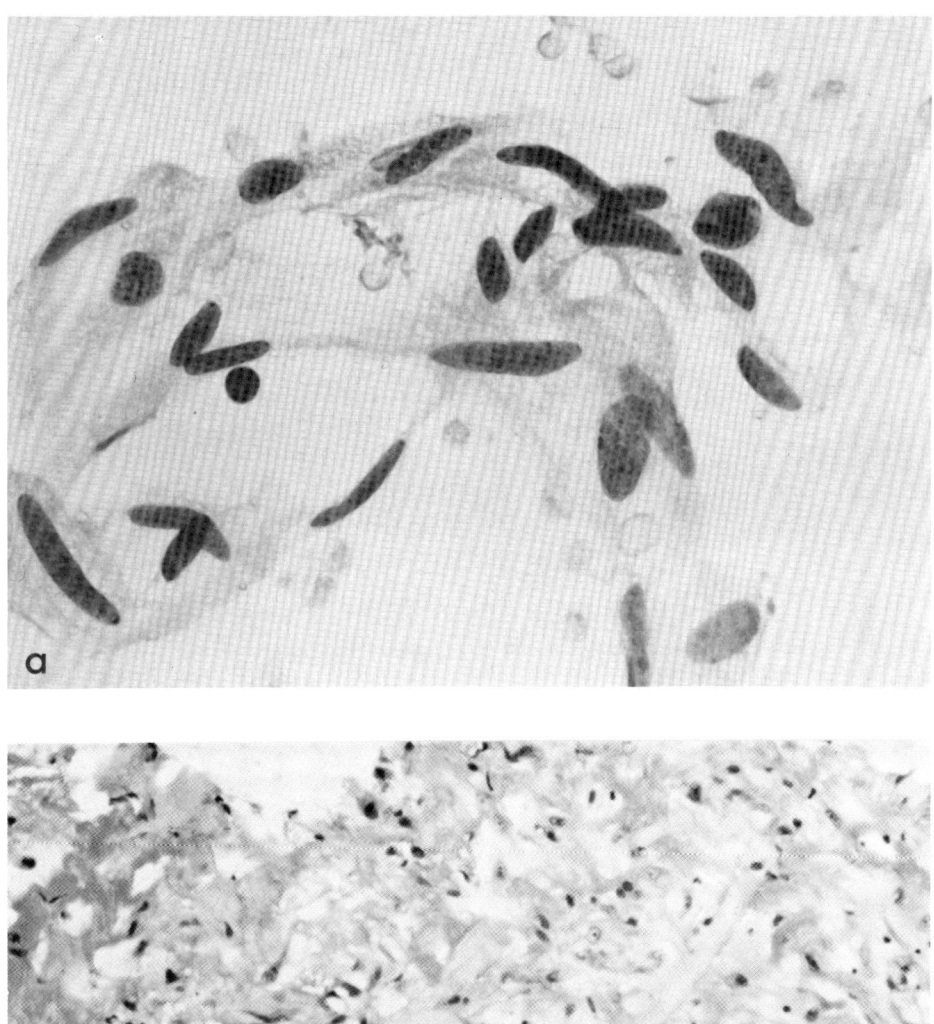

Fig. 9.13. A. Elongated spindle cells of fibroblastic origin, with long cytoplasmic processes. The nuclei are cigar shaped. The cells superficially resemble anaplastic carcinoma. The nuclei have a bland chromatin pattern. Papanicolaou preparation. × 630. **B.** Large-needle biopsy specimen showing granulation tissue. Hematoxylin and eosin preparation. × 160.

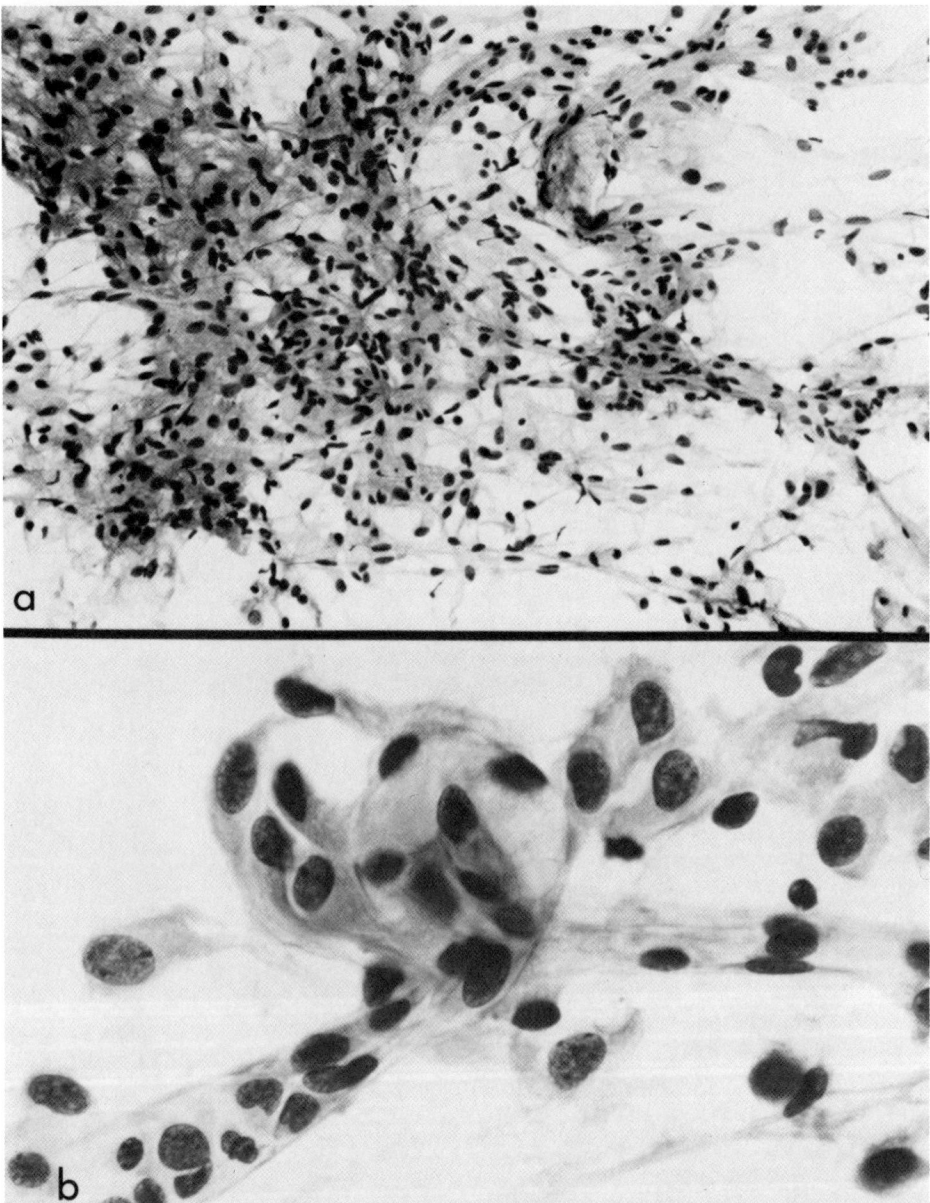

Fig. 9.14. A. Tissue fragments of proliferating fibroblasts resembling spindle cell carcinoma. Papanicolaou preparation. × 160. **B.** Although the nuclei are pleomorphic, the chromatin is rather bland. Papanicolaou preparation. × 630.

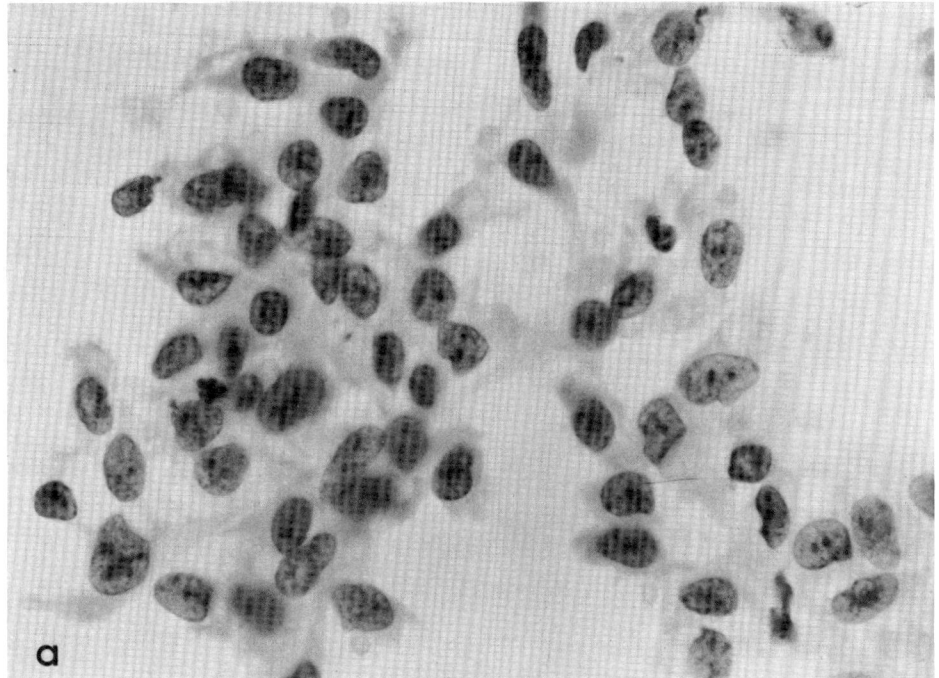

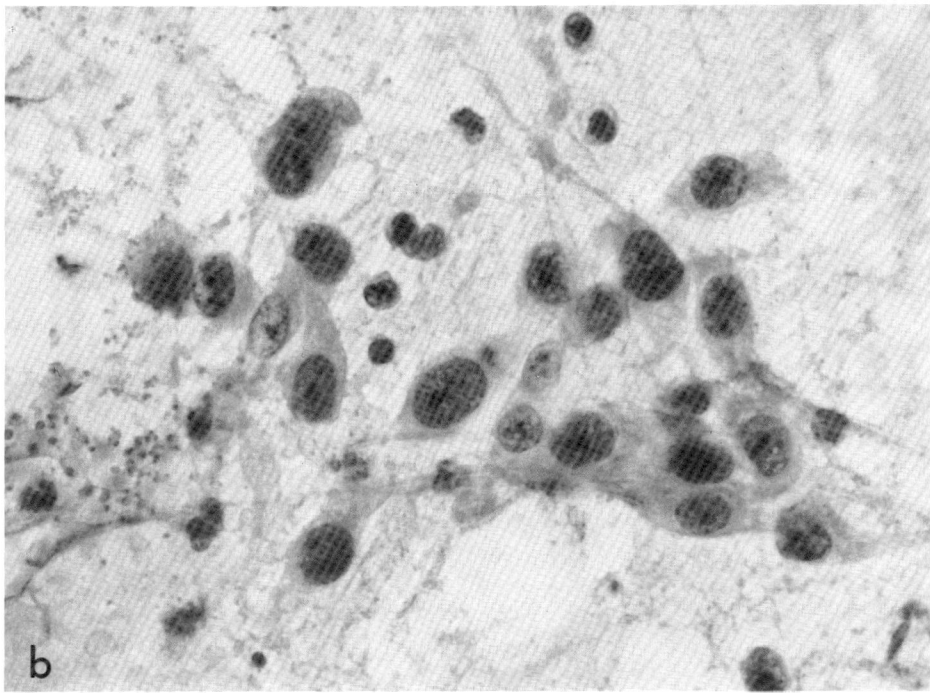

Fig. 9.15. Poorly cellular aspirate with only a few groups of pleomorphic giant and spindle cells. **A.** The nuclei are large with prominent macronucleoli. Cytologic diagnosis of anaplastic carcinoma was not consistent with the clinical findings in a 70-year-old patient with a history of lobectomy for nodular goiter. The excision of thyroid lobe showed only nodular goiter. The exact origin of these cells is not known, but they are thought to be fibroblasts. Papanicolaou preparation. × 630. **B.** Note similarity to anaplastic carcinoma cells. Papanicolaou preparation. × 630.

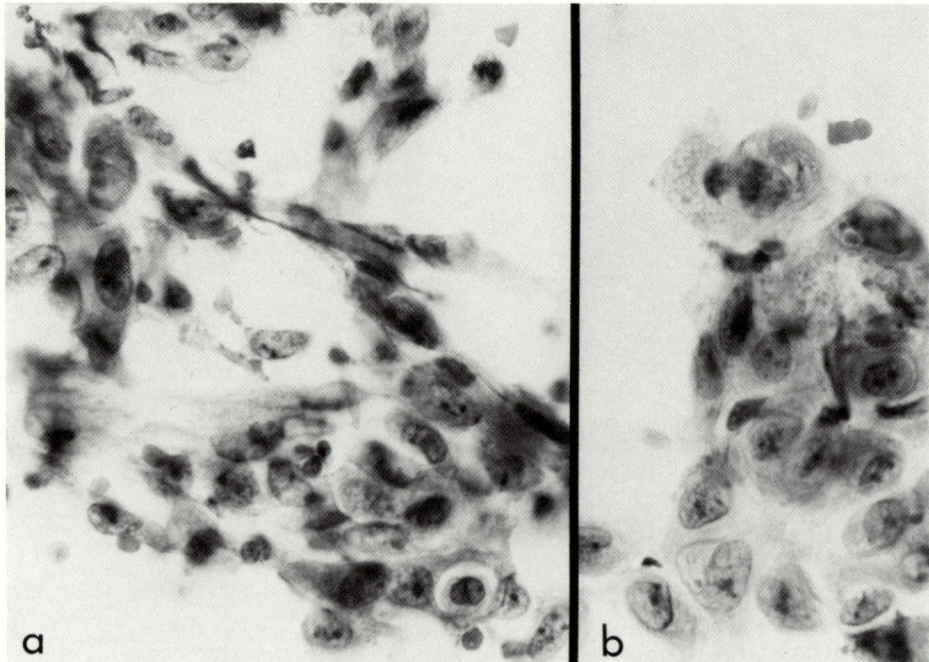

Fig. 9.16. A., B. Very pleomorphic cells, highly suggestive of anaplastic carcinoma, but believed to represent either histiocytes or fibroblasts. Thyroidectomy showed old hemorrhage and granulation tissue. Papanicolaou preparation. × 630.

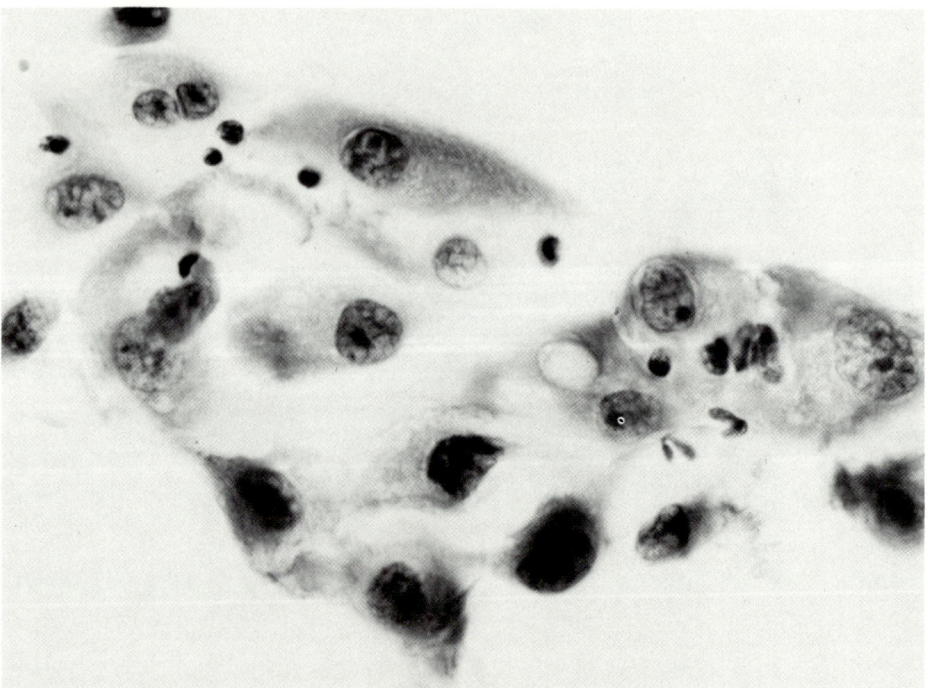

Fig. 9.17. Pleomorphic follicular cells with bizarre nuclei. The patient had 131 I therapy for Graves' disease. Without taking the clinical history into account, these cells may be misinterpreted as anaplastic carcinoma. Papanicolaou preparation. × 630.

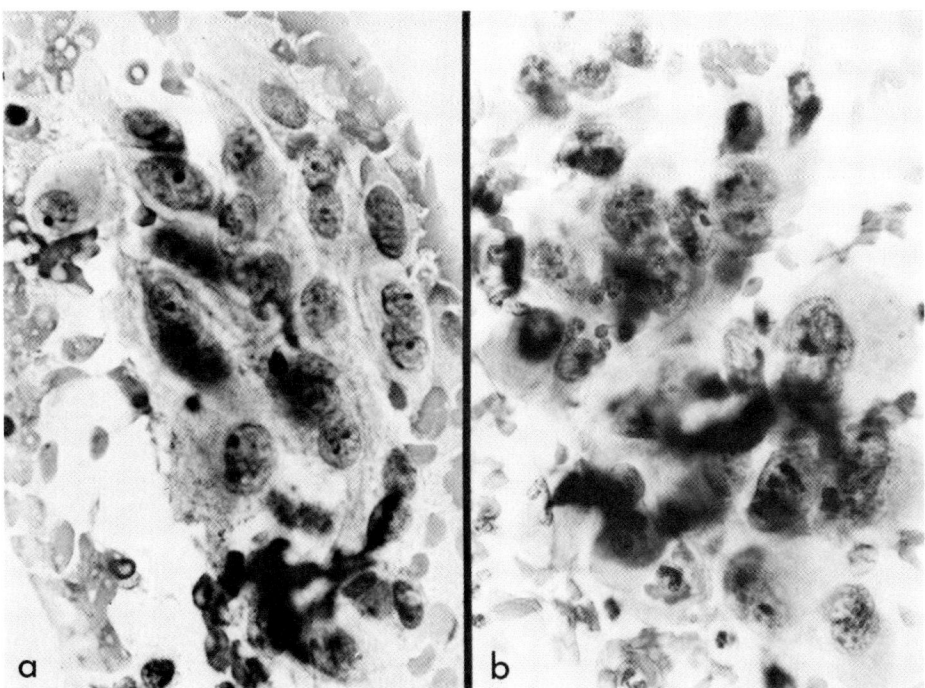

Fig. 9.18. A. Thyroid cells from the vicinity of an infarcted nodule. Papanicolaou preparation. × 630. **B.** Anaplastic carcinoma cells. Papanicolaou preparation. × 630. The two cell types are virtually indistinguishable.

REFERENCES

1. Albores-Saavedra J, Nadji M, Civantos F, Morales AR: Thyroglobulin in carcinoma of the thyroid: an immunohistochemical study. *Hum Pathol* 14:62–66, 1983.

2. Aldinger KA, Samaan NA, Ibanez M, Hill CS Jr: Anaplastic carcinoma of the thyroid: a review of 84 cases of spindle and giant cell carcinoma of the thyroid. *Cancer* 41:2267–2275, 1978.

3. Burt AD, Kerr DJ, Brown IL, Boyle P: Lymphoid and epithelial markers in small cell anaplastic thyroid tumors. *J Clin Pathol* 38:893–896, 1985.

4. Cameron RG, Seemayer TA, Wang NS, Almed MN, Tabah E: Small cell malignant tumors of the thyroid: a light and electron microscopic study. *Hum Pathol* 6:731–740, 1975.

5. Carcangiu ML, Steeper T, Zampi G, Rosai J: Anaplastic thyroid carcinoma. *Am J Clin Pathol* 83:135–158, 1985.

6. Esmaili JM, Hafez GR, Warner TFCS: Anaplastic carcinoma of the thyroid with osteoclast-like giant cells. *Cancer* 52:2112–2128, 1983.

7. Hashimoto H, Koga S, Watanabe H, Enjojl M: Undifferentiated carcinoma of the thyroid gland with osteoclast-like giant cells. *Acta Pathol Jpn* 30:323–334, 1980.

8. Kapp DS, Livolsi VA, Sanders ME: Anaplastic carcinoma: etiological considerations. *Yale J Biol Med* 55:521–528, 1982.

9. Kruseman ACN, Bosman FT, Henegouw JCV, Cramer-Knijnenberg G, Dela Reviera GB: Medullary differentiation of anaplastic thyroid carcinoma. *Am J Clin Pathol* 77:541–547, 1982.

10. Mambo NC, Irwin S: Anaplastic small cell neoplasms of the thyroid: an immunoperoxidase study. *Hum Pathol* 15:55–60, 1964.

11. McConahey WM, Taylor WF, Gorman CA, Woolner LB: Retrospective study of 820 patients treated for papillary carcinoma of the thyroid at the Mayo Clinic between 1946 and 1971. In Andreoli M, Monaco F, Robbins J: *Advances in Thyroid Neoplasia*. Rome, Field Educational Italia, 1981, pp. 245–262.

12. Meissner WA: *Tumors of the Thyroid Gland*. Second Series, Fasicle 4, Supplement. Washington, DC, Armed Forces Institute of Pathology, 1984, pp. 531–532.

13. Nel CJC, Van Heerden JA, Goellner JR, et al: Anaplastic carcinoma of the thyroid: a clinicopathologic study of 82 cases. *Mayo Clin Proc* 60:51–58, 1985.

14. Nishiyama RH, Dunn LL, and Thompson NW: Anaplastic spindle cell and giant cell tumors of the thyroid gland. *Cancer* 30:113–127, 1972.

15. Rayfield EJ, Nishiyama RH, Sisson JC: Small cell tumors of the thyroid: a clinicopathologic study. *Cancer* 28:1023–1030, 1971.

16. Schneider V, Frable WJ: Spindle and giant cell carcinoma of the thyroid. *Acta Cytol* 24:184–189, 1980.

17. Willems JS, Löwhagen T, Palombini L: The cytology of a giant cell osteoclastoma-like malignant thyroid neoplasm: a case report. *Acta Cytol* 23:214–216, 1979.

10
Medullary Carcinoma

Medullary carcinoma of thyroid arises from calcitonin-producing cells known as C-cells, clear cells, or parafollicular cells[23] (Figs. 10.1 and 10.2). In 1951, Horn[6] recognized this carcinoma as a separate entity from other differentiated carcinomas of thyroid by noting the differences in histologic patterns and biological behavior. In 1959, the term "medullary carcinoma" was coined by Hazard et al,[5] who identified the amyloid in the stroma of this neoplasm. Since then, medullary carcinoma has continued to arouse interest, and many advances have been made in understanding this disease.

Medullary carcinomas reportedly comprise 3.5–10% of all thyroid carcinomas.[1,4,11,22,25] Roughly 10–15% occur in patients who have a genetically mediated syndrome transmitted as an autosomal dominant trait. Familial medullary carcinoma may be seen in several members of a family. This carcinoma may be also associated with other endocrine tumors.[11,20,24] It is seen in patients of all ages, but is most common between the third and fifth decades. The incidence is slightly higher in women.

Medullary carcinoma of thyroid is characterized by high levels of serum calcitonin, which serves as the most sensitive indicator of its presence. In its early stages, this tumor metastasizes to the lymph nodes and to distant organs. Its biological behavior is more aggressive than that of other differentiated carcinomas of thyroid.

PATHOLOGY

Grossly, medullary carcinoma presents as a sharply defined, round, firm, non-encapsulated lesion (Fig. 10.3). Williams[22] has described its microscopic pathology in great detail. Recognized patterns, which may be seen alone or in combination (Fig. 10.4), include:

207

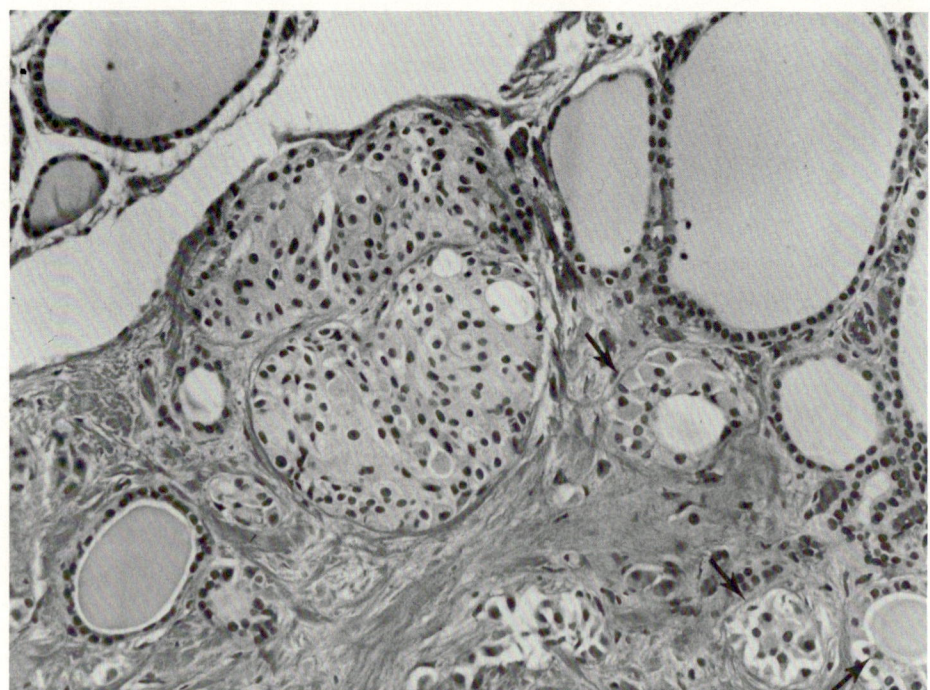

Fig. 10.1. Section of a thyroid from a familial medullary carcinoma showing C-cell hyperplasia *(arrow)*. Hematoxylin and eosin preparation. × 157.

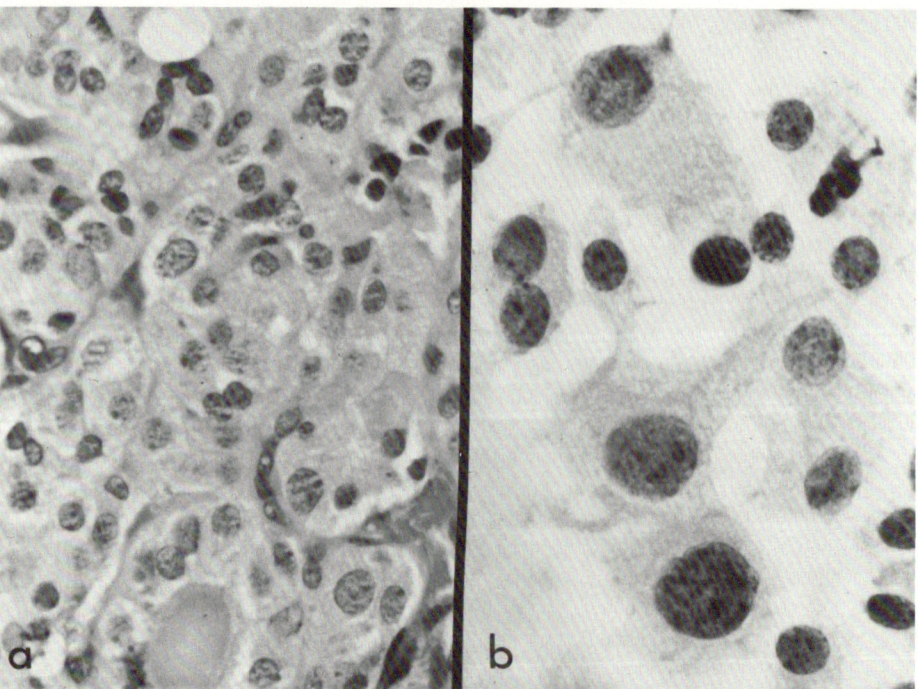

Fig. 10.2. A. Higher magnification of C-cells from Fig. 10.1. Note large cells with abundant cytoplasm and eccentric nuclei. Hematoxylin and eosin preparation. × 400. **B.** Imprint of the surgical specimen showing discrete C-cells with plasmacytoid appearance. Papanicolaou preparation. × 630.

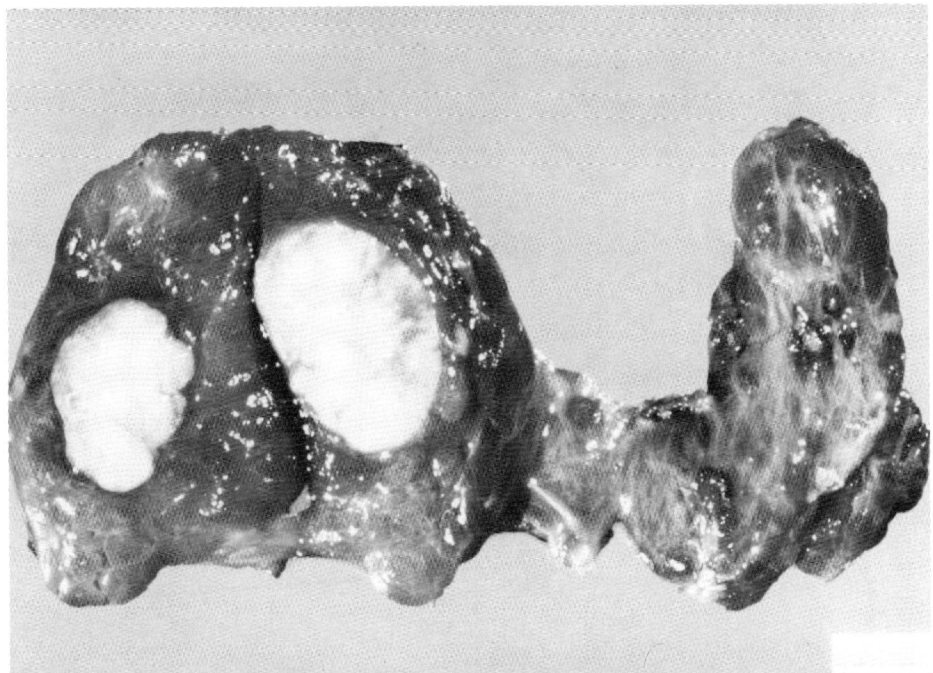

Fig. 10.3. Medullary carcinoma of the thyroid involving the right lobe. Note discrete, well demarcated tumor.

1. Carcinoid type, consisting of nests of small, round to cuboidal cells with scanty cytoplasm
2. Organoid pattern, characterized by masses of polyhedral cells with abundant clear to pale cytoplasm
3. Spindle cell pattern

Unusual patterns include papillary type, anaplastic variants, giant cell type, and mixed follicular and medullary carcinomas.[5,8,9,13,14,16] Psammoma bodies have also been described.

Medullary carcinoma cells are separated by variable stroma containing amyloid, which shows green birefringence under cross-polarized light when stained by Congo red; or green fluorescence under ultraviolet light when stained by thioflavin T. Since the advent of immunohistochemistry, calcitonin granules in the cytoplasm can be demonstrated by the immunoperoxidase staining technique (Fig. 10.5A). A detailed study of immunohistochemical features was reported by Uribe et al.[21] Ultrastructurally, the cytoplasm of medullary carcinoma cells demonstrates electron-dense granules[7] (Fig. 10.5B).

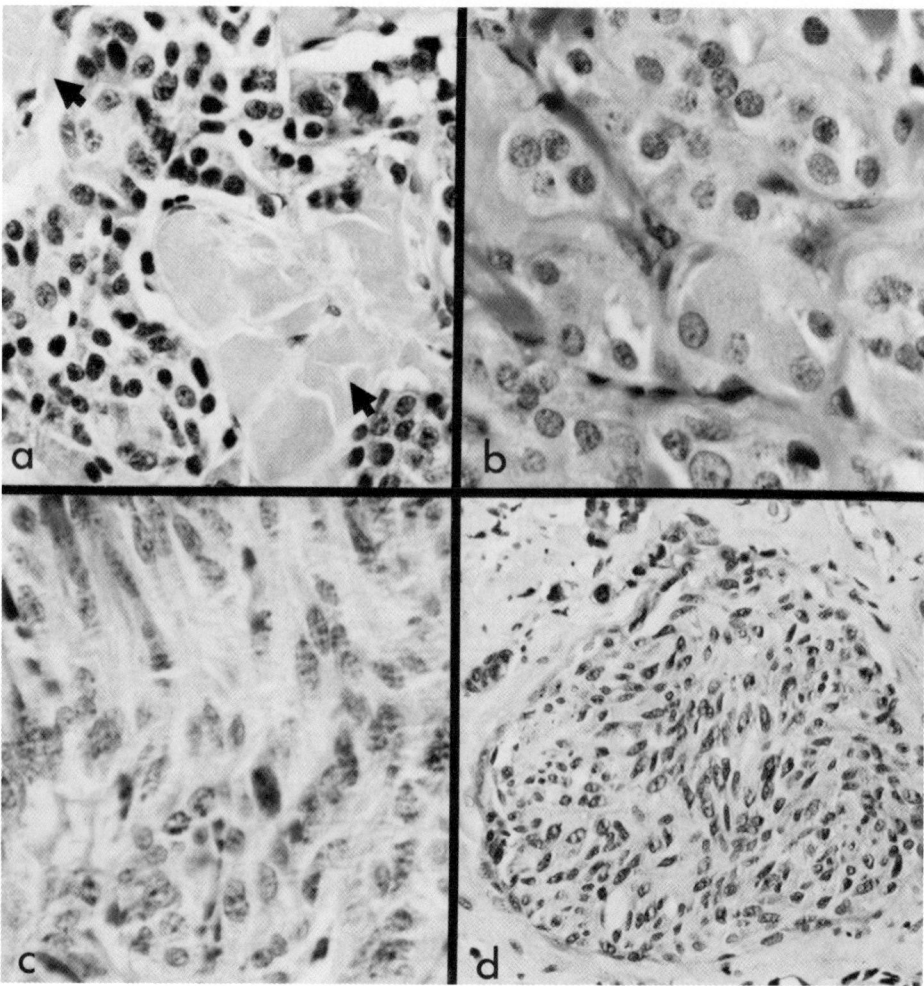

Fig. 10.4. Histologic patterns of medullary carcinoma. **A.** Small round cells. Note stromal amyloid. *(arrow)*. Hematoxylin and eosin preparation. × 400. **B.** Large oval to polygonal cells with abundant cytoplasm and eccentric nuclei. Hematoxylin and eosin preparation. × 400. **C.** Spindle cell pattern. Hematoxylin and eosin preparation. × 400. **D.** Nest of spindle and small round cells. Hematoxylin and eosin preparation. × 250.

CYTOPATHOLOGY

The cytopathologic features of medullary carcinoma vary depending on the histology; they are monomorphic if only one pattern is evident and pleomorphic if a combination of different patterns is seen[10] (Table 10.1).

The smear of an aspirate from medullary carcinoma of thyroid generally shows cancer cells, either isolated or in loosely cohesive groups (Fig. 10.6). Syncytial-type

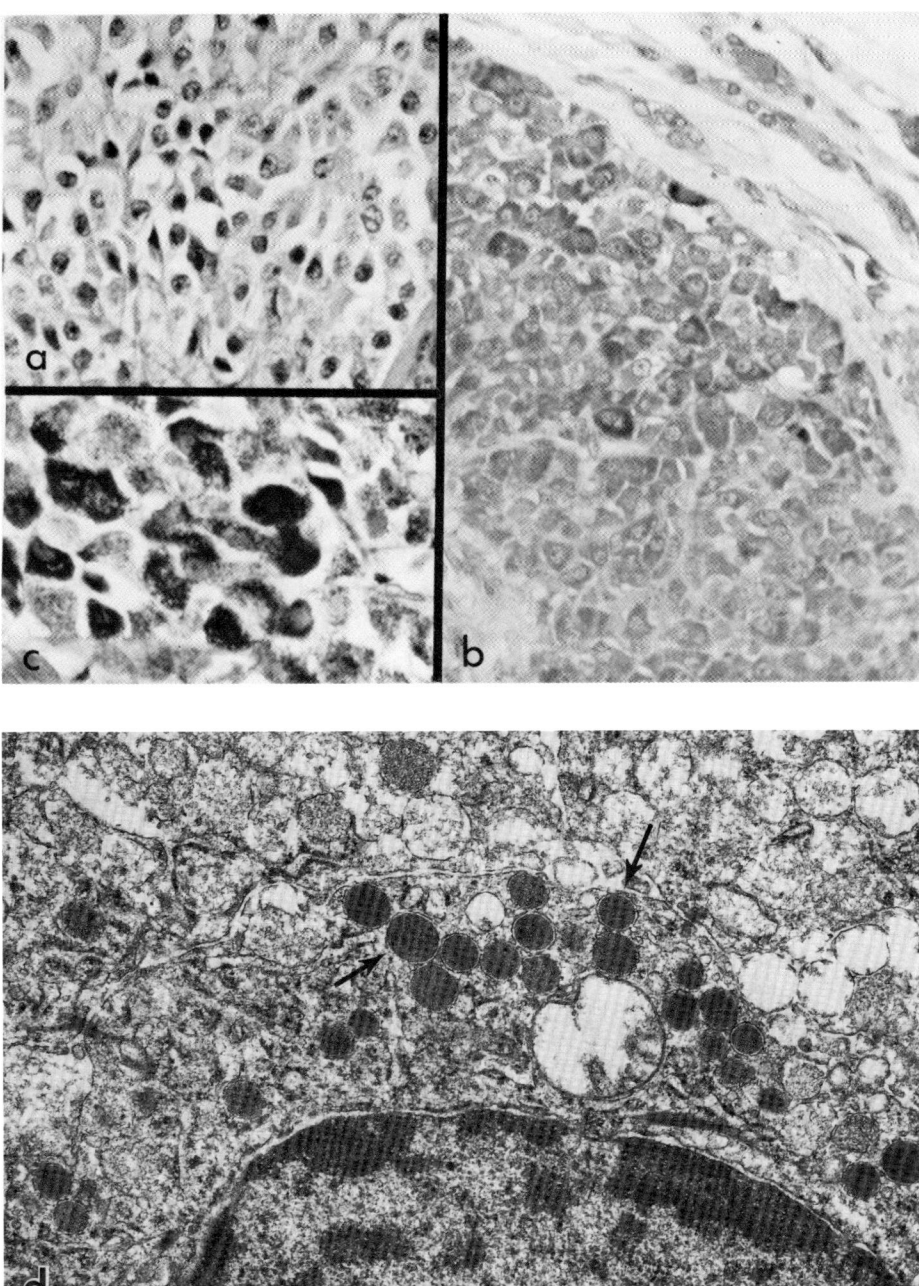

Fig. 10.5. A. Medullary thyroid carcinoma with polygonal cell pattern. Hematoxylin and eosin preparation. × 400. **B.** Calcitonin granules in cytoplasm, stained by immunoperoxidase technique. Avidin Biotin Complex method and Hematoxylin preparation. × 250. **C.** Higher magnification of **B**. Immunoperoxidase stain for calcitonin. Avidin Biotin Complex method and Hematoxylin preparation. × 400. **D.** Electron micrograph of medullary carcinoma showing spherical calcitonin granules with an electron-dense core and well-defined limiting membrane *(arrow)*. Uranyl acetate and lead citrate preparation. × 42,000.

211

TABLE 10.1. Cytopathologic Features of Medullary Carcinoma of Thyroid

Pattern	Isolated cells, loosely cohesive cell groups, or syncytial-type tissue fragments without follicular or papillary configuration; cell pattern monomorphic or pleomorphic
Cells	Varied types: small, round, cuboidal, oval to plasmacytoid, polygonal, racket shaped, triangular, or spindle; size variable
Nucleus	Round, oval, cigar shaped; occasionally multilobulated, giant, and bizarre; *always eccentric*; bi- and multinucleation common
	Chromatin coarsely granular; nucleoli inconsistent
	Intranuclear cytoplasmic inclusions
Cytoplasm	Pale, fibrillar, variable in amount, often drawn into delicate processes
	Intracytoplasmic calcitonin granules: stain pink in Romanowsky stain preparations, or are demonstrated by immunoperoxidase technique
Background	Extracellular amyloid: special stains necessary for confirmation

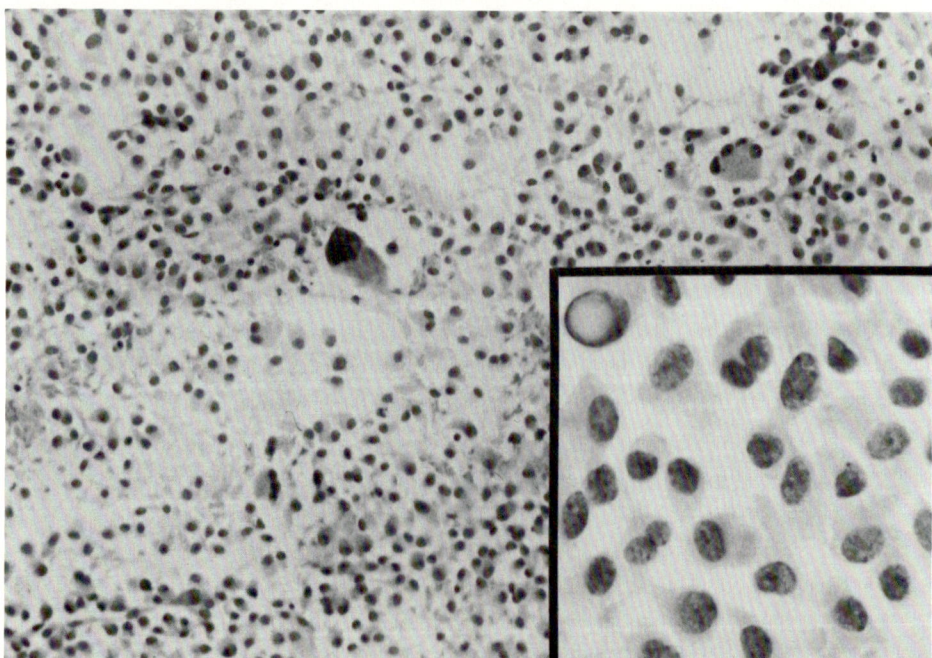

Fig. 10.6. Cellular smear showing discrete, isolated cells. Papanicolaou preparation. × 160.
Inset: Higher magnification. Papanicolaou preparation. × 630.

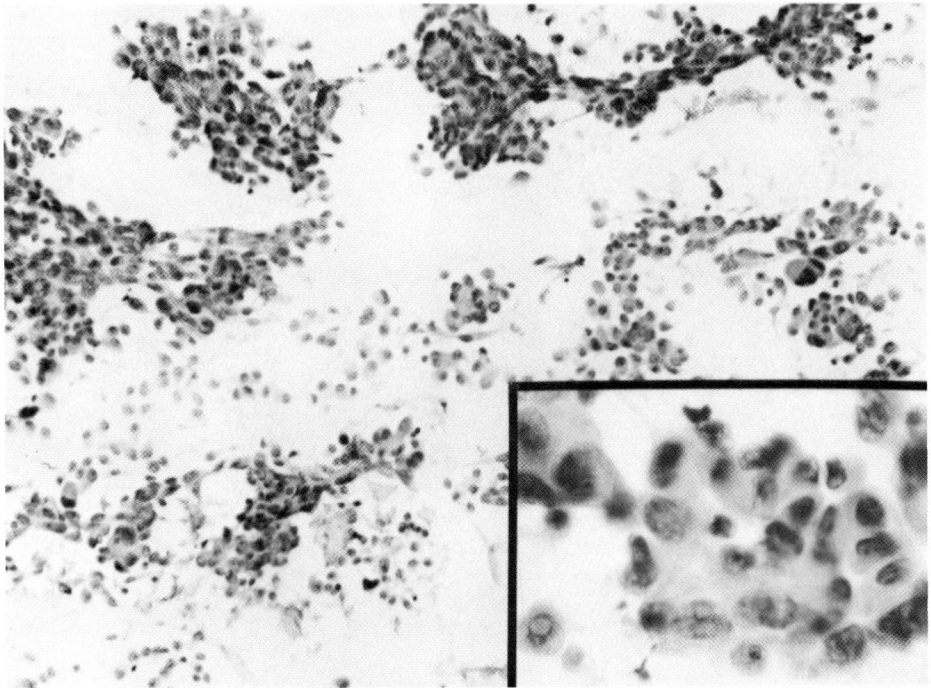

Fig. 10.7. Several syncytial-type tissue fragments of medullary carcinoma cells. This is an unusual pattern. Papanicolaou preparation. × 160. *Inset:* Higher magnification showing lack of architectural pattern. Papanicolaou preparation. × 630.

tissue fragments are infrequent (Fig. 10.7), and a papillary or follicular pattern is not identified. However, a pseudofollicular pattern may rarely be seen (Fig. 10.8).

Medullary carcinoma cells are very pleomorphic; any size or shape may be identified (Fig. 10.9). The carcinoma cells can be small, round to cuboidal, reminiscent of carcinoid cells, or oval to plasmacytoid. They may be triangular,polyhedral, racket shaped, or spindle shaped. Their size also varies: the small round cells are slightly larger than the follicular cells, and the larger cells are several microns in their largest dimension (Fig. 10.10). A pleomorphic cell pattern with different shapes and sizes is more commonly seen and is diagnostic of medullary carcinoma (Figs. 10.10 and 10.11), whereas a monomorphic pattern comprising only one type of cell is not frequently observed (Fig. 10.12).

The nuclei of medullary carcinoma cells are always eccentric, regardless of shape, cell size, or number of nuclei. Extreme marginal location of the nucleus is characteristic of the plasmacytoid cell type, and bi- and multinucleation occurs very frequently (Fig. 10.9) The nuclei are round, sometimes oval, and occasionally ovoid or elongated in spindle-shaped cells. Their chromatin is coarse. The presence of nucleoli is not a consistent finding. Bizarre nuclei, such as those seen in anaplastic

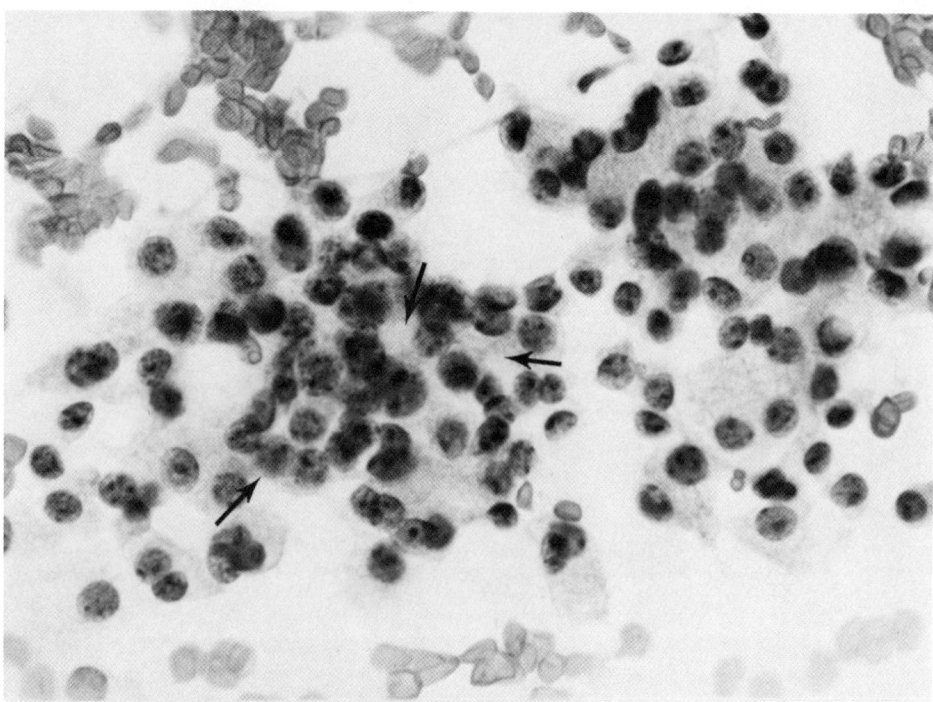

Fig. 10.8. Fine-needle biopsy specimen of medullary carcinoma showing pseudofollicular pattern *(arrows)*. The carcinoma cells are small and round, with scanty cytoplasm resembling carcinoid tumor. Papanicolaou preparation. × 630.

carcinomas, are rare (Fig. 10.13). A remarkable and consistent feature is the presence of intranuclear cytoplasmic inclusions[10,18] (Fig. 10.14).

The cytoplasm of medullary carcinoma cells is variable. In small round cells, it is very scant and hardly discernible, whereas in plasmacytoid or large polyhedral cells it is abundant (Fig. 10.10). It generally stains pale and has a fibrillar quality (Fig. 10.15). The cytoplasm is often drawn out in a delicate process, which may be rudimentary in cuboidal cells, uni- or bipolar in spindle cells, or multiple in triangular or polyhedral cells (Fig. 10.15). Söderström et al[19] called these dendritic processes. A group of spindle cells with delicate intertwined cytoplasmic processes is a characteristic finding in smears from medullary carcinoma (Fig. 10.11).

Another feature of diagnostic importance is the presence of azurophilic granules in the cytoplasm of medullary carcinoma cells. These are seen only in air-dried preparations stained by the Romanowsky method[12,15,19] (Plate 10.1). They are not stained by the Papanicolaou method. These granules are present in about 5–10% of the cell population and probably represent cytoplasmic calcitonin. The latter can be specifically demonstrated by the immunoperoxidase technique (Plate 10.2).

One of the characteristic features of medullary carcinoma is the presence of stromal amyloid. It can be seen in cytologic preparations as fluffy, finely granular, or dense acellular material in the background (Plate 10.3). The amyloid has the same staining characteristics as the colloid in Papanicolaou-stained preparations and cannot be

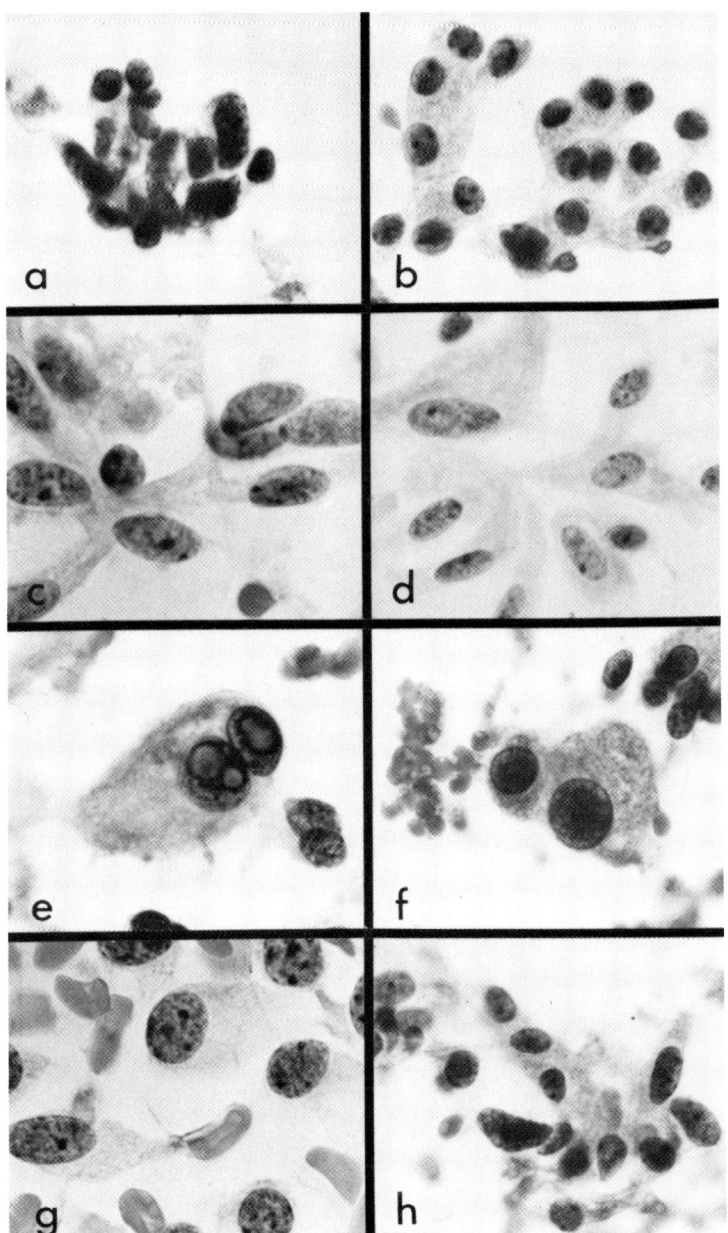

Fig. 10.9. Various types of cells seen in medullary carcinoma. **A.** Small cells with dense nuclei and scanty cytoplasm. Papanicolaou preparation. × 630. **B.** Small cuboidal cells. Papanicolaou preparation. × 630. **C.** Short spindle-shaped cells with plump nuclei. Papanicolaou preparation. × 630. **D.** Delicate spindle-shaped cells with cytoplasmic processes. Papanicolaou preparation. × 630. **E.** Large oval cell with binucleation and intranuclear cytoplasmic inclusions. Papanicolaou preparation. × 630. **F.** Triangular cells and small, round carcinoid-type cells. Papanicolaou preparation. × 630. **G.** Plasmacytoid cells with rudimentary cytoplasmic process. Papanicolaou preparation. × 630. **H.** Medium-sized cuboidal and oval cells with eccentric nuclei and cytoplasmic processes. Papanicolaou preparation. × 630. Note that, regardless of the shape of the cells, the nuclei are always eccentric. The chromatin is very coarse.

215

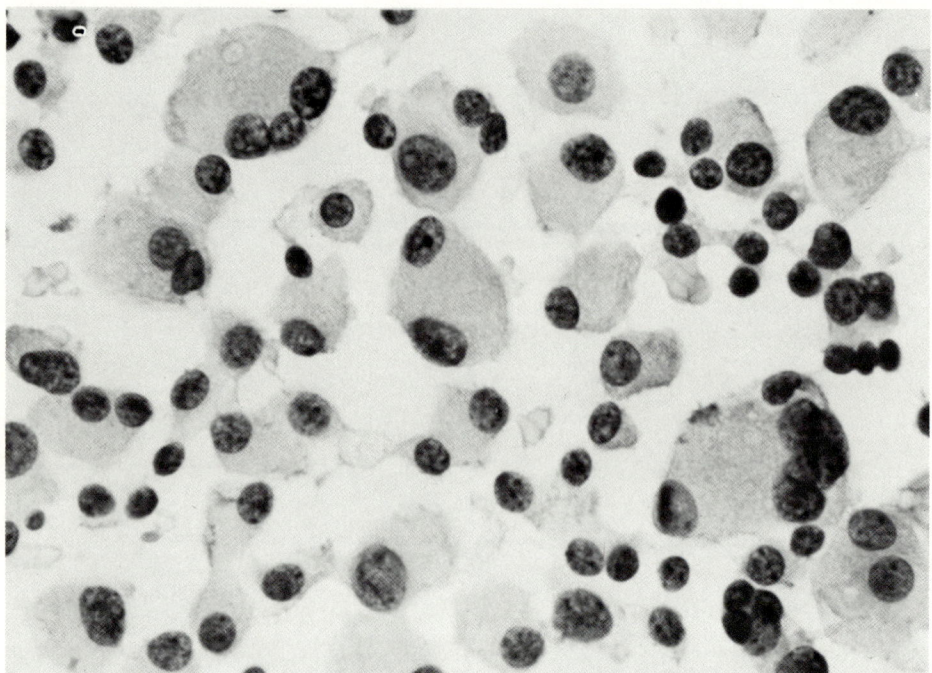

Fig. 10.10. Medulary carcinoma cells showing marked pleomorphism in size and shape. Note the admixture of carcinoid type cells, plasmacytoid cells, polyhedral and triangular cells with eccentric nuclei, and multinucleation. Papanicolaou preparation. × 630.

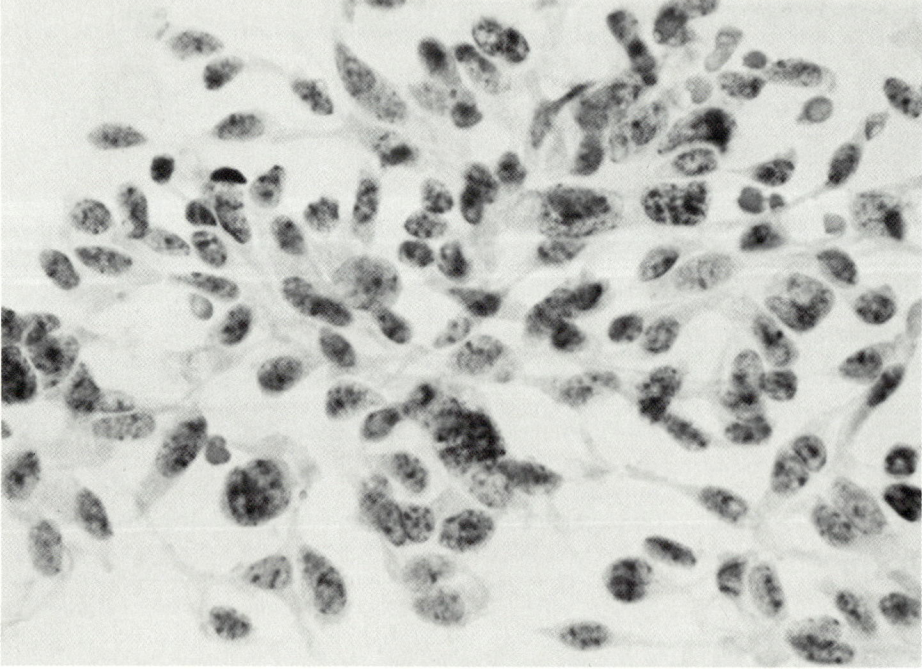

Fig. 10.11. Medullary carcinoma showing predominantly spindle-shaped cells, with delicate cytoplasmic processes sprinkled with round cells. Papanicolaou preparation. × 630.

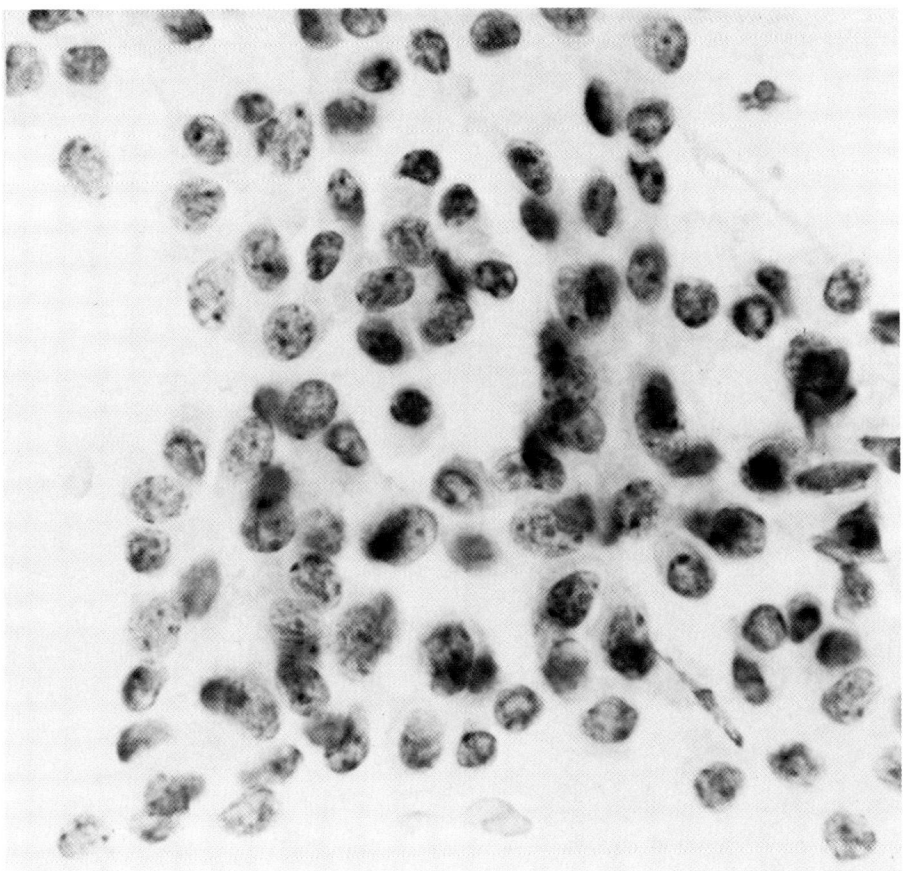

Fig. 10.12. Medullary carcinoma with cuboidal cells presenting a monomorphic pattern. Papanicolaou preparation. × 630.

differentiated from it without special stains such as Congo red or thioflavin T (Plate 10.3). Although the presence of intracellular amyloid has been described by Söderström and colleagues, it is not appreciated by Papanicolaou stain. The use of special stains to identify amyloid in cytologic preparations is time-consuming and not recommended.

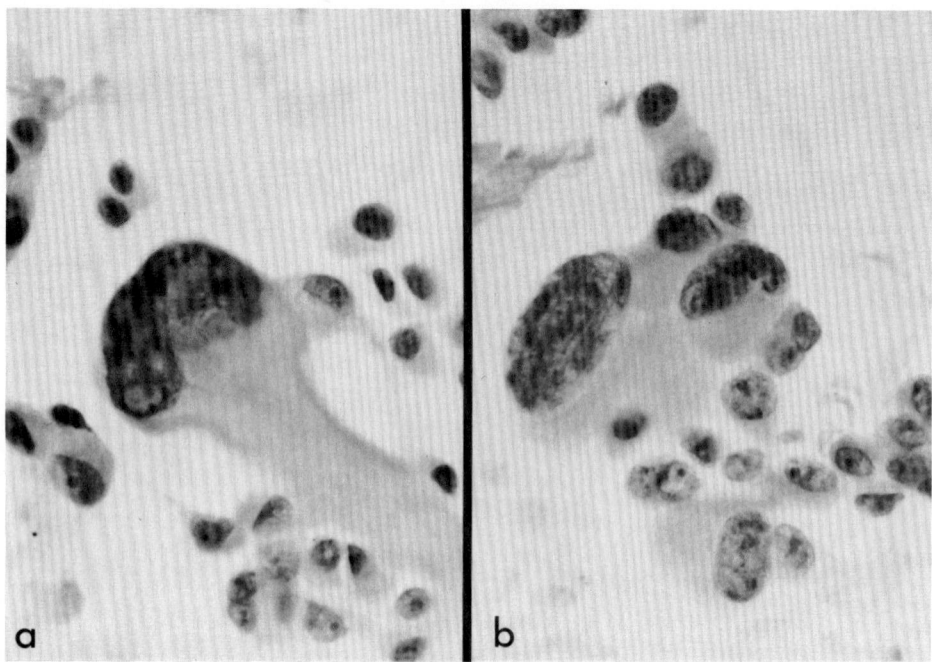

Fig. 10.13. A., B. Medullary carcinoma cells with bizarre nuclei. Note presence of large nucleoli. Papanicolaou preparation. × 630.

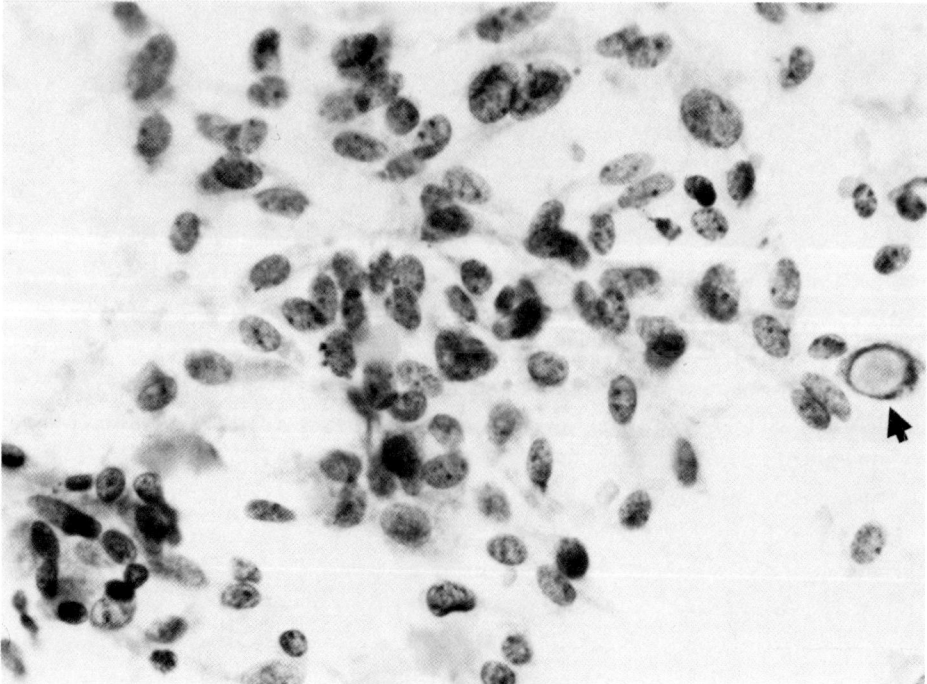

Fig. 10.14. Medulllary carcinoma cells with pleomorphic cell pattern. Note large intranuclear cytoplasmic inclusions *(arrow)*. Papanicolaou preparation. × 630.

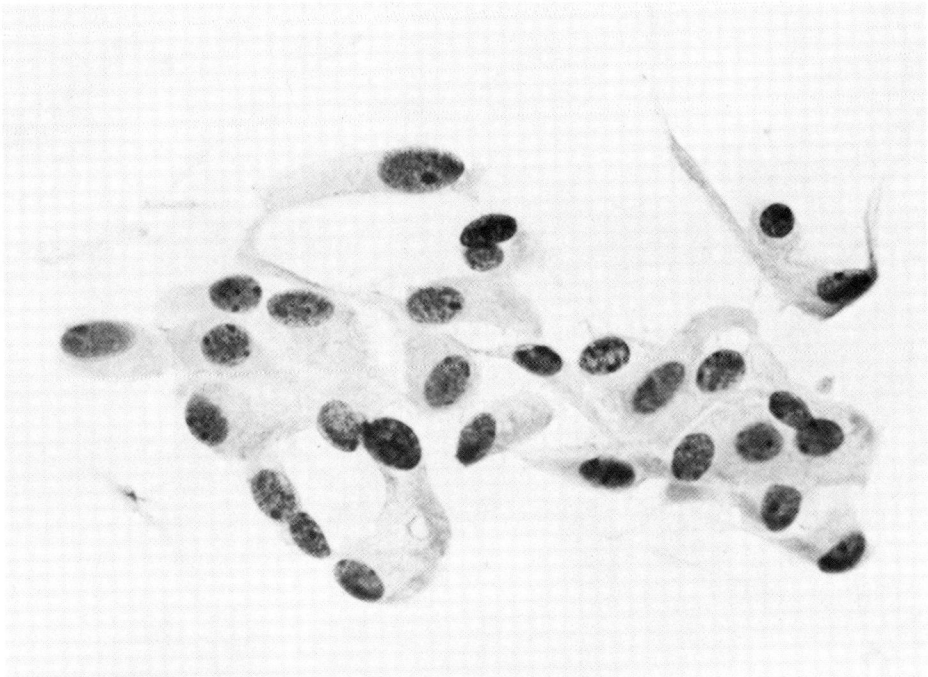

Fig. 10.15. Medullary carcinoma cells with abundant and fibrillar cytoplasm with cytoplasmic processes. Papanicolaou preparation. × 630.

DIAGNOSTIC ACCURACY

In our 9 years of experience with fine-needle aspirates of the thyroid nodules, 571 cases were diagnosed as primary thyroid malignancies by surgery, of which 27 (45%) were medullary carcinomas. Of these 27 cases, 20 were accurately typed from cytologic specimens. Three were interpreted as undifferentiated carcinoma, one as follicular variant of papillary carcinoma, and two as cellular follicular adenomas (Table 10.2). Typing errors are generally due to inexperience and unfamiliarity with the varied cytopathologic features of medullary carcinoma. Our errors were made within the first 2 years of our experience interpreting with biopsy specimens.

Medullary carcinoma also tends to be overdiagnosed cytologically. The monomorphic cell population of Hürthle cell carcinomas, the single cell pattern in papillary carcinomas, and the spindle cells in anaplastic carcinomas all may be mistaken for medullary carcinoma. In our series, 33 cases were typed cytologically as medullary carcinoma, of which 20 were confirmed, 8 were diagnosed as Hürthle cell carcinoma, 4 as papillary carcinoma, and 1 as nodular goiter (Table 10.2). A cytologic diagnosis of medullary carcinoma must be confirmed by other means, such as:

1. Immunoperoxidase stain for calcitonin granules
2. Large-needle biopsy (size permitting)[3,17]
3. Serum calcitonin levels

TABLE 10.2. Cytohistologic Correlation of Medullary Carcinoma of Thyroid

| | Histologic Diagnosis | | | |
| | Medullary Carcinoma | Hürthle Cell Carcinoma | Papillary Carcinoma | Nodular Goiter |
Cytologic Diagnoses	(n = 27)	(n = 8)	(n = 4)	(n = 1)
Medullary carcinoma	20	8	4	1
Hürthle cell carcinoma	0	0	0	0
Undifferentiated carcinoma	3	0	0	0
Papillary carcinoma	1	0	0	0
Follicular adenoma	2	0	0	0
Acellular	1	0	0	0

The immunoperoxidase stain for calcitonin performed on cytologic samples is quite specific. In our last 10 cases, it correlated 100% with increased serum calcitonin levels, as well as with histologic findings.

DIAGNOSTIC DIFFICULTIES IN MEDULLARY CARCINOMA AND DIFFERENTIAL DIAGNOSIS

A frequently encountered pleomorphic cell pattern is diagnostic of medullary carcinoma (Fig. 10.10 and 10.11). A monomorphic pattern, comprised of only one type of cell, is not common. It may be mistaken for other types of thyroid neoplasms, and vice versa (Table 10.3). Neoplasms such as Hürthle cell carcinomas are often confused with medullary carcinoma.

TABLE 10.3. Differential Diagnosis of Medullary Carcinoma

1. Hürthle cell carcinoma
2. Papillary carcinoma (single cell pattern)
3. Follicular neoplasms
4. Anaplastic carcinoma
5. Stromal cells in nodular goiter

Medullary Carcinoma Versus Hürthle Cell Carcinoma

In our experience, cells aspirated from some Hürthle cell carcinomas exhibit a morphologic resemblance to plasmacytoid cells of medullary carcinoma (Figs. 10.16–10.19; Table 10.4). This observation is shared by Söderström et al[19], but not by Geddie et al.[2] However, Söderström and colleagues[19] believed that the distinction between a Hürthle cell neoplasm and a medullary thyroid carcinoma could be made easily by the dusty, blue granulation of Hürthle cells in Romanowsky-stained preparations and the cytoplasmic pink granules of medullary carcinoma cells. Aprominent cherry-red macronucleolus favors the diagnosis of Hürthle cell carcinoma. Whenever an aspirate shows a monomorphic pattern of oval to plasmacytoid cells without other cytologic features of medullary carcinoma or Hürthle cell carcinoma, it is prudent to recommend tests to rule out medullary carcinoma.

TABLE 10.4. Differentiating Features Between Hürthle Cell Carcinoma and Medullary Carcinoma

Features	Hürthle Cell Carcinoma	Medullary Carcinoma
General pattern	Single cells	Single cells
Cell shape	Oval to plasmacytoid	Oval to plasmacytoid
Size	Variable	Variable
Cell borders	Well defined	Poorly defined
Cytoplasm	Granular or dense	Pale or fibrillar
Bi- and multinucleation	Common	Common
Eccentric location of nuclei	Common	Consistent
Nuclear chromatin	Finely granular	Coarsely granular
Intranuclear cytoplasmic inclusions	Rare	Always present
Colloid	May be present	Absent
Amyloid	Absent	Present
Romanowsky-stained preparation	Blue dusty	Azurophilic
	Granules in cytoplasm	Granules in cytoplasm
Immunoperoxidase stain for calcitonin	Negative	Positive

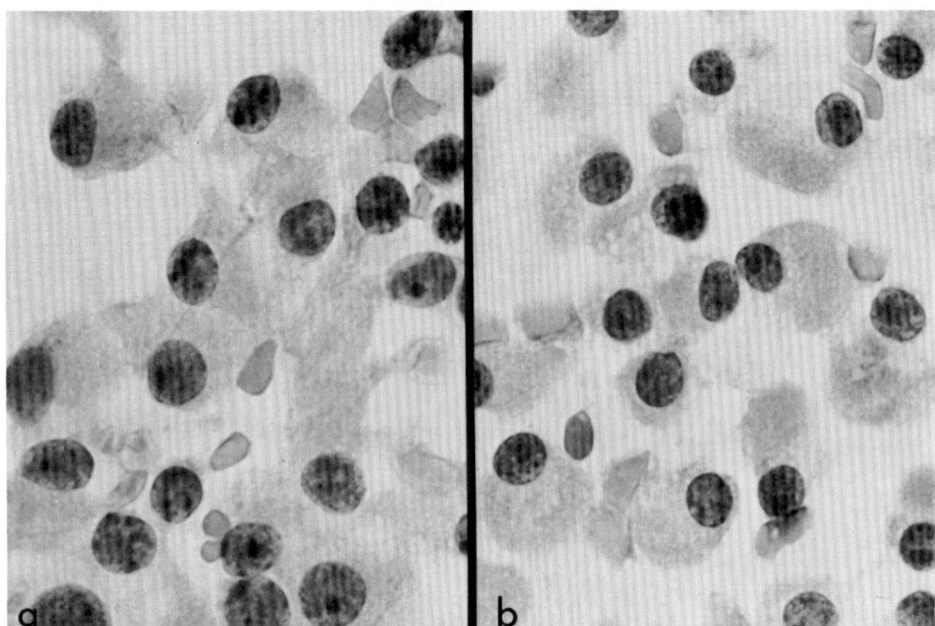

Fig. 10.16. A. Hürthle cell carcinoma. Papanicolaou preparation. × 630. **B.** Medullary carcinoma. Papanicolaou preparation. × 630. Hürthle cells are virtually indistinguishable from medullary carcinoma cells.

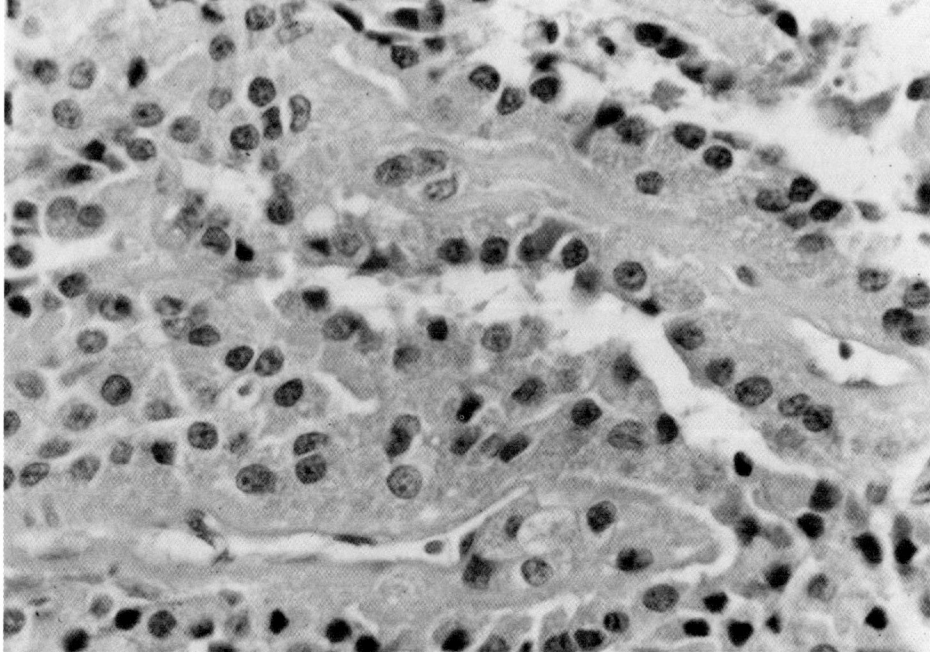

Fig. 10.17. Histologic section of Fig. 10.16 **A**, which was equally difficult to interpret and was misdiagnosed as medullary carcinoma. Serum calcitonin levels were within normal limits. Hematoxylin and eosin preparation. × 400.

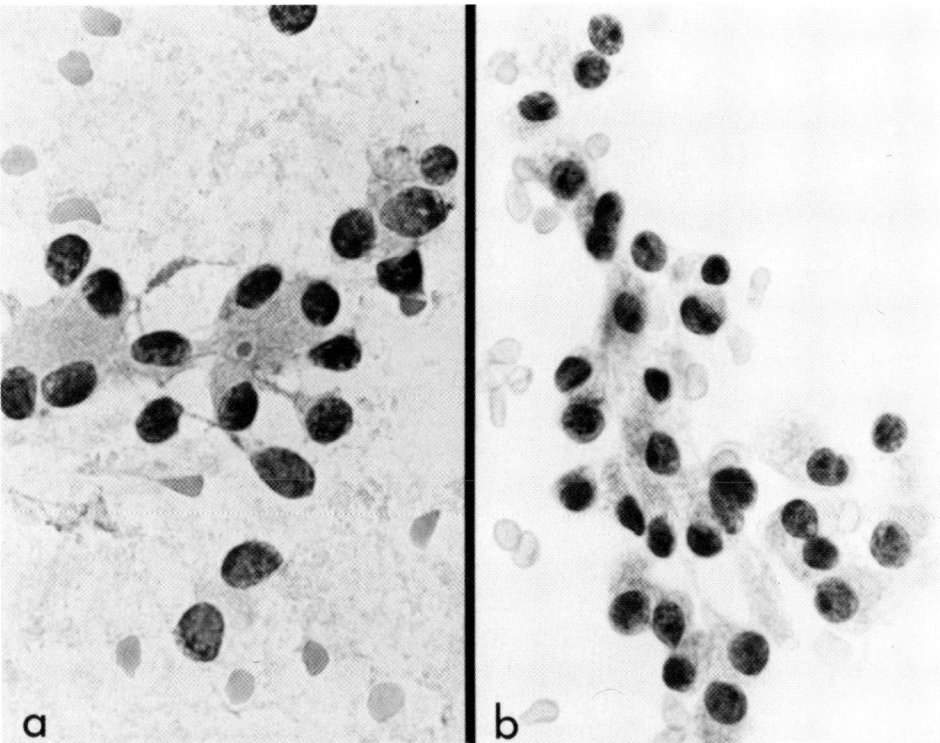

Fig. 10.18. A. Hürthle cell carcinoma. Papanicolaou preparation. × 630. **B.** Medullary carcinoma. Papanicolaou preparation. × 630. Hürthle cells in **A** did not show macronucleolei due to partial air-drying. Note the strong resemblance to medullary carcinoma cells in **B**.

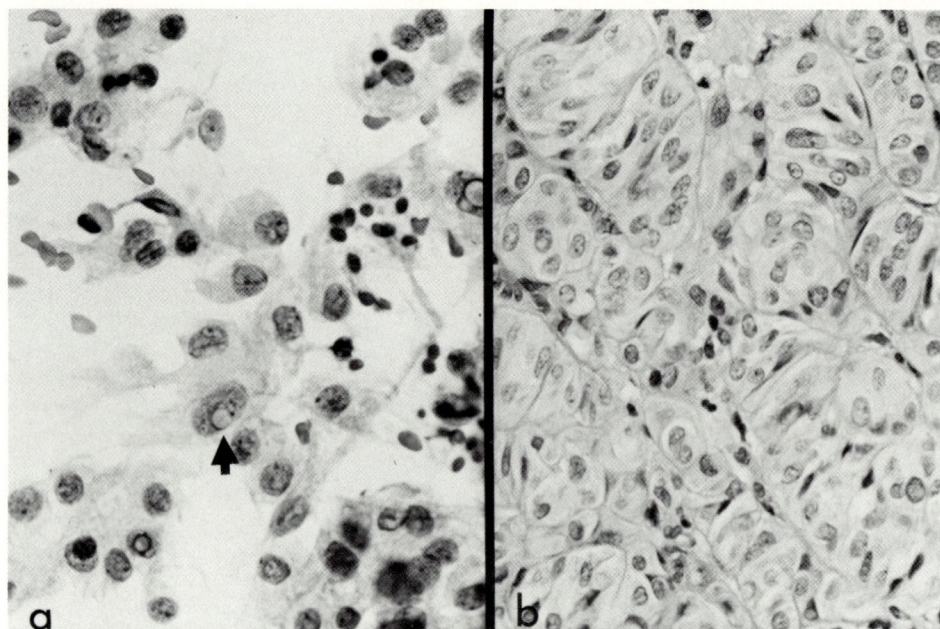

Fig. 10.19. Hürthle cell carcinoma with morphologic similarity to medullary carcinoma. **A.** Discrete plasmacytoid cells with intranuclear cytoplasmic inclusions *(arrow)* that can easily be misinterpreted as medullary carcinoma. Papanicolaou preparation. × 630. **B.** The histologic distinction between Hürthle cell carcinoma and medullary carcinoma was difficult. Serum calcitonin levels were within normal limits. No amyloid was demonstrated. Hematoxylin and eosin preparation. × 400.

Medullary Carcinoma Versus Papillary Carcinoma

Most papillary carcinomas of thyroid are easily recognized by the varied architectural patterns of the tissue fragments (Figs. 10.20–10.24; Table 10.5) (see Chapter 8, Papillary Carcinoma). Very infrequently, aspirates from papillary carcinomas present a single cell pattern with a large population of cuboidal, short columnar, or spindle-shaped cells similar to those seen in medullary carcinoma. Other diagnostic features of papillary carcinoma may not be present. Intranuclear cytoplasmic inclusions are seen in both carcinomas and are not helpful in differentiating the two. Powdery nuclear chromatin, micronucleoli, and a chromatin ridge, if present, suggest papillary carcinoma.

TABLE 10.5. Differentiating Features Between Medullary Carcicoma and Papillary Carcinoma with a Single Cell Pattern

Features	Papillary Carcinoma	Medullary Carcinoma
General pattern	Single cells, syncytia frequent	Single cells, syncytia infrequent
Cell shape	Cuboidal, short columnar	Cuboidal, short columnar
Size	Variable	Variable
Cell borders	Well difined	Poorly defined
Cytoplasm	Variable—pale, clear, vacuolated	Pale fibrillar
Cytoplasmic processes	Absent	Present
Bi- and multinucleation	Rare, almost absent	Common
Location of nuclei	Eccentric	Extreme, marginal
Nuclear chromatin	Fine powdery	Coarsely granular
Nucleoli	Multiple micronucleoli	Not consistent
Intranuclear cytoplasmic inclusions	Almost always present	Always present
Colloid	Scant to absent	Absent
Amyloid	Absent	Present
Giemsa-stained preparations	No cytoplasmic granulation	Azurophilic granules
Immunoperoxidase stain for calcitonin	Negative	Positive

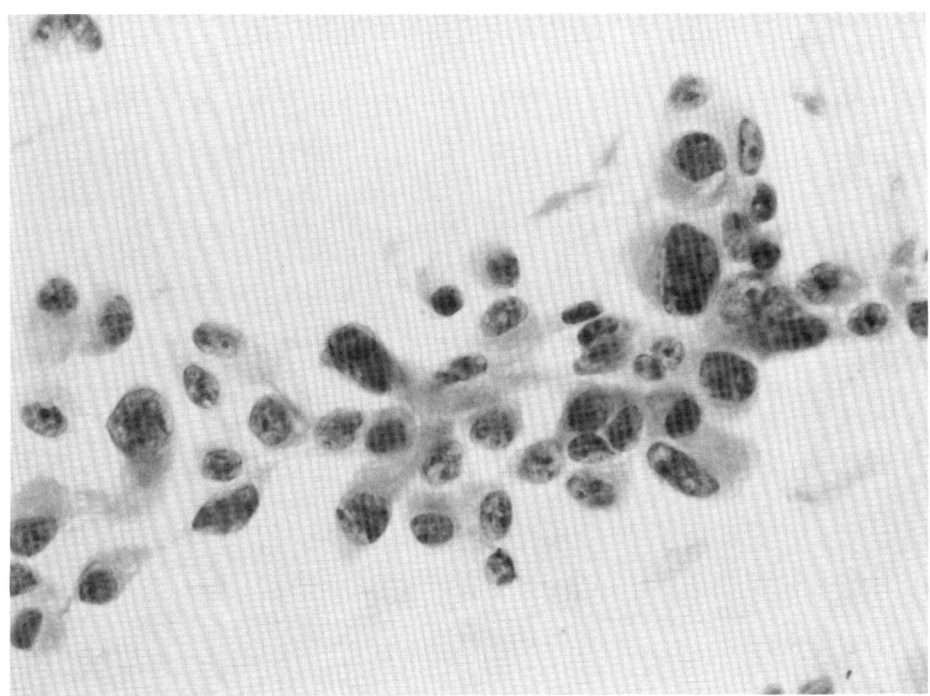

Fig. 10.20. Medullary carcinoma cells that can easily be misinterpreted as papillary carcinoma cells. Papanicolaou preparation. × 630.

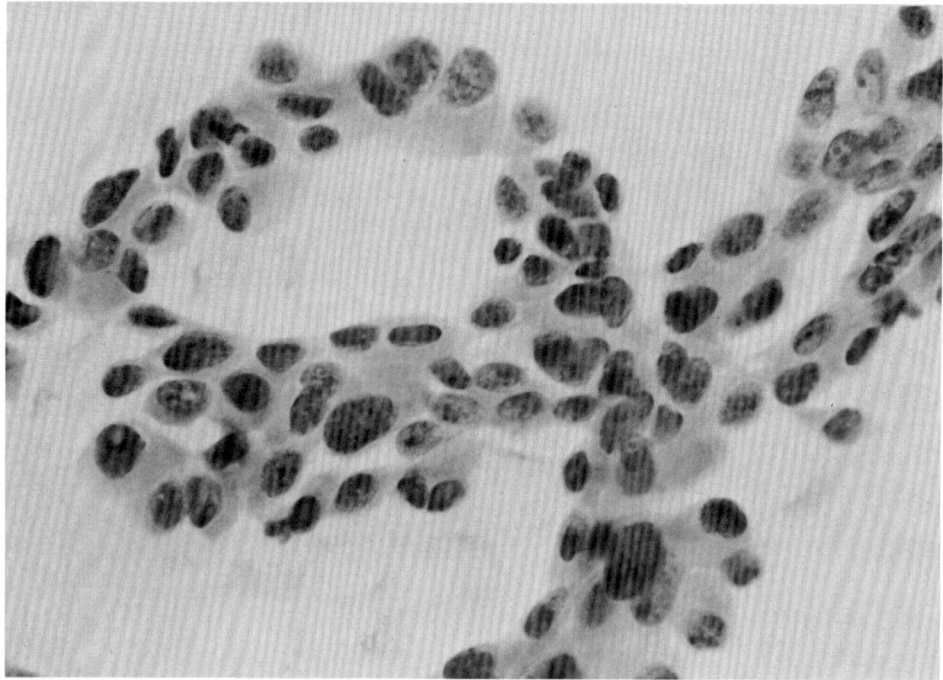

Fig. 10.21. This tissue fragment of medullary carcinoma cells resembles a monolayered tissue fragment of papillary carcinoma and can easily be misinterpreted as such. Papanicolaou preparation. × 630.

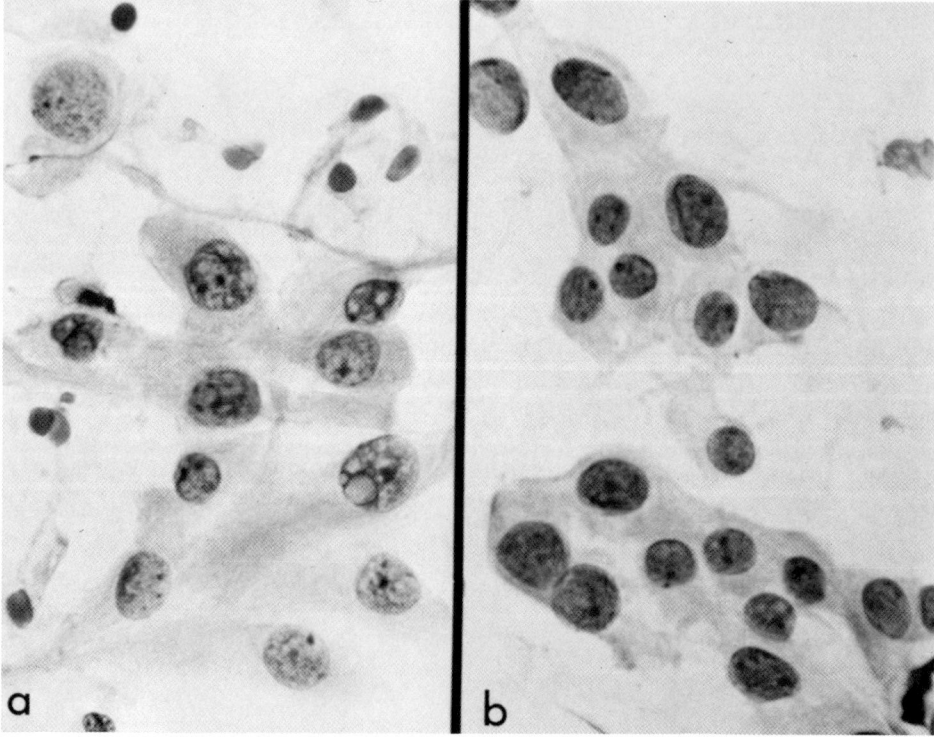

Fig. 10.22. Reversal of cytologic patterns. **A.** These cells of medullary carcinoma strongly resemble papillary carcinoma cells with powdery chromatin and nucleoli with intranuclear cytoplasmic inclusions. Papanicolaou preparation. × 630. **B.** These cells of papillary carcinoma have very coarse chromatin and fibrillar cytoplasm, resembling medullary carcinoma cells. Papanicolaou preparation. × 630.

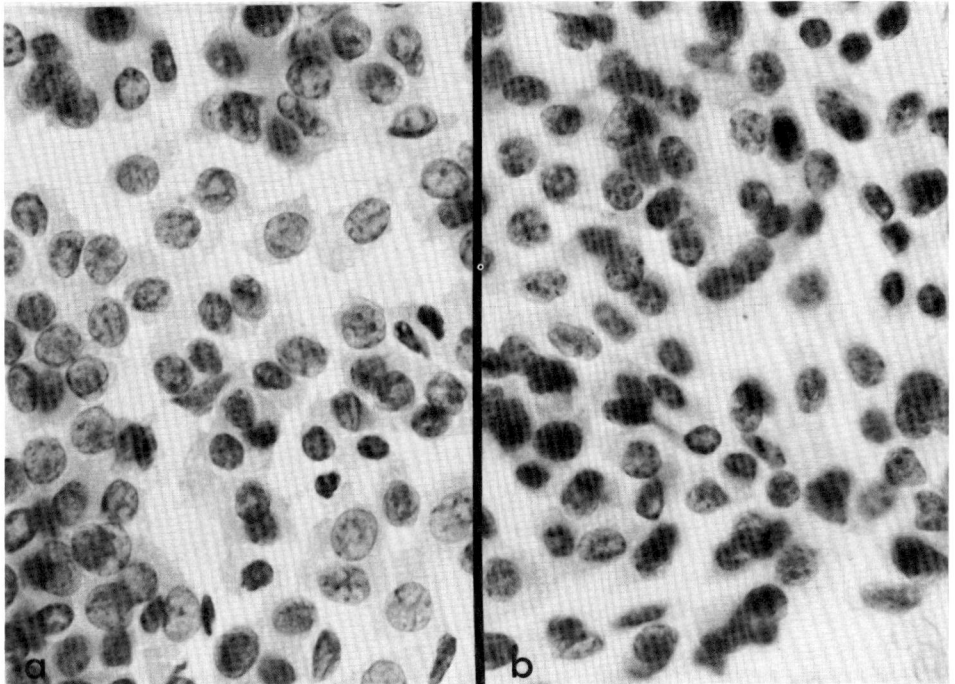

Fig. 10.23. A. Unusual single cell pattern of papillary carcinoma. Papanicolaou preparation. × 630. **B.** Medullary carcinoma. Papanicolaou preparation. × 630. The pattern in **A** can easily be misinterpreted as that of medullary carcinoma. Note the similarities of medullary carcinoma cells with cuboidal cell pattern.

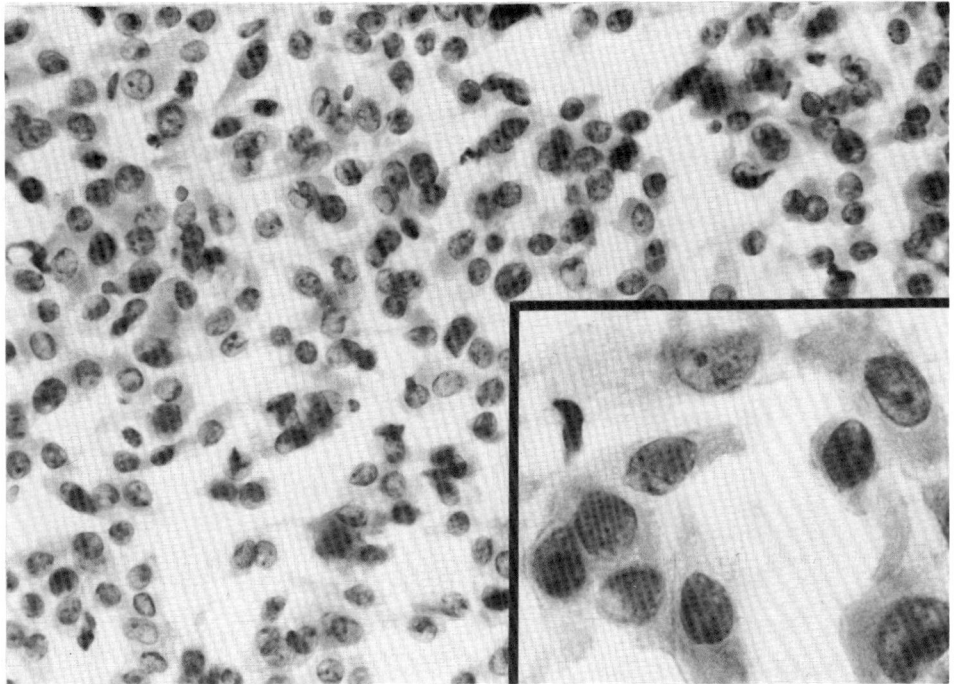

Fig. 10.24. This infrequent single cell pattern with columnar cells in papillary carcinoma may be mistyped as medullary carcinoma. Papanicolaou preparation. × 400. *Inset:* Higher magnification. Papanicolaou preparation. × 1000.

Medullary Carcinoma Versus Follicular Neoplasm

A common cytologic presentation of medullary carcinoma is that of isolated or loosely cohesive cells (Figs. 10.25 and 10.26). The infrequent cytologic presentation of syncytial-type tissue fragments with pseudofollicular pattern and small, round to cuboidal cells with nuclei containing coarse chromatin may be mistyped as follicular adenoma or carcinoma. The presence of intranuclear cytoplasmic inclusions favors a diagnosis of medullary carcinoma or a follicular variant of papillary carcinoma. Recognition of medullary carcinoma may be extremely difficult unless cytoplasmic processes are identified.

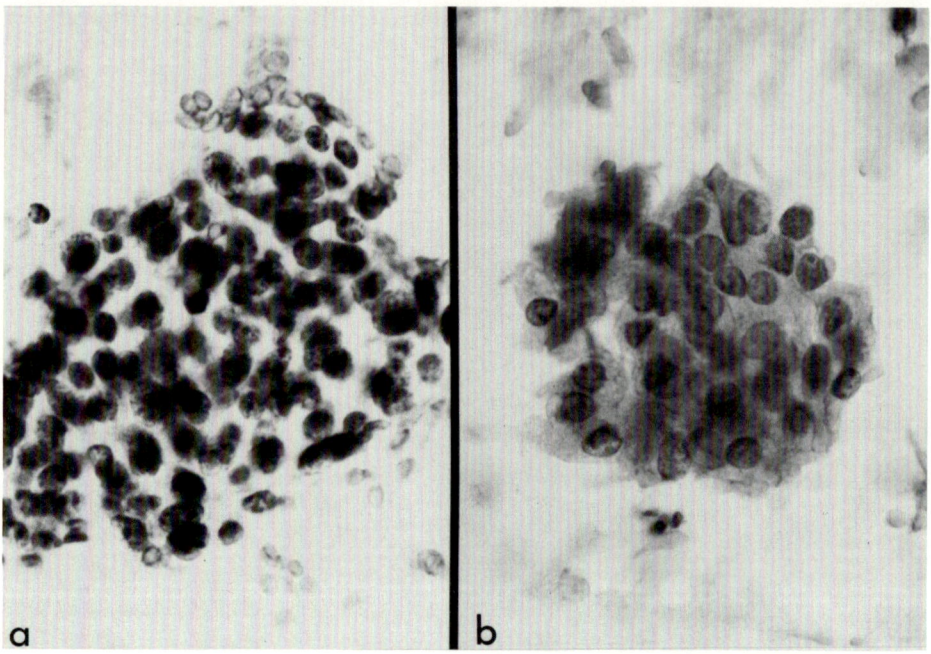

Fig. 10.25. A., B. Syncytial-type tissue fragments in medullary carcinoma. Both cases were mistyped as follicular neoplasm. Papanicolaou preparation. × 630.

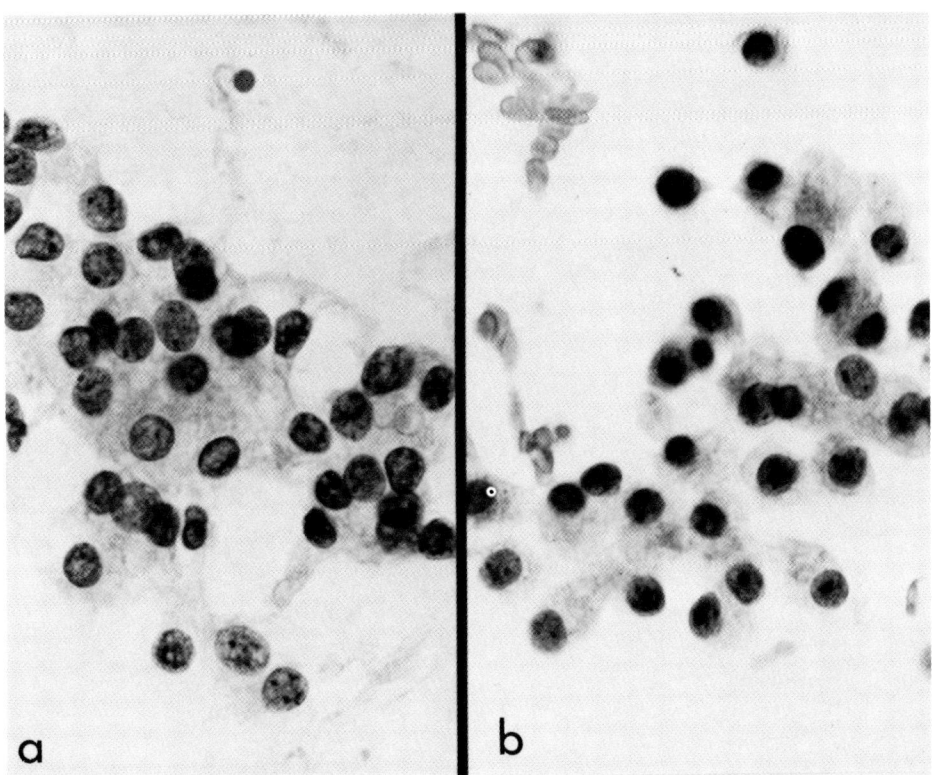

Fig. 10.26 **A.** Syncytial-type tissue fragment of follicular cell carcinoma. Papanicolaou preparation. × 630. **B.** Syncytial-type tissue fragment of small cuboidal and plasmacytoid cells of medullary carcinoma. Papanicolaou preparation. × 630. Note the morphologic similarities between **A** and **B.**

Medullary Carcinoma Versus Anaplastic Carcinoma

The monomorphic spindle cell pattern of medullary carcinoma (Fig. 10.27; Table 10.6) may be mistyped as anaplastic carcinoma, particularly when occasional nuclei appear bizarre. On the other hand, in the absence of usual cytopathologic features, such as pleomorphic and bizarre nuclei and tumor diathesis, the aspirate of anaplastic carcinoma may be mistyped as medullary carcinoma. Intranuclear cytoplasmic inclusions are seen in both types of cancer cells. The presence of other features of medullary carcinoma, as described earlier, are helpful in making a correct diagnosis. Intertwined cytoplasmic processes are not a feature of anaplastic carcinoma.

TABLE 10.6. Differentiating Features Between Medullary Carcinoma and
Anaplastic Carcinoma

Features	Anaplastic Carcinoma	Medullary Carcinoma
General pattern	Isolated cells	Isolated cells
Cell shape	Spindle	Spindle
Size	Variable	Variable
Cell borders	Well defined	Poorly defined
Cytoplasm	Variable	Scanty
Cytoplasmic processes	Absent	Strikingly uni- or bipolar, intertwined with those of other cells
Location of nuclei	Variable	Eccentric, marginal
Nuclear chromatin	Clumped and coarse with excessive parachromatin clearing, bizarre shapes	Round to oval nuclei, bland, occasional bizarre nuleus
Nucleoli	Multiple, irregular micro- and macronucleoi	Not consistent
Intranuclear cytoplasmic inclusions	May be present	Always present
Colloid	Absent	Absent
Amyloid	Absent	Present
Romanowsky-stained preparations	No azurophilic granules	Azurophilic granules present
Immunoperoxidase stain for calcitonin	**Negative**	**Positive**
Tumor diathesis	May be present	Absent

Medullary Carcinoma Versus Stromal Cells in Nodular Goiter

Although an aspirate of medullary carcinoma with its characteristic presentation will
not be typed as nodular goiter, the converse may not be true (Figs. 10.28 and 10.29).
In a nodular goiter, the fibroblasts from the supporting stroma or the granulation
tissue from an old hemorrhage sometimes appear very similar to the spindle cells of
medullary carcinoma. Features of nodular goiter, if present in other areas of the
smears, should aid in correct interpretation.

SUMMARY

Medullary thyroid carcinoma presents a characteristic cellular pattern with a wide
variety of cell shapes and sizes. The eccentric nuclear position, intranuclear

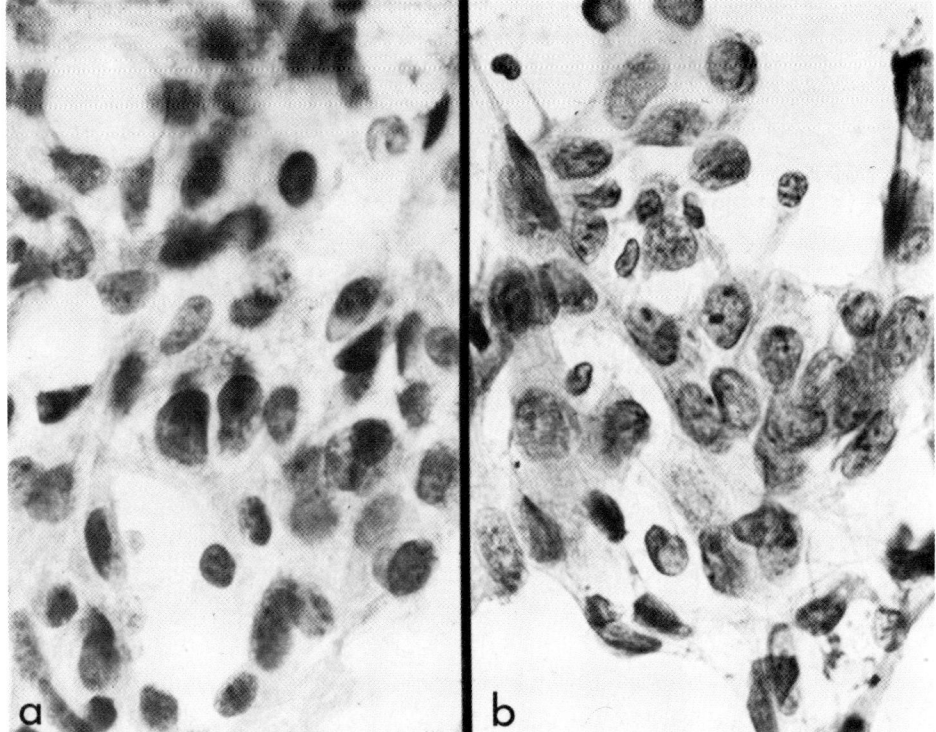

Fig. 10.27 A. Medullary carcinoma. Papanicolaou preparation. × 650. **B.** Anaplastic carcinoma. Papanicolaou preparation. × 650. The malignant cells in **A** were interpreted as anaplastic carcinoma. Note the bland nuclear pattern in **A** in contrast with obvious malignant nuclei in **B**.

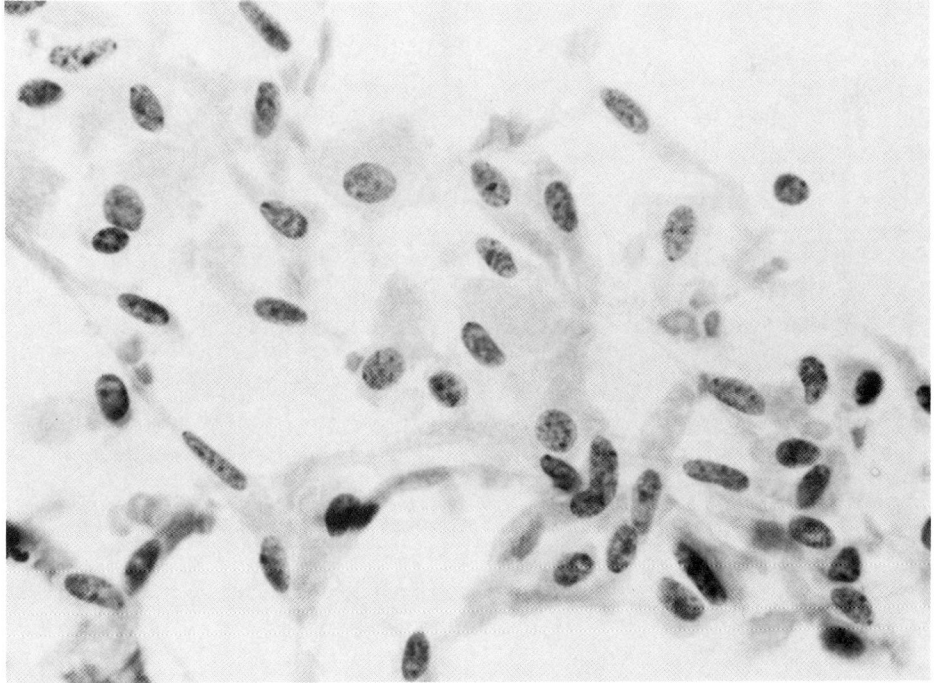

Fig. 10.28. Elongated stromal cells in nodular goiter with long cytoplasmic processes may be misinterpreted as medullary carcinoma. Papanicolaou preparation. × 630.

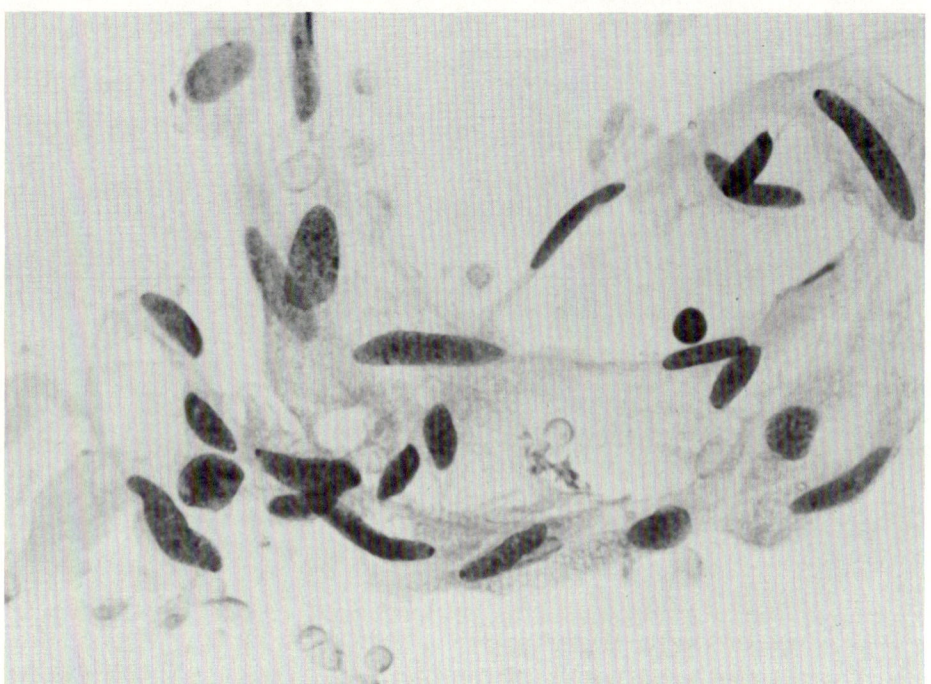

Fig. 10.29. Medullary carcinoma cells with morphologic similarity to fibroblasts seen in Fig. 10.28. Papanicolaou preparation. × 630.

cytoplasmic inclusions, fibrillar cytoplasm, cytoplasmic processes, and azurophilic granules (by Romanowsky stain) are diagnostic. Diagnosis can be confirmed by demonstrating calcitonin granules with immunoperoxidase staining technique; by large-needle biopsy; and by serum calcitonin levels.

REFERENCES

1. Fletcher JR: Medullary (solid) carcinoma of the thyroid gland: a review of 249 cases. *Arch Surg* 100:257–262, 1970.

2. Geddie WR, Bedard YC, Strawbridge HTG: Medullary carcinoma of the thyroid in fine needle aspiration biopsies. *Am J Clin Pathol* 82:552–558, 1984.

3. Hamburger JI, Miller JM, Kini SR: Clinical-pathological evaluation of thryoid nodules. In *Handbook & Atlas*, Southfield, MI, 1979, pp. 10–12.

4. Harach HR, Williams ED: Glandular (tubular and follicular variant of medullary carcinoma of the thyroid. *Histopathology* 7:83–9, 1983.

5. Hazard JB, Hawk WA, Crile G Jr: Medullary (solid) carcinoma of the thyroid: a clinicopathological entity. *J Clin Endocrinol Metab* 19:152–161, 1959.

6. Horn RC Jr: Carcinoma of the thyroid. Description of a distinctive morphologic variant: a report of seven cases. *Cancer* 4:697–707, 1951.

7. Ibanez ML: Medullary carcinoma of the thyroid gland. In Sommers SC: *Pathology Annual*. New York, Appleton-Century-Crofts, 1974, pp. 263–290.

8. Kakudo K, Miyauchi A, Ogihana T, et al.: Medullary carcinoma of the thyroid, giant cell type. *Arch Pathol Lab Med* 102:445–447, 1978.

9. Kakudo K, Miyavehi A, Takai SI et al: C-cell carcinoma of the thyroid—papillary type. *Acta Pathol Jpn* 29:633–659, 1979.

10. Kini SR, Miller JM, Hamburger JI, Smith MJ: Cytopathology of medullary carcinoma of the thyroid. *Arch Pathol Lab Med* 108:156–159, 1984.

11. Livolsi VA: Calcitonin; the hormone and its significance. *Prog Surg Pathol* 1:71–109, 1980.

12. Ljungberg O: Cytologic diagnosis of medullary carcinoma of thyroid. *Acta Cytol* 16:253–255, 1972.

13. Ljungberg O, Bondeson L, Bondeson AG: Differentiated thyroid carcinoma, intermediate type; a new tumor entity with features of follicular and parafollicular cell carcinoma. *Hum Pathol* 15:218–228, 1984.

14. Ljungberg O, Ericsson UB, Bondeson L, Thorell J: A compound follicular–parafollicular carcinoma of the thyroid; a new tumor entity. *Cancer* 52:1053–1061, 1983.

15. Löwhagen R, Spencer E: Cytologic presentation of thyroid lesions in aspiration biopsy smears. *Acta Cytol* 18:192–197, 1974.

16. Mendelsohn G, Bignes SH, Eggleston JC, Baylin SB, Wells SA Jr: Anaplastic variants of medullary thyroid carcinoma; a light microscopic and immunohistochemical study. *Am J Surg Pathol* 4:333–341, 1980.

17. Miller JM, Kini SR, Hamburger JI: *Needle Biopsy of the Thyroid*. New York, Praeger Publishers, 1983, pp. 104–107.

18. Schaffer R, Miller HA, Pfeifer U, Ormanns W: Cytological findings in medullary carcinoma of the thyroid. *Pathol Res Pract* 178:461–466, 1984.

19. Söderström N, Telenius-Berg M, Ackerman M: Diagnosis of medullary carcinoma of the thyroid by fine needle aspiration biopsy. *Acta Medica Scand* 197:71–76, 1975.

20. Steiner AL, Goodman AD, Powers SF: Study of a kindred with pleochromocytoma, medullary thyroid carcinoma, hyperparathyroidism and Cushing's disease; multiple endocrine neoplasia type 2. *Medicine* 47:371–409, 1968.

21. Uribe M, Fenogho-Prciser CM, Grimes M, Feind C: Medullary carcinoma of the thyroid gland. *Am J Surg Pathol* 9:577–594, 1983.

22. Williams ED: Medullary carcinoma of the thyroid. In Harrison CV, Weinbrank K: *Recent Advances in Pathology*. New York, Churchill Livingstone, 1975, pp. 152–164.

23. Williams ED: Histogenesis of medullary carcinoma of the thryoid. *J Clin Pathol* 19:114–118, 1966.

24. Williams ED, Pollack DJ: Multiple mucosal neuromata with endocrine tumors; a syndrome allied to Von Reckling-Hausen's disease. *J Pathol Bact* 91:71–80, 1966.

25. Woolner LB, Beahers OH, Black BM, McConahey WM, Keating FR: Classification and prognosis of thyroid carcinoma. *Am J Surg* 102:354–387, 1961.

11

Thyroiditis

Thyroiditis, an inflammatory condition of the thyroid, can be classified according to its etiology, duration, or morphology. As etiologic factors are not clearly established in most cases, classification by morphology and duration is accepted by most[12] (Table 11.1).

Any type of thyroiditis can be mistaken for a tumor. Clinical and gross features such as rapid asymmetric enlargement, nodularity, firmness, and fixation to adjacent structures are common to both inflammation and neoplasm. Without biopsy, the distinction between thyroiditis and tumor may be difficult or impossible clinically.

SUPPURATIVE THYROIDITIS

Suppurative thyroiditis is a rare inflammatory disease[18] caused by bacterial, fungal, and (very rarely) parasitic infection. More information can be found in the literature review by Berger et al.[2] The aspirates show neutrophilic infiltrate and cellular debris. The differential diagnoses include anaplastic carcinoma, which presents with acute pain and necrosis, as well as granulomatous thyroiditis.

GRANULOMATOUS THYROIDITIS

Granulomatous thyroiditis is a spontaneously remitting inflammatory disease considered to be of viral origin.[10,12,23] Synonyms for this disease include de Quervain's thyroiditis, pseudotuberculous thyroiditis, viral thyroiditis, nonsuppurative thyroiditis, struma granulomatosa, and giant cell thyroiditis. It is reportedly common in women from the second to the fifth decade. Patients present with a spectrum of clinical symptoms ranging from fatigue with slight tenderness on palpation of the

235

TABLE 11.1. Classification of Thyroiditis

Acute suppurative
Subacute Thyroiditis
    Granulomatous
    Lymphocytic
Chronic thyroiditis
    Lymphocytic (Hashimoto's autoimmune)
    Riedel's
    Specific, eg, tuberculous

thyroid gland, to an abrupt onset with chills, fever, severe neck pain, and symptoms of hyperthyroidism. Results of laboratory studies may include a high erythrocyte sedimentation rate, normal white blood cell count, and low radioiodine level. There may be increased blood levels of thyroxine and triiodothyronine, depending on the severity of the disease. The disease generally lasts from 2 to 5 months, although recurrence is common. However, it is self-limiting, and thyroid functions gradually return to normal.

Usually the entire gland is involved, but initially the disease may be focal. In such circumstances, a nodule may be diagnosed. Only one portion of the gland is involved, thus producing an asymmetric nodular involvement. The characteristic microscopic features show destruction of the thyroid parenchyma with foreign-body–type giant cells around the colloid that result in granuloma formation (Figs. 11.1 and 11.2).[16,23] The inflammatory infiltrate consists of neutrophils and eosinophils, as well as lymphocytes and plasma cells. Lymphoid nodules with germinal center cells have not been described. The intervening stroma shows fibrosis.

Cytopathology

Fine-needle biopsy is not routinely used to confirm the diagnosis of granulomatous thyroiditis because the clinical picture and laboratory data are characteristic. Biopsies are performed in patients with an unusual presentation to rule out suppurative thyroiditis or anaplastic carcinoma. Because aspiration biopsy of granulomatous thyroiditis is so infrequently done, one rarely encounters a case in routine cytopathology practice, and our experience is limited to only six cases. A good review is given by Chang et al.[4]

The cytopathologic features of granulomatous thyroiditis are presented in Table 11.2. The cellularity of the aspirate will vary, depending on the stage of the disease. In the initial stages, the aspirate is cellular and is characterized by several large multinucleated foreign-body–type giant cells containing up to several hundred nuclei (Fig. 11.3). Some giant cells resemble Langhans' type in their nuclear arrangement (Fig. 11.4). The nuclei are generally small, round to oval, with a sharp nuclear membrane, finely granular chromatin, and one or more micronucleoli. These giant cells have abundant, granular to dense, cytoplasm. They are often seen in the vicinity of either follicular epithelial cells or colloid droplets (Fig. 11.5).

Other inflammatory cells include spindle-shaped or plump epithelioid cells (Fig. 11.5), lymphocytes, and plasma cells. Germinal center cells are not identified. In the

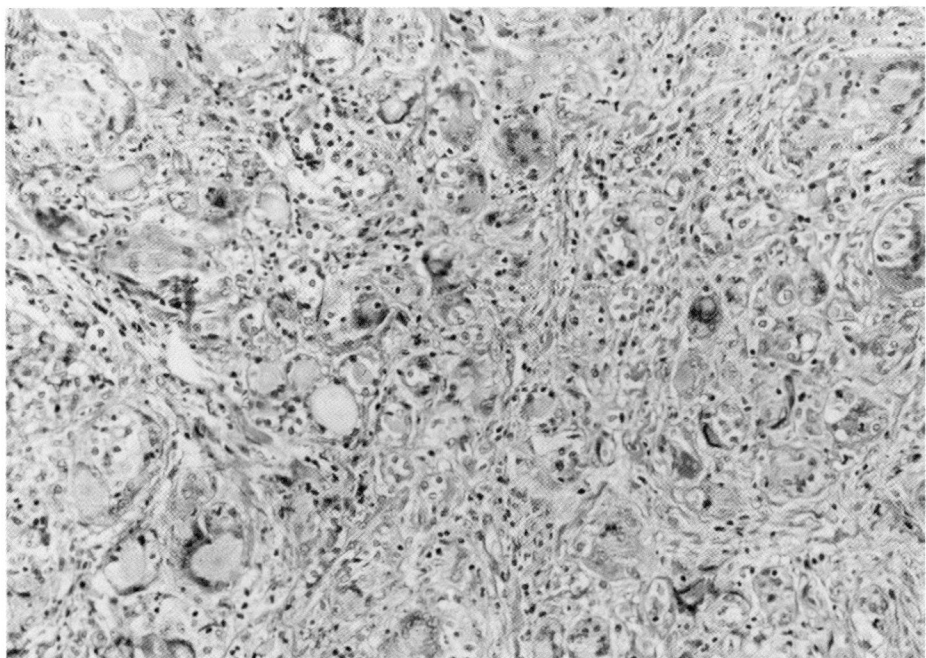

Fig. 11.1. Granulomatous thyroiditis. The thyroid follicles are filled with multinucleated giant cells. Hematoxylin and eosin preparation. × 160.

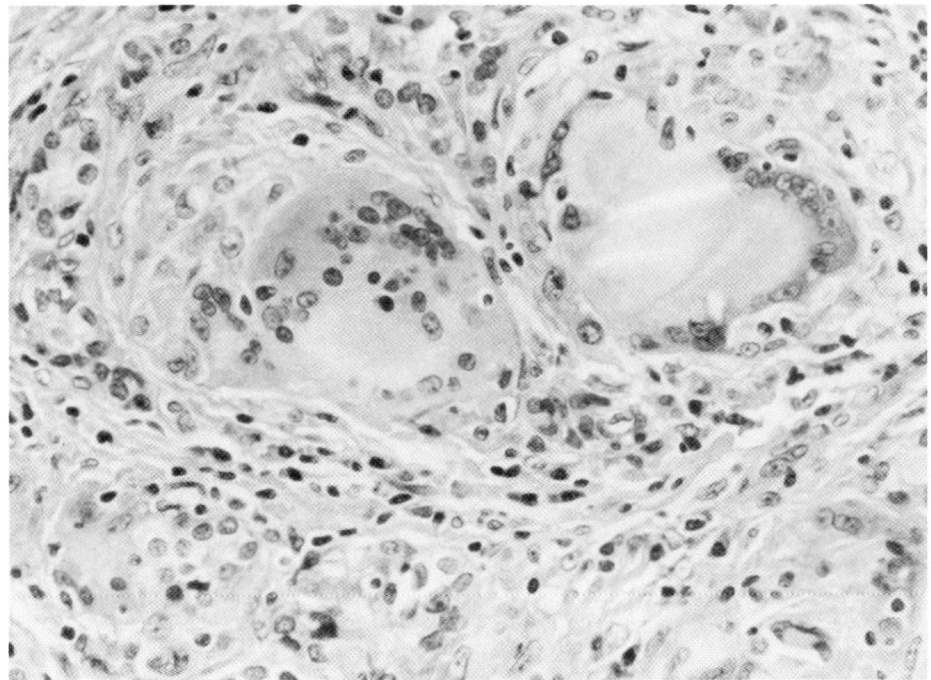

Fig. 11.2. Higher magnification of Fig. 11.1. Large multinucleated foreign-body–type giant cells. Hematoxylin and eosin preparation. × 400.

TABLE 11.2. Cytopathologic Features of Granulomatous Thyroiditis

Large, multinucleated foreign-body–type giant cells in the vicinity of colloid droplets or follicular cells
Epithelioid cells, lymphocytes, plasma cells, polymorphonuclear leukocytes may be present; germinal center cells absent
Follicular and Hürthle cells with or without nuclear atypia
Cellular and inflammatory debris may be present
Stromal cells during healing phase

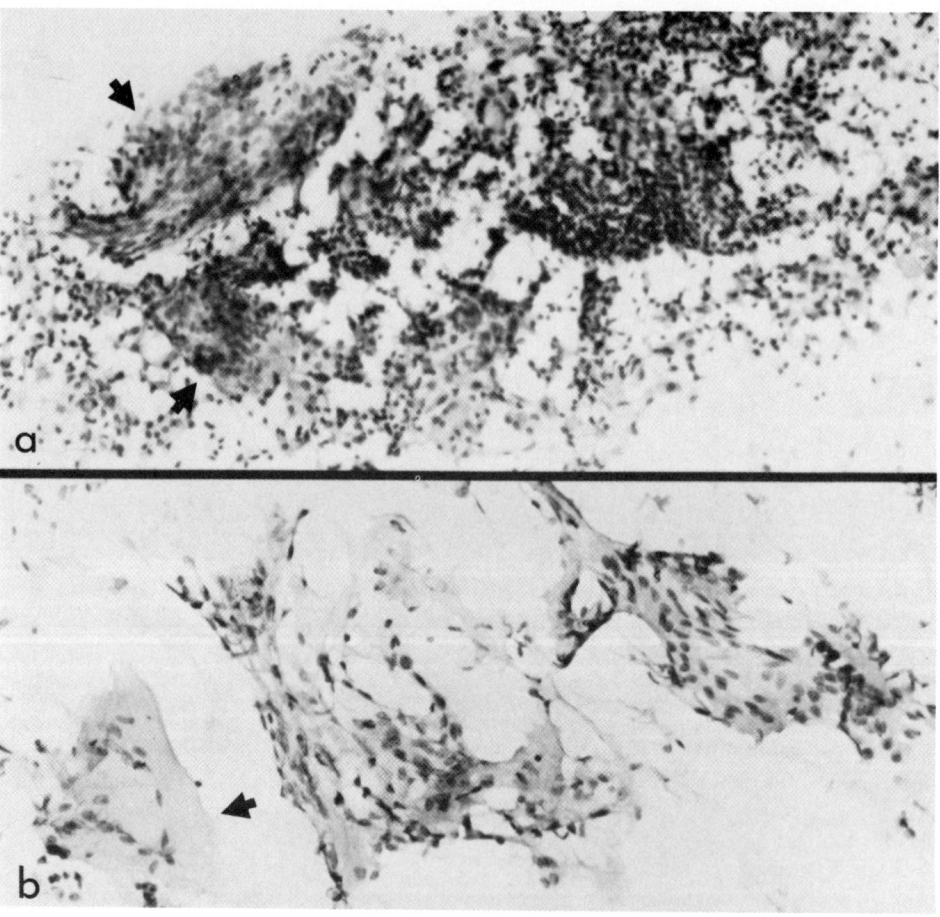

Fig. 11.3. Low-power view of aspirates from granulomatous thyroiditis. **A.** Cellular aspirate with inflammatory cells and enormously larger multinucleated foreign-body–type giant cells. *(arrow)*. Papanicolaou preparation. × 160. **B.** Sparsely cellular aspirate with stromal tissue fragment and foreign-body–type giant cells *(arrow)*. Papanicolaou preparation. × 160.

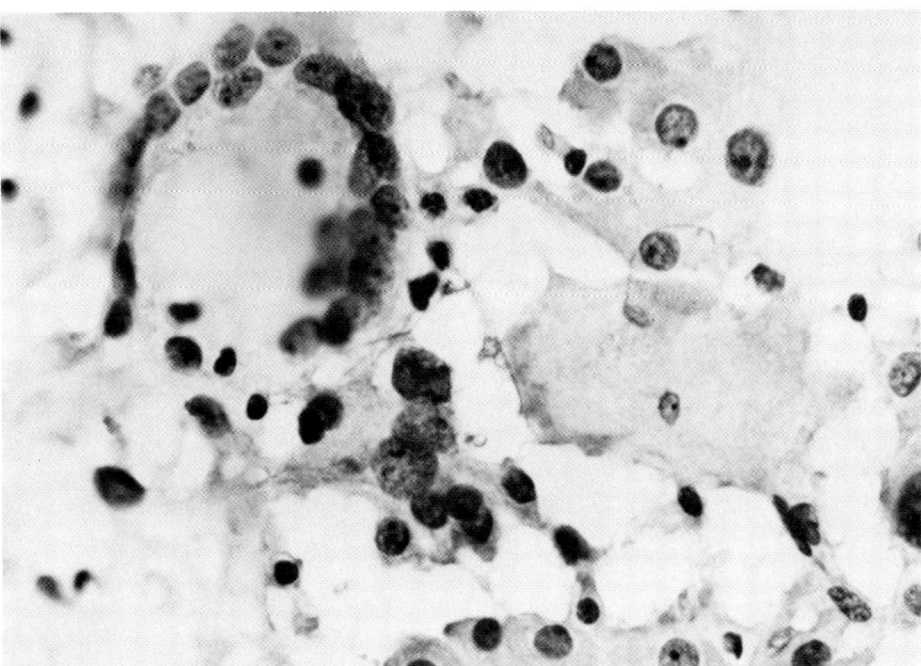

Fig. 11.4. Granulomatous thyroiditis. A Langhans' type giant cell in close proximity to colloid droplet. Papanicolaou preparation. × 630.

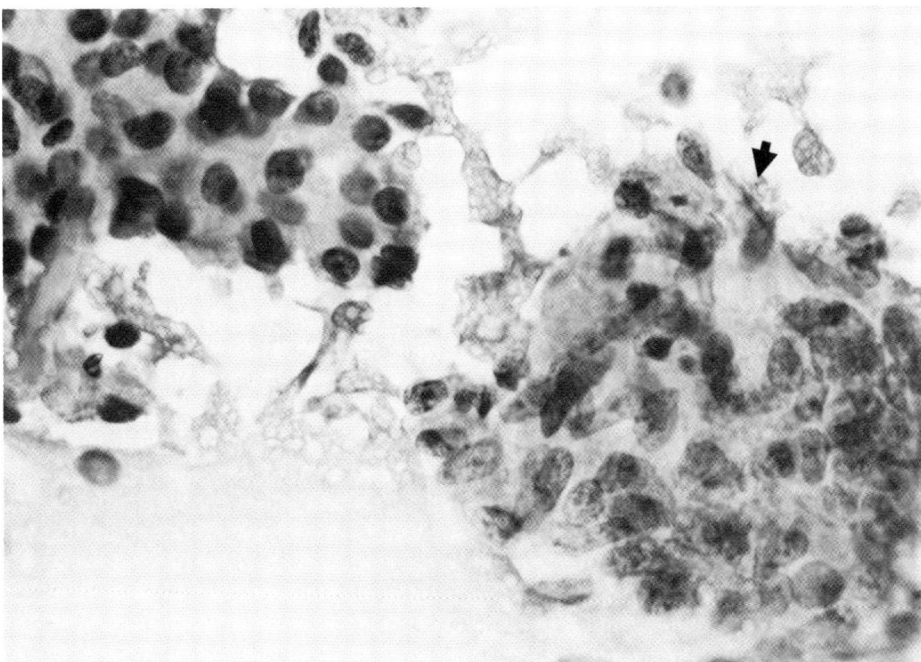

Fig. 11.5. Granulomatous thyroiditis. A granuloma formed by epithelioid cells *(arrow)* is seen in the vicinity of follicular cells. Papanicolaou preparation. × 400.

early stages, neutrophils and eosinophils may be seen, along with cellular and inflammatory debris. Stromal cells are often aspirated, especially in the later stages, with a sparse inflammatory and epithelial component (Fig. 11.3). Giant cells may be absent during the healing phase. Nuclei of fibroblasts form stromal tissue fragments and can appear very active; they may be mistaken for anaplastic carcinoma.

Differential Diagnosis

The cytologic pattern of an aspirated sample from granulomatous thyroiditis has characteristic features, especially the presence of large giant cells. However, multinucleated giant cells can also be seen in chronic lymphocytic thyroiditis or papillary carcinoma. The differentiating features between chronic lymphocytic thyroiditis and granulomatous thyroiditis are discussed later in this chapter, in the section on Hashimoto's thyroiditis.

Anaplastic carcinoma is important as a differential diagnosis clinically, because both diseases present with a painfully enlarged thyroid. Cytologic differentiation between the two is not difficult. Occasionally, proliferating stromal fibroblasts may be mistaken for spindle cell type anaplastic carcinoma, the nuclei of which are bizarre and not bland, like those of fibroblasts.

SUBACUTE LYMPHOCYTIC THYROIDITIS

This relatively recently recognized entity is also referred to as painless thyroiditis. Some cases show changes identical to those of granulomatous thyroiditis, but most show a predominant lymphocytic infiltrate. This type of thyroiditis is very common in the United States and is frequently seen in the postpartum state. Autoantibodies are generally negative, and the value of the biopsy is debated. More information can be found in the literature.[11]

INVASIVE FIBROUS THYROIDITIS

Invasive fibrous thyroiditis, the most rare form of thyroiditis,[17] primarily affects women. Synonyms for this disease include Riedel's thyroiditis, chronic sclerosing thyroiditis, and Riedel's struma. Originally described by Riedel in 1896, it is a progressive disease characterized by complete destruction of the thyroid gland by proliferating fibrosis that extends into the adjacent soft tissue. The process causes pressure symptoms in the neck, with fixation of the neck organs. Clinically, this form of thyroiditis must be differentiated from the fibrous variant of Hashimoto's disease (see below) and granulomatous thyroiditis. Fine-needle biopsy yields no cellular material.

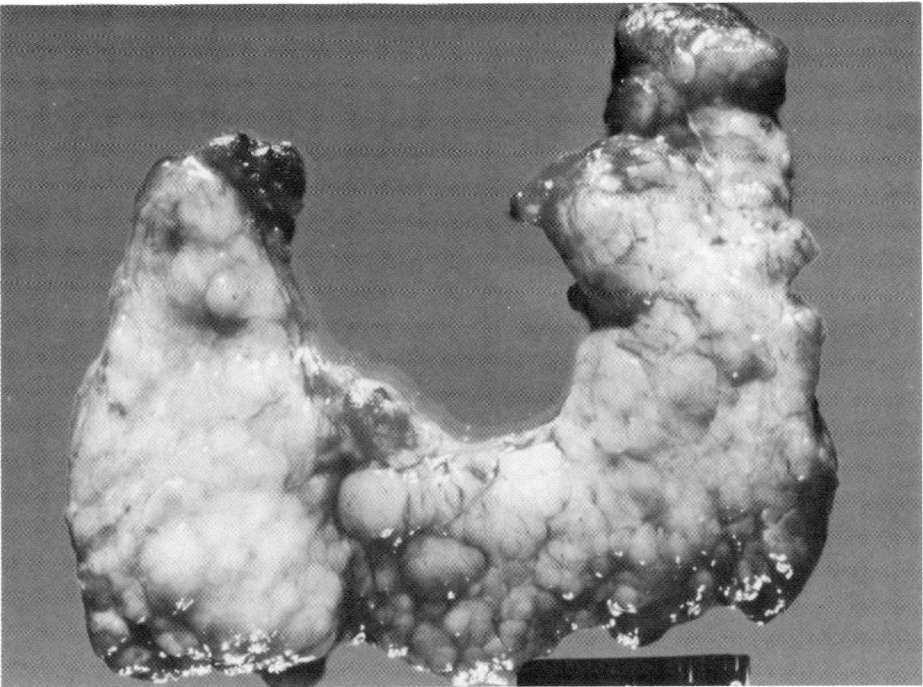

Fig. 11.6. Hashimoto's thyroiditis. The thyroid is diffusely enlarged, pale, and with an accentuated lobular pattern.

LYMPHOCYTIC (HASHIMOTO'S) THYROIDITIS

Hashimoto's thyroiditis, first described in 1912, is the most common form of thyroiditis. Seen predominantly in women of all ages, its synonyms include struma lymphomatosa, lymphadenoid goiter, autoimmune thyroiditis, and chronic lymphocytic thyroiditis. Clinically, the disease is characterized by a diffuse goiter with or without nodularity. It is considered an autoimmune process, as indicated by increased titers of antithyroglobulin and/or antimicrosomal antibodies. Imaging quite often shows patchy uptake or cold defects. Hashimoto's thyroiditis may be progressive, and it is an important cause of hypothyroidism.

Pathology

Grossly, the thyroid is symmetrically enlarged two to four times normal size (Fig. 11.6), and both lobes are involved, as well as the pyramidal lobe, if present. The capsule is smooth and tense. The gland feels firm and rubbery. The cut surface is pale and meaty, with an accentuated lobular pattern. Degeneration is not seen.

Microscopically (Figs. 11.7–11.10), all the lobules are involved and are well demarcated by increased fibrous tissue. Progressive destruction of the thyroid parenchyma is seen, along with interlobular and interfollicular lymphoplasmacytic infiltrate and lymphoid follicles with germinal centers.

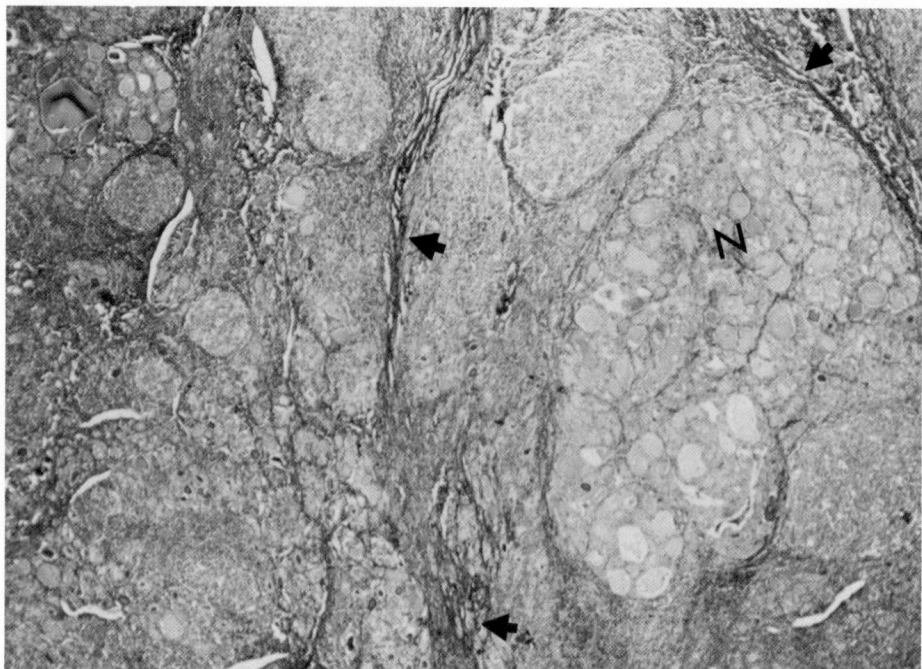

Fig. 11.7. Hashimoto's thyroiditis. Heavy inflammatory infiltrate, lymphoid follicles with germinal centers, and follicular nodules *(N)*. Note prominent perilobular fibrosis *(arrow)*. Hematoxylin and eosin preparation. × 63.

The epithelial changes are varied and are characterized by oxyphilic change of the follicular epithelium (Hürthle cell change) that can be focal, diffuse, or sometimes extensive with nodule formation. Oxyphilic change of the epithelium is considered a hallmark of Hashimoto's disease. The follicular epithelium may be hyperplastic with papillary change, or the follicles may be small and atrophic, with inspissated colloid or devoid of colloid. Nuclei of the oxyphilic or regular follicular epithelium often show considerable atypia. Multinucleated foreign-body–type giant cells may be seen infrequently. Although Hashimoto's thyroiditis involves the entire thyroid, focal changes limited to one lobe or part of the lobe may be seen. In later stages, there may be marked fibrosis (fibrous variant).

The intensity of the changes described above varies from lobe to lobe, as well as within a lobe. Variations from a typical pattern of Hashimoto's thyroiditis occur in children, where oxyphilia is not a prominent feature, but the lymphocytic infiltration is diffuse and extensive. This is referred to as the juvenile type, and Woolner et al[25] called it a lymphoid form.

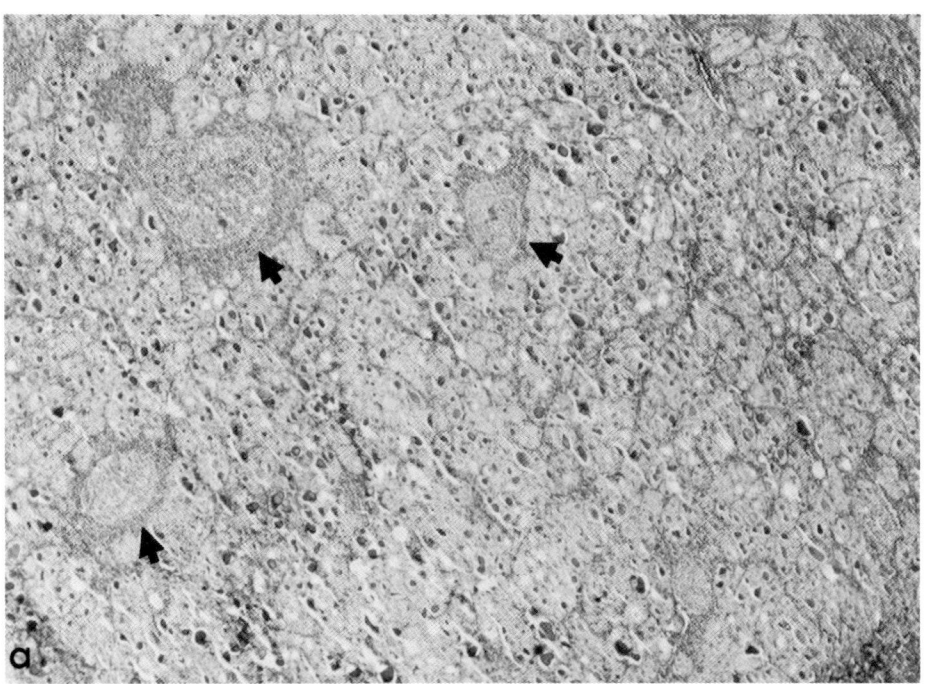

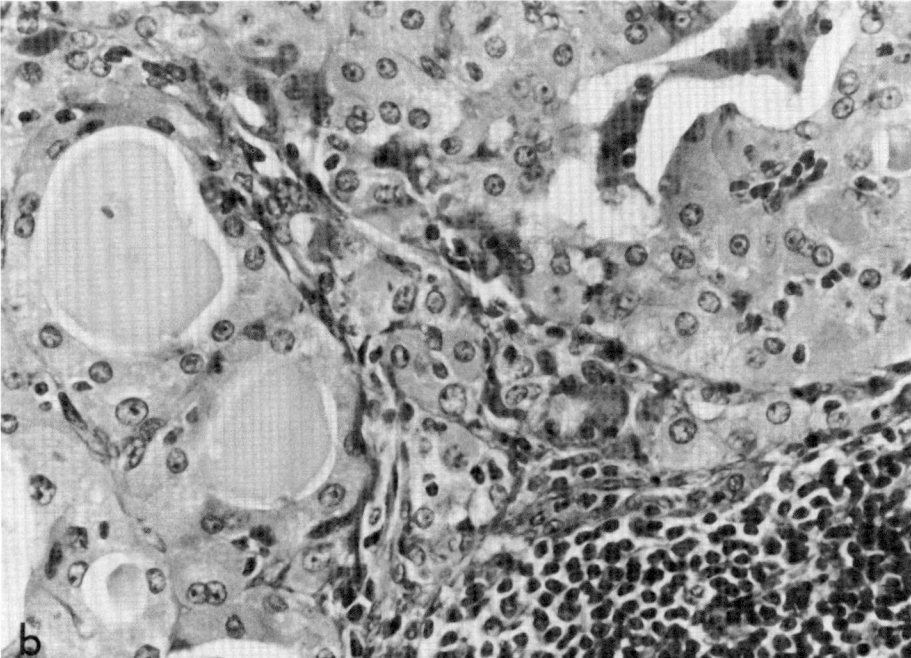

Fig. 11.8. A. Hashimoto's thyroiditis with an involutional or Hürthle cell nodule and lymphoid follicles *(arrows)*. Hematoxylin and eosin preparation. × 63. **B.** Higher magnification of **A** showing Hürthle cell metaplasia and lymphoid infiltrate. Hematoxylin and eosin preparation. × 400.

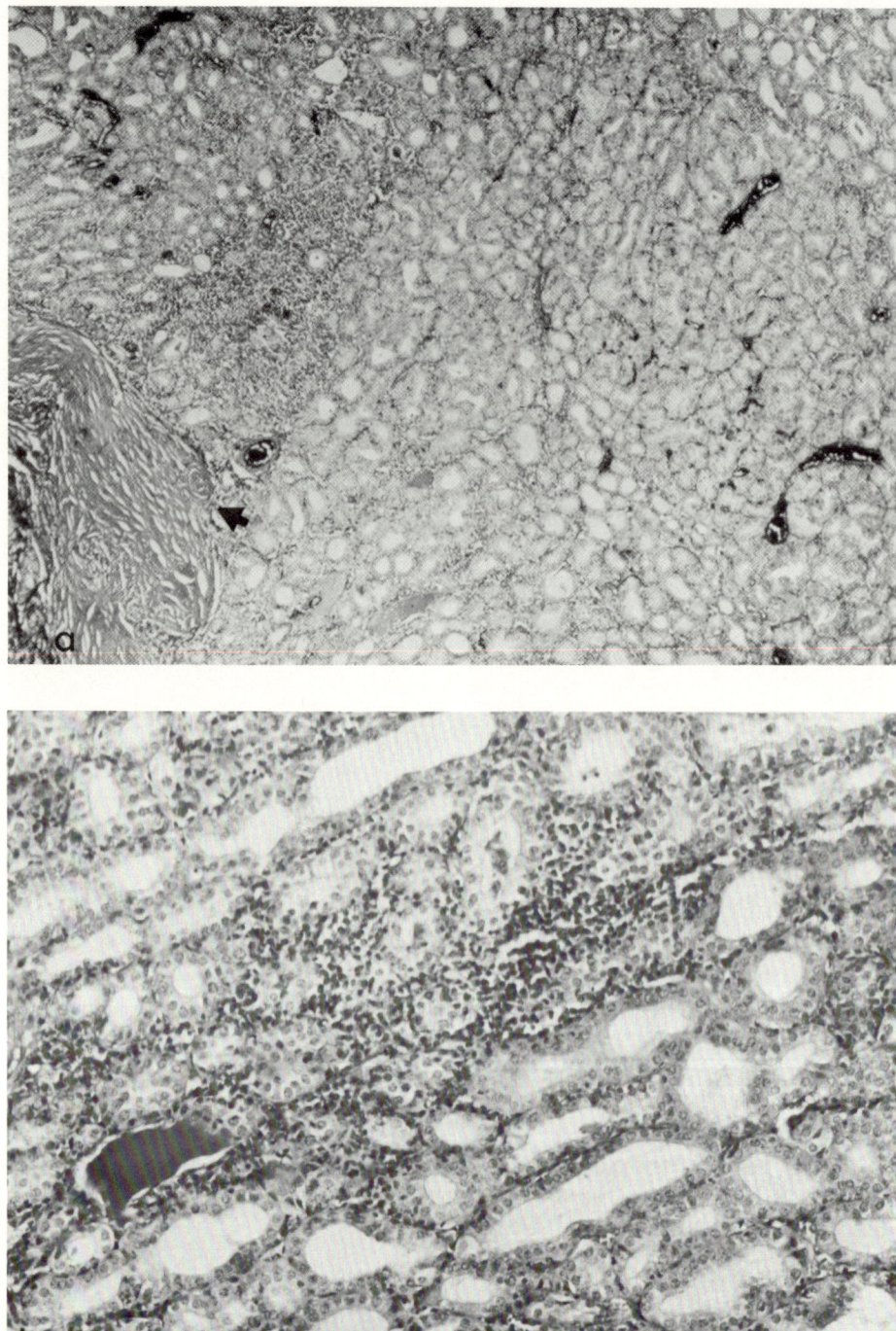

Fig. 11.9. A. Hashimoto's thyroiditis with follicular hyperplasia and fibrosis *(arrow)*. Hematoxylin and eosin preparation. × 160. **B.** Higher magnification of **A** showing hyperplastic follicles without colloid. Hematoxylin and eosin preparation. × 400.

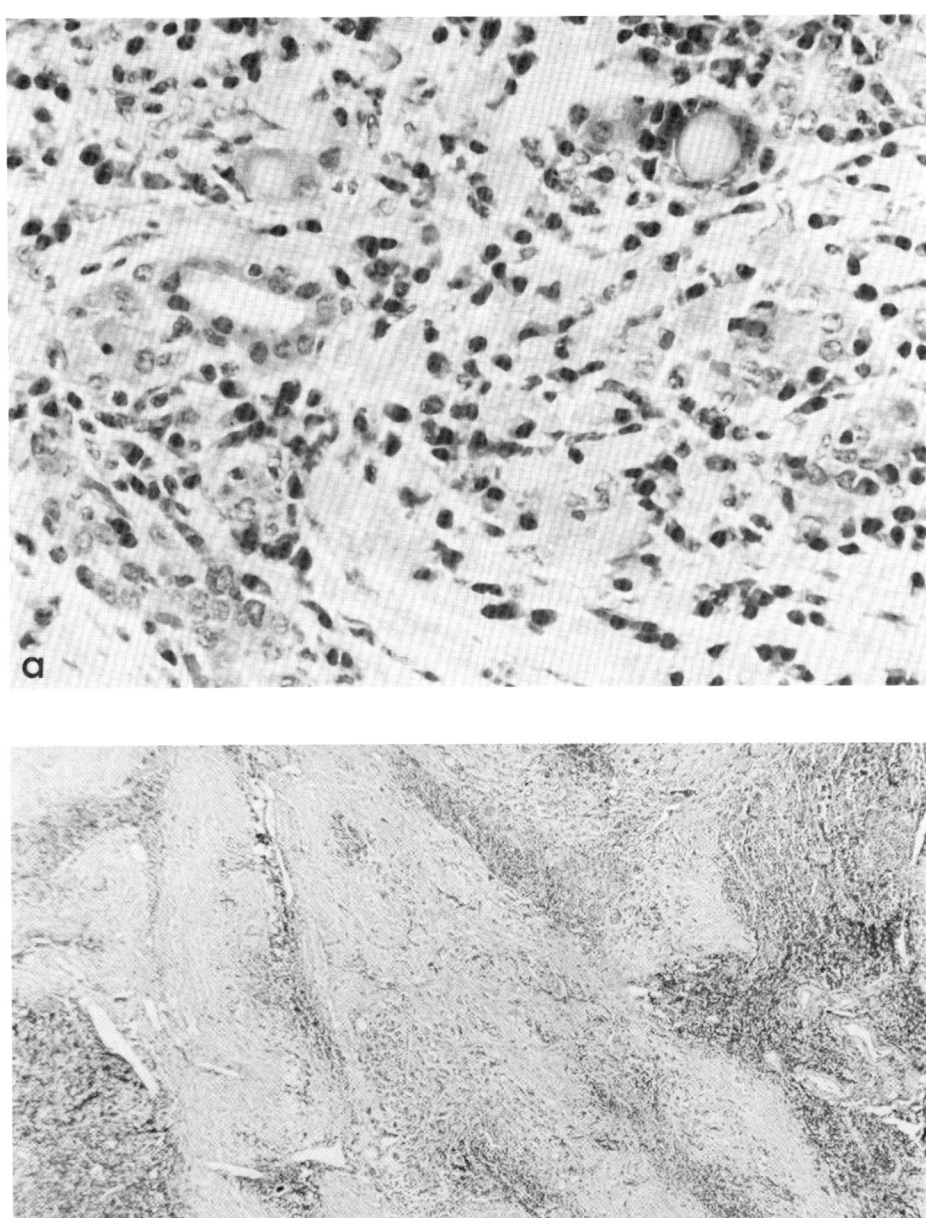

Fig. 11.10. **A.** Hashimoto's thyroiditis with parenchymal atrophy, lymphoid infiltrate, and fibrosis. Hematoxylin and eosin preparation. × 400. **B.** Fibrous variant of Hashimoto's thyroiditis with extensive fibrosis. Hematoxylin and eosin preparation. × 63.

Cytopathology

Aspirates of the thyroid gland involved by Hashimoto's disease are polymorphic with an admixture of inflammatory cells and epithelial cells in varying proportions[1,15] (Fig. 11.11; Table 11.3). The cellularity is variable, according to the stage of the disease and the extent of involvement. Usually, the inflammatory cells are comprised of lymphocytes, plasma cells, and lymphoid follicle center (germinal center) cells. These last cells are characterized by the entire range of transforming lymphocytes, including immunoblasts and histiocytes with phagocytic debris (Fig. 11.12A). The lymphoid cells, being very fragile, are often distorted and are seen as stretched fibers, frequently in dark, tangled masses[8] (Fig. 11.12B). Aspirate of the lymphoid variety, as described by Woolner, grossly resembles a buffy coat of centrifuged blood.

TABLE 11.3. Cytopathologic Features of Lymphocytic (Hashimoto's) Thyroiditis

1. Inflammatory cell component
   Lymphocytes
   Plasma cells
   Germinal center cells, eg, transforming lymphocytes, immunoblasts, and histiocytes
      with or without phagocytized debris
2. Multinucleated foreign-body–type giant cells
3. Epithelial cell component
   Hürthle cells, mostly in tissue fragments
   Considerable pleomorphism in size of cells and nuclei
   Follicular cells in tissue fragments with and without nuclear atypia; follicular pattern
      uncommon
4. Colloid scant or absent

Cytologic preparations of such aspirates show a dense population of lymphoid cells, resembling an imprint or lymph node aspirate (Fig. 11.13). Multinucleated foreign-body–type giant cells are seen only infrequently (Fig. 11.14).

Epithelial cells, generally seen in tissue fragments, are either Hürthle cell or regular follicular cell type, or both (Fig. 11.15). The component cells are very cohesive and rather sticky, although epithelial cells can occur singly. The Hürthle cells are pleomorphic in size and shape. Likewise, their nuclei vary considerably, often staining hyperchromatic and pyknotic. Prominent cherry-red nucleoli, a feature so characteristic of Hürthle cell neoplasm, is not commonly seen. The follicular cells may be their usual size or hyperplastic, and are aspirated in tight clusters. When the cells are of normal size with scanty cytoplasm, they are difficult to differentiate from lymphocytes (Fig. 11.16). Tissue fragments of follicular epithelium rarely show a good follicular pattern. Their nuclei often show pronounced atypia. In fact, an atypical nuclear pattern of both Hürthle cells and regular follicular cells is more common in Hashimoto's thyroiditis. Colloid is scant or absent. In the latter stages with increasing fibrosis, the aspirate is often acellular or poorly cellular, showing only a few lymphocytes. Stromal tissue fragments may be occasionally seen.

There are frequent deviations from the usually encountered patterns described above that may result in interpretative traps for the cytopathologist. These are discussed in detail in the following sections of this chapter.

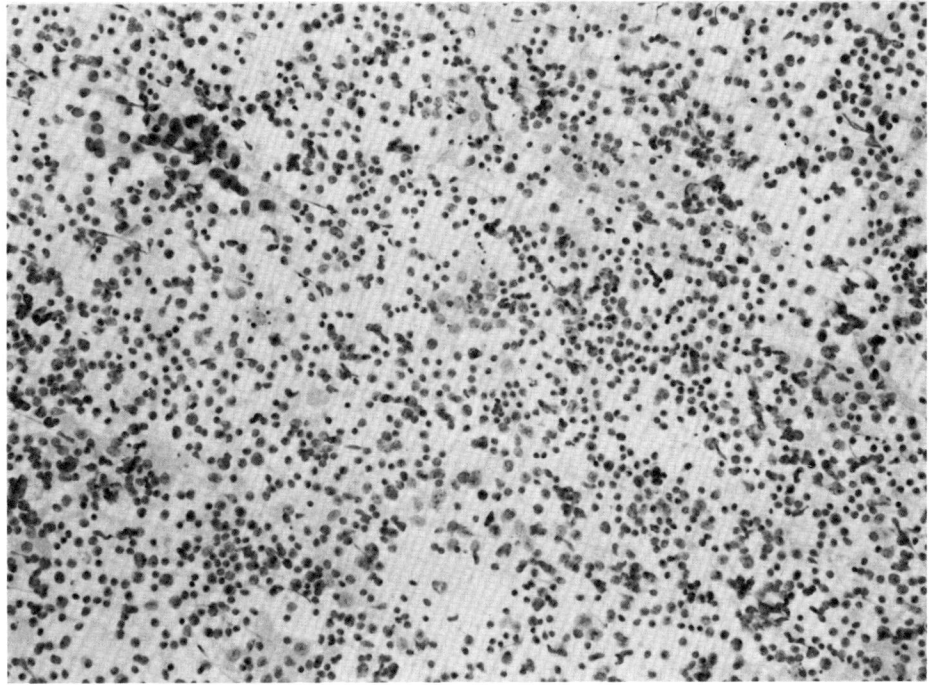

Fig. 11.11. Aspiration biopsy specimen of Hashimoto's thyroiditis showing an admixture of inflammatory and epithelial cells. Papanicolaou preparation. × 160.

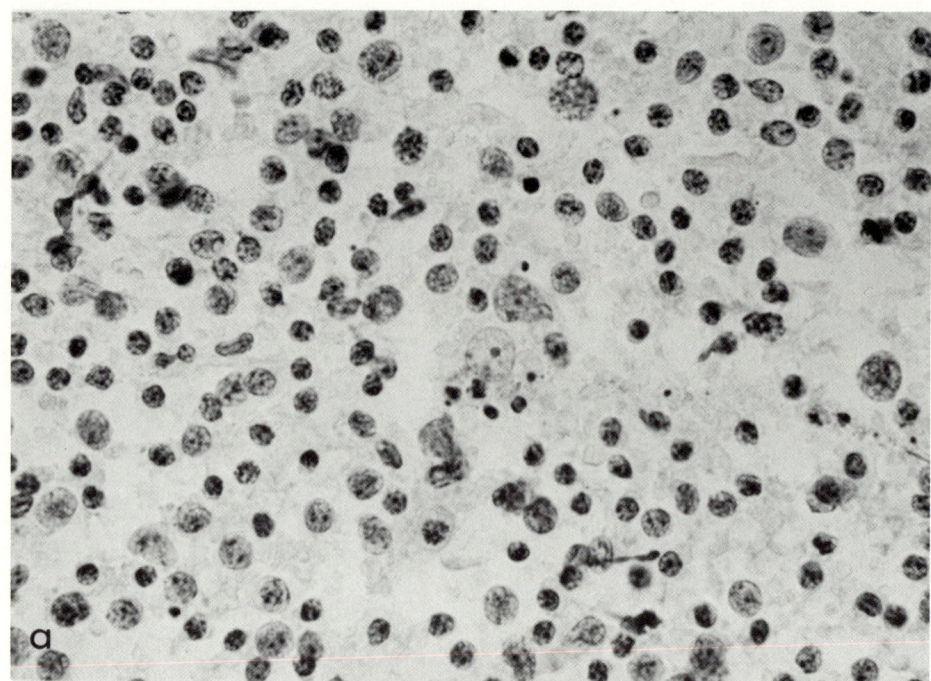

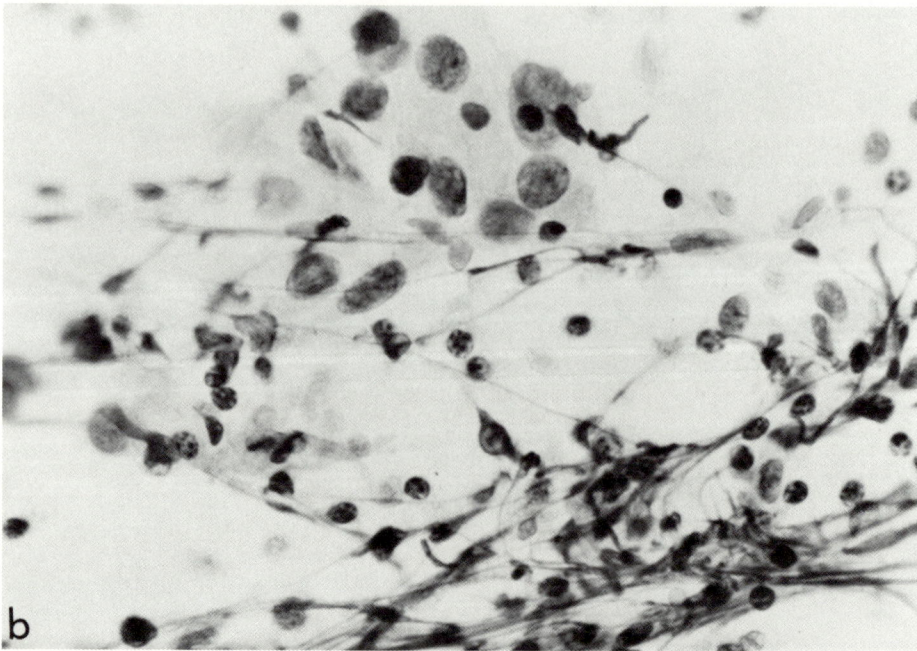

Fig. 11.12. A. Polymorphic cell population representing a germinal center of lymphoid follicles. Papanicolaou preparation. × 630. **B.** Hashimoto's thyroiditis showing stretched lymphocytes and Hürthle cells. Papanicolaou preparation. × 630.

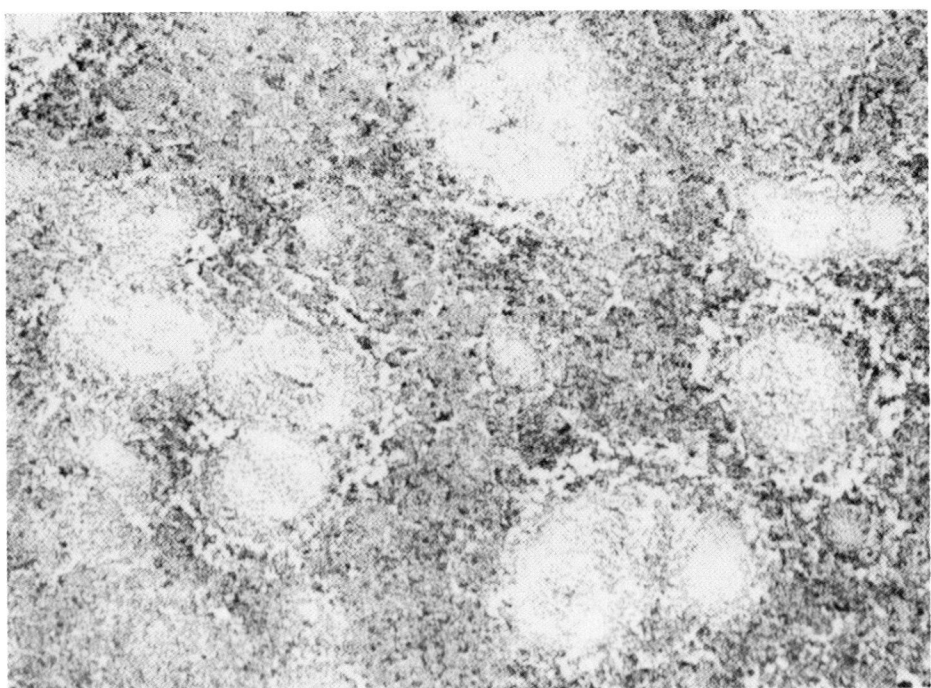

Fig. 11.13. Hashimoto's thyroiditis, lymphoid variety showing a heavy inflammatory component resembling an imprint of a lymph node. The light and dark areas duplicate the follicular pattern of the lymph node. Papanicolaou preparation. × 63.

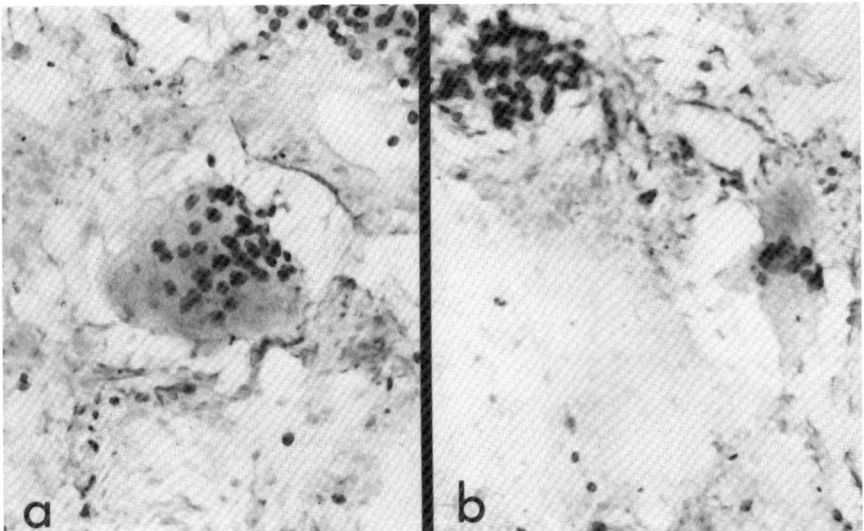

Fig. 11.14. A., B. Multinucleated foreign-body–type giant cells. This is not a usual pattern. Papanicolaou preparation. × 630.

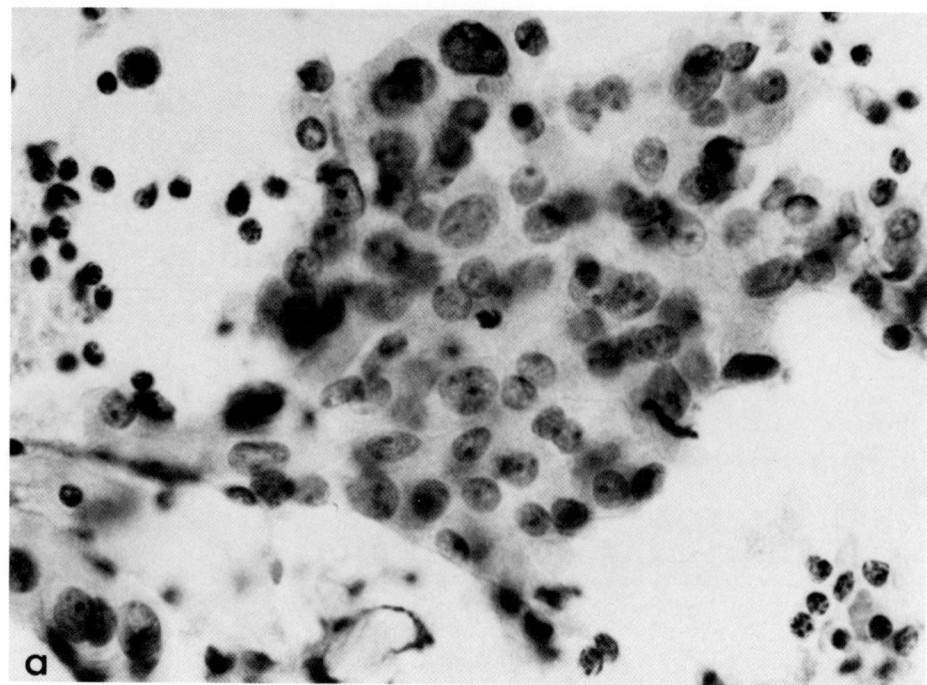

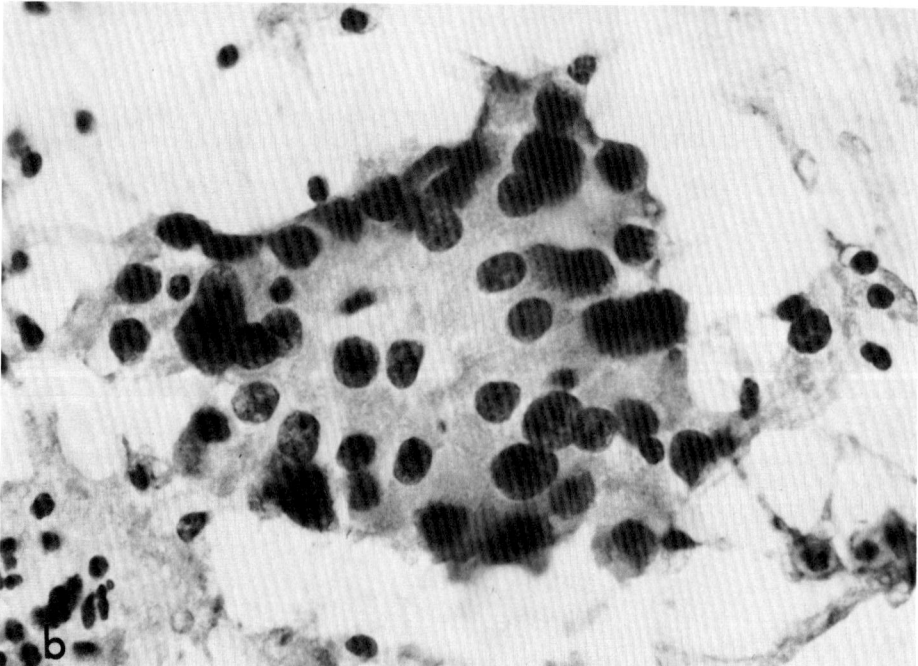

Fig. 11.15. A. Hashimoto's thyroiditis with epithelial component. A tissue fragment of follicular cells with atypical nuclei and lymphoplasmacytic cells in the background. Papanicolaou preparation. × 630. **B.** Tissue fragement of Hürthle cells with pleomorphic nuclei. Note compact chromatin and absence of macronucleoli. Papanicolaou preparation. × 630.

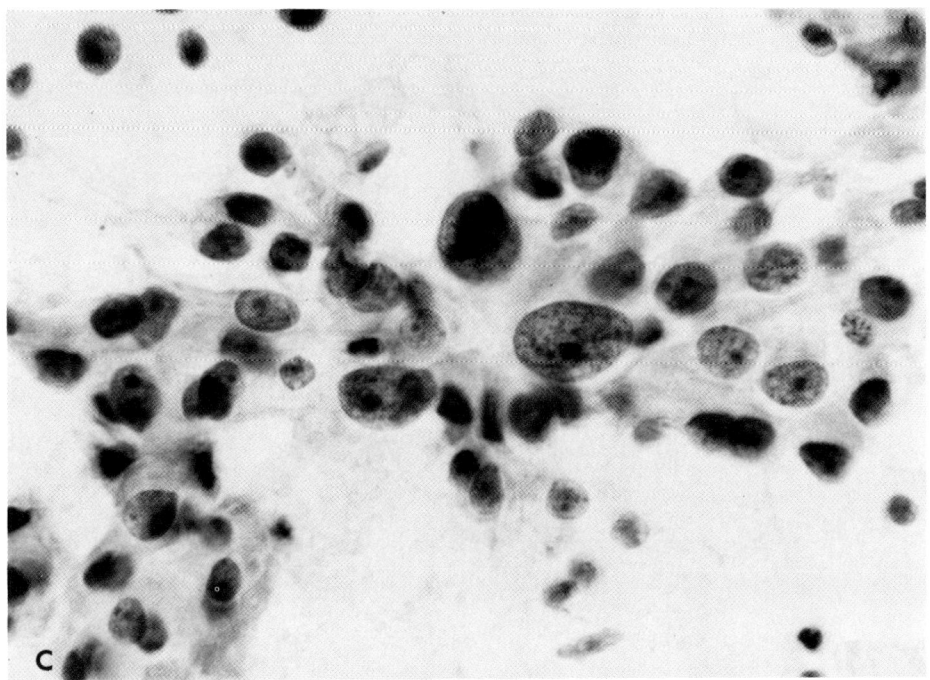

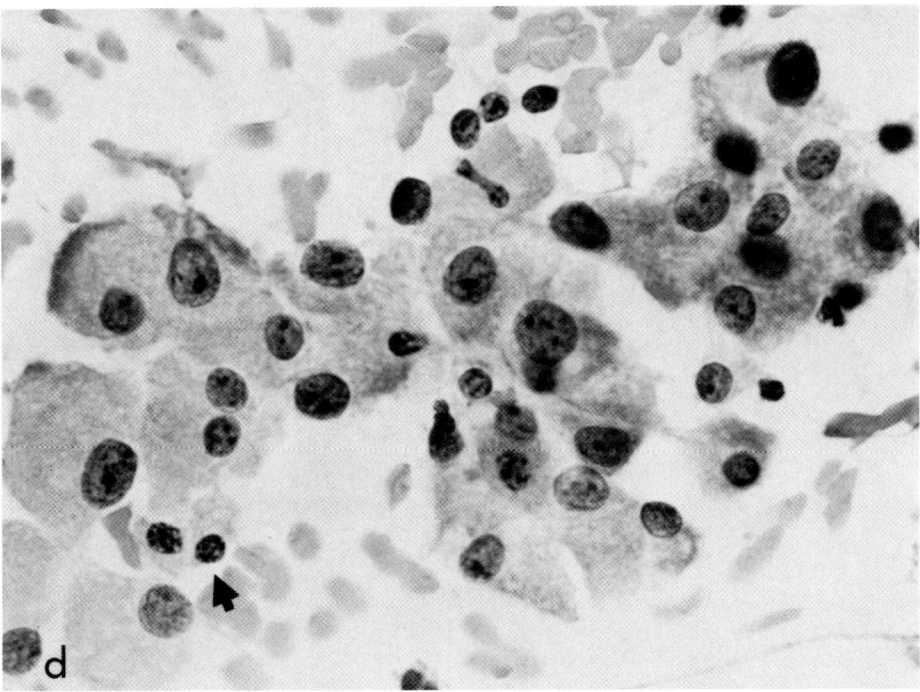

Fig. 11.15. C. Tissue fragment of Hürthle cells with pleomorphic nuclei, an occasional one containing macronucleolus. Inflammatory cells are sparse. Such an aspirate may be mistyped as Hürthle cell tumor. Papanicolaou preparation. × 630. **D.** Discrete Hürthle cells, many showing macronucleoli. The chromatin pattern is compact. Note plasma cells in the background *(arrow)*. In the presence of inflammatory cells, such an aspirate must not be interpreted as Hürthle cell neoplasm. Papanicolaou preparation. × 630.

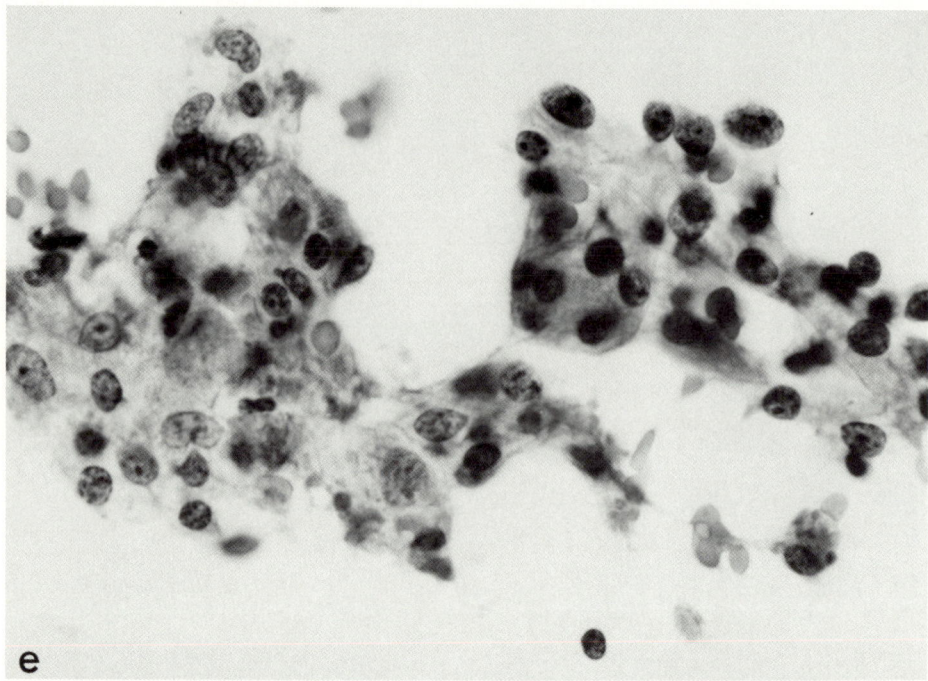

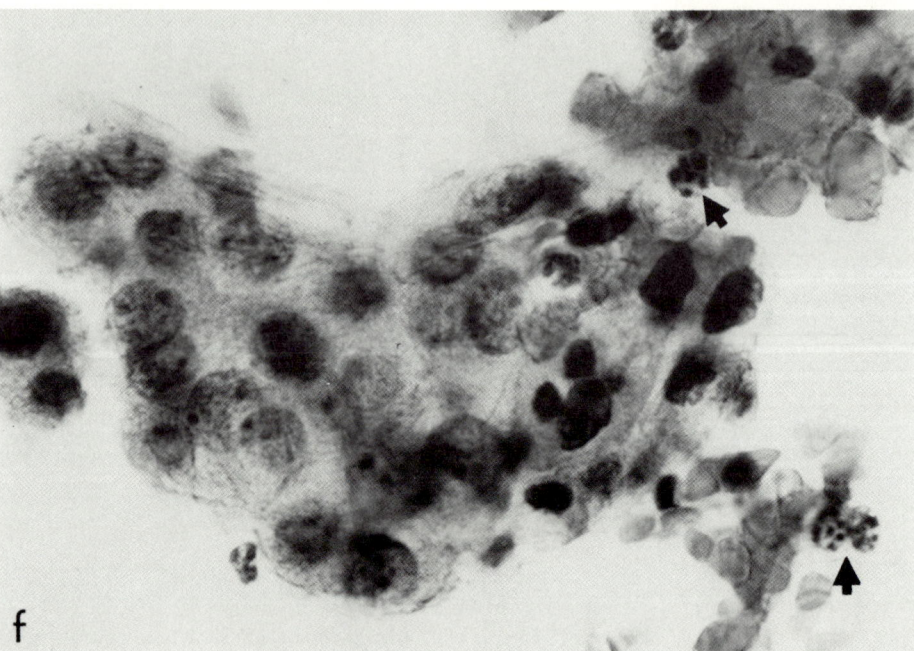

Fig. 11.15. E. Tissue fragments of follicular cells with nuclear atypia. Lymphocytes are very scarse. This aspirate can easily be mistyped as follicular neoplasm. Papanicolaou preparation. × 630. **F.** Tissue fragments of follicular epithelium with pronounced nuclear atypia suspected of being follicular carcinoma. Note plasma cells *(arrow)*. Thyroidectomy revealed extensive Hashimoto's thyroiditis. Papanicolaou preparation. × 1000.

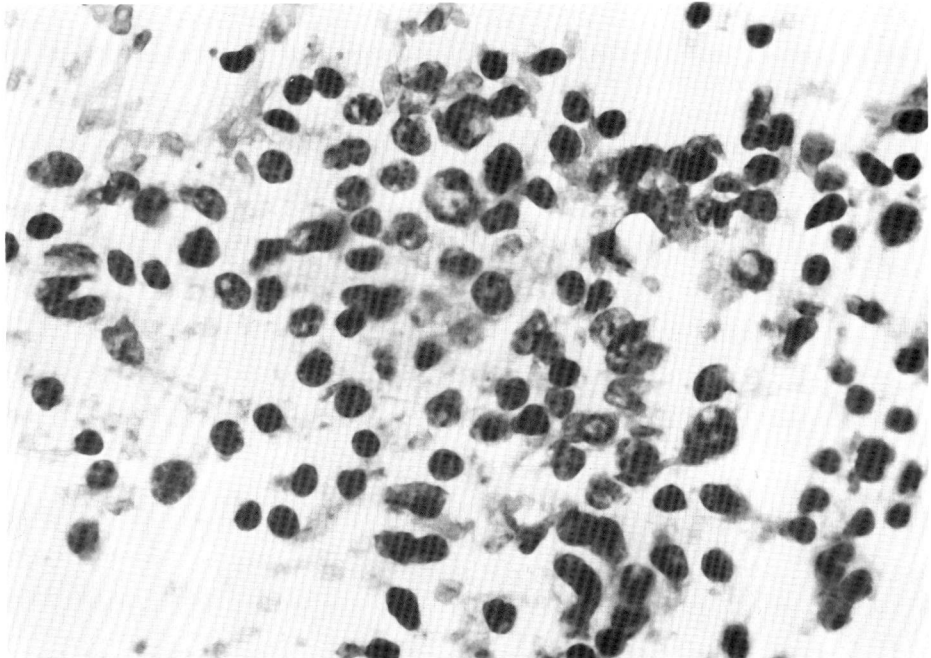

Fig. 11.16. Epithelial cell cluster obscured by lymphoplasmacytic cells. It is difficult to differentiate both the components. Papanicolaou preparation. × 630.

Diagnostic Accuracy

Hashimoto's thyroiditis as a disease entity presents complex diagnostic problems, not only because its cytologic changes mimic various types of neoplasia, but also because benign or malignant neoplasms occur frequently in its background. Hashimoto's thyroiditis can simulate symptoms and signs commonly associated with the neoplastic process. Features such as asymmetric enlargement, firmness, and nodularity of the thyroid gland are seen in Hashimoto's thyroiditis with or without a coexisting neoplasm. Imaging defects can be seen in both. It is extremely difficult to differentiate cases of Hashimoto's thyroiditis with neoplasm from those that do not harbor any tumors.[26] Thus, a fair number of patients with thyroiditis are subjected to surgery. Thomas and Rutledge[22] reported a high incidence of chronic thyroiditis in surgical specimens. Hashimoto's thyroiditis, with its characteristic clinical presentation and specific laboratory data, does not justify a thyroidectomy for diagnosis or treatment. In doubtful cases, aspiration biopsy is very useful.

It is most difficult for us to judge the diagnostic accuracy of Hashimoto's thyroiditis because, in our practice, typical cases are not subject to biopsy. In patients with a clinical diagnosis of Hashimoto's thyroiditis, an aspiration biopsy is performed primarily to rule out a neoplastic process under the following circumstances:

Enlarging goiter with suppression therapy

Nodularity with or without cold imaging defects

Enlarging tender goiter

Also, some patients are asymptomatic and present with palpable nodules that are cold on imaging. A diagnosis of Hashimoto's thyroiditis is made on a cytologic basis after an aspiration biopsy has been performed, followed by routine studies done for Hashimoto's thyroiditis.

Cytologic errors in Hashimoto's thyroiditis can be grouped into two main areas:

1. False-positive diagnoses, ie, diagnoses of neoplastic disease made when cytologic changes of Hashimoto's thyroiditis mimic neoplasia. A diagnosis of coexisting thyroiditis may or may not have been made.

2. False-negative diagnoses, ie, failure to identify a neoplastic process coexistent with thyroiditis.

Our initial experience in this field revealed many false-positive as well as false-negative results, reflecting inexperience in cytologic interpretations and the failure to appreciate subtle differentiating features. In later years, errors have been considerably minimized. Thus, the statistics presented here reflect two time periods: 1976–1978 (Table 11.4) and 1979–1985 (Table 11.5).

The first period includes 117 cases (Table 11.4) in which aspiration biopsy was performed because of cold nodules.[15] The diagnosis of Hashimoto's thyroiditis was made clinically, cytologically, or histologically. Thirteen cases were misinterpreted as follicular or Hürthle cell neoplasms. Three cases of malignant lymphoma were diagnosed as thyroiditis. A papillary carcinoma in the background of thyroiditis was identified easily and accurately.

During the second period (Table 11.5), 398 patients had a cytologic diagnosis of Hashimoto's thyroiditis, of which 89 cases had a diagnosis of coexistent neoplasm. Histologic confirmation was available for only a small number of patients (Table

TABLE 11.4. Cytohistologic Data on 117 Patients with Hashimoto's Thyroiditis[15] (1976–1978)

Cytologic Diagnosis	No. of Patients	No. of Biopsies	Histologic Diagnosis
Lymphocytic thyroiditis	87*	20	17 lymphocytic thyroiditis 3 malignant lymphoma
Lymphocytic thyroiditis and papillary carcinoma	7	7	7 papillary carcinoma with lymphocytic thyroiditis
Lymphocytic thyroiditis and cellular adenoma	6	4	4 cellular adenomas with lymphocytic thyroiditis
Lymphocytic thyroiditis and possible lymphoma	4	3	1 lymphocytic thyroiditis 2 malignant lymphoma
Cellular adenoma	3	3	3 lymphocytic thyroiditis
Hüthle cell tumor	3	3	3 lymphocytic thyroiditis
Suspected follicular carcinoma	7	7	7 lymphocytic thyroiditis
Total	117		

*One patient developed malignant lymphoma 7 years after the diagnosis of lymphocytic thyroiditis.

11.5). It is noteworthy that coexistent diagnoses of follicular neoplasms or Hürthle cell neoplasms were only sparingly made, whereas the diagnosis of malignant lymphoma or papillary carcinoma in the presence of Hashimoto's thyroiditis was made more frequently.

Hashimoto's Thyroiditis Versus Other Diseases

Diagnostic difficulties can occur when Hashimoto's thyroiditis is mistaken for other diseases. A cytologic diagnosis of Hashimoto's thyroiditis is easily made when an aspirate presents lymphoplasmacytic cells along with epithelial cells, and both components are present in fair proportions. However, potential errors can occur if an inflammatory or an epithelial component predominates, and the usual presentation is absent. Thus, cytologic changes of Hashimoto's thyroiditis can be mistaken for other types of thyroiditis or various types of neoplasms (Table 11.6). The differentiating features are summarized in Table 11.7.

TABLE 11.5. Cytohistologic Data on 398 Patients with Hashimoto's Thyroiditis (1979–1985)

Cytologic Diagnosis	No. of Patients	No. of Patients with Large Needle Biopsy	No. of Patients with Surgery	Histologic Diagnosis
Lymphocytic thyroiditis	307	45		Hashimoto's thyroiditis
Lymphocytic thyroiditis and papillary carcinoma	18		18	16 papillary carcinoma and Hashimoto's thyroiditis 2 Hashimoto's thyroiditis
Lymphocytic thyroiditis and suspected papillary carcinoma	9	1	3	1 papillary carcinoma and Hashimoto's thyroiditis 3 Hashimoto's thyroiditis
Lymphocytic thyroiditis and malignant lymphoma	21	21	18	18 malignant lymphoma and Hashimoto's thyroiditis 1 lymphocytic thyroiditis 2 atypical lymphoid hyperplasia
Lymphocytic thyroiditis and suspected malignant lymphoma	10	9	4	3 malignant lymphoma and Hashimoto's thyroiditis 6 Hashimoto's thyroiditis
Lymphocytic thyroiditis and cellular adenoma	1		1	Cellular adenoma and Hashimoto's thyroiditis
Lymphocytic thyroiditis and (?)cellular adenoma	15	4		2 nodular goiter 2 cellular adenoma
Lymphocytic thyroiditis and follicular carcinoma	2	2	2	1 follicular carcinoma and Hashimoto's thyroiditis 1 atypical adenoma and Hashimoto's thyroiditis
Lymphocytic thyroiditis and (?)Hürtle cell tumor	11	2		1 Hashimoto's thyroiditis 1 cellular adenoma
Lymphocytic thyroiditis and Hürtle cell carcinoma	1	1	1	Hashimoto's thyroiditis and atypical Hürtle cell nodule
Lymphocytic thyroiditis and carcinoma, type unknown	1	1	1	Malignant thymoma
Cellular adenoma	1	1		Hashimoto's thyroiditis
Hüthle cell tumor	1	1		Hashimoto's thyroiditis
Total	398			

TABLE 11.6. Cytopathologic Changes of Hashimoto's
Thyroiditis Commonly Misdiagnosed as

Granulomatous thyroiditis
Hürthle cell neoplasm
Follicular neoplasm (adenoma or carcinoma)
Papillary carcinoma
Malignant lymphoma

Hashimoto's Thyroiditis Versus Granulomatous Thyroiditis

Multinucleated foreign-body–type giant cells are seen only infrequently in aspirates of Hashimoto's thyroiditis. When present, they are sparse. If there is an unusually large number of such giant cells, granulomatous thyroiditis may be suspected. In the latter, giant cells are enormous in size and contain several nuclei, whereas those from Hashimoto's thyroiditis tend to be modest in size, with fewer nuclei. Lymphocytes are present in both, but germinal center cells are not present in granulomatous thyroiditis. Hürthle cell changes with nuclear atypia may be seen in both. Clinical data are necessary to corroborate the cytologic findings.

Hashimoto's Thyroiditis Versus Hürthle Cell Neoplasm

A pronounced Hürthle cell change in thyroiditis can give rise to palpable nodules that are often suspected of a neoplasm clinically and on imaging (Figs. 11.17 and 11.18; Plate 11.1). Aspiration biopsy specimen of such nodules will show a large population of Hürthle cells and very few lymphocytes, which can be easily overlooked (see Chapter 7, Hürthle Cell Lesions). It must also be noted that this diagnostic pitfall sometimes extends to histologic specimens as well.

Hürthle cells in aspirates of Hashimoto's thyroiditis are more often seen in cohesive groups. The cells, as well as their nuclei, are pleomorphic, atypical, and frequently pyknotic, lacking the prominent macronucleolus of neoplastic Hürthle cells. The monomorphic pattern characteristic of a neoplasm is not generally appreciated in involutional nodules, but exceptions do occur (Fig. 11.18).

Hashimoto's Thyroiditis Versus Follicular Neoplasm

Follicular hyperplasia in Hashimoto's thyroiditis results in nodule formation (Figs. 11.19 and 11.20; Plates 11.2 and 11.3). Fine-needle biopsy specimens of such nodules show mostly tissue fragments of follicular epithelium, with or without nuclear atypia. The follicular cells appear very cohesive and are architecturally difficult to differentiate from syncytial-type tissue fragments of follicular neoplasm. A follicular pattern, however, is not common in thyroiditis. The presence of any inflammatory cells, such as lymphocytes or plasmacytes, suggests a non-neoplastic nodule (Fig. 11.21). Stretched out lymphoid cells often serve as a clue in identification of the aspirate as that of Hashimoto's thyroiditis.

TABLE 11.7. Differential Diagnosis of Hashimoto's Thyroiditis

	Hashimoto's Thyroiditis	Granulomatous Thyroiditis	Hürthle Cell Tumor	Follicular Neoplasms	Papillary Carcinoma	Malignant Lymphoma
INFLAMMATORY CELLS:						
Lymphocytes	Alway present	Present	Absent	Absent	Present if associated with thyroiditis	Monomorphic population of poorly differentiated lymphoid cells
Plasma cells	Present	Sometimes	Absent	Absent	Present if associated with thyroiditis	
Germinal center cells	Usually present	Absent	Absent	Absent	Present if associated with thyroiditis	Lymphocytes, plasma cells, and germinal center cells may be present in other slides or separate from lymphoma cell population

	Hashimoto's Thyroiditis	Granulomatous Thyroiditis	Hürthle Cell Tumor	Follicular Neoplasms	Papillary Carcinoma	Malignant Lymphoma
INFLAMMATORY CELLS:						
Neutrophils	Absent	Present in early stages	Absent	Absent	Absent	Absent
Foreign-body–type multinucleated giant cells	Sometimes	Always present; large, with several nuclei in close proximity to epithelial cells or colloid	Absent	Absent	Present	Absent
Epithelioid cells	Absent	Present	Absent	Absent	Absent	Absent
EPITHELIAL CELLS:						
Hürthle cells	Usually present, mostly in cohesive groups, some isolated; pleomorphic in size; nuclei usually hyperchromatic, atypical, lack cherry-red macronucleus, often obscured by lymphocytes	Often present, nuclear atypia may or may not be present	Monomorphic cells, isolated or loosely cohesive groups; well-defined cell borders; binucleation common; cherry-red macronucleoli characteristic	Absent	May be present as part of coexisting thyroiditis	Hürthle cells or follicular cells may be present separate from lymphoma cells

TABLE 11.7. Continued

EPITHELIAL CELLS:

	Hashimoto's Thyroiditis	Granulomatous Thyroiditis	Hürthle Cell Tumor	Follicular Neoplasms	Papillary Carcinoma	Malignant Lymphoma
Follicular cells	Usually present, mostly in tissue fragments without follicular pattern, occasional single cells; papillary configuration may be seen; nuclei variable in size, may be markedly atypical; nuclear morphology of papillary carcinoma lacking	Present with or without nuclear atypia	Absent	Syncytial-type tissue fragments with or without follicular pattern; nuclei uniformly enlarged	Syncytial-type tissue fragments with or without follicular pattern; papillary or monolayered tissue fragments; single cells may be present; typical nuclear cytomorphology; psammoma bodies help in diagnosis	
Intranuclear cytoplasmic inclusions	Rarely seen	Absent	May be present in Hürthle cell carcinoma	Absent	Very frequent	Absent
Colloid	Generally absent	Inspissated droplets	Absent	Scant or absent	Scant or absent	Absent
Degenerative Changes	Generally absent	Absent	May be present	May be present	Often	May be present
Karyorrhexis	Absent	Absent	Absent	Absent	Absent	Often
Stromal cells	Occasional	Often			Often	

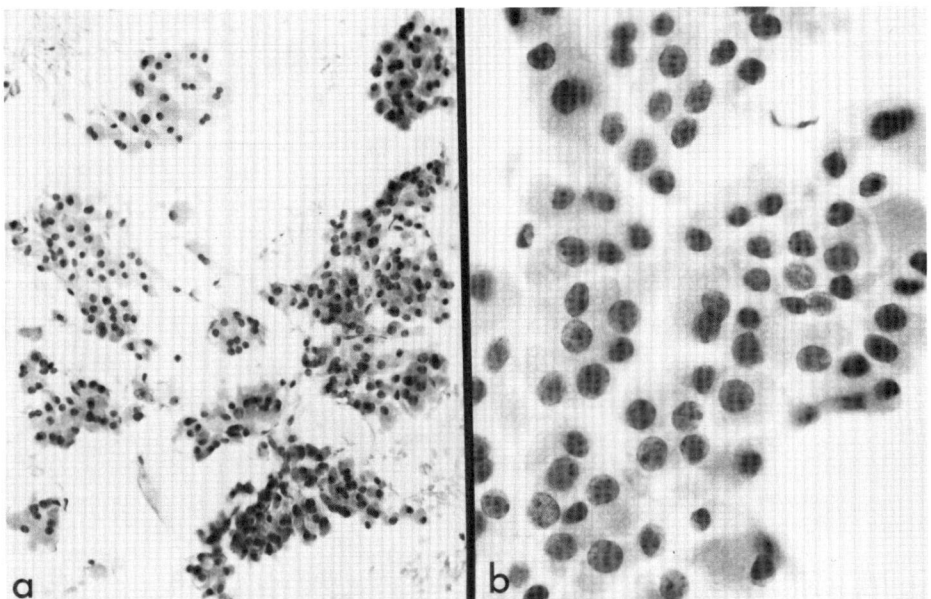

Fig. 11.17. A. Cellular aspirate showing several tissue fragments of Hürthle cells. Papanicolaou preparation. × 160. **B.** Higher magnification of **A** showing loosely cohesive Hürthle cells lacking macronucleoli. Lymphocytes were not identified in the aspirate. Papanicolaou preparation. × 630. A diagnosis of Hürthle cell tumor was not confirmed by large-needle biopsy, which showed Hashimoto's thyroiditis.

Hashimoto's Thyroiditis Versus Papillary Carcinoma

Papillary hyperplasia of the follicular epithelium may be seen occasionally in Hashimoto's thyroiditis and can be mistaken for papillary carcinoma. Earlier, we reported that the diagnosis of papillary carcinoma can easily be made in the background of Hashimoto's thyroiditis.[15] Since then, we have had some cases in which this diagnosis was not confirmed histologically. Clinically, a papillary hyperplasia in thyroiditis can present with nodularity, and on biopsy specimen it can exhibit papillary tissue fragments. Generally, however, such an hyperplastic process fails to show the typical nuclear morphology of papillary carcinoma. Intranuclear cytoplasmic inclusions may be rarely encountered, leading to a false-positive diagnosis. Errors may be made when minimal criteria for the diagnosis of papillary carcinoma are not met (see Chapter 8, Papillary Carcinoma).

Hashimoto's Thyroiditis Versus Malignant Lymphoma

Aspiration biopsy of the lymphoid variety of Hashimoto's thyroiditis will yield an aspirate containing a dense population of lymphocytes that can be easily mistaken for malignant lymphoma (Plate 11.4). This is discussed in Chapter 12, Malignant Lymphoma.

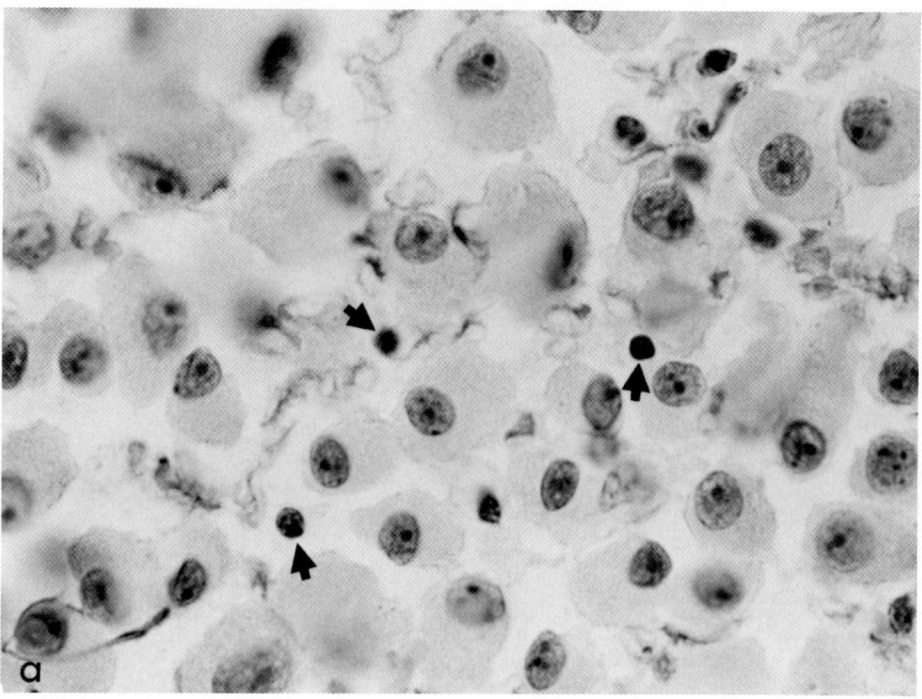

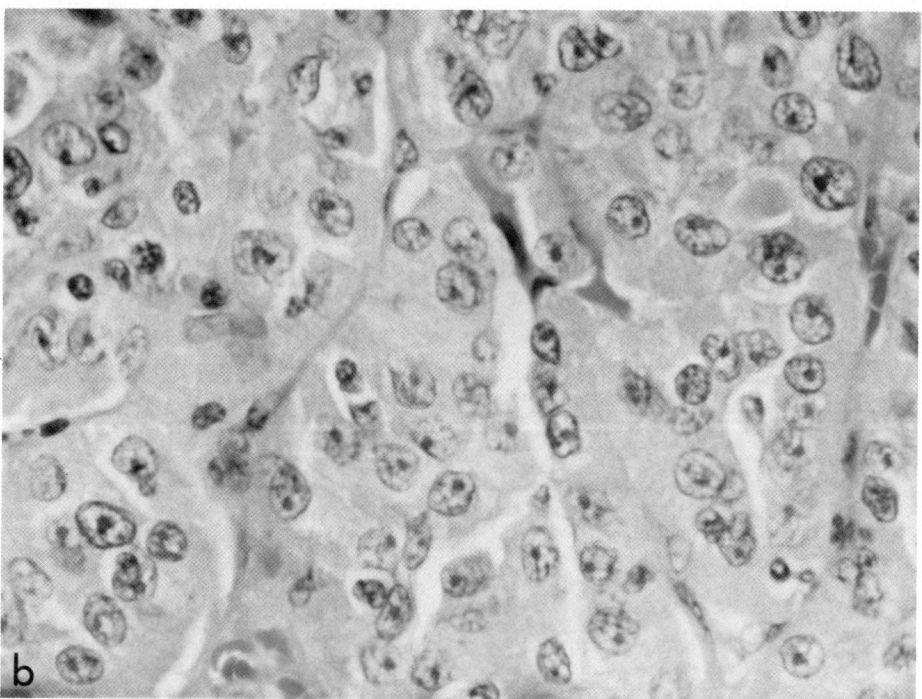

Fig. 11.18. A. These Hürthle cells with high nuclear/cytoplasmic ratio and prominent macronucleoli were highly suggestive of Hürthle cell carcinoma in spite of lymphocytes *(arrow)*. Papanicolaou preparation. × 630. **B.** Large-needle biopsy specimen, which was equally convincing of Hürthle cell carcinoma. Note the trabecular pattern with crowding. Hematoxylin and eosin preparation. × 630.

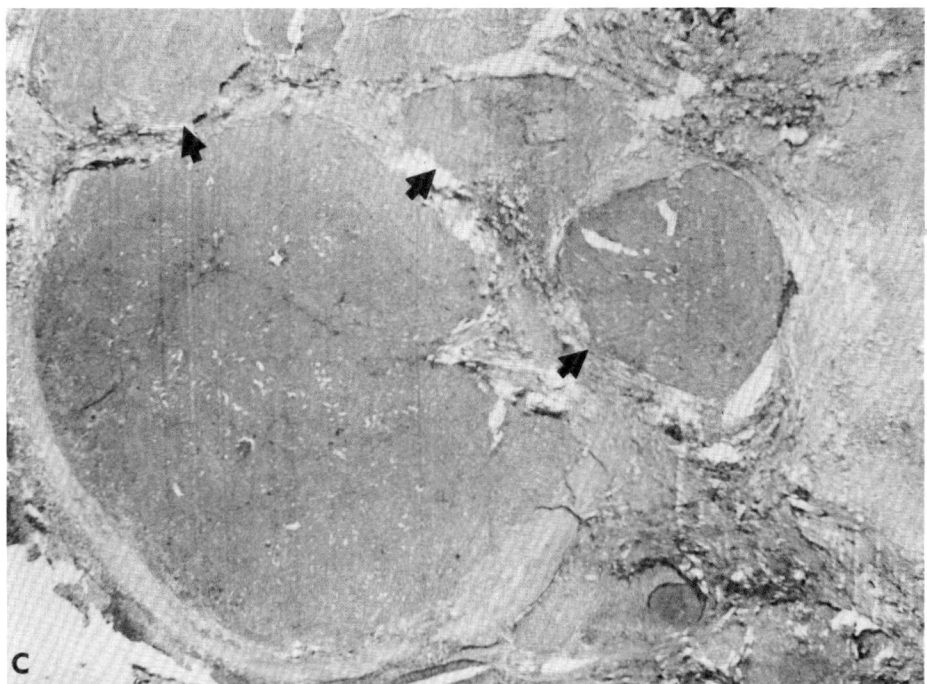

Fig. 11.18. C. Thyroidectomy showed extensive Hashimoto's thyroiditis with encapsulated Hürthle cell nodule extending outside the capsule *(arrows)*, with histomorphology the same as in **B**. Final diagnosis by the pathologist was atypical Hürthle cell nodule. Hematoxylin and eosin preparation. × 43.

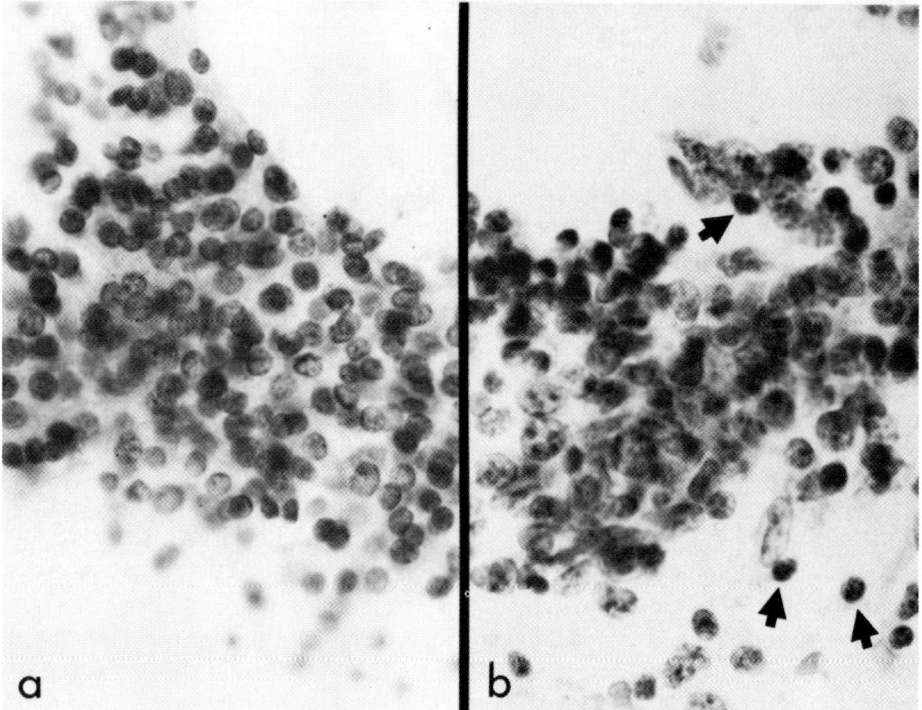

Fig. 11.19. Similarities between cells of follicular neoplasm and follicular hyperplasia in Hashimoto's thyroiditis. **A.** Follicular neoplasm. Papanicolaou preparation. × 630. **B.** Follicular hyperplasia in Hashimoto's thyroiditis. Papanicolaou preparation. × 630. Without lymphocytes in the background *(arrow)*, distinction between the two is not possible.

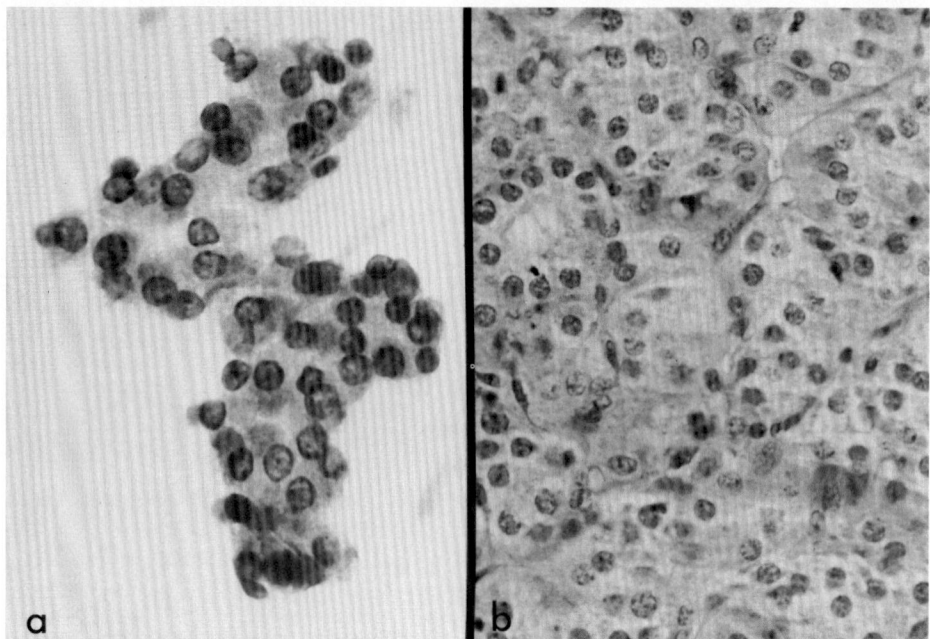

Fig. 11.20. Hyperplastic follicular nodule. **A.** Aspirate showing tissue fragments of follicular epithelium with follicular pattern. In the absence of lymphoid cells, these cannot be differentiated from a follicular neoplasm. Papanicolaou preparation. × 630. **B.** Large-needle biopsy specimen showing follicular hyperplasia. Hashimoto's thyroiditis was seen elsewhere in the section. Hematoxylin and eosin preparation. × 400.

Hashimoto's Thyroiditis and Associated Neoplasms

There is considerable controversy over the causal relationship between Hashimoto's thyroiditis and other thyroid neoplasms. Some pathologists have disregarded any association between Hashimoto's thyroiditis and other thyroid neoplasms (Table 11.8). The controversy stems from several inconsistencies, including the lack of uniformity in terminology and criteria for Hashimoto's thyroiditis among pathologists.

In a review of 1150 surgical pathology reports on thyroidectomies from our series, lymphocytic infiltrate was noted in 190 cases and was diagnosed by different pathologists variously as Hashimoto's thyroiditis, chronic lymphocytic thyroiditis, nonspecific lymphocytic infiltrate, or nonspecific thyroiditis. Although Woolner et al[25] classified various histologic types of Hashimoto's thyroiditis and concluded that the disease process can be diffuse or focal and that Hürthle cell change may not be consistent, some pathologists require a diffuse disease process and Hürthle cell change for the diagnosis of Hashimoto's thyroiditis. As antibody titers of all patients who undergo thyroid surgery are not routinely obtained, the findings of Hashimoto's thyroiditis and other neoplasms cannot be correlated. Livolsi and Marino[17] have justly remarked that adequate serologic and clinical documentation of Hashimoto's thyroiditis in patients with thyroid carcinoma is sorely lacking. Also, there is no direct correlation of clinical levels of thyroid-stimulating hormone, free thyroxine index (FTI), and antibody titers with the severity of histologic changes. Some have attributed the lymphocytic infiltrate in papillary thyroid carcinomas to host response,[22] but Carcangiu et al[3] have questioned this viewpoint.

Although a detailed discussion of this debate is beyond the scope of this monograph, it is enough to say here that there does seem to be an association between Hashimoto's thyroiditis and neoplasms. The problem is identifying the two disease processes.[9] Although we believe that malignant lymphoma and papillary carcinoma can be identified in the background of thyroiditis, we cannot say the same about Hürthle cell neoplasm or follicular cell neoplasm. The latter are difficult to diagnose in the presence of lymphocytes. The cytologic changes in the follicular epithelial component of thyroiditis are almost identical to those seen in follicular neoplasms. The differentiating features are very subtle, and experience is needed to appreciate them. On the other hand, papillary carcinoma presents specific diagnostic criteria that can be appreciated even in the background of thyroiditis. Nevertheless, caution must be exercised not to make a diagnosis too readily on the basis of insufficient criteria (see Chapter 8, Papillary Carcinoma). When malignant lymphoma is seen, it almost always arises in the background of Hashimoto's thyroiditis. The cytologic features and diagnostic pitfalls are described in Chapter 12, Malignant Lymphoma.

The apparent ease with which a papillary carcinoma or malignant lymphoma can be diagnosed in the background of thyroiditis and the difficulties presented by follicular or Hürthle cell neoplasms are understandable. Malignant lymphomas and most papillary carcinomas are nonencapsulated neoplastic processes (Fig. 11.21A). Involvement is, at times, diffuse and multicentric. Thus, the aspiration biopsy will yield samples that represent both disease processes. Also, several diagnostic features of papillary carcinoma allow easy recognition of both disease processes. On the other hand, follicular or Hürthle cell neoplasms are discrete, well demarcated, encapsulated lesions. Aspiration biopsy will sample only the lesion bordered by the capsule and not the adjacent parenchyma (Fig. 11.21B). Therefore, the coexisting process of Hashimoto's disease, if it exists, will be identified only in surgically removed specimens. Involutional Hürthle cell nodules or hyperplastic follicular nodules of Hashimoto's thyroiditis are nonencapsulated lesions, even though they are discrete and large. They almost always show lymphocytic infiltrate and even germinal centers. Thus, aspiration biopsy will show mostly epithelial cells and lymphoplasmacytic cells (Fig. 11.21C). These are usually few in number and easily overlooked. Hence, we recommend extreme caution in the diagnosis of follicular and Hürthle cell neoplasms in the presence of lymphocytes. If any doubt exists, it is our practice to alert the clinician and suggest additional investigations. These include laboratory studies to confirm thyroiditis, if they have not been done, and a large-needle biopsy, if the nodule size permits. Because thyroid neoplasms are slow-growing, it is not necessary to hasten surgical intervention.

Hashimoto's Thyroiditis and Papillary Carcinoma

Of the malignant neoplasms associated with Hashimoto's thyroiditis, papillary carcinoma (Fig. 11.22) is the most frequent. In a review of 329 papillary carcinomas of the thyroid, lymphocytic infiltration was noted cytologically in 36 cases (10%), and histologically in 92 cases (28%). The disparity is explained by Fig. 11.21, as

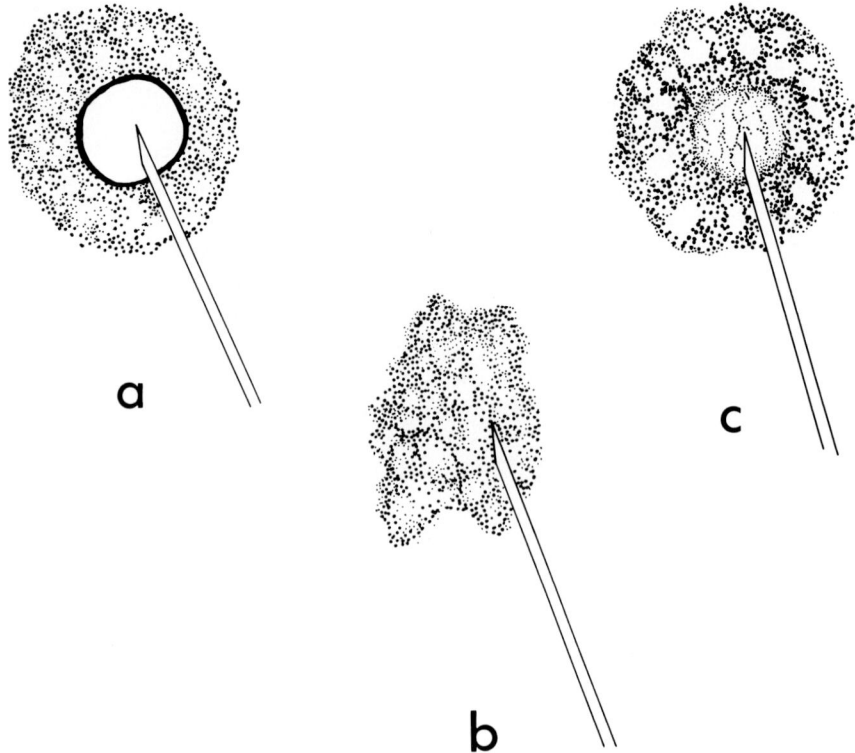

Fig. 11.21. Hashimoto's thyroiditis with associated neoplasms and hyperplastic or involutional nodules. **A.** Hashimoto's thyroiditis coexistent with discrete encapsulated neoplasms, e.g., follicular adenoma, minimally invasive follicular carcinoma, Hürthle cell tumors, follicular variant of papillary carcinoma, or discrete but nonencapsulated papillary carcinoma. The aspirates will represent only the neoplasm, and not the surrounding thyroid parenchyma. Coexistent Hashimoto's thyroiditis cannot be identified cytologically and is diagnosed only after thyroidectomy. **B.** Hashimoto's thyroiditis coexistent with malignant lymphoma or papillary carcinoma. The neoplastic process is quite often diffuse and multicentric. Thus, the aspiration biopsy specimen contains representative samples of both disease processes. **C.** Hashimoto's thyroiditis and hyperplastic or involutional nodules. Although these appear discrete and palpable when enlarged, they are nonencapsulated and often have lymphoplasmacytic infiltrate extending into the nodule. Aspiration biopsy specimen shows large population of epithelial cells (follicular or Hürthle) and a few lymphoplasmacytic cells as well. Presence of the latter indicates a non-neoplastic process.

mentioned earlier. With adequate cellularity showing several of the cytologic features of papillary carcinoma, both diseases may be diagnosed accurately (Figs. 11.23–11.26). The diagnostic pitfalls have been described above.

Hashimoto's Thyroiditis and Malignant Lymphoma

The association between these two diseases has been recognized by most authors. Cytologic identification of both diseases is certainly a challenge to the cytopathologist. Large groups of poorly differentiated lymphoid cells without an admixture of polymorphic germinal center cells should alert the examiner, even though areas on

TABLE 11.8. Incidence of Neoplasms in Hashimoto's Thyroiditis

Authors (yr)	Hashimoto's Thyroiditis	Hashimoto's Thyroiditis plus Neoplasms, Benign and Malignant	Hashimoto's Thyroiditis plus Carcinoma	Hashimoto's Thyroiditis plus Malignant Lymphoma	Hashimoto's Thyroiditis plus Malignancy	Hashimoto's Thyroiditis plus Adenoma
Chesky et al[5] (1962)	432	48	43 (10%)	5(1.1%)	(11.1%)	
Woolner et al[25] (1959)	605		18 (3%)	12 (2%)	(5%)	
Dailey et al[7] (1954)	278	73 (36.2%)	35 (17.7%)		(17.7%)	38 (18.5%)
Pollock and Sprang[19] (1985)	52	6 (11.5%)	5 (10%)	(1.2%)	(11.5%)	
Hirabayashi and Lindsay[13] (1965)	752		169 (22.5%)		(22.5%)	
Schlicke et al[20] (1960)	103		9 (8.7%)		(8.7%)	
Shands[21] (1960)	44	18 (32%)	3 (7%)		(7.0%)	
Crile[6] (1978)	373			1 (0.37%)	(0–0.37%)	
Holmes[14] (1977)	60	10 (6.6%)	2 (3.3%)	(3.5%)	(8.3%)	

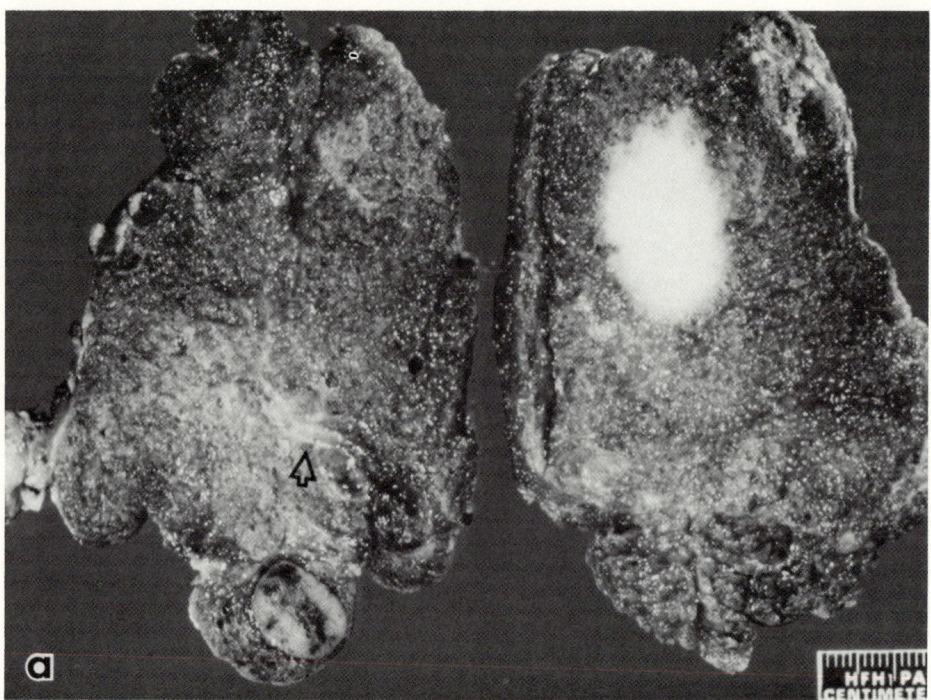

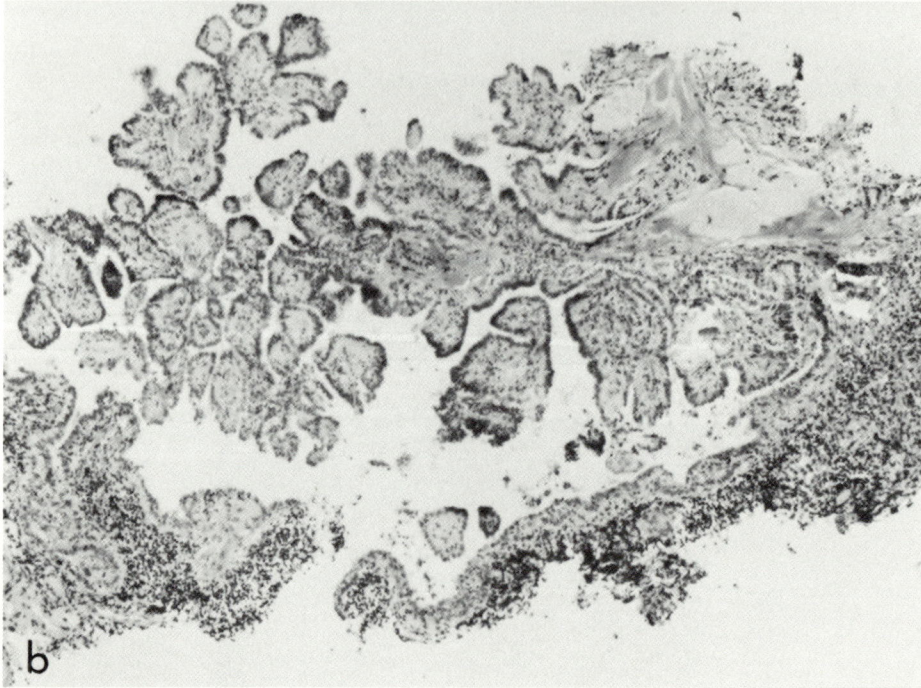

Fig. 11.22. A. Hashimoto's thyroiditis with fibrosis *(arrow)* and nonencapsulated lesion—a papillary carcinoma involving the left lobe. **B.** Large-needle biopsy specimen showing papillary carcinoma in the background of Hashimoto's thyroiditis. Hematoxylin and eosin preparation. × 63.

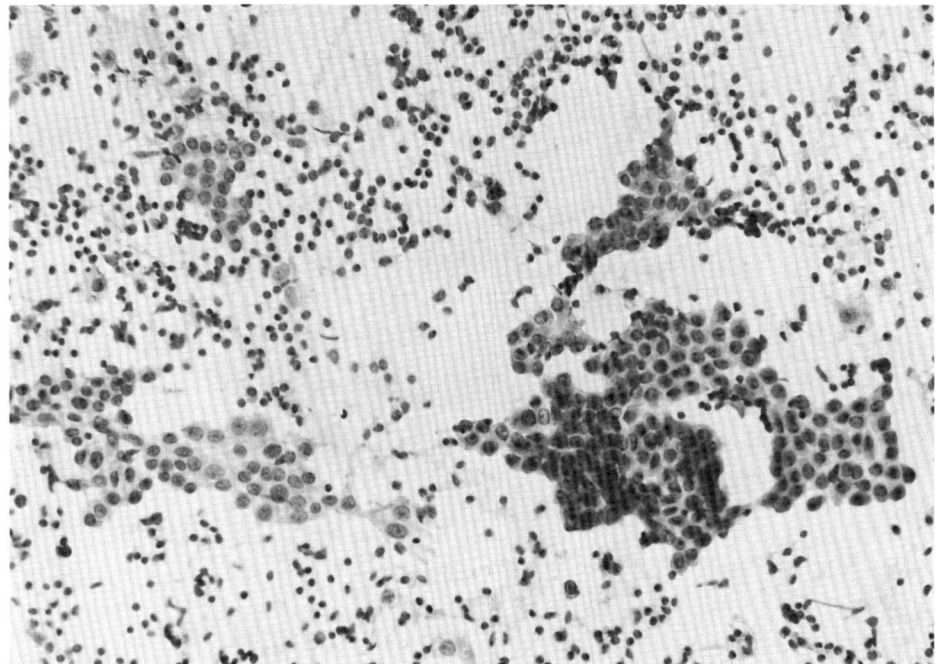

Fig. 11.23. Papillary carcinoma and Hashimoto's thyroiditis showing several monolayered tissue fragments and lymphoid cells. Papanicolaou preparation. × 400.

the same slide or sample smears on other slides display characteristic features of Hashimoto's thyroiditis.

Hashimoto's Thyroiditis and Benign Neoplasms

Most of the literature has focused on the association between Hashimoto's thyroiditis and malignant neoplasms (Table 11.8), and only a few authors have mentioned other neoplasms, such as follicular adenoma or Hürthle cell tumors.

We find it difficult to diagnose follicular or Hürthle cell neoplasms cytologically. Lymphocytic infiltrate is frequently seen in thyroid parenchyma adjacent to a benign neoplasm. Without clinical or laboratory data, the association between the neoplasm and lymphoid infiltrate is difficult to diagnose.

Summary

Hashimoto's thyroiditis is a clinical disease entity that presents with a diffusely enlarged goiter accompanied by altered laboratory data and varied histologic changes. Because a lymphocytic infiltrate may be seen in conditions other than Hashimoto's thyroiditis, cytologically the aspirates are best reported as lymphocytic thyroiditis.

This disease presents important diagnostic pitfalls. Not only is it a great imitator of various neoplasms, but the latter are very frequently present in its background.

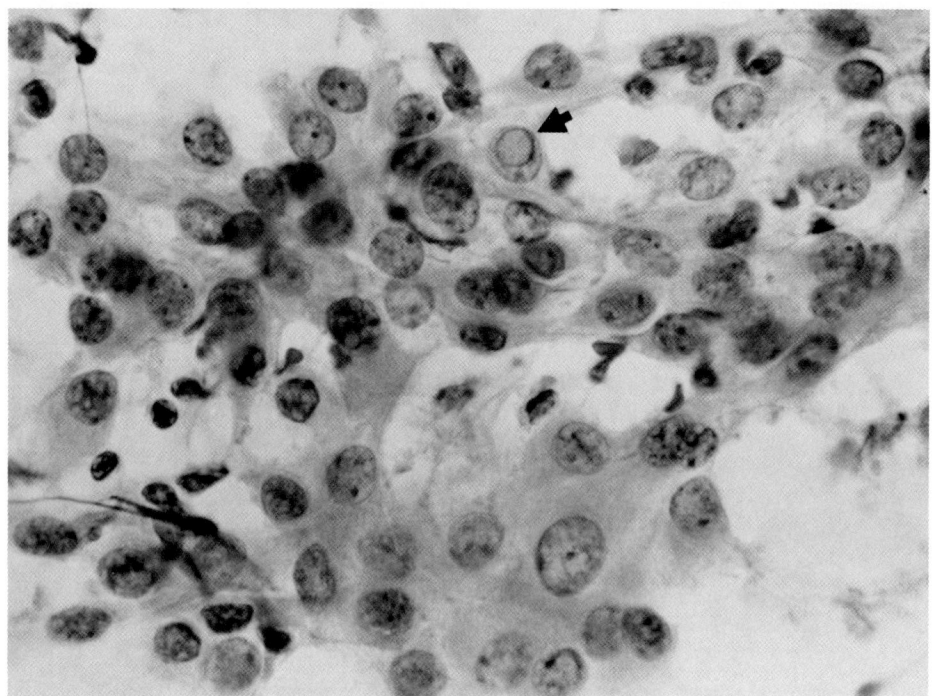

Fig. 11.24. Higher magnification of Fig. 11.23 showing enlarged nuclei, powdery chromatin, and intranuclear cytoplasmic inclusions *(arrow)*. Papanicolaou preparation. × 630.

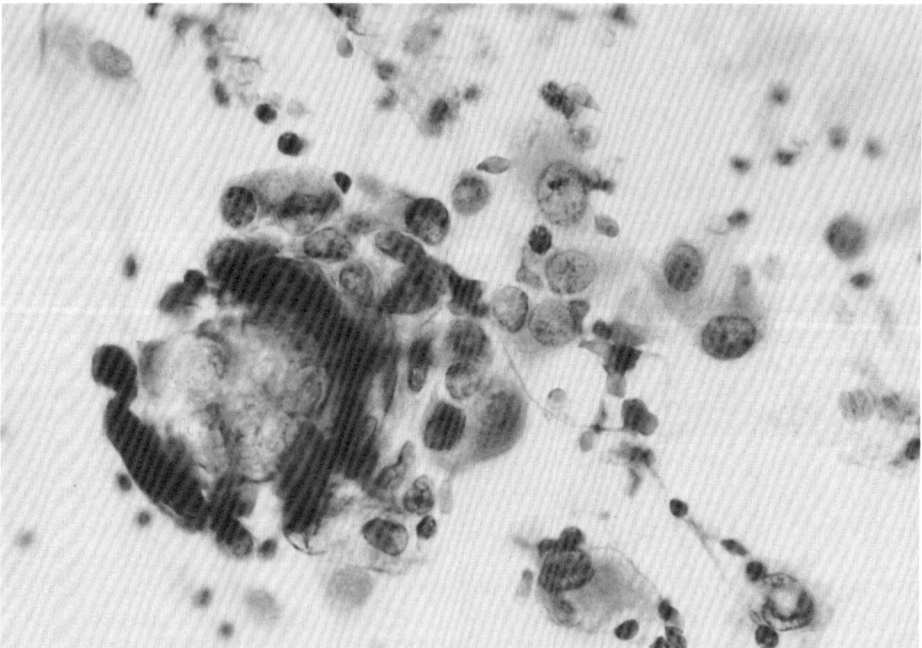

Fig. 11.25. Characteristic psammoma body surrounded by carcinoma cells, with nuclear morphology of papillary carcinoma in the background of lymphocytes, suggests the diagnosis of papillary carcinoma and lymphocytic (Hashimoto's) thyroiditis. Papanicolaou preparation. × 630.

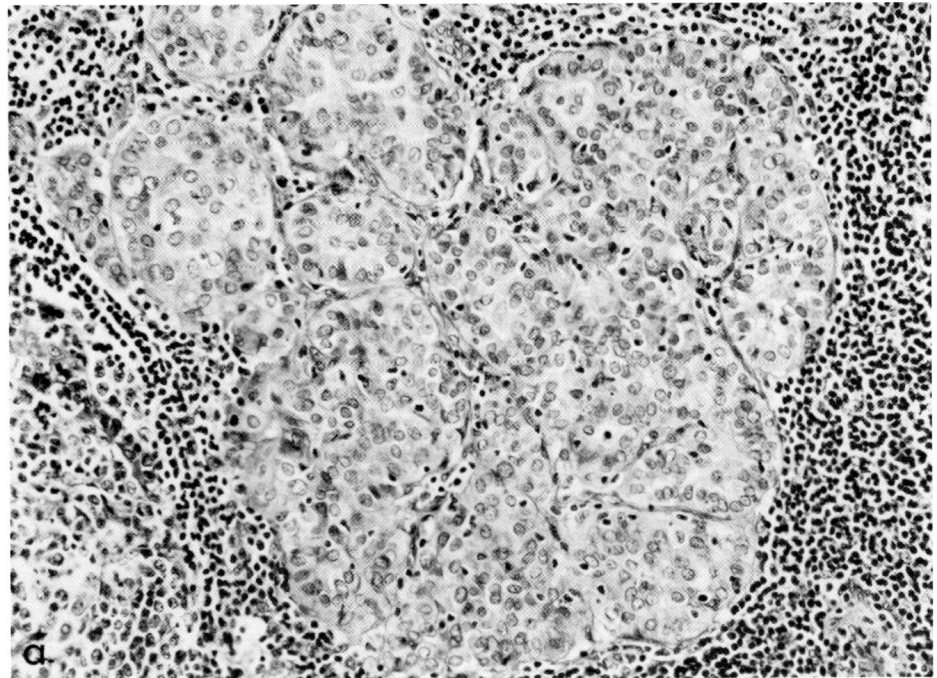

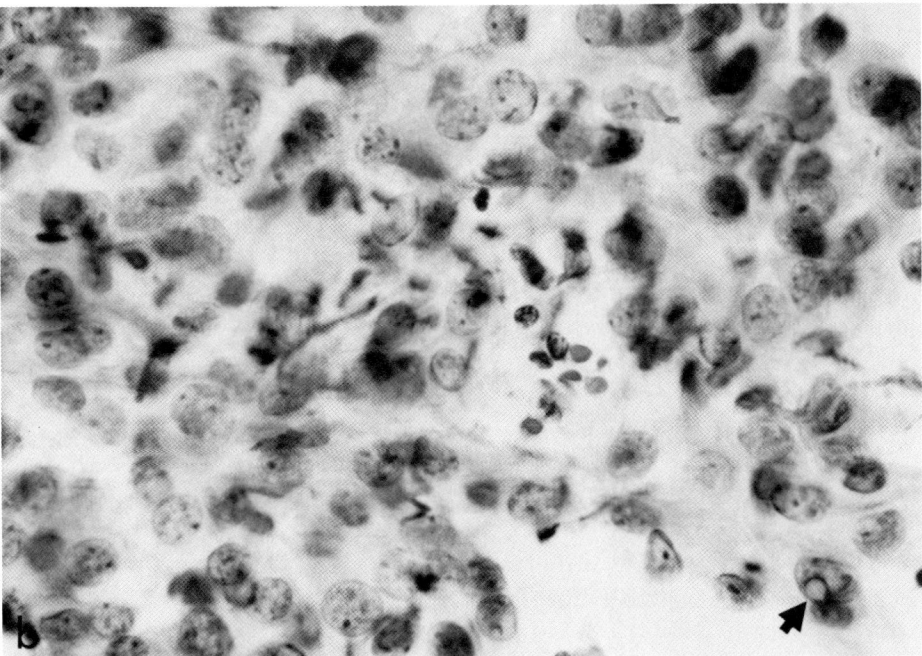

Fig. 11.26. **A.** Papillary carcinoma and Hashimoto's thyroiditis. The carcinoma cells are forming large syncytial-type masses with follicular pattern. The cells are oxyphilic. In the absence of psammoma bodies and obvious papillary configuration and nuclear changes, this case would be difficult to diagnose as papillary carcinoma in the background of thyroiditis. Hematoxylin and eosin preparation. × 250. **B.** Aspirate of case shown in **A** equally difficult to interpret without typical features of papillary carcinoma. Note intranuclear cytoplasmic inclusions, powdery chromatin, and micronucleoli. Papanicolaou preparation. × 630.

REFERENCES

1. Baker BA, Gharib H, Markowitz H: Correlation of thyroid antibodies and cytologic features in suspected autoimmune thyroid disease. *Am J Med* 74:941–944, 1983.

2. Berger SA, Zonszein J, Villamera P, Mittaman N: Infectious diseases of the thyroid gland. *Rev Infect Dis* 5:108–122, 1983.

3. Carcangiu ML, Zampi G, Rosai V: Papillary thyroid carcinoma: a study of its many morphologic expressions and clinical correlates. *Pathol Annu* 20(part 1):1–44, 1985.

4. Chang FC, Chen FW, Kau S: Diagnostic criteria of granulomatous thyroiditis by needle aspiration cytopathology. *J Formosan Med Assoc* 82:496–502, 1983.

5. Chesky VE, Hellwig CA, Welch JW: Cancer of the thyroid associated with Hashimoto's disease: an analysis of 48 cases. *Am Surg* 28:678–685, 1962.

6. Crile G Jr: Strume lymphomatosa and carcinoma of the thyroid. *Surg Gynecol Obstet* 147:350-352, 1978.

7. Dailey WE, Lindsay S, Skahen R: Relation of the thyroid neoplasms to Hashimoto's disease of the thyroid gland. *Arch Surg* 70:291, 1954.

8. Droese M: *Cytological Aspiration of the Thyroid.* Stuttgart, F.K. Schattauer-Verlag, 1980, p. 83.

9. Friedman M, Shimauka F, Roo U, et al: Diagnosis of chronic lymphocytic thyroiditis (nodular presentation) by needle aspiration. *Acta Cytol* 25:513–522, 1981.

10. Greene JN: Subacute thyroiditis. *Am J Med* 51:97–108, 1971.

11. Hamburger JI, Meier DA: Are silent thyroiditis and postpartum silent thyroiditis forms of chronic thyroiditis or different? In: Hamburger JI, Miller JM: *Controversies in Clinical Thyroidology.* New York, Springer-Verlag, 1981, pp. 21–67.

12. Hay ID: Thyroiditis: a clinical update. *Mayo Clin Proc* 60:836–843, 1985.

13. Hirabayashi RN, Lindsay S: The relation of thyroid carcinoma and chronic thyroiditis. *Surg Gynecol Obstet* 121:243, 1965.

14. Holmes HB Jr, Krenter A, O'Brien PH: Hashimoto's thyroiditis and its relationship to other thyroid diseases. *Surg Gynecol Obstet* 144: 887-890, 1977.

15. Kini SR, Miller JM, Hamburger JI: Problems in the cytologic diagnosis of the "cold" thyroid nodule in patients with lymphocytic thyroiditis. *Acta Cytol* 25:506–512, 1981.

16. Lindsay S, Dailey ME: Granulomatous or giant cell thyroiditis: a clinical and pathologic study of 37 patients. *Surg Gynecol Obstet* 98:197–211, 1954.

17. Livolsi VA, Marino MJ: Histopathologic differential diagnosis of the thyroid. *Pathol Annu* 16(part 2):357–506, 1981.

18. Millar AJW: Acute suppurative thyroiditis: a case report. *S Afr Med J* 58:617–618, 1980.

19. Pollock WF, Sprang DH Jr: The rationale of thyroidectomy for Hashimoto's thyroiditis: a premalignant lesion. *West J Surg* 66:17, 1985.

20. Schlicke CP, Hill JE, Schultz GF: Carcinoma in chronic thyroiditis. *Surg Gynecol Obstet* 111:552, 1960.

21. Shands WC: Carcinoma of the thyroid in association with struma lymphomatosa (Hashimoto's disease). *Ann Surg* 151:675, 1960.

22. Thomas CG, Rutledge R: Surgical intervention in chronic (Hashimoto's) thyroiditis. *Am Surg* 193:769–776, 1981.

23. Volpe R: Subacute thyroiditis. *Prog Clin Biol Res* 74:115–134, 1981.

24. Volpe R: Hashimoto's thyroiditis. *Curr Ther* 3:68–76, 1977.

25. Woolner LB, McConahey WM, Beh OH: Struma lymphomatosa and related thyroidal disorders. *J Clin Endocrinol Metab* 19:53, 1959.

26. Wortsman J, Dietrich J, Apesus J, Folse R: Hashimoto's thyroiditis simulating cancer of the thyroid. *Arch Surg* 116:386–388, 1981.

12

Malignant Lymphoma

PRIMARY MALIGNANT LYMPHOMA OF THYROID

Primary malignant lymphoma of thyroid is a form of localized lymphoma. It is considered a rare disease,[3,4-8,15,23,24,26,27,31] but lately is being seen and reported with increasing frequency.[3,4,6,11,17,30] The incidence as reported in the literature varies from 1.6% to 8%. The incidence in our series of 571 primary thyroid malignancies was 5.5% (32 cases).

Most primary malignant lymphomas of thyroid are non-Hodgkin's type. Hodgkin's disease with primary involvement of thyroid is extremely rare.[1,9,22] A strong association with Hashimoto's thyroiditis has been reported.[3,4,6,10-13,15,30,31] It is believed that Hashimoto's thyroiditis, with its abnormal immune state, is predisposed to the development of malignant lymphoma.

The clinical presentation of primary malignant lymphoma of thyroid is distinctive. Patients are predominantly elderly women beyond their sixth decade. The youngest patient reported was 11 years old,[4] but the average age is 63–65 years. The female to male ratio is 4:1, although it differs in younger age groups.[11]

Patients generally give a history of preexisting goiter of variable duration. Presenting symptoms include a rapidly enlarging tender mass in the neck, often with pressure symptoms such as dysphagia, hoarseness, or tracheal compression. Imaging shows cold nodules, cold areas in diffuse goiters, or a patchy uptake. Because of associated Hashimoto's thyroiditis, antithyroid antibody levels are often elevated.

The prognosis depends upon several factors, such as the patient's age at the time of diagnosis, type of lymphoma, extent of the tumor beyond the thyroid capsule, invasion of the blood vessels, involvement of cervical lymph nodes, and diffuse versus nodular processes.[3,4] Most primary lymphomas are diagnosed late in the disease, always after thyroidectomy or at autopsy. The only study of prospective diagnoses is that by Hamburger et al.[11]

275

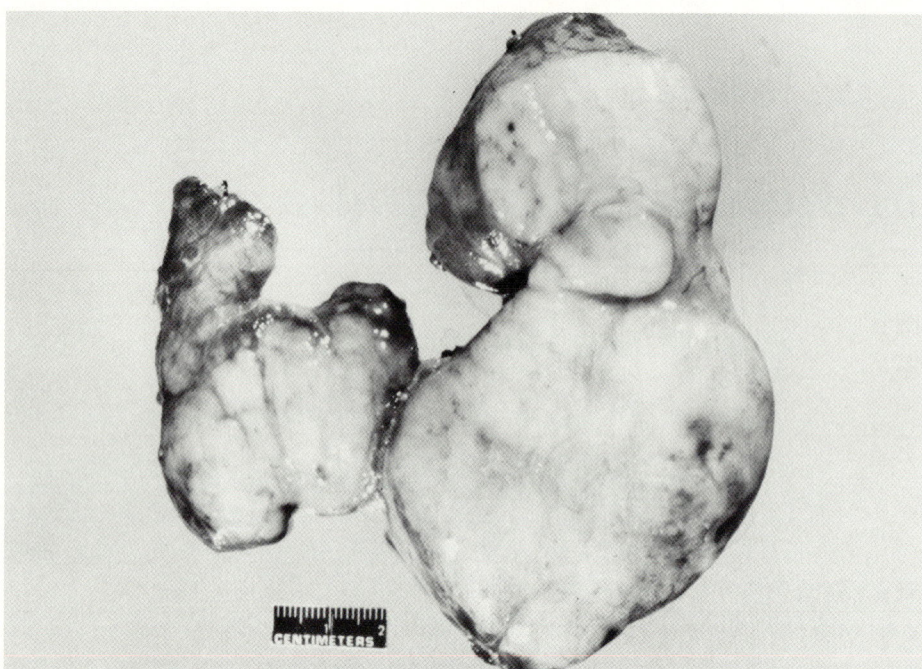

Fig. 12.1. Malignant lymphoma involving both lobes of the thyroid, which are asymmetrically enlarged. The cut surface is fleshy and bulging.

Pathology

Grossly, the thyroid (Fig. 12.1) is involved by an expanding, bulging, firm, homogeneous, fleshy mass; it is pink-tan in color, and the thyroid architecture is obliterated. Necrosis is not a usual feature. The tumor may involve the surrounding soft tissues.

Histologically, non-Hodgkin's type lymphomas are considered B-cell type, although the T-cell type has been reported.[8] They can be nodular or diffuse. Most are large cell type, whereas some may be lymphocytic or mixed (Rappaport classification).[21] All types have been described, eg, Burkitt's lymphoma, plasmacytoma, and signet ring cell lymphoma.[2–4,16,18,25]

Early cases of malignant lymphoma in the background of Hashimoto's thyroiditis are difficult to identify. These may be diagnosed as atypical lymphocytic thyroiditis because of insufficient criteria for definite diagnosis of malignant lymphoma. Compagno and Oertel[4] described 12 such cases.

Cytopathology

The cytopathologic diagnosis of primary malignant lymphoma of thyroid from the material obtained by an aspiration biopsy (Figs. 12.2–12.11) is not only challenging, but it also provides an opportunity to identify the disease in clinically unsuspected cases and in early stages when the disease can be controlled.

Aspirates tend to be very cellular (Table 12.1). The cell spreads show a dense population of cells, larger than the lymphocytes. The morphology depends upon the type of lymphoma, eg, lymphocytic, large cell type, mixed lymphocytic and large cell type, plasmacytic, etc. Lymphoma cells are usually discrete and round, with scanty pale cytoplasm. The nuclei are large, with finely granular chromatin that gives an open pattern in contrast with the compact nuclei of the mature lymphocytes. Nucleoli are always present, either small and multiple in a marginal location, or large in a central position. Mitotic activity occurs frequently. Karyorrhexis is a common feature of malignant lymphoma. Fragmented nuclei are often seen in the background and also as phagocytized debris in the histiocytes; these are referred to by Droese[7] as lymphoglandular bodies. In exfoliative cytology, lymphoma cells are characterized by a discrete pattern. But in the material obtained by an aspiration biopsy, it is not unusual to find a tissue fragment of lymphoma cells. These fragments of small, round cells with scanty cytoplasm should not be mistaken for carcinoma. Tumor diathesis may occasionally be seen in the background.

Lymphoma cells are usually seen in large aggregates or masses. In such areas, germinal center cells or epithelial cells are conspicuously absent. However, cytologic features of Hashimoto's thyroiditis may be present separate from lymphoma cells on the same smear, or on different smears representing other areas of the thyroid. Such a varied pattern is not infrequent when the thyroid is focally involved or when the malignant lymphoma is of the nodular type.

TABLE 12.1. Cytologic Features of Malignant Lymphoma

Monomorphic population of poorly differentiated lymphoid cells
Cells isolated, occasionally in tissue fragments
Absence of germinal center cells or epithelial cells
Karyorrhexis
Tumor diathesis infrequent

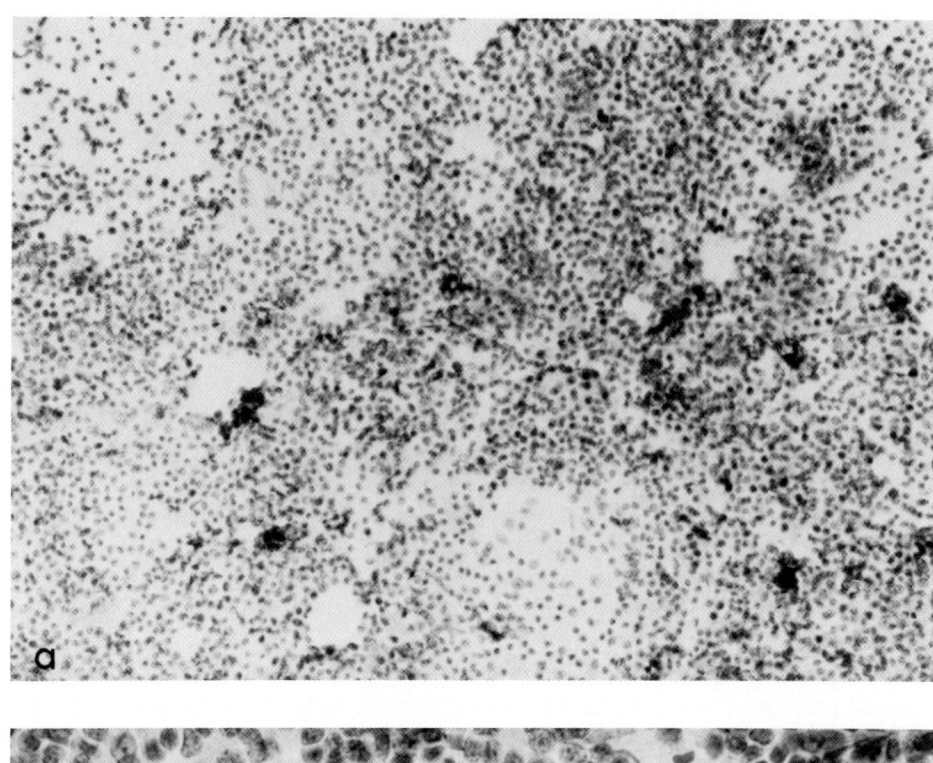

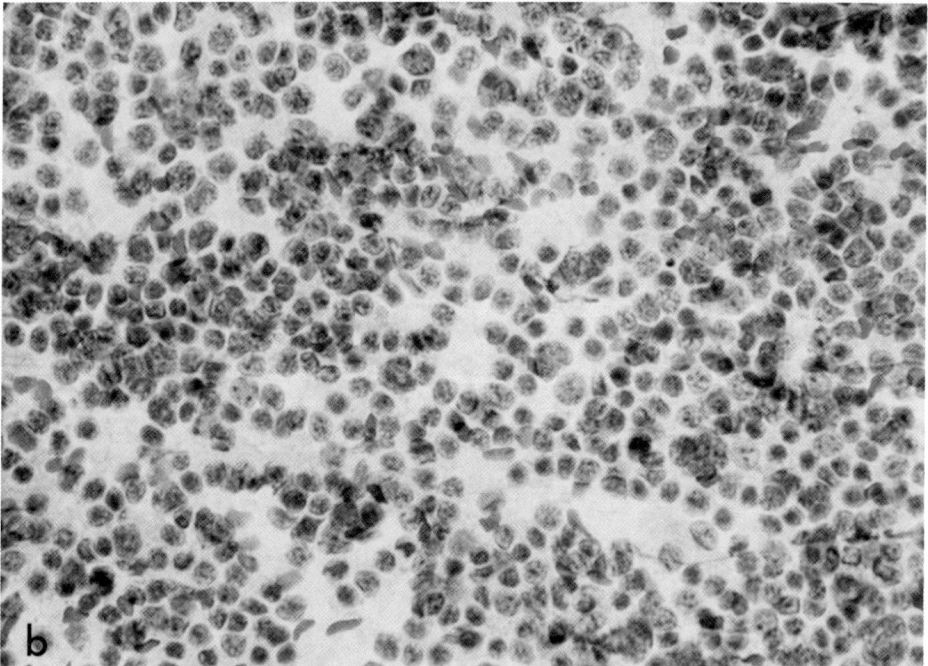

Fig. 12.2. A. Aspiration biopsy of malignant lymphoma showing a large population of discrete lymphoid cells. Papanicolaou preparation. × 160. **B.** Higher magnification of **A** showing a monomorphic pattern, with poorly differentiated lymphoid cells. Note absence of epithelial cells and germinal center cells. Papanicolaou preparation. × 630.

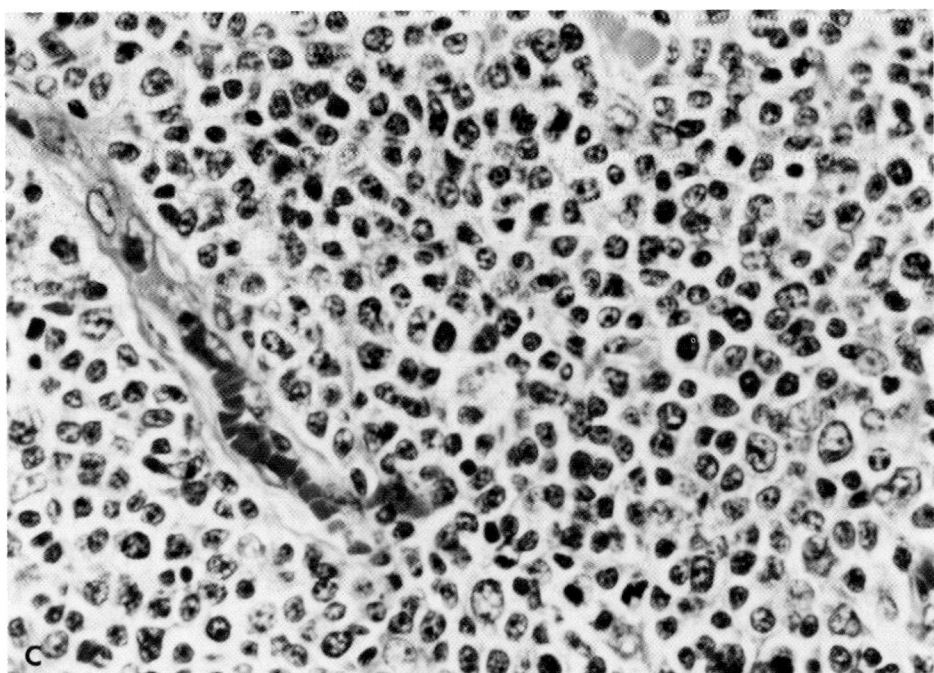

Fig. 12.2. C. Section of thyroid showing malignant lymphoma, diffuse large cell type. Hematoxylin and eosin preparation. × 630.

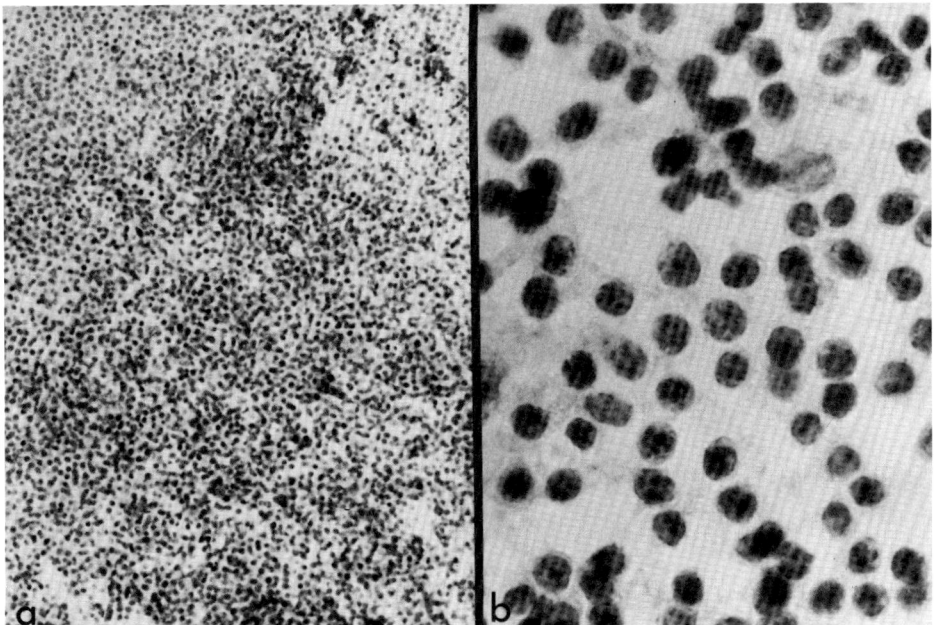

Fig. 12.3. Aspiration biopsy specimen of malignant lymphoma. A. Dense population of lymphoid cells, with absence of epithelial cells. Papanicolaou preparation. × 160. B. Higher magnification of A reveals the monomorphic nature of poorly differentiated lymphoid cells. Papanicolaou preparation. × 1000. Thyroidectomy confirmed poorly differentiated lymphocytic lymphoma.

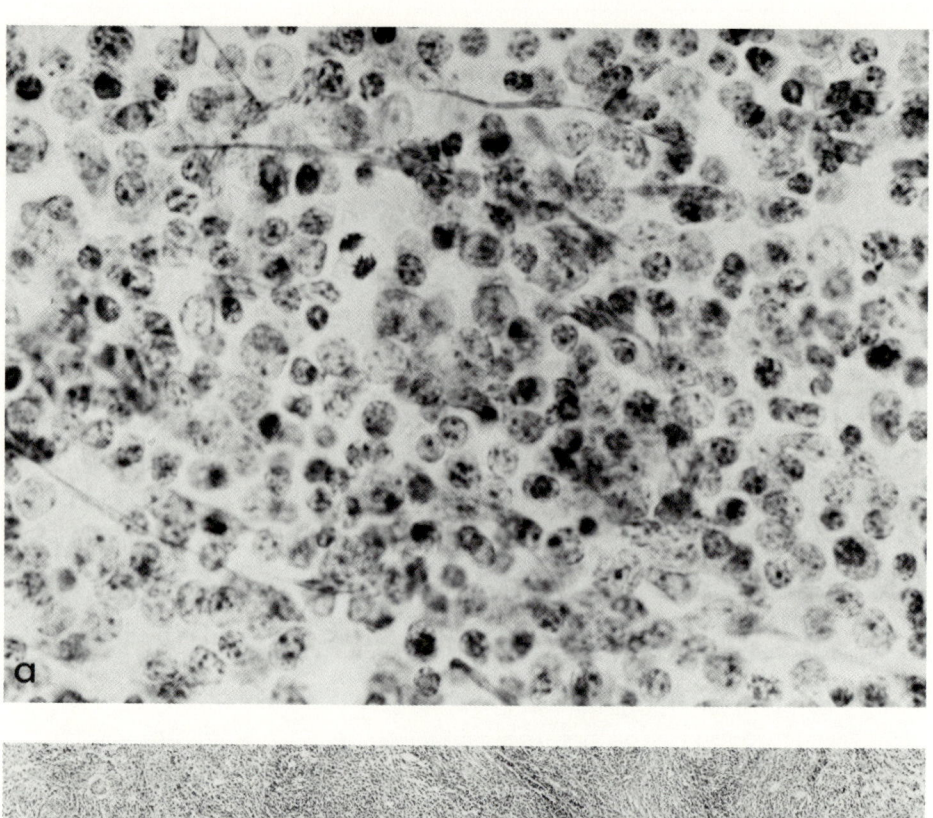

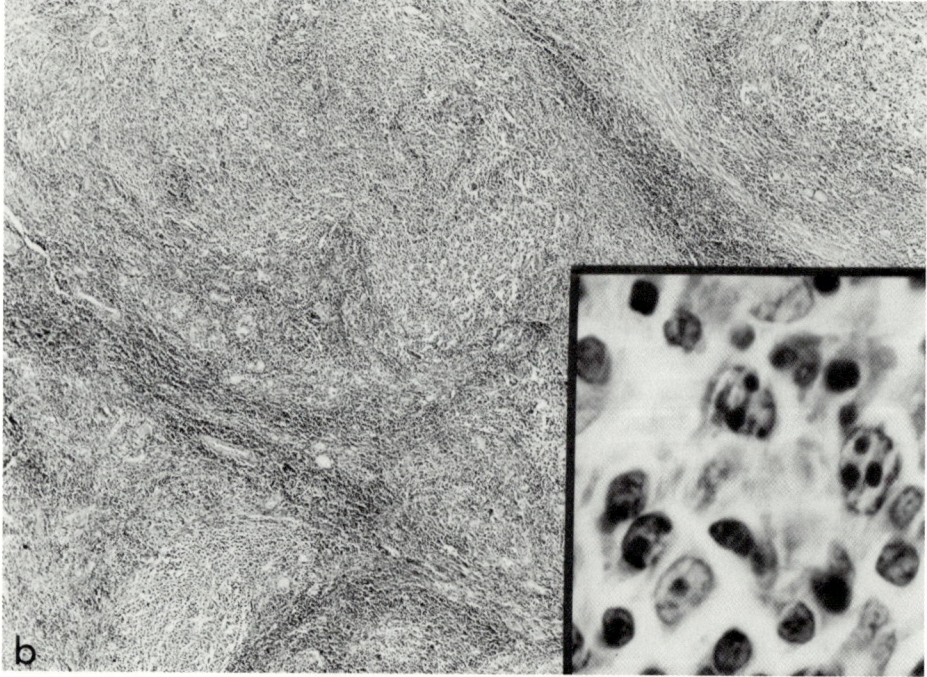

Fig. 12.4. A. Malignant lymphoma, with a large population of poorly differentiated lymphoid cells. Note the absence of germinal center cells. Papanicolaou preparation. Thyroidectomy confirmed nodular and diffuse malignant lymphoma in the background of Hashimoto's thyroiditis. **B.** Section of the thyroid showing nodular lymphoma. Hematoxylin and eosin preparation. × 63. *Inset:* Mixed lymphocytic and large cell type lymphoma. Hematoxylin and eosin preparation. × 1000.

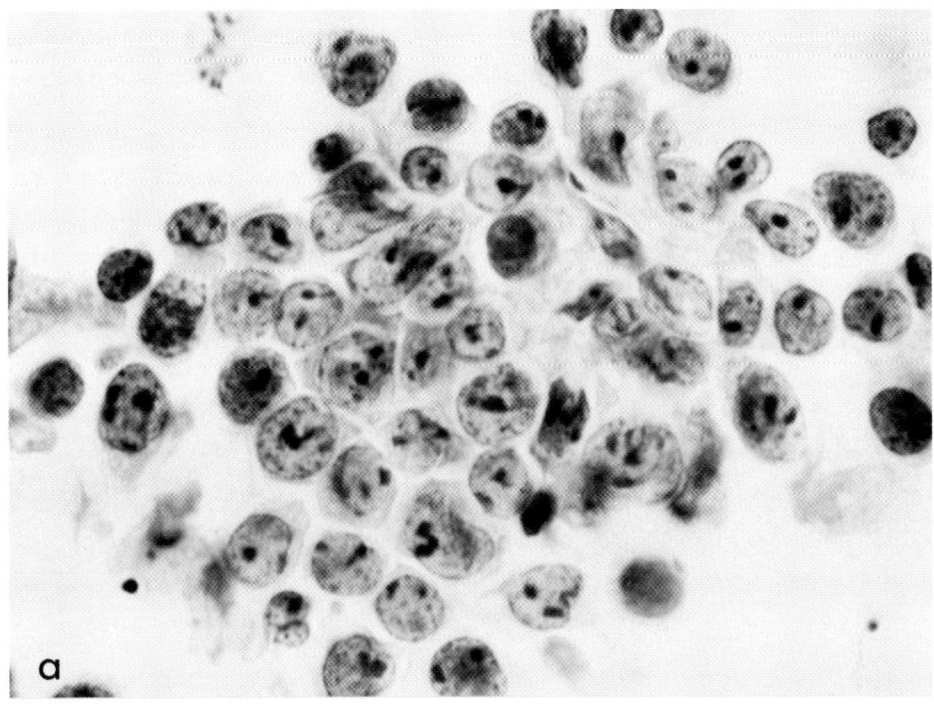

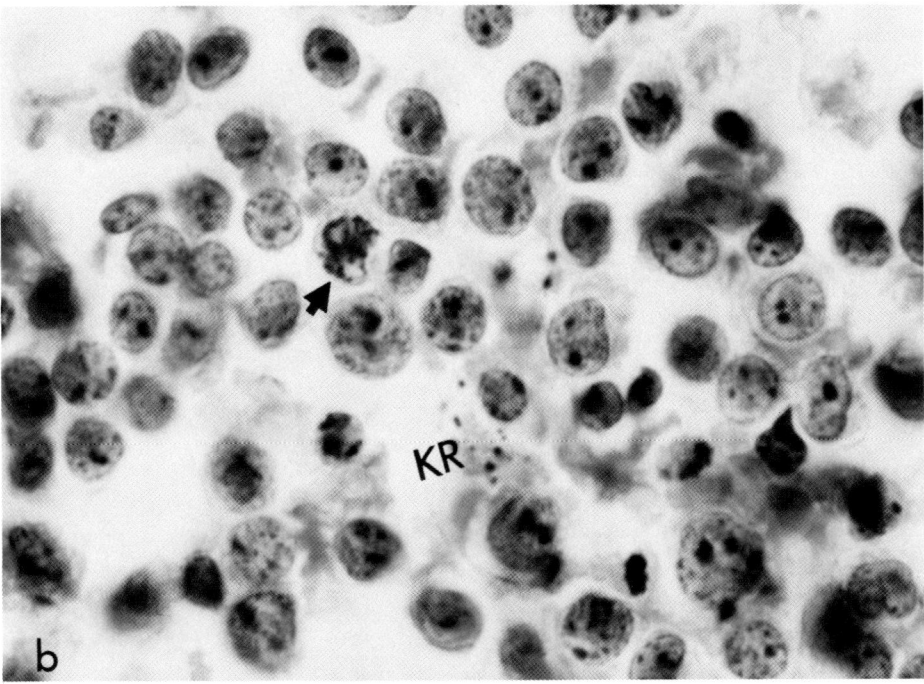

Fig. 12.5. **A.** Malignant lymphoma. Discrete mononuclear cells with scanty cytoplasm, large nuclei with open chromatin pattern, and multiple nucleoli. Papanicolaou preparation. × 1000. **B.** Another field from the smear in **A** showing mitosis *(arrow)* and karyorrhexis *(Kr)*. Papanicolaou preparation. × 1000. Thyroidectomy confirmed malignant lymphoma, Burkitt's type, and associated Hashimoto's thyroiditis.

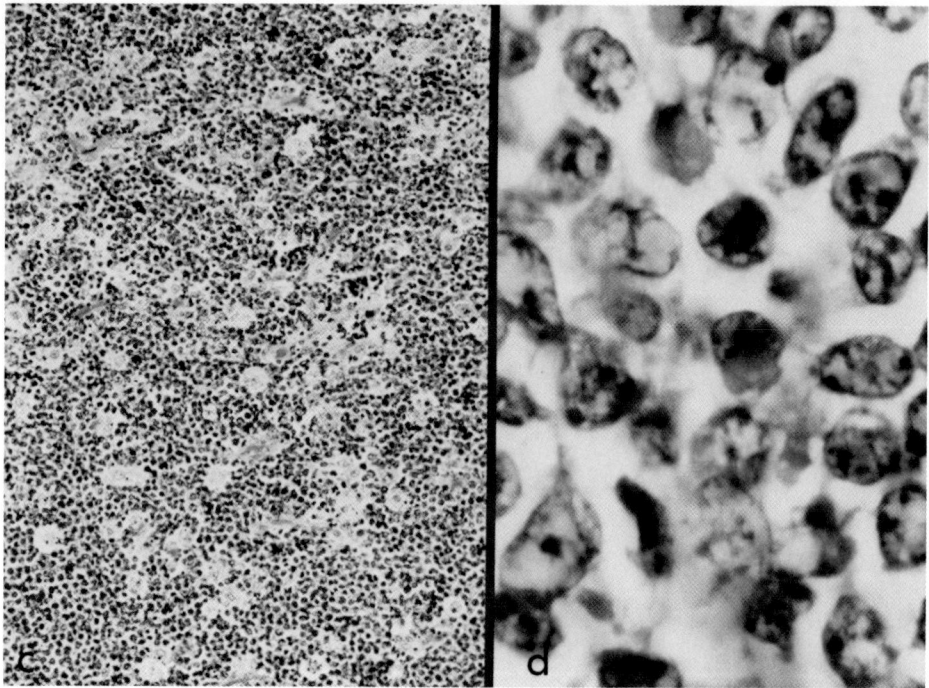

Fig. 12.5. C. Section of the thyroid showing a "starry-sky" pattern. Hematoxylin and eosin preparation. × 63. **D.** Higher magnification of Burkitt's lymphoma. Hematoxylin and eosin preparation. × 1000.

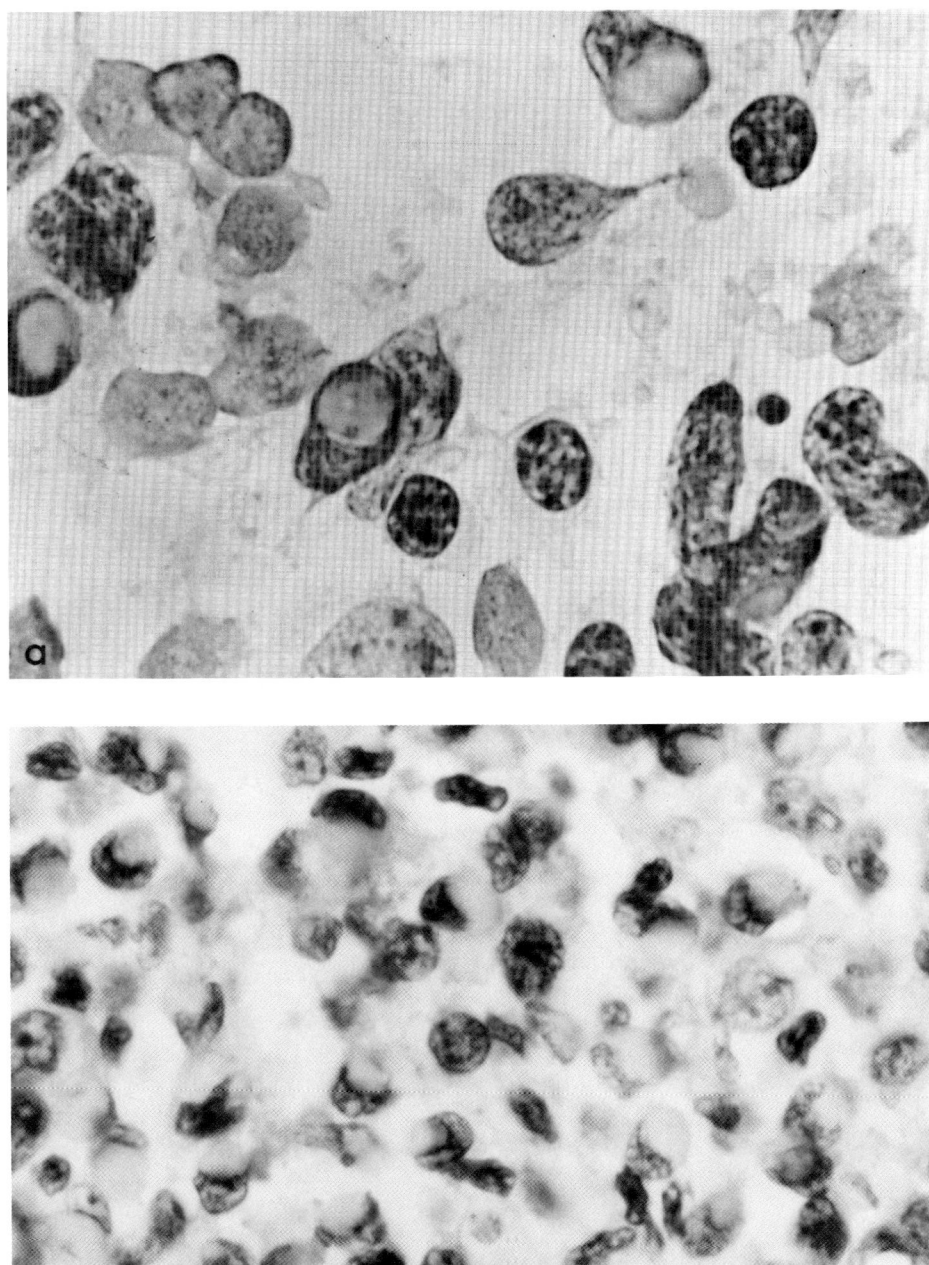

Fig. 12.6. A. Aspiration biopsy specimen of malignant lymphoma, signet ring cell type. Note cytoplasmic secretions. Papanicolaou preparation. × 1000. Thyroidectomy revealed signet ring cell lymphoma and Hashimoto's thyroiditis. **B.** Section of the thyroid showing signet ring cell lymphoma. Hematoxylin and easin preparation. × 1000.

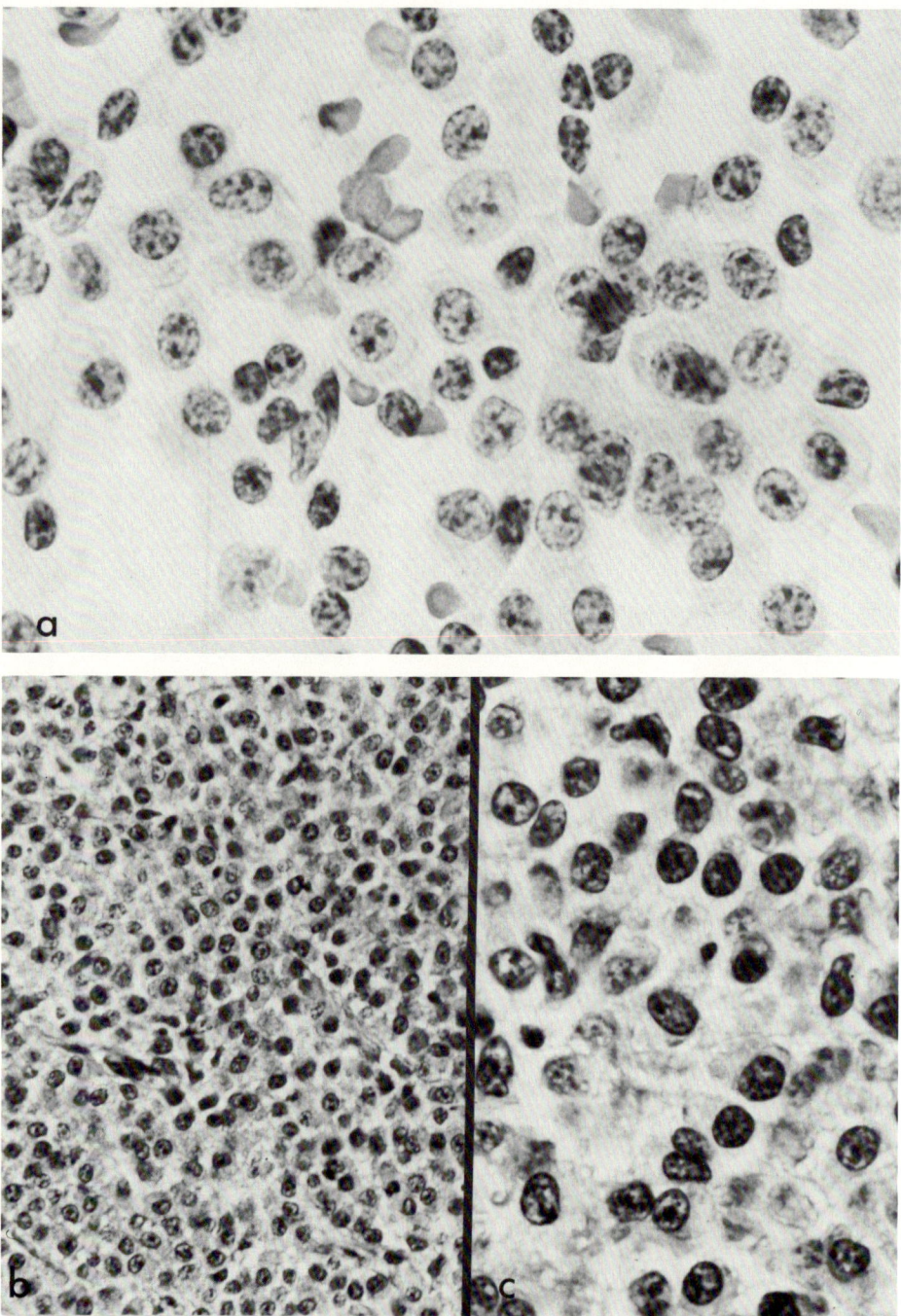

Fig. 12.7. A. Aspiration biopsy specimen of solitary plasmacytoma of thyroid, with large population of poorly differentiated plasma cells. Papanicolaou preparation. × 1000. **B.** Large-needle biopsy specimen confirmed plasmacytoma. Hematoxylin and eosin preparation. × 400. **C.** Higher magnification of plasmacytoma. Hematoxylin and eosin preparation. × 1000.

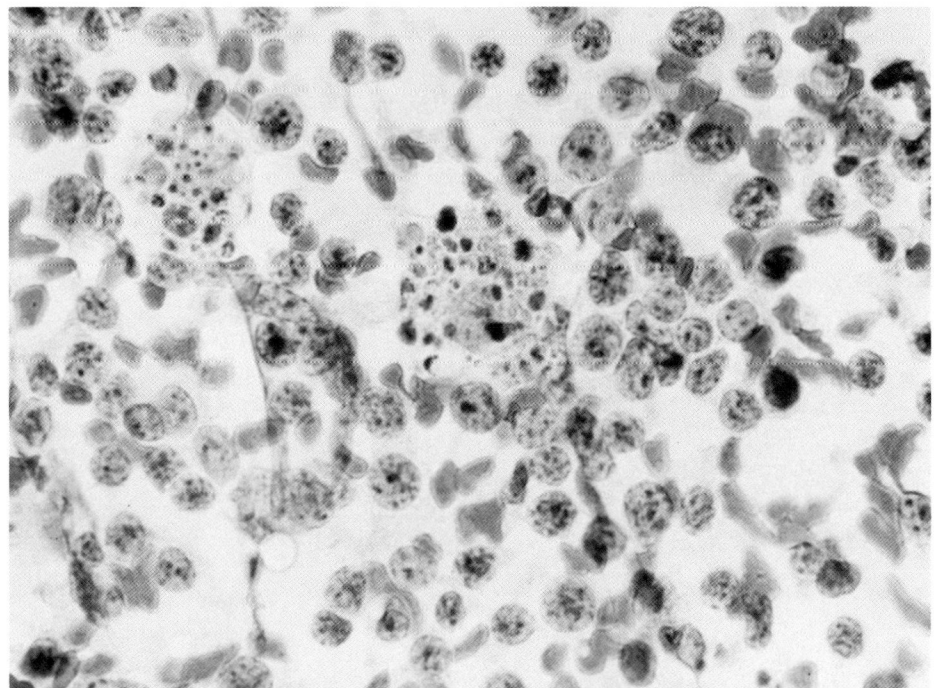

Fig. 12.8. Malignant lymphoma with histiocytes containing karyorrhectic debris. These are not indicative of germinal center cells. The cell population is monomorphic and represents poorly differentiated lymphoid cells. Papanicolaou preparation × 630. An open biopsy specimen revealed diffuse, large cell type lymphoma infiltrating the soft tissues of the neck.

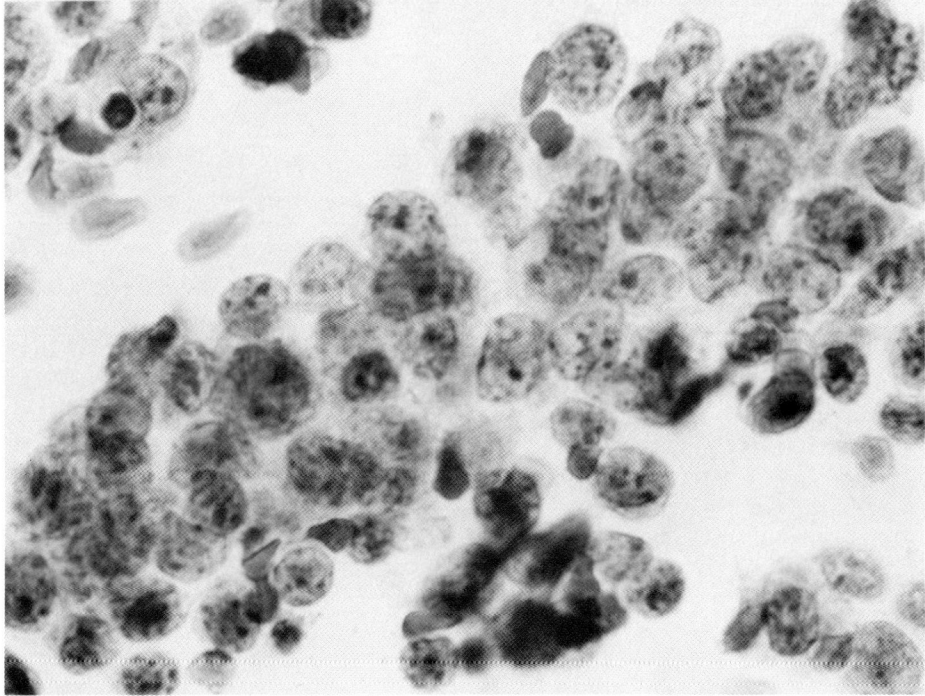

Fig. 12.9. Aspiration biopsy specimen of malignant lymphoma with tissue fragments of lymphoma cells. A diagnosis of poorly differentiated carcinoma was also considered. Papanicolaou preparation. × 1000. Thyroidectomy revealed diffuse, large cell type lymphoma and associated Hashimoto's thyroiditis.

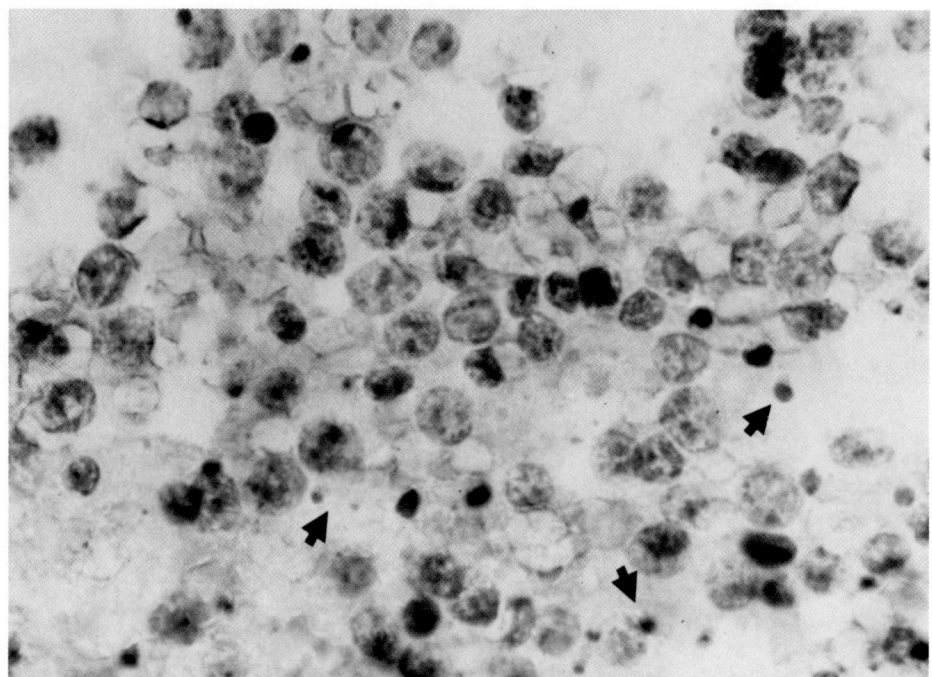

Fig. 12.10. Malignant lymphoma, poorly differentiated lymphocytic type. Note tumor diathesis and karyorrhexis *(arrows)*. Papanicolaou preparation. × 1000.

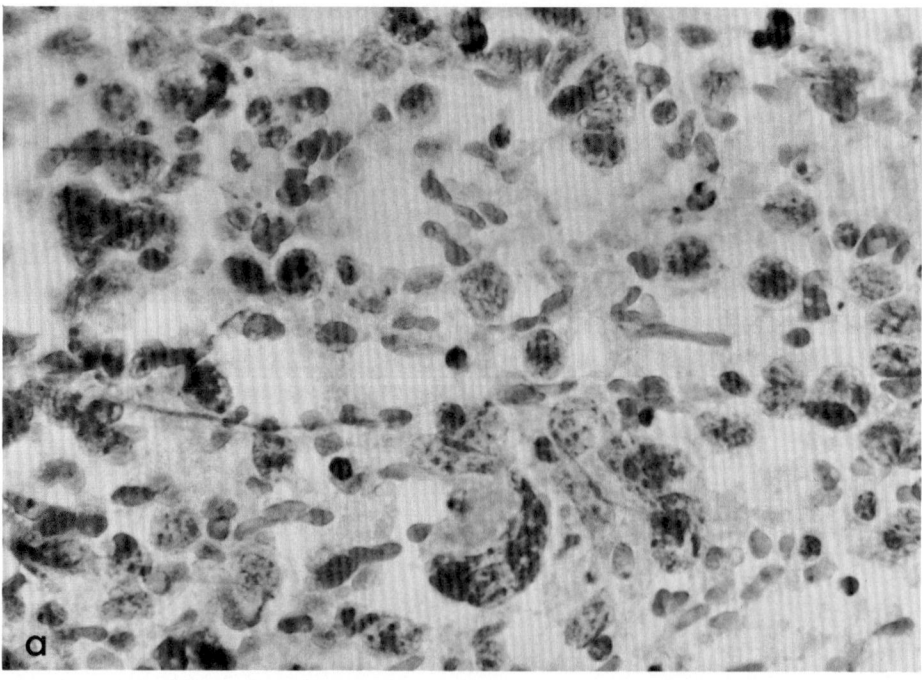

Fig. 12.11. **A.** Malignant lymphoma, large cell type. The tumor diathesis and large nuclear size suggested the differential diagnosis of poorly differentiated carcinoma and malignant lymphoma. Papanicolaou preparation. × 1000. Thyroidectomy confirmed diffuse, large cell type lymphoma and associated Hashimoto's thyroiditis.

286

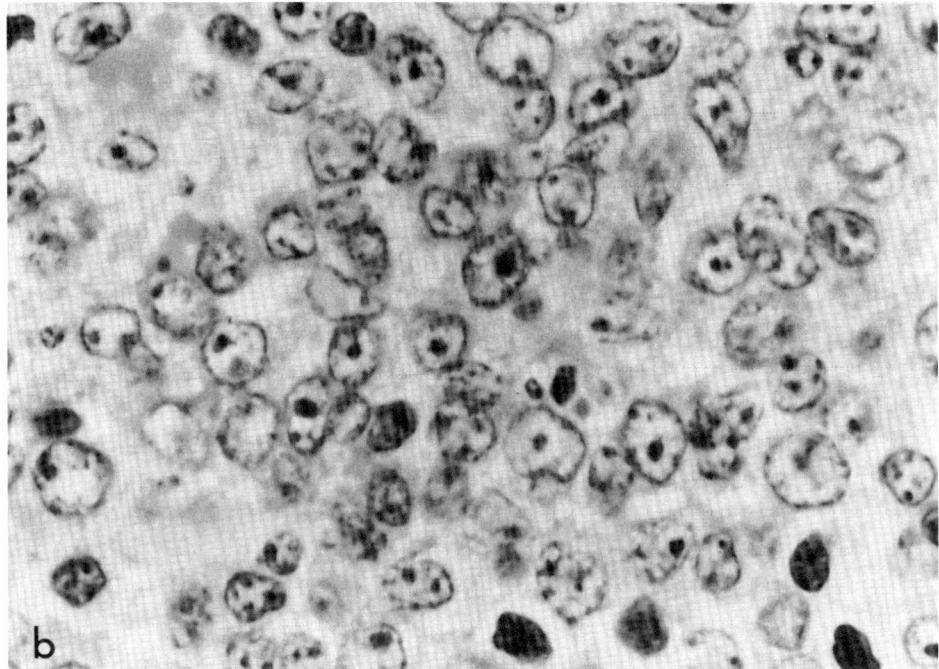

Fig. 12.11. B. Section of the thyroid showing large cell type lymphoma. Hematoxylin and eosin preparation. × 1000.

Diagnostic Accuracy

Accuracy in cytopathologic diagnosis of primary malignant lymphoma of thyroid depends on several factors, such as adequacy of the specimen and proper cytopreparatory technique, as well as the examiner's familiarity with the cytopathologic patterns. Lymphoma cells are very fragile and dry quickly unless wet fixed immediately for Papanicolaou stain. Drying artifacts prevent proper cytopathologic evaluation. Most thyroid lymphomas are diagnosed retrospectively. Thus, literature on ABC of malignant lymphoma of thyroid and its diagnostic pitfalls is very limited.[7,29] Inadequate specimens and/or inexperience are prime reasons for false-negative results. Due only to inexperience, our first three cases of malignant lymphoma were interpreted as lymphocytic thyroiditis[14] (Table 12.2).

TABLE 12.2. Cytologic Diagnosis of 32 Primary Non-Hodgkin's Type Malignant Lymphoma of the Thyroid

Malignant lymphoma	2
Malignant lymphoma and lymphocytic thyroiditis	18
Suspected malignant lymphoma and lymphocytic thyroiditis	3
(?)Carcinoma, (?)malignant lymphoma, lymphocytic thyroiditis	2
Lymphocytic thyroiditis*	3
Unsatisfactory (acellular)*	4
Total	32

*Diagnosis of malignant lymphoma based on large-needle biopsy specimen.

287

Of 23 cases cytologically diagnosed as malignant lymphoma, 20 were confirmed; 2 were difficult to diagnose histologically, but had a final diagnosis of atypical-lymphoid hyperplasia; and 1 was Hashimoto's thyroiditis. Of 10 cases of suspected malignant lymphoma, only 3 were confirmed (Table 12.3). Typing errors are occasionally involved between large cell lymphoma and poorly differentiated carcinoma. Some false-positive results must be anticipated in the cytologic diagnosis of malignant lymphoma if false-negative results are to be avoided, and in order to maintain a high sensitivity for its diagnosis.

TABLE 12.3. Histologic Diagnoses of 35 Cases of Cytologically Diagnosed
             Malignant Lymphoma or Suspected Malignant Lymphoma

| | | Histologic Diagnosis | | |
Cytologic Diagnosis	No.	Malignant Lymphoma	Atypical Lymphoid Hyperplasia	Hashimoto's Thyroiditis
Malignant lymphoma	23	20	2	1
(?)Malignant lymphoma, (?)carcinoma	2	2	—	—
Suspicious malignant lymphoma	10	3	—	7

Diagnostic Difficulties and Differential Diagnosis

Just as the diagnosis of malignant lymphoma of the thyroid is difficult histologically, either by large-needle biopsy specimen[28] or surgically excised specimen, cytologic diagnosis may pose similar problems because of the following reasons:

1. Lymphomas often infiltrate the thyroid parenchyma, and follicles become trapped. The aspirate may show follicular epithelium, regular or oxyphilic type, in association with lymphoma cells. However, this should not be mistaken for Hashimoto's thyroiditis. The immaturity of the lymphoid cells seen in large clusters should be a diagnostic clue.

2. In nodular lymphomas, when involvement is focal, multiple punctures will show lymphoma cells on some cell spreads and evidence of Hashimoto's thyroiditis on others. Such a diverse pattern is often present. A cytologic pattern of Hashimoto's disease on one of the specimens should not be a deterrent to calling it a lymphoma.

3. Lymphoma cells, especially the large cell type, are large and may be mistaken for carcinoma.

4. Phagocytic histiocytes with karyorrhectic debris are seen frequently. These should not be mistaken for germinal center cells.

5. Aspiration biopsy may yield a few tissue fragments of neoplastic lymphoid cells. As traditional diagnostic criteria of malignant lymphoma in exfoliative cytopathology include a single cell pattern, the presence of a tissue fragment should not be considered a feature contradicting the diagnosis of malignant lymphoma.

The differential diagnoses include lymphoid variety of Hashimoto's thyroiditis, atypical lymphoid hyperplasia, poorly differentiated "insular" carcinoma of the thyroid, and, rarely, a metastatic small cell carcinoma of the lung (Table 12.4).

TABLE 12.4. Differential Diagnosis of Malignant Lymphoma

1. "Lymphoid" variety of Hashimoto's thyroiditis
2. Atypical lymphoid hyperplasia
3. Poorly differentiated carcinoma or "insular" type
4. Metastatic carcinoma, small cell type (eg, lung)

Malignant Lymphoma Versus Hashimoto's Thyroiditis

In the lymphoid variety of Hashimoto's thyroiditis, the aspirates generally exhibit a dense population of lymphoid cells, without an admixture of epithelial cells. The presence of polymorphic germinal center cells favors the diagnosis of Hashimoto's thyroiditis. However, it is at times very difficult to rule out malignant lymphoma on a cytologic basis. A repeat aspiration biopsy or a core-needle biopsy is recommended.

Malignant Lymphoma Versus Atypical Lymphoid Hyperplasia

Differentiation between malignant lymphoma and atypical lymphoid hyperplasia is extremely difficult, not only cytologically, but histologically as well. Whetheratypical lymphoid hyperplasia represents an early stage in the evolution of malignant lymphoma in the background of thyroiditis is a subject beyond the scope of this monograph. Compagno and Oertel[4] have also referred to this problem. Cytologically, such cases may be diagnosed as malignant lymphoma or suspected malignant lymphoma. Figure 12.12 illustrates one of three such cases in our experience.

Malignant Lymphoma Versus Poorly Differentiated Carcinoma

Malignant lymphoma cells of large cell type are sometimes mistyped as poorly differentiated carcinoma, and vice versa. This difficulty is sometimes extended to histologic specimens as well. Tumor diathesis may be present in both cases. A large-needle biopsy is generally recommended for confirmation of the diagnosis.

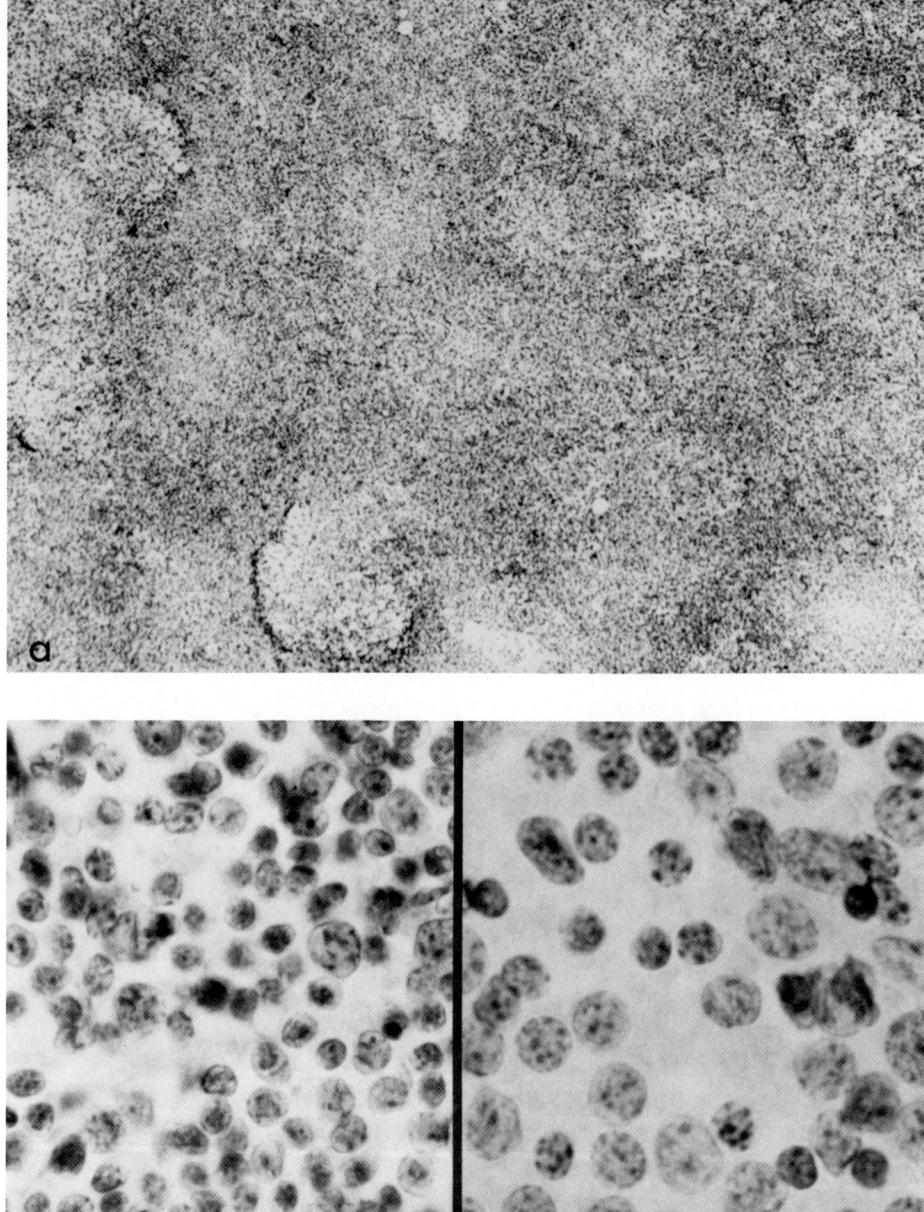

Fig. 12.12. A. Aspirate showing dense population of lymphoid cells with an admixture of epithelial cells. Papanicolaou preparation. × 160. **B.** Same aspirate as in **A** at higher magnification. Papanicolaou preparation. × 630. **C.** Still higher magnification of same aspirate as in **A.** Papanicolaou preparation. × 1000. The higher magnifications in **B** and **C** show all the cells to be poorly differentiated lymphoid cells, suggesting the diagnosis of malignant lymphoma. Thyroidectomy showed extensive Hashimoto's Thyroiditis, with atypical lymphoid hyperplasia.

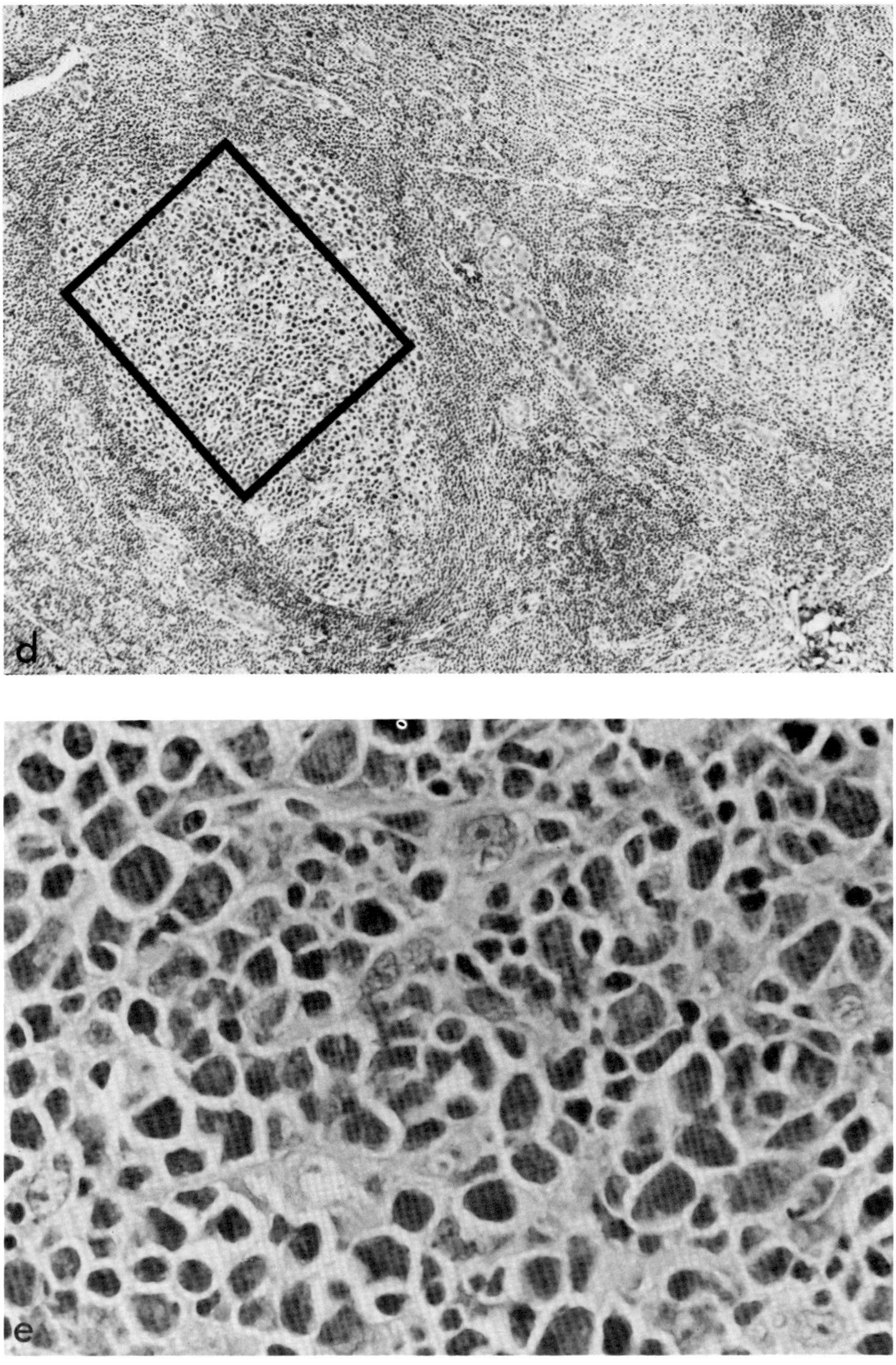

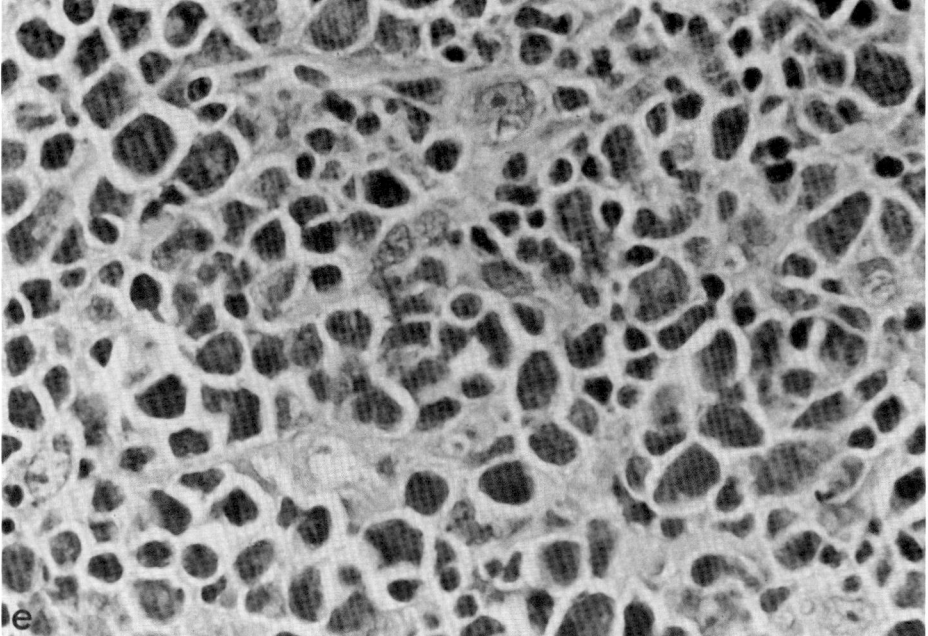

Fig. 12.12. **D.** Section of thyroid showing large lymphoid modules with germinal centers composed of very atypical cells. Hematoxylin and eosin preparation. × 63. **E.** Higher magnification of the germinal center from **D.** Hematoxylin and eosin preparation. × 1000.

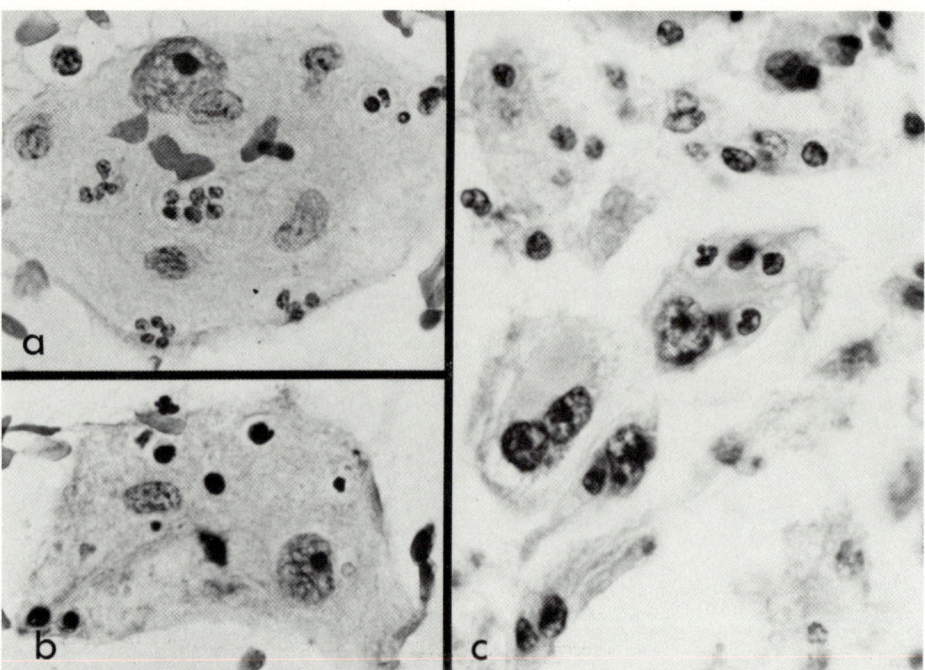

Fig. 12.13. Aspiration biopsy specimen of thyroid involved by generalized malignant histiocytosis. **A., B.** Large malignant histiocyte with erythroleukophagocytosis. Papanicolaou preparation. × 630. **C.** Cervical lymph node with sinusoids filled with malignant histiocytes exhibiting erythroleukophagocytosis. Hematoxylin and eosin preparation. × 630.

Malignant Lymphoma Versus Metastatic Carcinoma

On rare occasions, small cell carcinoma of the lung metastatic to the thyroid may be mistaken for malignant lymphoma. Clinical history and other diagnostic studies, including a large-needle biopsy, are necessary for establishing a diagnosis.

The increasing incidence of primary malignant lymphoma of thyroid has been recognized only in recent years. An early diagnosis of this disease made possible by aspiration cytology can certainly accomplish the goals of early cancer detection, ie, effective treatment and control of the disease. This is one of the greatest contributions of aspiration cytology of thyroid.

SECONDARY INVOLVEMENT OF THYROID BY MALIGNANCY OF HEMATOPOIETIC SYSTEM

The thyroid gland is reported to be frequently involved by malignancies of the lymphoid tissue.[19] In a series of 300 autopsies on patients dying of lymphomas,

Hodgkin's or non-Hodgkin's type, Naylor[20] found that leukemias and multiple myelomas formed an overall incidence of thyroid involvement in 17.7%. None of the patients in Naylor's series experienced thyroid enlargement during life; the secondary involvement was identified only on microscopic examination. Figure 12.13 shows cytologic presentation of a thyroid gland that was secondarily involved by malignant histiocytosis.

REFERENCES

1. Abel WG, Finnerly J: Primary Hodgkin's disease of thyroid. *NY State J Med* 69:314–315, 1969.

2. Allevato PA, Kini SR, Rebuck JW, Miller JM, Hamburger JI: Signet ring cell lymphoma of the thyroid: a case report. *Hum Pathol* 16:1066–1068, 1985.

3. Burke JS, Butler JJ, Fuller LM: Malignant lymphomas of the thyroid: a clinico-pathologic study of 35 patients including ultrastructural observations. *Cancer* 39:1587–1602, 1977.

4. Compagno J, Oertel JE: Malignant lymphoma and other lymphoproliferative disorders of the thyroid gland: a clinico-pathologic study of 245 cases. *Am J Clin Pathol* 74:1–11, 1980.

5. Cox M: Malignant lymphoma of the thyroid. *J Clin Pathol* 17:591–601, 1964.

6. Devine RM, Edis AJ, Banks PM: Primary lymphoma of the thyroid: a review of the Mayo Clinic experience through 1978. *World J Surg* 5:33–38, 1981.

7. Droese M: *Cytological Aspiration Biopsy of the Thyroid Gland.* Stuttgart, F.K. Schattauer-Verlag, 1980, p. 231.

8. Dunbar JA, Lyall MH, MacGillivray JB, Potts RC: T-cell lymphoma of the thyroid. *Br Med J* 2:679, 1977.

9. Frigin GA, Buss DH, Paschal B, Woodruff RD, Myers RT: Hodgkin's disease manifested as a thyroid nodule. *Hum Pathol* 13:774–776, 1982.

10. Goudie RB, Angouridakis CE: Autoimmune thyroiditis associated with malignant lymphoma of thyroid (abstr). *J Clin Pathol* 23:77, 1970.

11. Hamburger JI, Miller JM, Kini SR: Lymphoma of the thyroid. *Ann Intern Med* 99:685–693, 1983.

12. Heimann R, Vannineuse A, DeSloover C, Dur P: Malignant lymphomas and undifferentiated small cell carcinoma of the thyroid: a clinico-pathological review in the light of the Kiel classification for malignant lymphomas. *Histopathology* 2:201–213, 1978.

13. Hohm LE, Blomgren H, Lowhagen T: Cancer risks in patients with chronic lymphocytic thyroiditis. *N Engl J Med* 312:601–604, 1985.

14. Kini SR, Miller JM, Hamburger JI: Problems in cytologic diagnosis of the "cold" thyroid nodule in patients with lymphocytic thyroiditis. *Acta Cytol* 25:506–512, 1981.

15. Lindsay S, Dailey ME: Malignant lymphoma of the thyroid gland and its relation to Hashimoto's disease: a clinical and pathologic study of 8 patients. *J Clin Endocrinol Metab* 15:1332–1353, 1955.

16. Lopez M, DiLauro L, Marolla P, Madonna V: Plasmacytoma of the thyroid gland. *Clin Oncol* 9:61–66, 1983.

17. Miller JM, Kini SR, Rebeck J, Hamberger JL: Is lymphoma of the thyroid a disease

which is increasing in frequency? In Hamburger JI, Miller JM: *Controversies in Clinical Thyroidology*. New York, Springer-Verlag, 1981, pp. 267–297.

18. More JRS, Dawson DW, Ralston AJ, Craig L: Plasmacytoma of the thyroid. *J Clin Pathol* 21:661–667, 1968.

19. Mortensen JD, Woolner LB, Bennett WA: Secondary malignant tumors of the thyroid gland. *Cancer* 9:306–309, 1956.

20. Naylor B: Secondary lymphoblastomatous involvement of the thyroid gland. *Arch Pathol* 67:432–437, 1959.

21. Rappaport H: *Tumors of the Hematopoietic System*. Fascicle 8, *Atlas of Tumor Pathology*. Washington, DC, Armed Forces Institute of Pathology, 1966.

22. Roberts TW, Howard RG: Primary Hodgkin's disease of the thyroid. *Ann Surg* 157:625, 1963.

23. Schwarze EW, Papadimetriou CS: Non-Hodgkin's lymphoma of the thyroid. *Pathol Res Proc* 167:346–362, 1980.

24. Selzer G, Kahn L, Albertyn L: Primary malignant tumors of the thyroid gland: a clinico-pathologic study of 254 cases. *Cancer* 40:1501–1510, 1977.

25. Shimaoka K, Garlani S, Yaukada Y, Barcos M: Plasma cell neoplasm involving the thyroid. *Cancer* 41:1140–1146, 1978.

26. Sirota DK, Segal RL: Primary lymphomas of the thyroid gland. *JAMA* 242:1743–1746, 1979.

27. Taylor I: Malignant lymphoma of the thyroid. *Br J Surg* 63:932–933, 1976.

28. Vickery Al Jr: Needle biopsy pathology. *J Clin Endocrinol Metab* 10:275–293, 1981.

29. Willems JS, Lowhagen T: The role of fine needle aspiration cytology in the management of thyroid disease. *J Clin Endocrinol Metab* 10:267–273, 1981.

30. Williams ED: Malignant lymphoma of the thyroid. *Clin Endocrinol Metab* 10:379–398, 1981.

31. Woolner LB, McConahey WM, Beahrs OH, Black BM: Primary malignant lymphoma of the thyroid. *Am J Surg* 111:502–523, 1966.

13

Metastatic Carcinoma to Thyroid

The thyroid gland is a rare site for metastatic malignancy. According to the literature, its incidence varies from 0.19% to 24.2% among patients with cancer, mostly as identified in autopsy series.[7,10,11,15] At the Mayo Clinic,[5] 30 cases were reported from a series of 1161 thyroid cancers over a period of 25 years. Our own series included 22 cases of 593 thyroid cancers over a period of 9 years. A thyroid nodule occurring in a patient with a history of cancer may be a diagnostic problem for the clinician because it may represent a benign lesion, a metastatic implant from cancer elsewhere in the body, or a primary thyroid cancer. Rarely, a metastatic cancer may masquerade as primary thyroid cancer.[1,3,4,8,9,13] Trokoudes et al[14] reported a case of metastatic breast carcinoma to thyroid that presented with symptoms and signs of subacute thyroiditis. Although the thyroid gland can harbor metastatic tumor from any site of the body, four sites are listed as the most common sources, accounting for 70% of reported cases.[1—15] These are lung, kidney, breast, and malignant melanoma. The thyroid gland may also be involved by contiguous spread from cancers of the neighboring organs, such as esophagus or larynx.

PATHOLOGY

Willis[15] described three histologic patterns of metastatic tumor to the thyroid: (1) multiple small discrete areas less than 2 mm; (2) single discrete large nodule; and (3) diffuse with widespread involvement (Figs. 13.1–13.3).

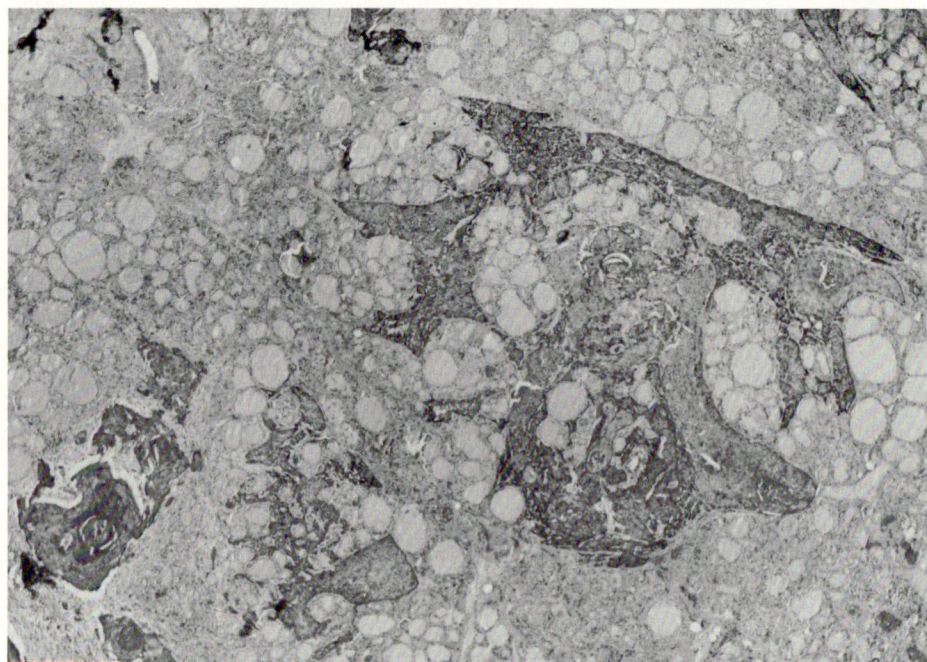

Fig. 13.1. Infiltrating pattern of a metastatic carcinoma (squamous cell carcinoma from lung) involving the thyroid. Note the tumor is infiltrating between the thyroid follicles. The nodules are less than 2 mm. Hematoxylin and eosin preparation. × 20.

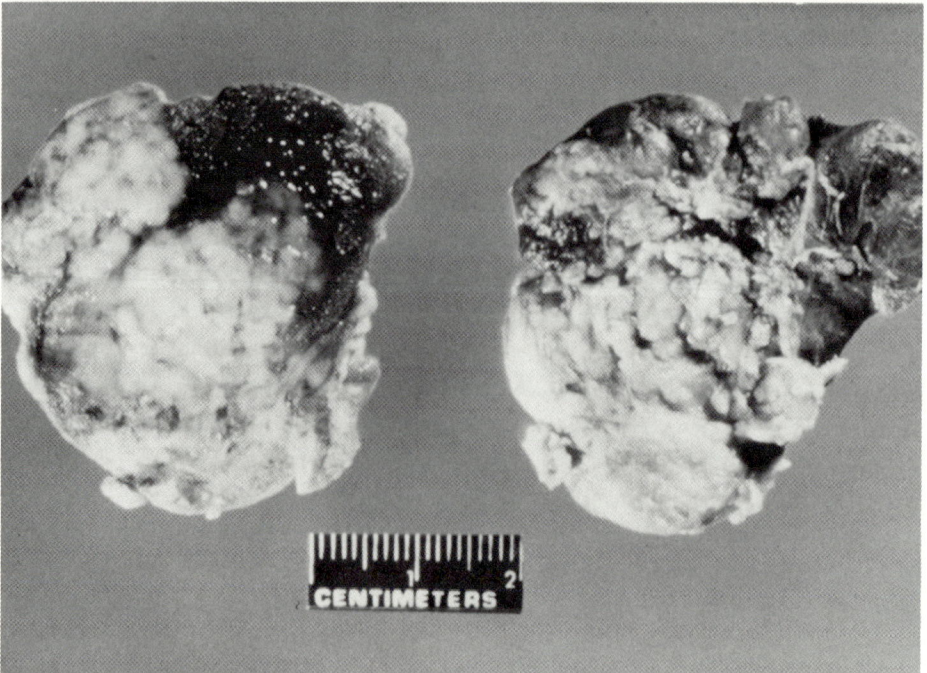

Fig. 13.2. Discrete, large metastatic nodule from malignant melanoma.

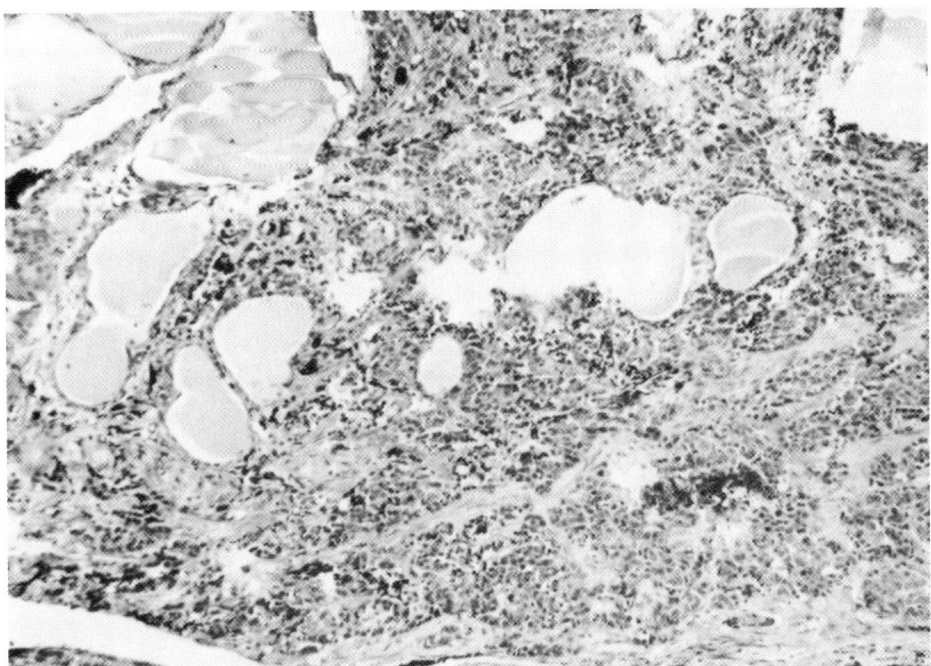

Fig. 13.3. Section of thyroid, diffusely involved by anaplastic, small cell, undifferentiated carcinoma of lung. Hematoxylin and eosin preparations. × 100.

CYTOPATHOLOGY

The cytologic pattern of a metastatic tumor (Figs. 13.4–13.12) depends on the manner in which the thyroid is involved by secondary neoplasms (Table 13.1). The cellular material basically reveals two patterns. With nodules less than 2 mm in size, the cytologic samples show an admixture of benign follicular cells and cancer cells (Fig. 13.4). Tumor diathesis is rare or absent. With a single discrete large palpable nodule or with diffuse widespread involvement, the aspirates show only the cancer cells (Figs. 13.5–13.11). Follicular epithelial cells are absent, and tumor diathesis is frequent. Recognizing a metastatic cancer is easy if carcinoma cells are functionally differentiated with keratin or with mucin production. Typical cytomorphology of anaplastic small cell carcinoma of lung, showing compact nuclear chromatin and molding or cigar-shaped nuclei and a "picket-fence" arrangement of colonic carcinoma cells, is a clue to the correct identification of a metastatic tumor. Without

TABLE 13.1. Cytohistologic Pattern of Metastatic Tumors to Thyroid and Their Differential Diagnosis

Histologic Pattern	Cytologic Pattern	Differential Diagnosis
Multiple, discrete small nodules less than 2 mm in diameter	Admixture of benign follicular cells and cancer cells; tumor diathesis usually absent	Degenerating follicular cells in nodular goiter
Single, large discrete nodule	Large population of malignant cells; no thyroid follicular cells; tumor diathesis usually present	1. Primary anaplastic carcinoma, when cytoplasm of metastatic lesion shows no functional differentiation 2. Primary malignant lymphoma, non-Hodgkin's type, if metastatic tumor is small cell, undifferentiated carcinoma
Diffuse and widespread involvement	Same as above	Same as above

these differentiating features, a poorly differentiated metastatic carcinoma is difficult to differentiate from primary metastatic carcinoma of thyroid.

The cytohistologic patterns of metastatic tumors and their differential diagnoses are listed in Table 13.1. The features that help differentiate primary from secondary tumors are listed in Table 13.2.

False-positive diagnoses may be given when degenerated follicular cells in the background of nodular goiter exhibit retrogressive changes with atypical nuclei, mimicking the cytologic pattern seen in discrete small nodules (Figs. 13.11 and 13.12).

TABLE 13.2. Primary Versus Secondary Tumor of Thyroid: Differentiating Features

1. History of primary cancer elsewhere in body
2. Presence of unremarkable thyroid follicular cells mixed with cancer cells
3. Functional differentiation of cytoplasm of cancer cells, eg, keratin or mucin production
4. Cytomorphology
   Small cells with hyperchromatic nuclei, scanty cytoplasm and nuclear molding, eg, anaplastic small cell cancer of the lung
   Cigar-shaped nuclei with "picket-fence" pattern, eg, colonic cancer

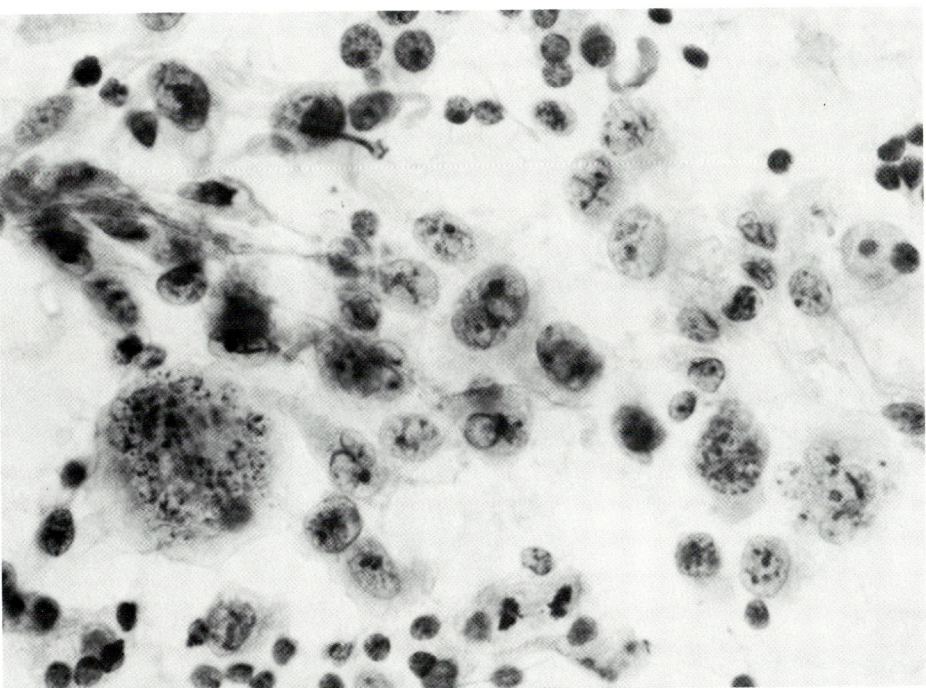

Fig. 13.4. Aspirate from metastatic carcinoma involving, in the form of small nodules less than 2 mm, showing an admixture of cancer cells and benign follicular cells. Papanicolaou preparation. × 630.

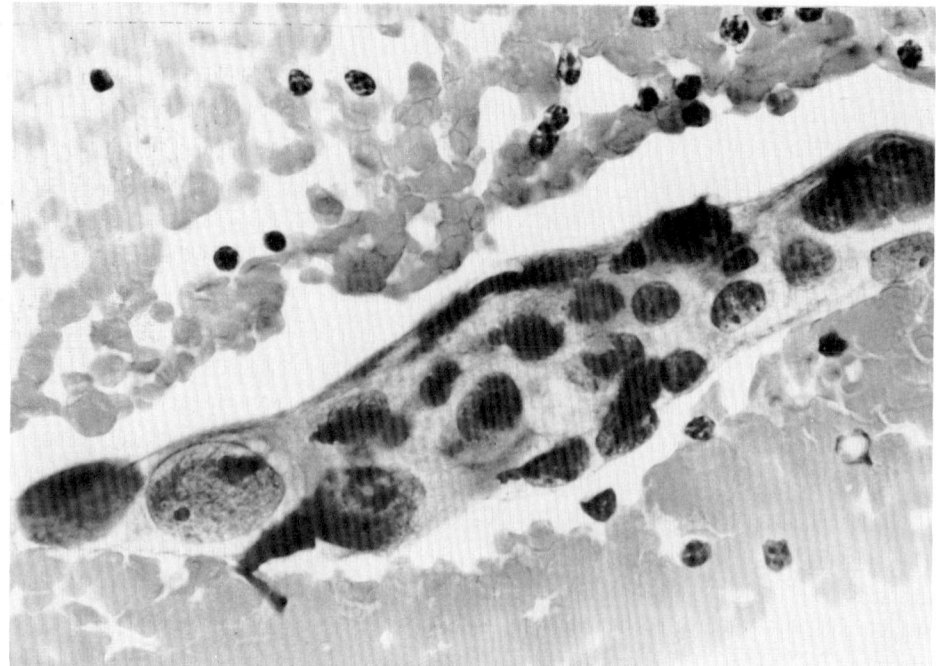

Fig. 13.5. Metastatic sebaceous carcinoma of meibomian glands. Papanicolaou preparation. × 630.

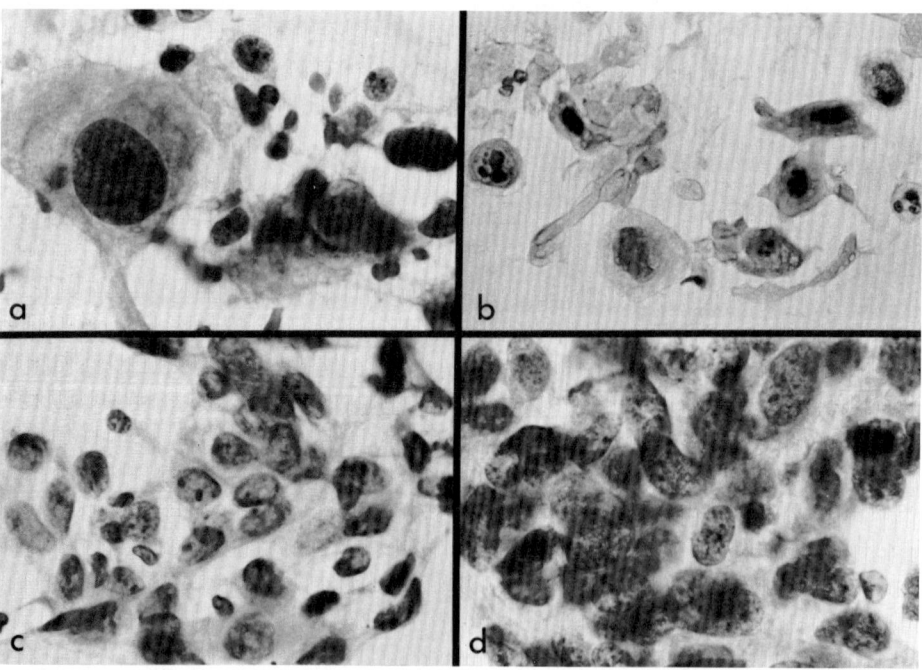

Fig. 13.6. Metastatic squamous carcinoma to thyroid gland. A., B. Keratinized squamous cell carcinoma with pleomorphic cells, easily identified as metastatic carcinoma. Papanicolaou preparation. × 630. C., D. Poorly differentiated squamous carcinoma masquerading as goiter; difficult to differentiate from primary anaplastic carcinomas of thyroid. Papanicolaou preparation. × 630.

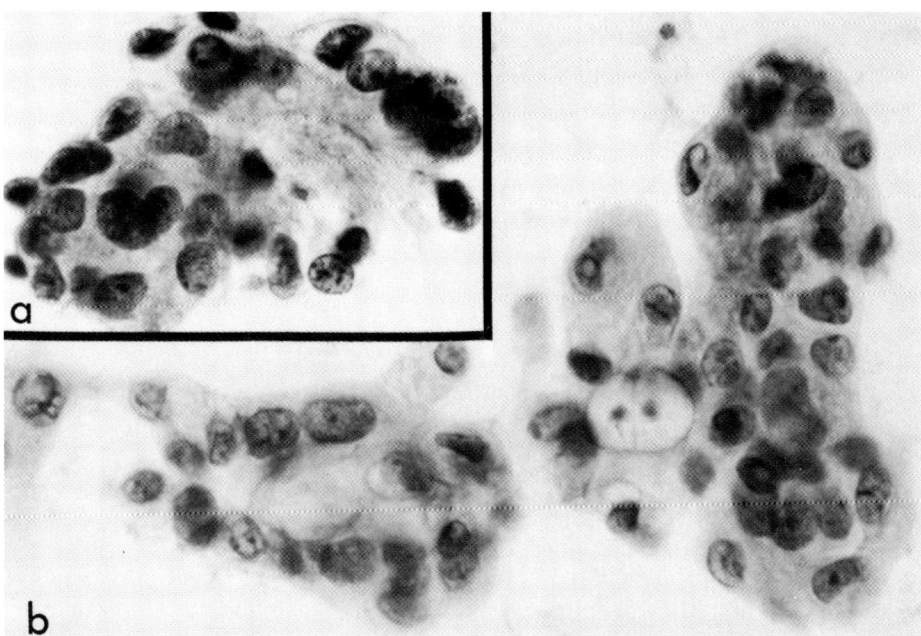

Fig. 13.7. Metastatic colonic adenocarcinoma to thyroid. **A.** Typical "picket-fence" arrangement of nuclei of colonic adenocarcinoma. Papanicolaou preparation. × 630. **B.** Syncytial-type tissue fragments of carcinoma cells with an acinar pattern. Papanicolaou preparation. × 630.

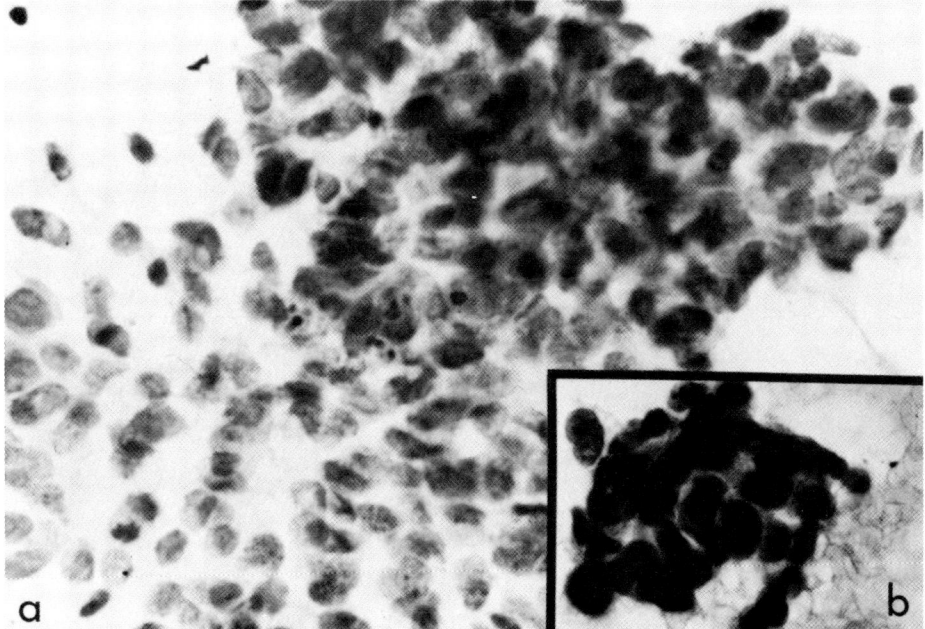

Fig. 13.8. **A., B.** Metastatic small cell, undifferentiated carcinoma from lung. This lung carcinoma clinically presented as a goiter. Papanicolaou preparation. × 630.

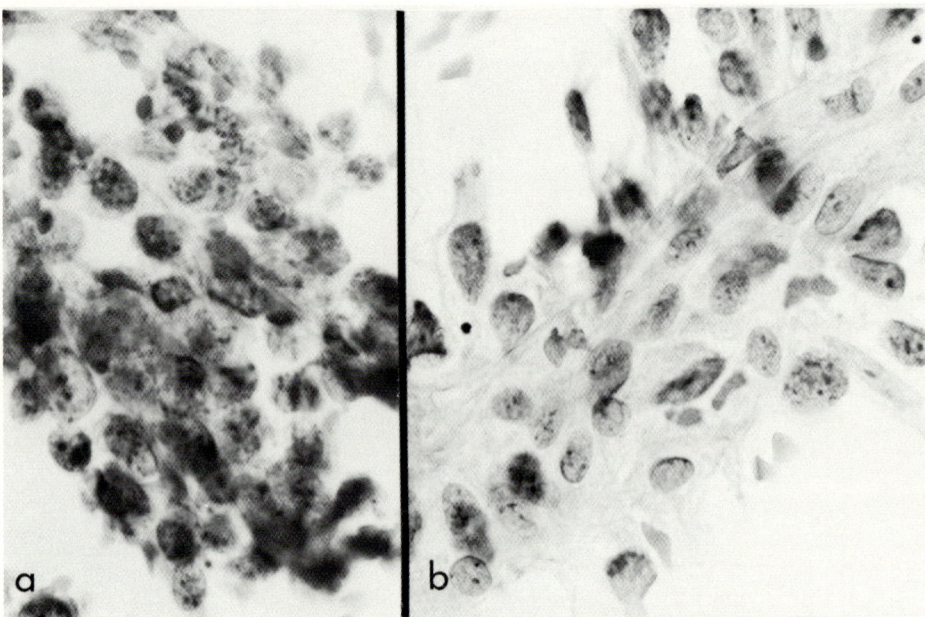

Fig. 13.9. Metastatic carcinosarcoma from esophagus infiltrating thyroid, masquerading as goiter. **A.** Poorly differentiated carcinoma cells. Papanicolaou preparation. × 630. **B.** Spindle cell component. Papanicolaou preparation. × 630.

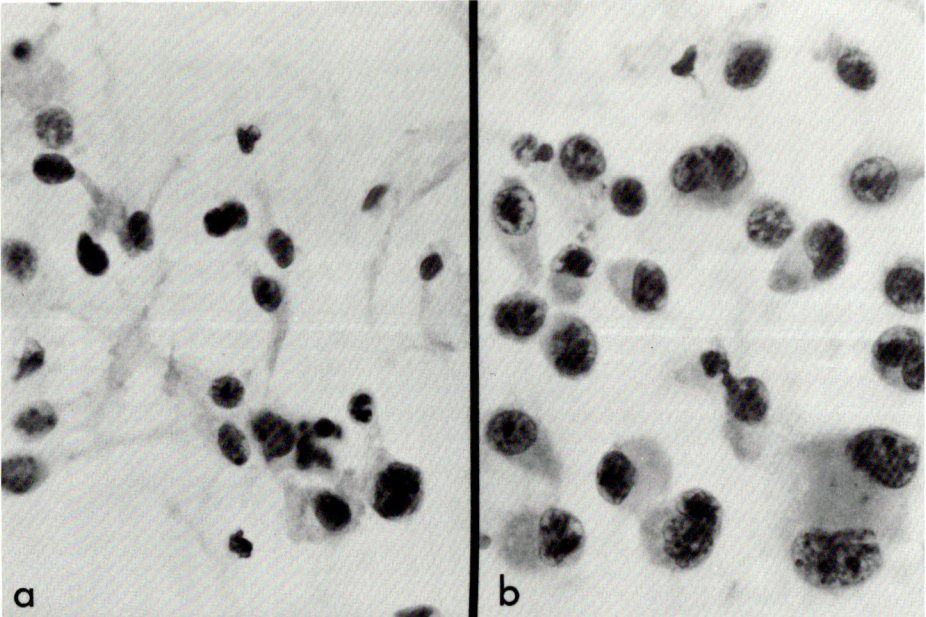

Fig. 13.10. A. Metastatic renal cell carcinoma. Note large cells with pale, but abundant, cytoplasm. Papanicolaou preparation. × 630. **B.** Metastatic malignant melanoma. Papanicolaou preparation. × 630.

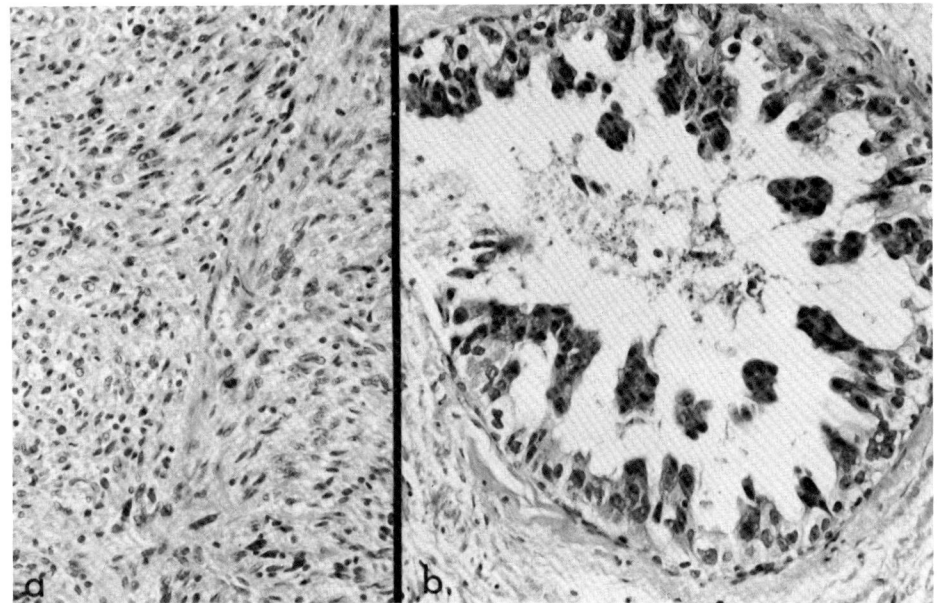

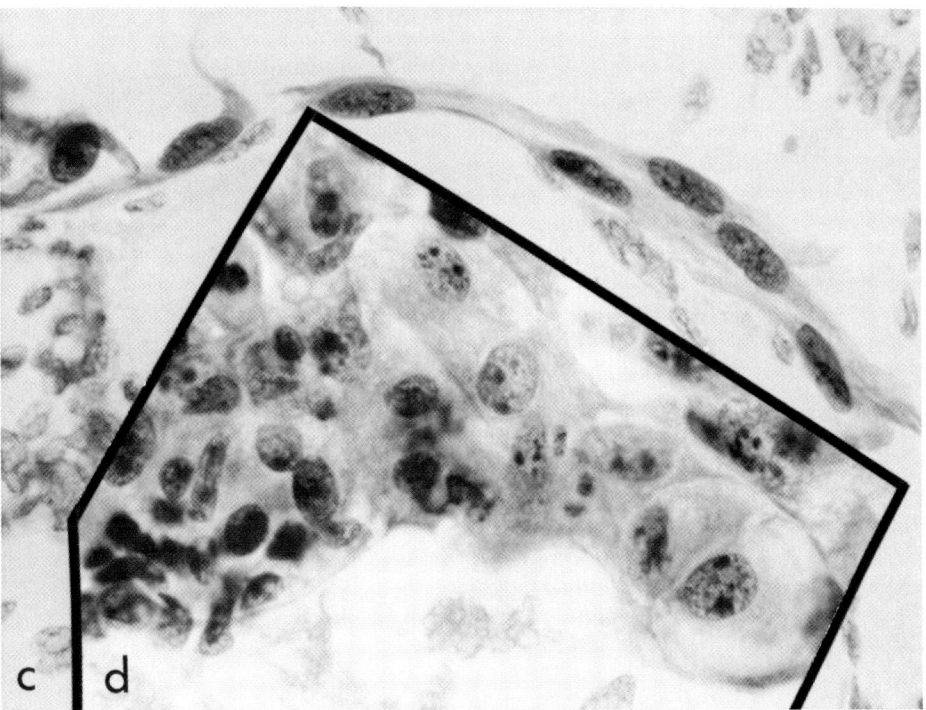

Fig. 13.11. A patient with a history of leiomyosarcoma of inferior vena cava and mastectomy for carcinoma of breast developed a cold nodule of thyroid. **A.** Section of leiomyosarcoma. Hematoxylin and eosin preparation. × 160. **B.** Section of breast with adenocarcinoma. Hematoxylin and eosin preparation. × 160. **C.** Spindle-shaped cells with large atypical nuclei, suggesting metastatic leiomyosarcoma. Patient had metastatic implants of sarcoma on skin elsewhere. Papanicolaou preparation. × 630. **D.** Large epithelial cells with atypical nuclei, suggesting metastatic adenocarcinoma from breast. Papanicolaou preparation. × 630. Whether this case represents a double metastasis is not known, as histologic confirmation is not available.

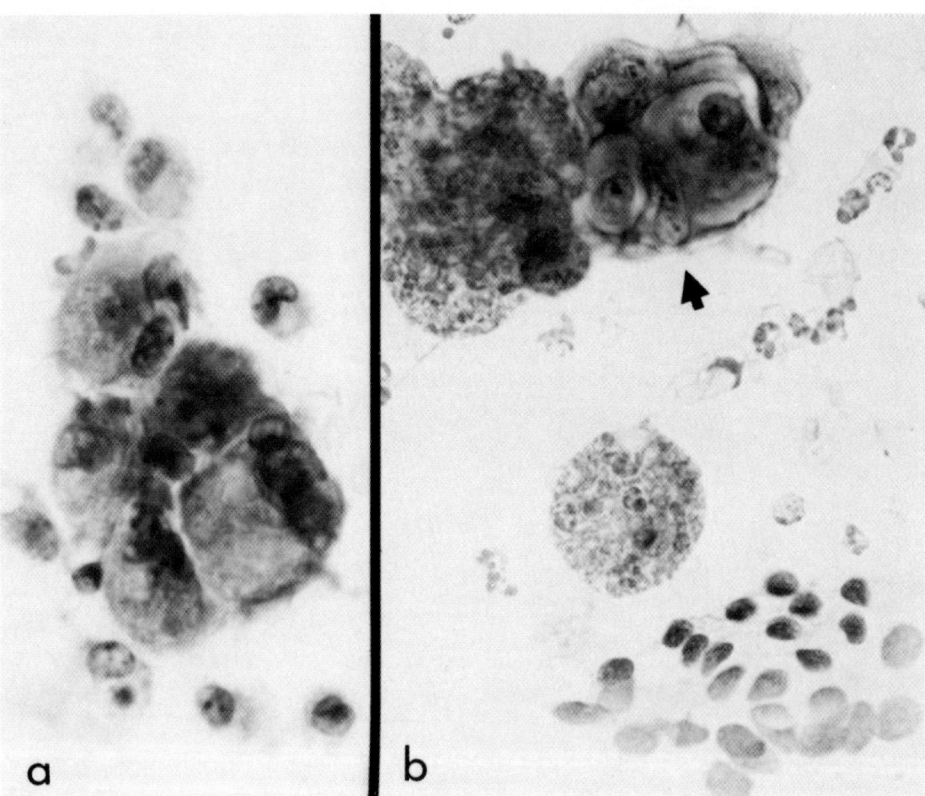

Fig. 13.12. A. Atypical cells in background of nodular goiter in an elderly woman were considered as metastatic carcinoma. Papanicolaou preparation. × 630. Thyroidectomy did not confirm the diagnosis. In retrospect, these are degenerating follicular cells. **B.** Metastatic breast carcinoma *(arrow)* in background of benign follicular cells and hemosiderin-containing histiocytes. Papanicolaou preparation. × 630.

REFERENCES

1. Elliott RHE Jr, Frantz VK: Metastatic carcinoma masquerading as primary thyroid cancer. *Am J Surg* 151:551–556, 1960.

2. Friberg S Jr, Kinnman J: Renal adenocarcinoma with metastasis to the thyroid gland. *Acta Otolaryngol* 67:552–562, 1969.

3. Gault EW, Leung THW, Thomas DP: Clear cell renal carcinoma masquerading as thyroid enlargement. *J Clin Pathol* 113:21–25, 1974.

4. Harcourt-Webster JN: Secondary neoplasm of the thyroid presenting as a goiter. *J Clin Pathol* 18:282–287, 1965.

5. Ivy HK: Cancer metastatic to the thyroid: a diagnostic problem. *Mayo Clin Proc* 59:856–859, 1984.

6. Lernard TWJ, Wadehra V, Farndon JR: Fine needle aspiration biopsy in diagnosis of metastasis to thyroid gland. *J R Soc Med* 77:196–197, 1984.

7. Mortensen JD, Woolner LB, Bennett WA: Secondary malignant tumors of the thyroid gland. *Cancer* 9:306, 1956.

8. Pillary SP, Angarn IB, Baker LW: Tumor metastasis to the thyroid gland. *S Afr Med J* 51:509–512, 1977.

9. Rosen IB, Bedard YC, Walfish PG, Bain J: Metastasis of cancer to the thyroid gland as a cause of goiter. *Can Med Assoc J* 118:1265–1268, 1978.

10. Shimaoka K, Sokal JE, Pickern J: Metastatic neoplasms in the thyroid gland. *Cancer* 15:557–565, 1962.

11. Silverberg SG, Vidone RA: Metastatic tumors in the thyroid. *Pacific Med Surg* 68:117–119, 1954.

12. Thomson JA, Kennedy JS, Browne MK, Hutchison J: Secondary carcinoma of the thyroid gland. *Br J Surg* 62:692–693, 1975.

13. Treadwell T, Alexander BB, Owen M, McConnel TH, Ashworth CT: Clear cell renal carcinoma, masquerading as a thyroid nodule. *South Med J* 74:878–879, 1981.

14. Trokoudes KM, Rosen IB, Strawbridge HTG, Bain J: Carcinomatous pseudothyroiditis: a problem in differential diagnosis. *Can Med Assoc J* 119:896–898, 1978.

15. Willis RA: *The Spread of Tumors in the Human Body*. London, Butterworth, 1951, pp. 271–275.

14

Cysts of Thyroid

Cysts of thyroid are common. In solitary thyroid lesions removed surgically, the incidence varies from 6% to 35%.[2–4,8,11–13,19] They usually occur as a result of degeneration, necrosis, or hemorrhage within an adenomatous nodule and sometimes within a neoplasm. Existence of true primary cyst of the thyroid is doubtful.[20] Intrathyroidal cysts lined by squamous or columnar epithelium occur occasionally.[11,15]

The majority of cysts of thyroid are benign. The incidence of malignancy reported in various series ranges from 0% to 33%[1,3,6–9,12–14,17–19,21] (Table 14.1). Although purely cystic carcinomas are rare, partial cystic degeneration occurs more often. Cystic change appears to be more common in larger nodules, as degeneration and hemorrhage occur frequently in neoplasms greater than 4 cm.[7] Rarely, a cancer may develop in the cyst wall. The impression that cystic lesions are generally a favorable finding and unlikely to be associated with malignancy[3,9] is disputed by the findings of Hammer et al.[7]

Clinically, cysts can be diagnosed by a rounded nodule that appears tense or taut.[3] The sudden appearance of a nodule that enlarges rapidly and causes discomfort is nearly always a cyst with hemorrhage into a nodule.[3] Although ultrasonography can identify a purely cystic lesion,[2] it is less accurate in demonstrating a partially cystic nodule.[7,8,15,16,19] Hammer et al[7] reported a false-positive rate of 32%, and a false-negative rate of 29%. Aspiration biopsy has been found to be very useful for (1) identifying the lesion as a cyst; and (2) differentiating between benign and malignant cysts when sonography cannot make this determination. This differentiation is done by cytologic examination of the aspirated fluid.

Benign cysts arising from nodular goiter collapse after being drained. A small number may recur or bleed immediately due to negative pressure; this necessitates a second aspiration. If cysts recur, especially with hemorrhagic contents, malignancy should be suspected.

TABLE 14.1. Incidence of Carcinoma in Cysts of Thyroid

Authors (yr)	No.	Percent
Miller et al[13] (1983)	2/303	0.6
Ma and Ong[10] (1975)	1/62	1.6
Crile[3] (1966)	0/50	0
Goellner and Johnson[6] (1982)	9/158	5.6
Suen and Quenville[18] (1983)	2/59	3.0
Walfish et al[21] (1977)	3/13	23.0
Jensen and Rasmussen[8] (1976)	0/288	0
Hammer et al[7] (1982)	16/48	33.0

EXAMINATION OF CYST FLUID

Grossly, the volume of the aspirate varies from a few milliliters to 20 ml or more. The characteristics of the fluid reflect the duration of the cyst. Soon after hemorrhage, the specimen will resemble venous blood, but later, the aspirate changes from chocolate–opaque to olive–translucent and ultimately to a yellow–transparent fluid.[13] A nodule that has undergone degeneration and necrosis may yield a small amount of turbid, thick fluid. These gross characteristics have no significant bearing on the nature of the lesions. Cytopreparation depends on the type of specimen (see Chapter 3, Adequacy, Reporting System, and Cytopreparatory Technique).

CYTOPATHOLOGY OF CYST FLUID

The cytopathologic pattern of cyst fluid depends on several factors, such as duration; type of the cyst, ie, benign or malignant; and hemorrhage into the cyst. The fluid medium to which exfoliated cells are exposed may induce retrogressive changes that could simulate neoplasia, constituting important diagnostic pitfalls. True neoplasia can be masked by retrogressive changes as well. In that case, cyst fluid presents diagnostic problems on which very little attention has been focused. Most of the literature discusses the identification of a cyst rather than the diagnosis of the type of a cyst. A detailed description is found in the book by Droese.[5]

CYTOPATHOLOGY OF CYSTS DERIVED FROM ADENOMATOUS GOITER

Fluid from a long-standing cyst is thin, clear, and practically accellular. The absence of well-preserved follicular cells seems to be the rule, rather than the exception.

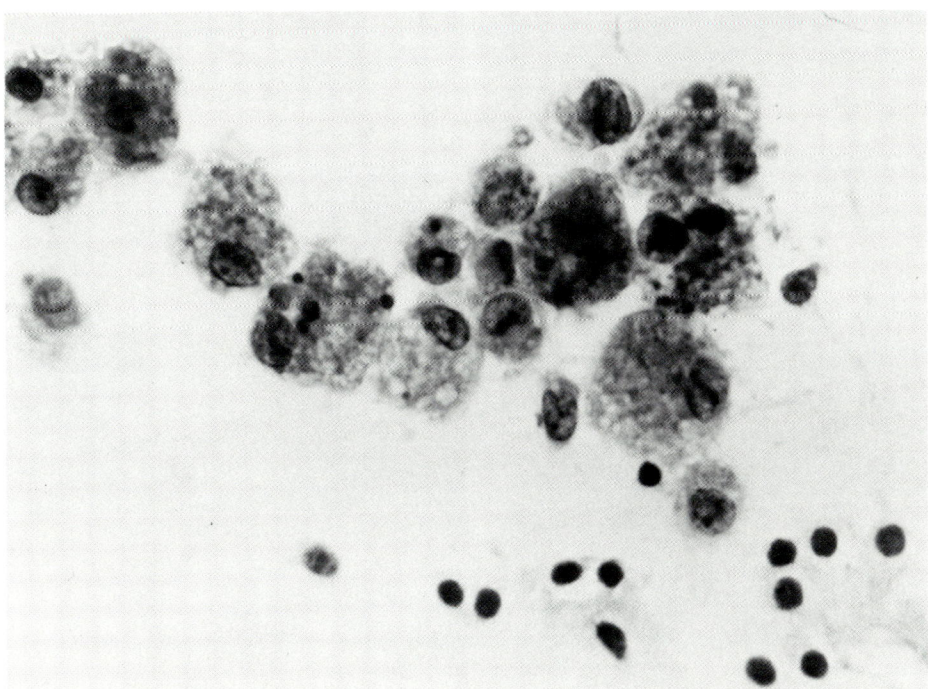

Fig. 14.1. Usual cytopathological pattern of cyst fluid showing several hemosiderin-containing histiocytes. Papanicolaou preparation. × 630.

Generally, the smears prepared from the sediment of the cyst fluid almost always show variable numbers of histiocytes, with or without hemosiderin pigment (Fig. 14.1). These cells have abundant granular or foamy cytoplasm, with round nuclei in a slightly eccentric location. The nuclear chromatin is finely granular, and nucleoli may be conspicuous. Multinucleated foreign-body–type giant cells are also present. Cholesterol crystals are often identified by the wet-mount technique (Fig. 14.2) (see Chapter 3, Adequacy, Reporting System, and Cytopreparatory Technique). Follicular epithelial cells are present only in cysts of recent origin, but these exhibit regressive changes that are extremely difficult to differentiate from malignant cells.[5] Degenerating cells show various morphologic changes. They may enlarge and acquire abundant granular cytoplasm resembling histiocytes. Some may exhibit phagocytic activity and contain hemosiderin pigment (Fig. 14.3). The nuclei also enlarge in size, but not in the same proportion as the cytoplasm (Fig. 14.4), and contain prominent nucleoli that suggest malignancy. The cytoplasm may be vacuolated or may contain a large, single vacuole. Large tissue fragments of benign follicular cells within the cyst cavity exposed to the fluid environment may resemble syncytial-type tissue fragments of neoplasms (Figs. 14.5 and 14.6; Plate 14.1).

The background may be hemorrhagic and contain granular, amorphous, and inflammatory debris. Also, during the process of centrifugation of the cyst fluid, the histiocytes may aggregate and resemble a tissue fragment (Plate 14.1).

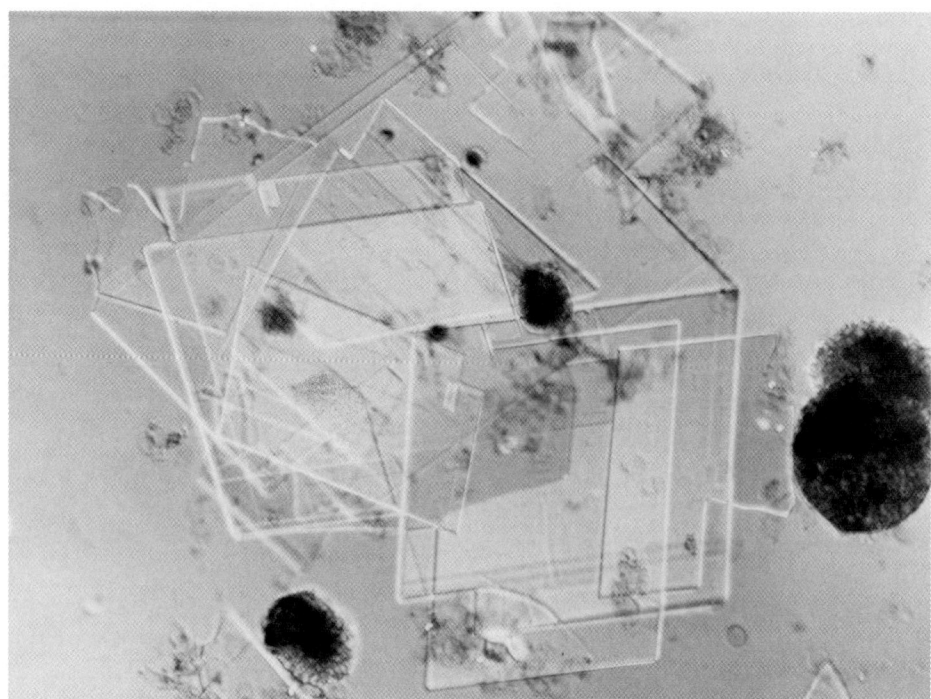

Fig. 14.2. Cyst fluid from degenerated nodular goiter with cholesterol crystals and hemosiderin-containing histiocytes. Toludine blue preparation. × 630.

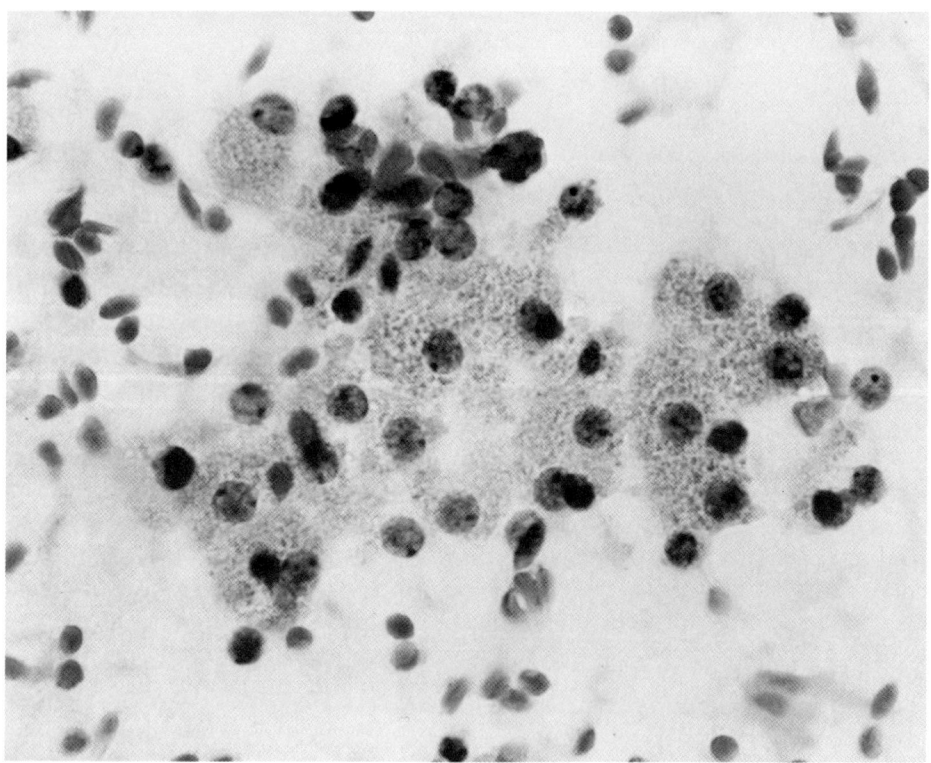

Fig. 14.3. Degenerating follicular cells with hemosiderin pigment. Papanicolaou preparation. × 630.

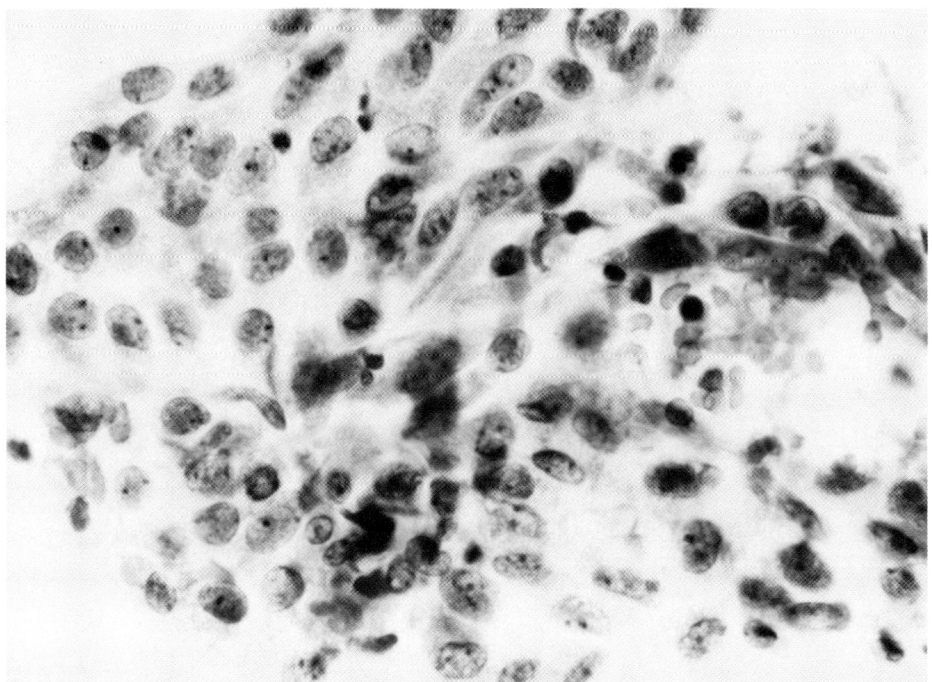

Fig. 14.4. Degenerating follicular cells from a cyst fluid showing marked nuclear atypia, suggesting a neoplasm. Thyroidectomy showed nodular goiter. Papanicolaou preparation. × 630.

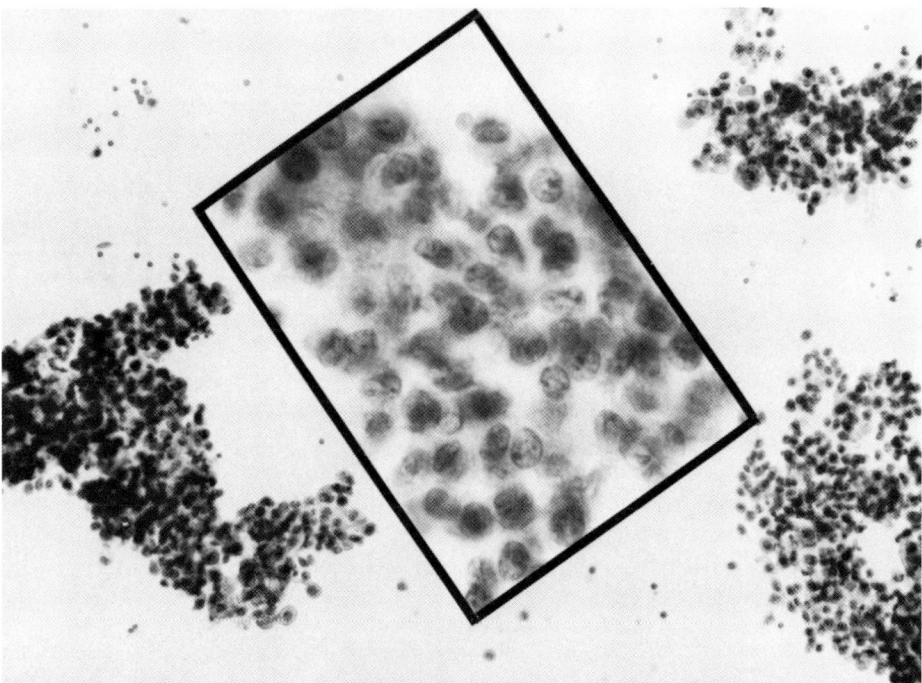

Fig. 14.5. Cyst fluid from nodular goiter showing large tissue fragments. Papanicolaou preparation. × 160. *Inset:* Poor nuclear detail in higher magnification, still suggestive of neoplasm. Papanicolaou preparation. × 630.

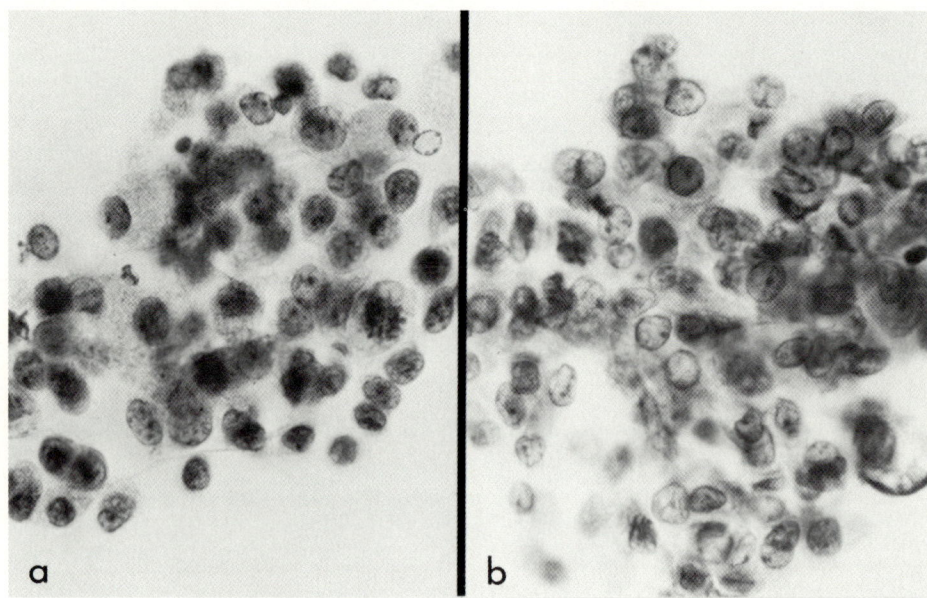

Fig. 14.6. **A.** Degenerating follicular cells from cystic nodular goiter, suggesting papillary carcinoma. Papanicolaou preparation. × 630. **B.** Papillary carcinoma cells from cystic papillary carcinoma. Note morphologic similarities with **A.** Papanicolaou preparation. × 630.

CYTOPATHOLOGY OF CYST FLUID FROM NEOPLASMS

Cystic change is very common in papillary carcinomas.[1] These carcinomas are also difficult to diagnose from aspirated fluid because of hemorrhage or scanty cellular material that is often altered by degenerative changes in the fluid medium[6] (Fig. 14.6). Walfish et al[21] and Miller et al[14] reported, respectively, false-negative rates of 16.7% and 45% in cystic papillary carcinomas. See Chapter 8, Papillary Carcinoma, for a discussion of the diagnostic problems of cystic papillary carcinoma.

Cystic change is also encountered in follicular neoplasms, as well as in Hürthle cell tumors,[12] especially if they are large. Cytologic diagnosis may be difficult for the same reasons as with papillary carcinomas.

The differential diagnosis of a thyroid cyst includes branchial cleft cyst and thyroglossal duct cyst. Both show keratinized and nonkeratinized squamous cells (Fig. 14.7). Carcinoma arising in thyroglossal duct cyst will present a cytopathologic pattern of that particular cancer, and the exact location of the neoplasm is usually established only after thyroidectomy.

SUMMARY

The majority of cyst fluids are poorly cellular, containing only a few histiocytes. Degenerated follicular cells from adenomatous goiter constitute an important

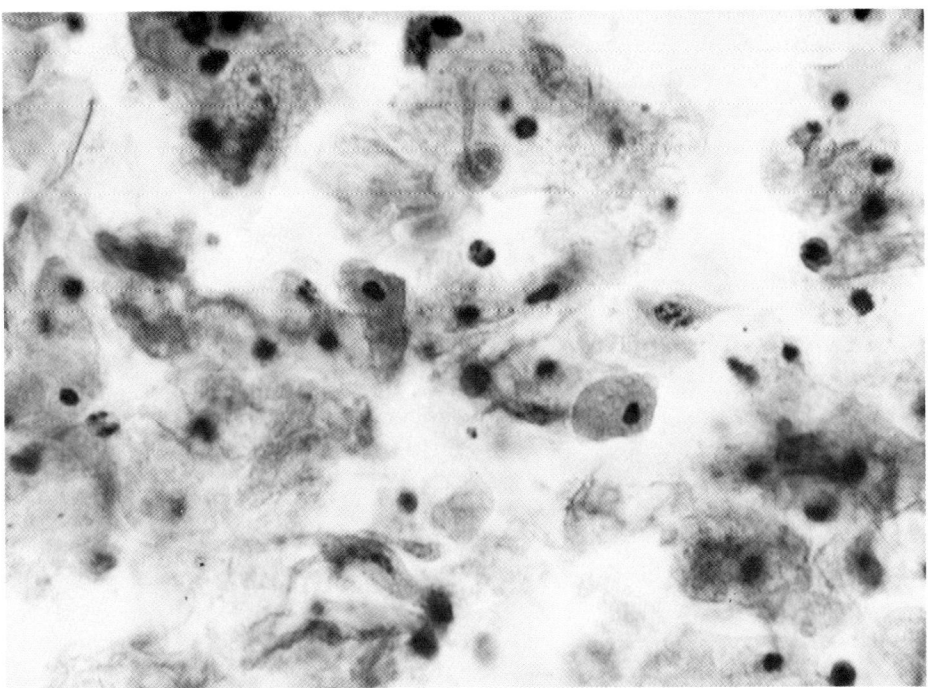

Fig. 14.7. Branchial cleft cyst fluid showing squamous cells. Papanicolaou preparation. × 630.

diagnostic pitfall. Papillary carcinomas have a tendency for cystic degeneration and may pose diagnostic difficulties.

REFERENCES

1. Carcangiu ML, Zampi G, Pupi A, Castagnoli AZ, Rosai J: Papillary carcinoma of the thyroid: a clinico-pathological study of 241 cases treated at the University of Florence, Italy. *Cancer* 55:805–808, 1985.

2. Clark OH, Greenspan FS, Coggs GC, Goldman L: Evaluation of solitary cold thyroid nodules by echography and thermography. *Am J Surg* 130:206–211, 1975.

3. Crile G Jr: Treatment of thyroid cysts by aspiration. *Surgery* 59:210–212, 1966.

4. Crockford PM, Bain G: Fine needle aspiration biopsy of the thyroid. *Can Med Assoc J* 110:1029–1032, 1974.

5. Droese M: *Cytologic Aspiration Biopsy of the Thyroid Gland.* Stuttgart, F.K. Schattauer-Verlag, 1980, pp. 55–79.

6. Goellner JR, Johnson DA: Cytology of cystic papillary carcinoma of the thyroid. *Acta Cytol* 26:787–799, 1982.

7. Hammer M, Wortsman J, Folse R: Cancer in cystic lesions of the thyroid. *Arch Surg* 117:1020–1023, 1982.

8. Jensen F, Rasmussen SN: The treatment of thyroid cysts by ultrasonically guided fine needle aspirate. *Acta Chir Scand* 142:209–211, 1976.

9. LeGierfo P, Ting M: Method for biopsy of the wall of a thyroid cyst. *Am J Surg* 146:383–384, 1983.

10. Ma MKG, Ong B: Cystic thyroid nodules. *Br J Surg* 62:205–206, 1975.

11. Meissner WA: *Tumors of the Thyroid Gland.* Fascicle 4, Second Series, *Atlas of Tumor Pathology.* Washington, DC, Armed Forces Institute of Pathology, 1969, p. 29.

12. Miller N, Cooperberg PL, Suen KCH, Thorsan SC: Needle aspiration biopsy in cystic papillary carcinoma of the thyroid. *Am J Roentgenol* 144:251–253, 1985.

13. Miller JM, Hamburger JI, Taylor CI: Is needle aspiration of the cystic thyroid nodule effective and safe treatment? In Hamburger JI, Miller JM: *Controversies in Thyroidology.* New York, Prager Publishers, 1983, pp. 209–236.

14. Miller JM, Zafar S, Karo JJ: The cystic thyroid nodule. *Diagn Radiol* 110:257–261, 1974.

15. Ohashi H, Sato A, Tanagbe Y, Shimokawa K, Ojima Akitsugu: Cystic goiter with squamous cell metaplasia—case report and comment on origin of squamous cell cyst. *Acta Pathol Jpn* 26:503–508, 1976.

16. Rosen IB, Walfish PG, Miskin M: The use of B-mode ultrasonography in changing indications for thyroid operations. *Surg Gynecol Obstet* 139:193–197, 1974.

17. Rosen IB, Wallace C, Strawbridge HG, Walfish PG: Re-evaluation of needle aspiration cytology in detection of thyroid cancer. *Surgery* 90:747–756, 1981.

18. Suen KC, Quenville NF: Fine needle aspiration biopsy of the thyroid gland: a study of 304 cases. *J Clin Pathol* 36:1036–1045, 1983.

19. Thijs LG, Winer JD: Ultrasonic examination of the thyroid gland—possibilities and limitations. *Am J Med* 60:96–105, 1976.

20. Vickery A Jr: Needle biopsy pathology. *Clin Endocrinol Metabol Dis* 10:283–292, 1981.

21. Walfish PG, Hazani E, Strawbridge HTH, Miskin M, Rosen IB: Combined ultrasound and needle aspiration cytology in the assessment and management of hypofunctioning thyroid nodule. *Ann Intern Med* 87:270–274, 1977.

15

Miscellaneous

This chapter is a potpourri of some unexpected cytopathologic patterns encountered in aspiration biopsy specimens of thyroid nodules. These patterns cover a broad range of uncommon and unusual lesions, some related to the thyroid and some nonthyroidal in origin. Infarction of thyroid nodule following aspiration biopsy and cold nodules in pediatric and adolescent patients are also covered in this chapter, as well as cytopathologic patterns of thyroid cancers metastatic to other body sites.

NON-NEOPLASTIC CELLS OF NONTHYROID ORIGIN

Aspiration biopsy of the thyroid gland may yield cells that are nonthyroidal in origin. Most often, these represent skeletal muscle fibers, adipose tissue, or fragments of epidermis. Occasionally, ciliated columnar cells from the trachea are encountered. Gay et al[18] described fragments of tracheal or laryngeal cartilage and hematopoietic cells from bone marrow of ossified laryngeal cartilage. Our experience with one case of thyroid aspirate showing megakaryocytes is illustrated in Fig. 15.1

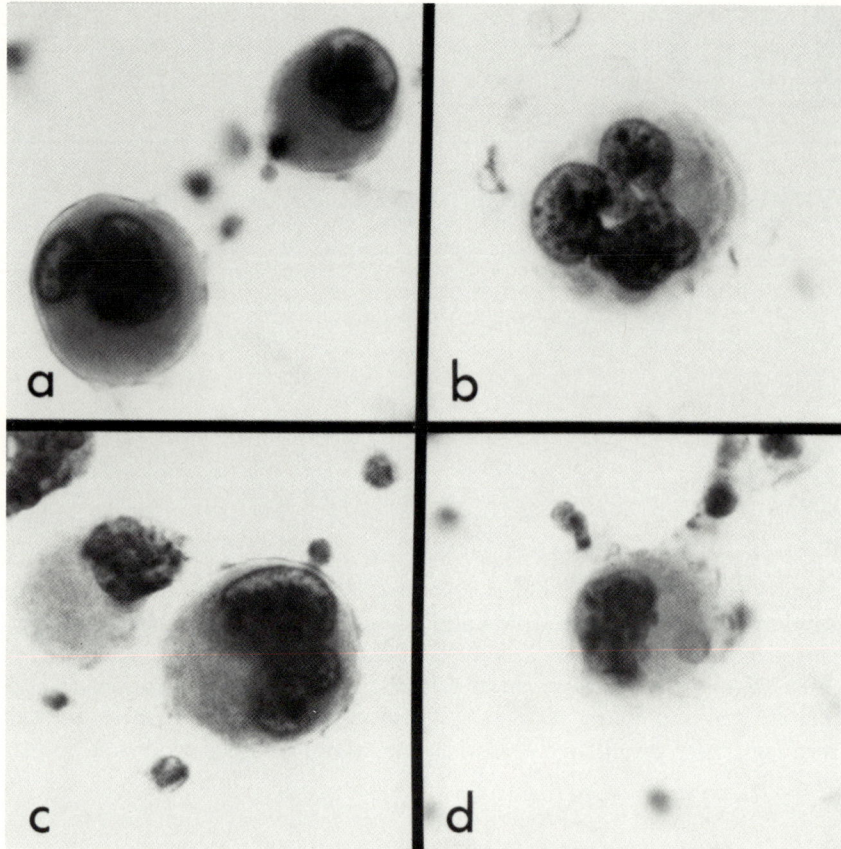

Fig. 15.1. A–D. Hematopoietic cells. An initial aspirate of the cold nodule in a 30-year-old woman showed large mononuclear cells and cells with multilobulated nuclei. Follicular epithelial cells were absent. Repeat aspirate revealed features consistent with cellular adenoma, later confirmed by thyroidectomy. In retrospect, these cells are consistent with megakaryocytes. Papanicolaou preparation. × 630.

ASPERGILLUS THYROIDITIS

Among the fungal diseases involving the thyroid gland, *Aspergillus* is reported to be the most common.[3,18] The thyroid is affected in approximately 20% of patients with disseminated *Aspergillosis*, based on autopsy studies.[5] Antemortem diagnosis is seldom made, and only one case has been reported so far.[21]

We have seen one case of *Aspergillus* thyroiditis diagnosed in an immunosuppressed patient with a kidney transplant, who presented with hypercalcemia and cold nodule of thyroid. *Aspergillus* was diagnosed by aspiration biopsy, and was later confirmed by thyroidectomy (Fig. 15.2).

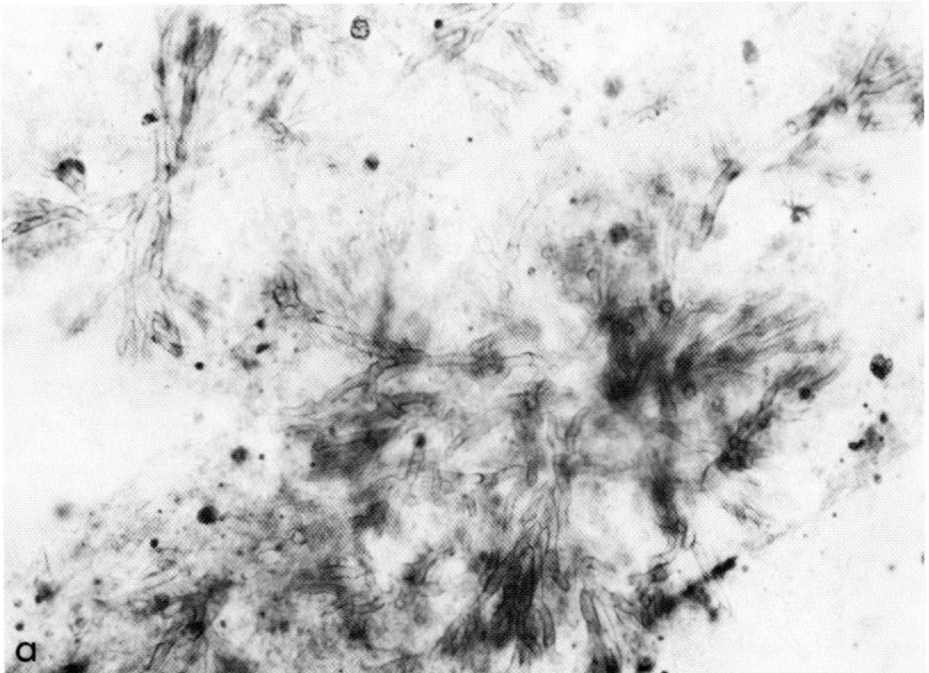

Fig. 15.2. A. Aspiration biopsy specimen of a cold nodule in an immunosuppressed patient, yielded turbid fluid that showed branching hyphae morphologically resembling *Aspergillus* species. Papanicolaou preparation. × 630.

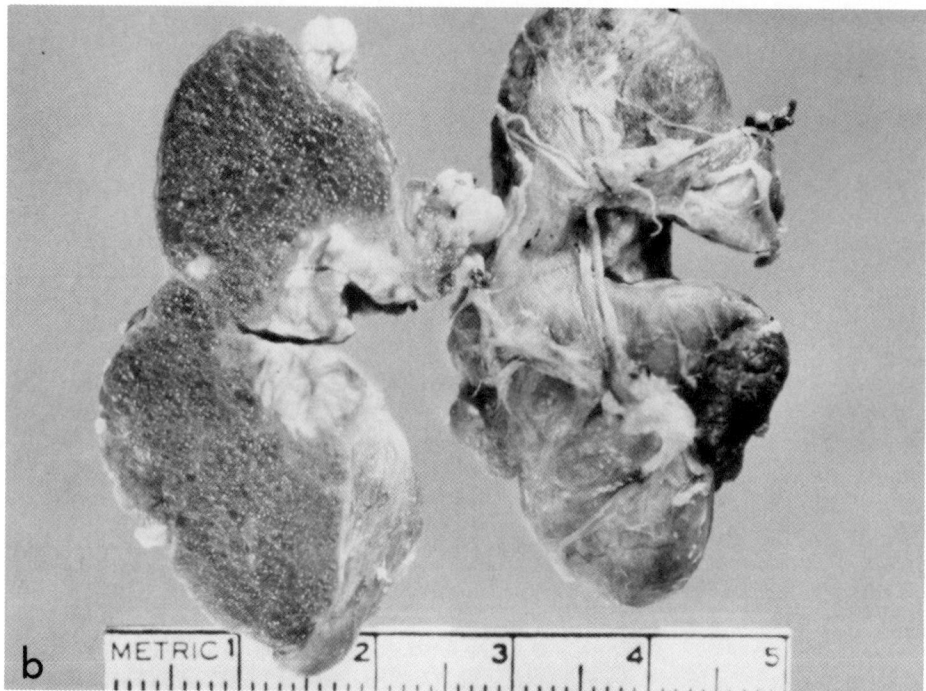

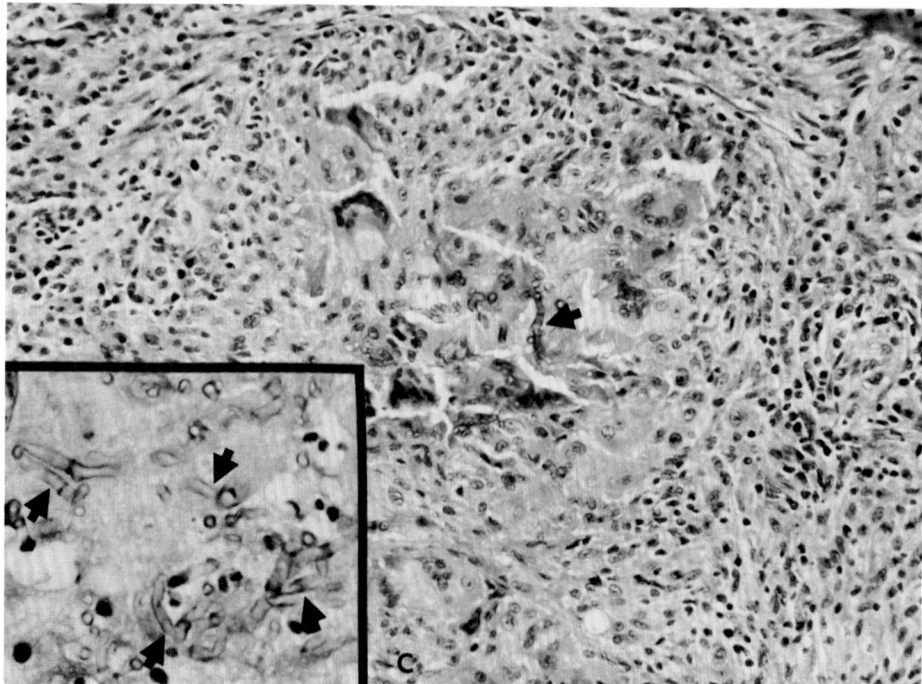

Fig. 15.2. B. Thyroidectomy was performed. An abscess was identified involving the right lobe. **C.** Histologic section showing granulomatous inflammation. Hematoxylin and eosin preparation. × 250. *Inset: Aspergillus* hyphae within granuloma *(arrows)*. Hematoxylin and eosin preparation. × 400.

SQUAMOUS CELL CARCINOMA OF THYROID

Squamous cell carcinoma of thyroid is a rare malignant neoplasm. It can occur in a pure form[19,31,35,41]; in combination with papillary or follicular, so-called adenosquamous, carcinomas[50,51]; or as a subgroup of anaplastic carcinoma, as indicated by Carcangiu et al.[8] The incidence of primary squamous carcinoma of thyroid is very low, and is reported to be 1.1% of all thyroid cancers.[19] Squamous cell carcinoma may arise from squamous epithelium in normal thyroid, and is derived from the ultimobranchial body or thyroglossal duct remnant.[34] It may also arise from metaplastic squamous cells, which are frequently seen in nodular goiter and thyroiditis, as well as papillary and follicular carcinomas.

Primary squamous cell carcinomas are known to follow a rapidly progressive course. They are generally radioresistant and offer a poor prognosis.

Squamous carcinoma aspirates show malignant squamous cells with or without keratinization (Fig. 15.3). Secondary involvement of thyroid by squamous carcinoma from other organs must be ruled out before diagnosing it as primary in thyroid.

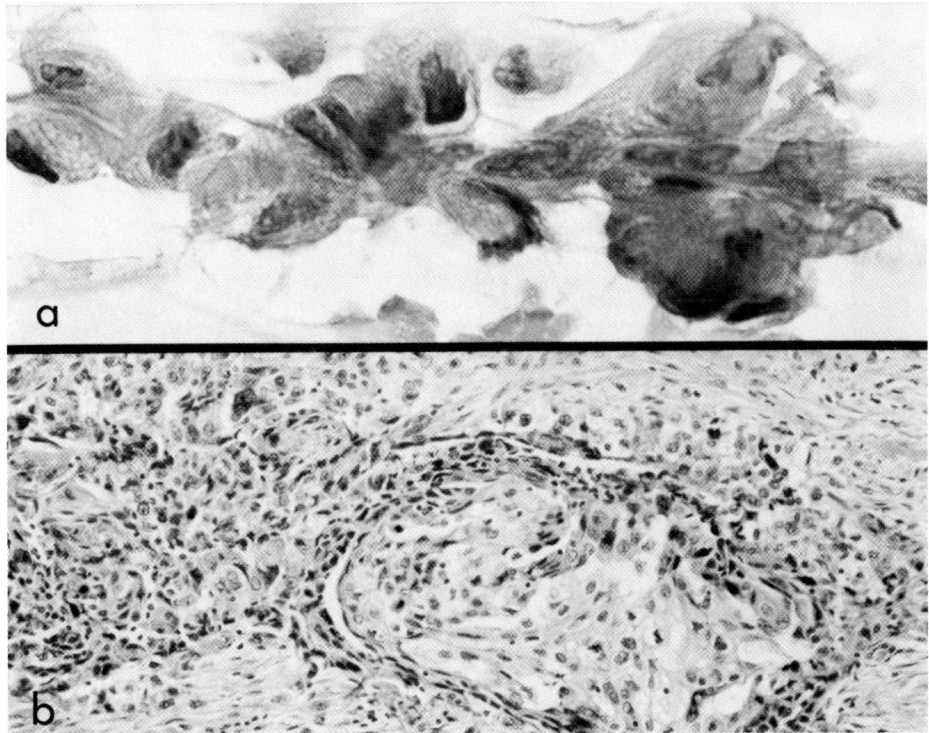

Fig. 15.3. A. Aspirate of primary squamous cell carcinoma of thyroid, showing a group of keratinized squamous cells. Papanicolaou preparation. × 630. **B.** Histologic section of squamous cell carcinoma. Hematoxylin and eosin preparation. × 100.

INTRATHYROIDAL THYMOMA

A thymoma can arise in the thyroid gland from aberrant thymic tissue.[22,39,47] It represents a distinct entity, separate from squamous carcinoma, from which it must be differentiated. This differentiation is necessary because squamous cell carcinomas have a poor prognosis.

Our experience with one case of thymoma is illustrated in Fig. 15.4. Cytologically, the lymphoid cells mixed with epithelial cells suggested a carcinoma in the background of lymphocytic thyroiditis. Cytologic diagnosis of the lesion as thymoma is difficult when the aspirate is obtained from intrathyroidal lesion.

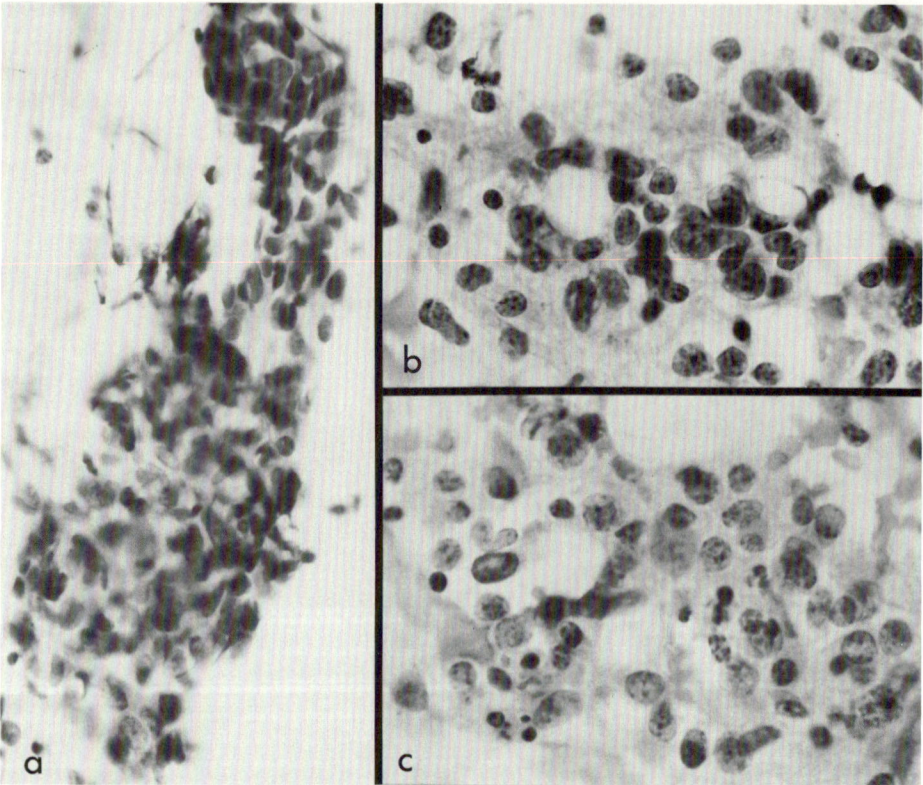

Fig. 15.4. A. Intrathyroidal thymoma. Aspirate showed syncytial-type tissue fragments of cells with ovoid nuclei, identification of which was difficult. Papanicolaou preparation. × 630. **B., C.** Note lymphocytes in the background, along with large cells having poorly defined cell borders, pale cytoplasm, and large round nuclei. The cytopathologic pattern suggested malignancy, but typing was difficult. Papanicolaou preparation. × 630.

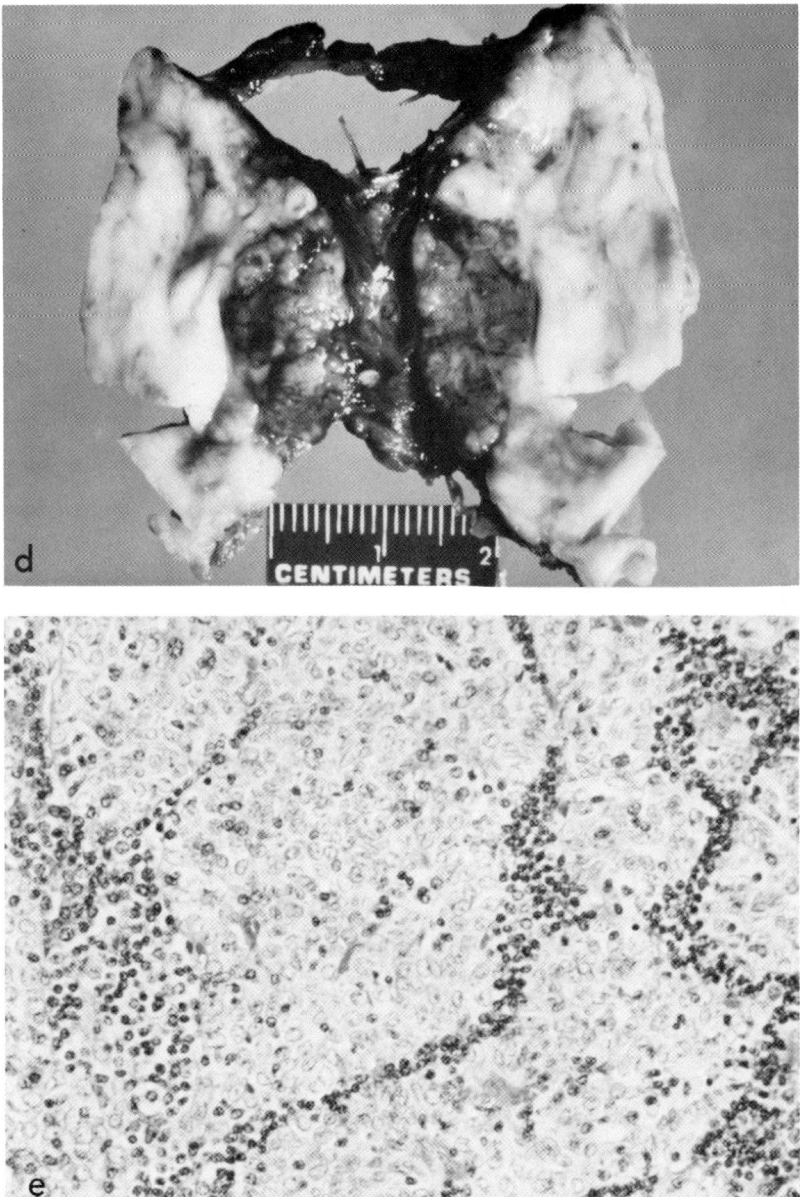

Fig. 15.4. D. Left thyroid lobe totally involved by a white, fleshy tumor. **E.** Section of the tumor showing typical pattern of epithelial thymoma. Hematoxylin and eosin preparation. × 250.

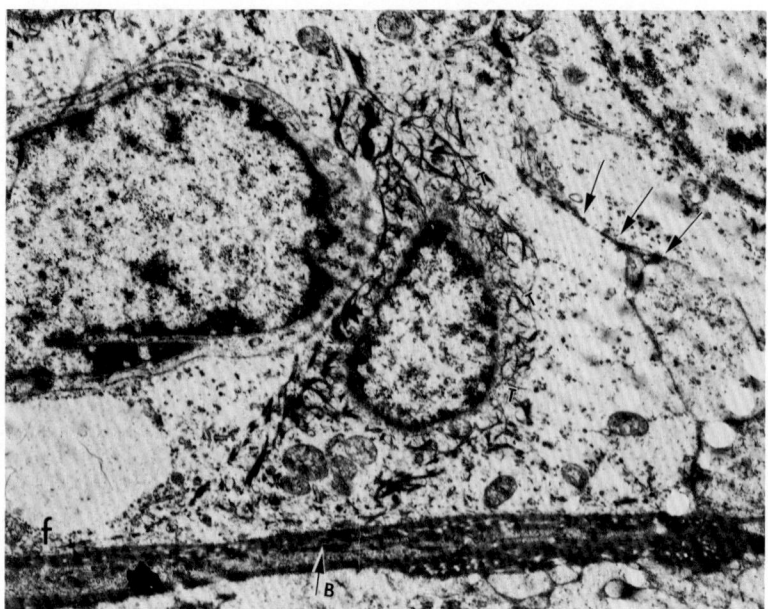

Fig. 15.4. F. Ultrastructurally, the neoplastic cells showed typical features of thymoma. This electron micrograph shows groups of squamoid epithelial cells invested by a basement membrane *(B)*. The cells have numerous perinuclear bundles of tonofilaments *(T)* and desmosomes *(arrows)*. Uranyl acetate and lead citrate preparation. × 43,200.

CELLULAR CHANGES IN THYROID SECONDARY TO RADIOIODINE

Histopathologic changes in thyroid following radioiodine (^{131}I) therapy are varied, depending on the dose of radiation as well as the duration.[41,58] These include initially neutrophilic infiltrate, necrosis of follicular cells, and giant cell reaction, followed by atrophy and fibrosis. Changes similar to Hashimoto's thyroiditis and development of adenomatous nodules have also been described.[13] Follicular cells may show marked cytoplasmic and nuclear pleomorphism. The cytologic specimens from thyroid previously subjected to radioiodine correspondingly show various changes. If the cytopathologist is unaware of the radiation therapy, the aspirates may be misinterpreted as malignant neoplasms.

The cellular changes described by Droese[15] include, in early stages, the presence of neutrophils, degenerating follicular cells, and histiocytes. Subsequently, the aspirate may contain large fragments of stroma. The epithelial cells and stromal cells may show cytomegaly, with marked pleomorphism in their size (Fig. 15.5). The cytoplasm can be dense or vacuolated, and may contain blue–black pigment granules, and the cells may have cytoplasmic processes. Likewise, the nuclei can be very atypical with coarse chromatin, and may contain nucleoli. Intranuclear clear inclusions have also been described[15] (Fig. 15.5B). The nuclei may be giant form and appear "naked" due to disintegration of the cytoplasm.

The differential diagnosis of these atypical cells includes anaplastic carcinoma.

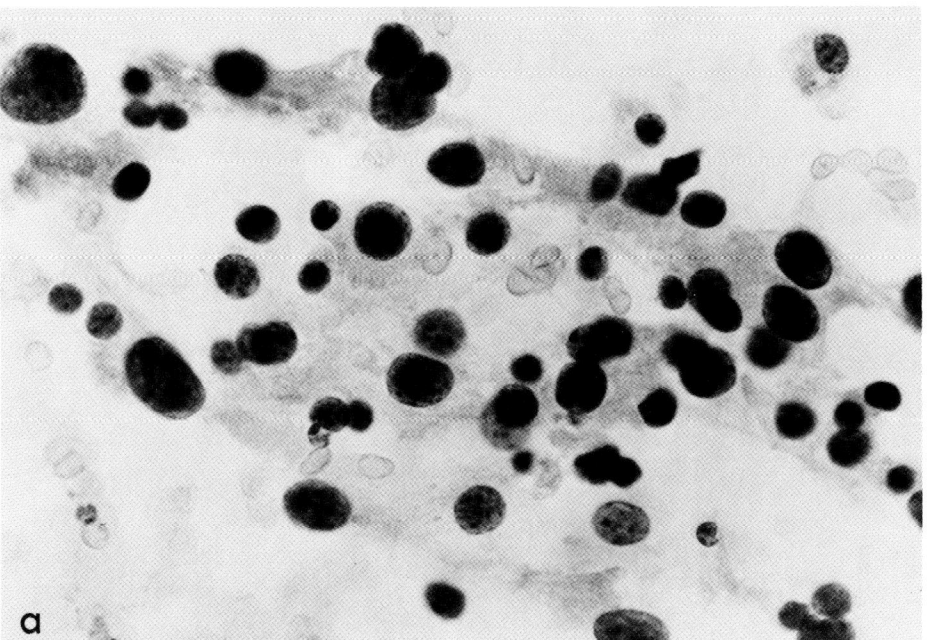

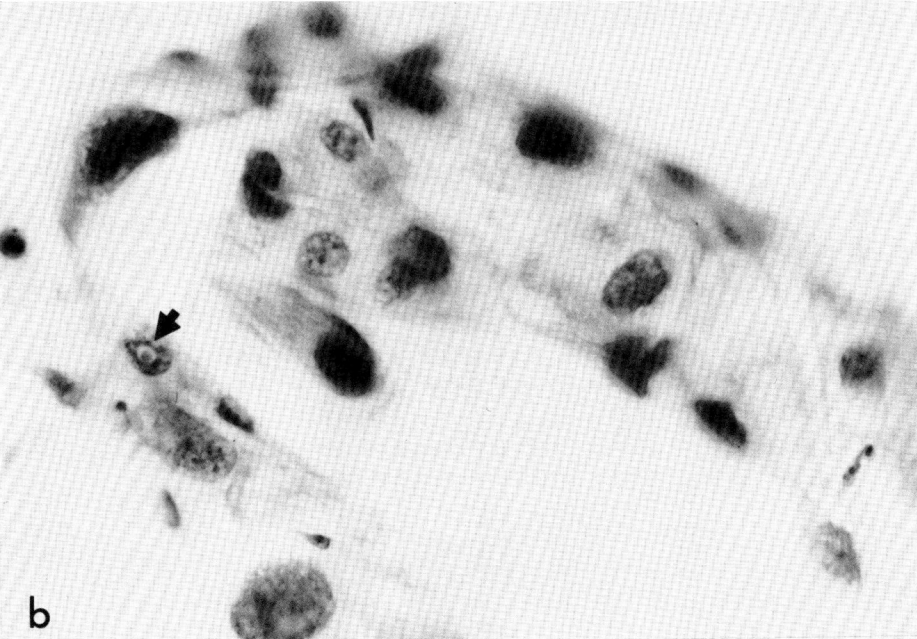

Fig. 15.5. A. Follicular cells aspirated from a thyroid treated with ^{131}I therapy. The nuclei are considerably enlarged in size, pyknotic, and many are "naked." Papanicolaou preparation. × 630. **B.** Group of very pleomorphic, spindle-shaped cells aspirated from thyroid, treated with ^{131}I therapy. Note intranuclear inclusion *(arrow)*. Papanicolaou preparation. × 630. Without this history available to the cytopathologist, a diagnosis of anaplastic carcinoma can easily be made.

MULTIPLE MALIGNANCIES IN THYROID

The presence of multiple tumors, benign and malignant, occult or apparent, in the same thyroid is not uncommon,[6] but the incidence is not known due to the sparsity of literature on the subject. O'Neill and Lomas[44] and Lamberg et al[33] reported concurrent medullary carcinoma and papillary carcinoma. Ayala et al[3] described one case of Hashimoto's thyroiditis with follicular carcinoma and malignant lymphoma. These reported cases have been identified following surgery. Cytologic diagnosis of multiple malignances has not been reported. Our experience includes two cases of Hashimoto's thyroiditis with papillary carcinoma and malignant lymphoma (Fig. 15.6), and one case of Hürthle cell carcinoma and papillary carcinoma identified in cytologic samples (Fig. 15.7).

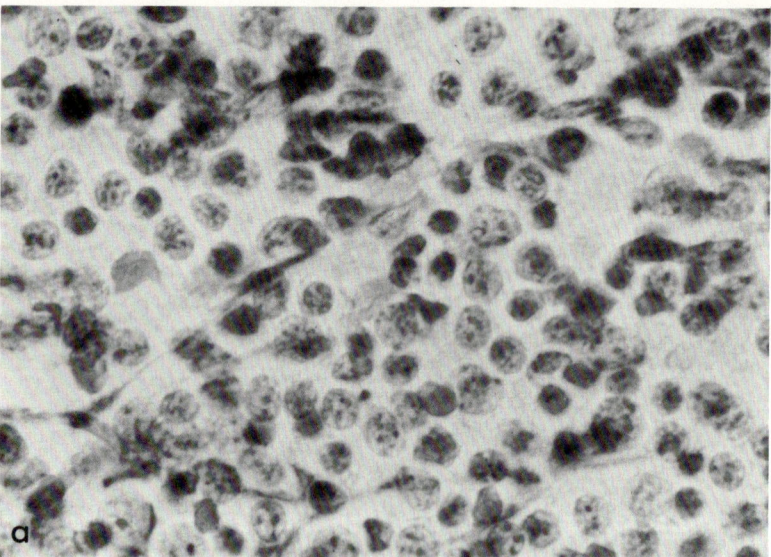

Fig. 15.6. A. Aspirate from a 30-year-old woman with diffusely enlarged thyroid with nodularity showing a large population of immature lymphoid cells, consistent with malignant lymphoma. Papanicolaou preparation. × 630.

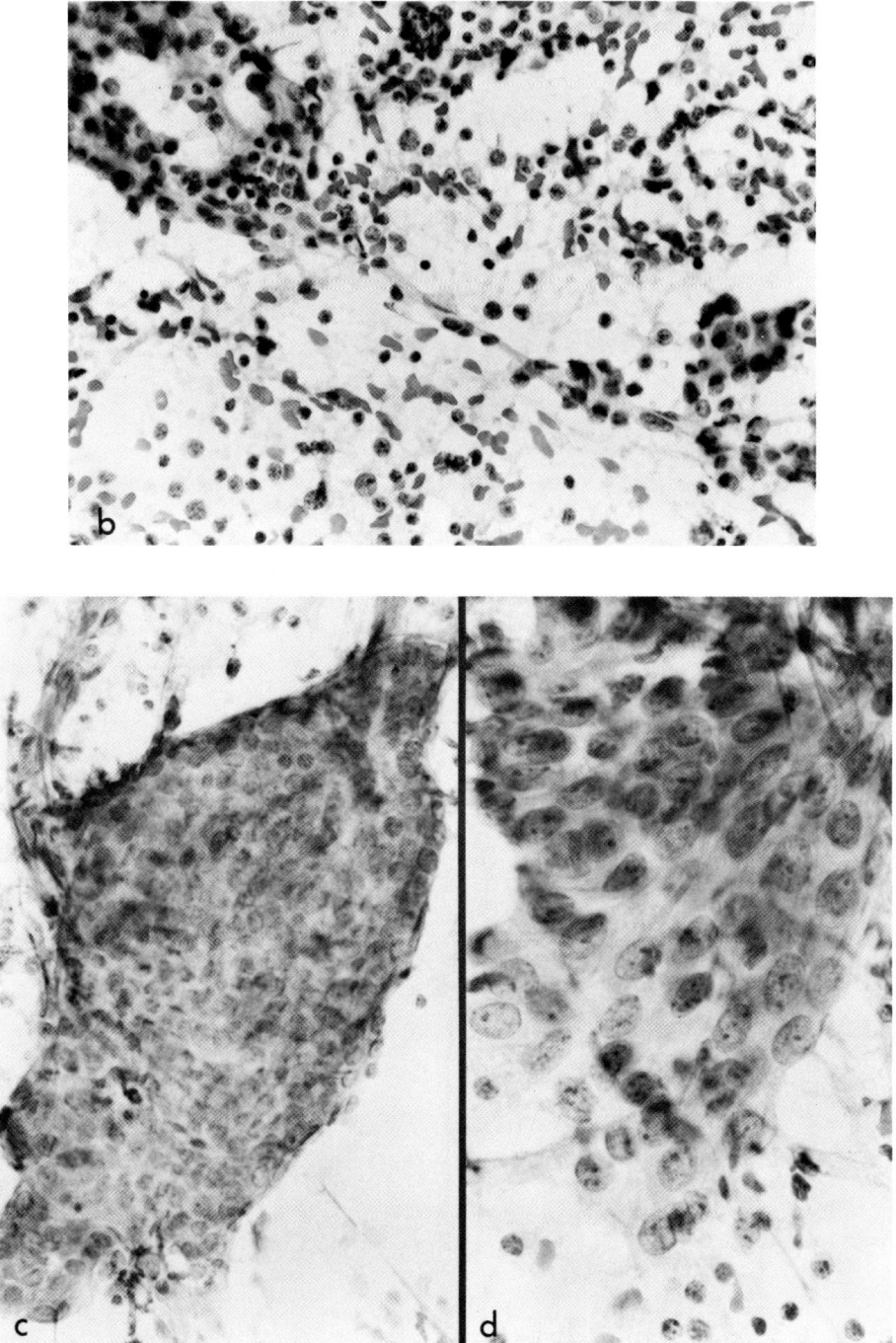

Fig. 15.6. B. Smears from other areas of thyroid showing features of lymphocytic (Hashimoto's) thyroiditis. Papanicolaou preparation. × 630. **C., D.** Aspirate also showed syncytial-type tissue fragments, with typical nuclear morphology of papillary carcinoma. Papanicolaou preparation. × 630.

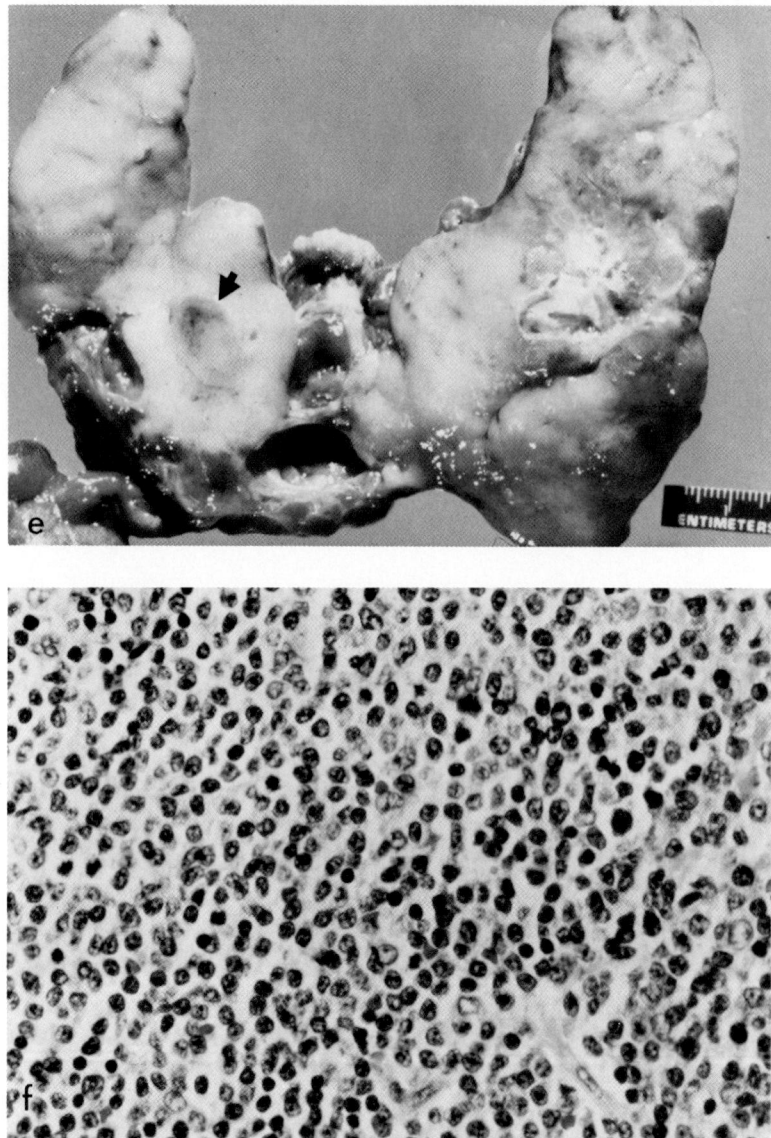

Fig. 15.6. E. Total thyroidectomy revealed both lobes enlarged and replaced by white, fleshy tumor. Note discrete nodule in the right lobe *(arrow)*. **F.** Histologic section confirming malignant lymphoma, diffuse mixed lymphocytic and large cell type. Hematoxylin and eosin preparation. × 400.

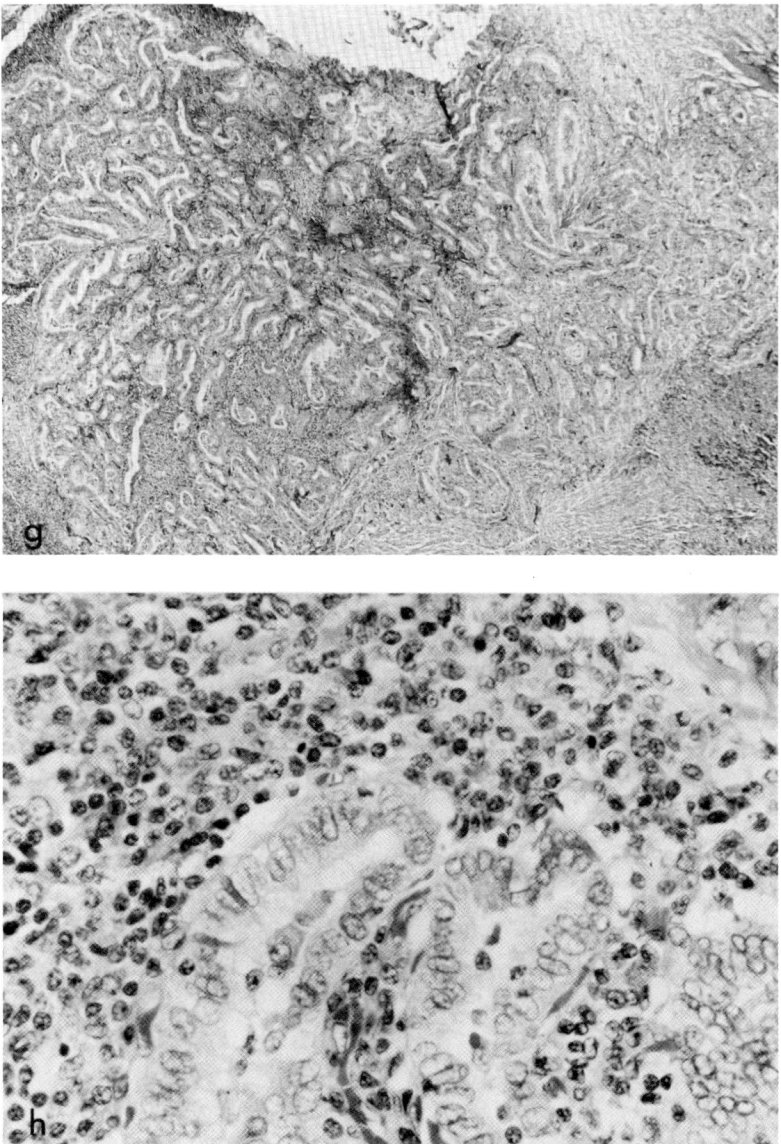

Fig. 15.6. G. Section of the discrete nodule showing a papillary carcinoma. Hematoxylin and eosin preparation. × 63. **H.** Higher magnification of **G** showing lymphoma cells and papillary carcinoma. Hematoxylin and eosin preparation. × 400.

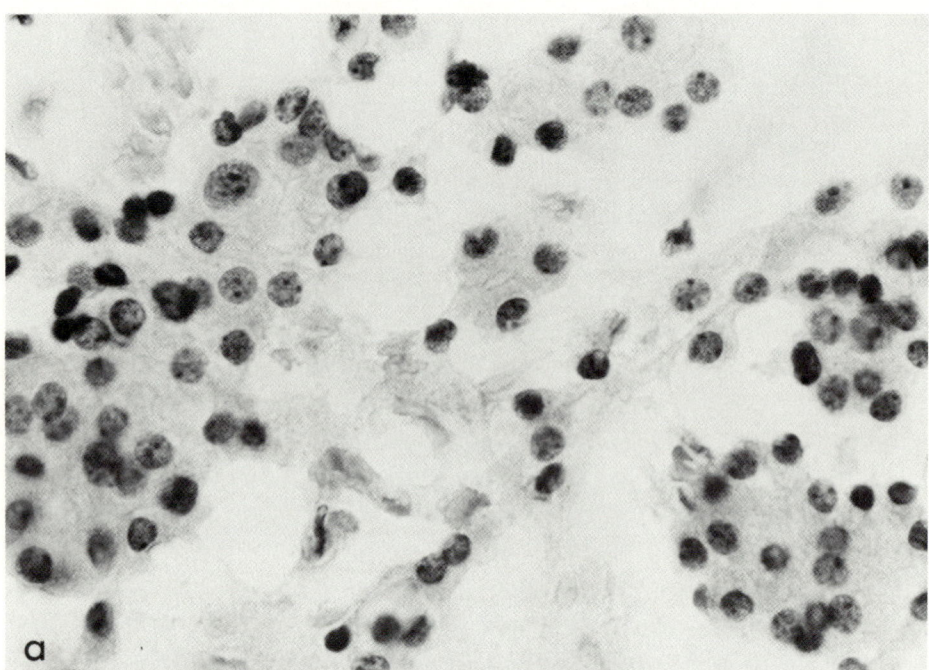

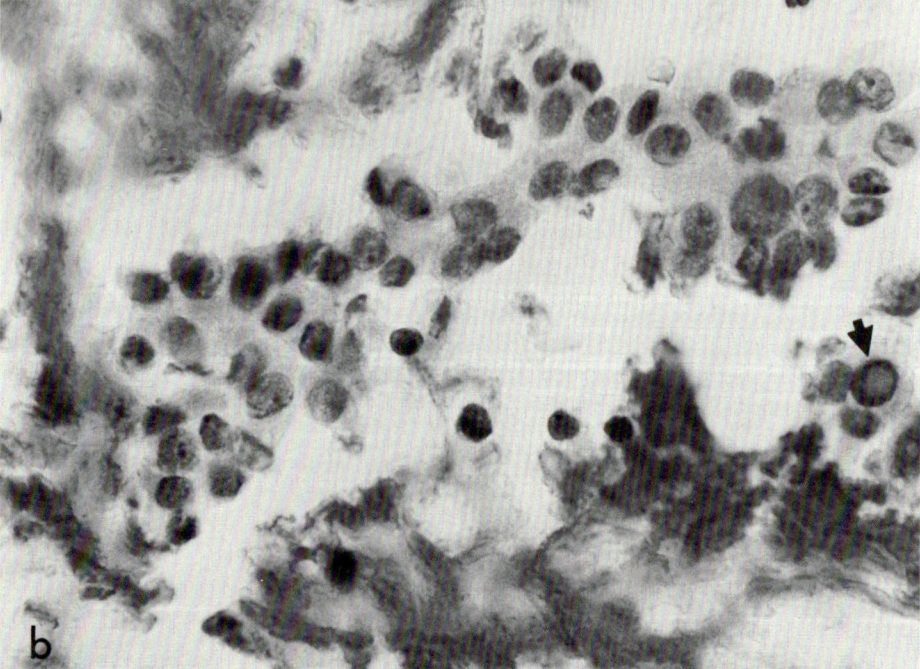

Fig. 15.7. A. Aspirate of a cold nodule showing small Hürthle cells, discrete and in tissue fragments, suggesting a diagnosis of Hürthle cell carcinoma. Papanicolaou preparation. × 630. **B.** Another field from the same smear as in **A** showing syncytial-type tissue fragments, with nuclei exhibiting typical morphology of papillary carcinoma. Note intranuclear cytoplasmic inclusions *(arrow)*. Papanicolaou preparation. × 630. Thyroid-ectomy confirmed both Hürthle cell carcinoma and papillary carcinoma.

THYROID CARCINOMA ARISING IN THYROGLOSSAL DUCT CYST

Thyroglossal duct cysts or fistulas are relatively common congenital anomalies, but a carcinoma arising from such a remnant is a rare entity[30,36,40,58] (Fig. 15.8). Only 95 cases have been reported in the literature, and the incidence is less than 1%. Although they have been described in patients of all ages, they are most often seen in the sixth to eighth decades, and are slightly more common in women. The clinical presentation is similar to that of benign cysts, and the diagnosis of carcinoma is usually made following an excision. Most are of papillary type, although follicular and squamous types have also been reported. Aspiration biopsy is a useful diagnostic technique for establishing a preoperative diagnosis.

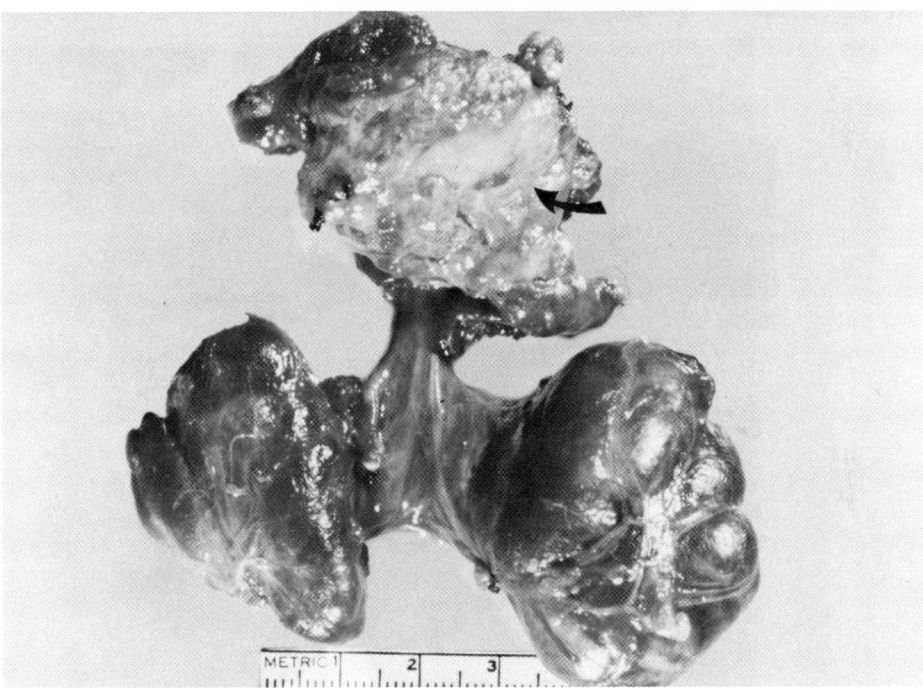

Fig. 15.8. Papillary carcinoma arising in a thyroglossal duct cyst, which was correctly identified from an aspiration biopsy specimen. However, the origin was determined only at the time of surgery.

NONTHYROID MASSES IN THYROID AREA

Lesions in front of the neck or those that move with deglutition are not necessarily thyroidal in origin. Enlarged cervical lymph nodes, soft tissue tumors along the lateral borders of thyroid, lesions of the trachea and larynx, thyroglossal duct cyst, branchial cleft cyst, and parathyroid lesions may all appear clinically to be originating in the thyroid gland. Anterior mediastinal masses extending proximally into the neck may also appear to arise from the thyroid gland. Clinically, radiologically, and even on imaging these lesions may simulate cold thyroid nodules.

Malignant Lymphoma Involving Cervical Lymph Nodes: Hodgkin's and Non-Hodgkin's Type

Because cervical lymph nodes often move with the thyroid, they are sometimes clinically mistaken for part of the thyroid. The same holds true for anterior mediastinal mass that extends into the neck, covering the thyroid. An aspiration biopsy specimen provides an accurate diagnosis in such instances. We have diagnosed five cases of Hodgkin's lymphoma that presented clinically as thyroid masses (Figs. 15.9 and 15.10). One case of poorly differentiated lymphocytic lymphoma arose from the anterior mediastinum, extended in front of the neck, and presented as goiter. It was correctly identified following an aspiration biopsy (Fig. 15.11).

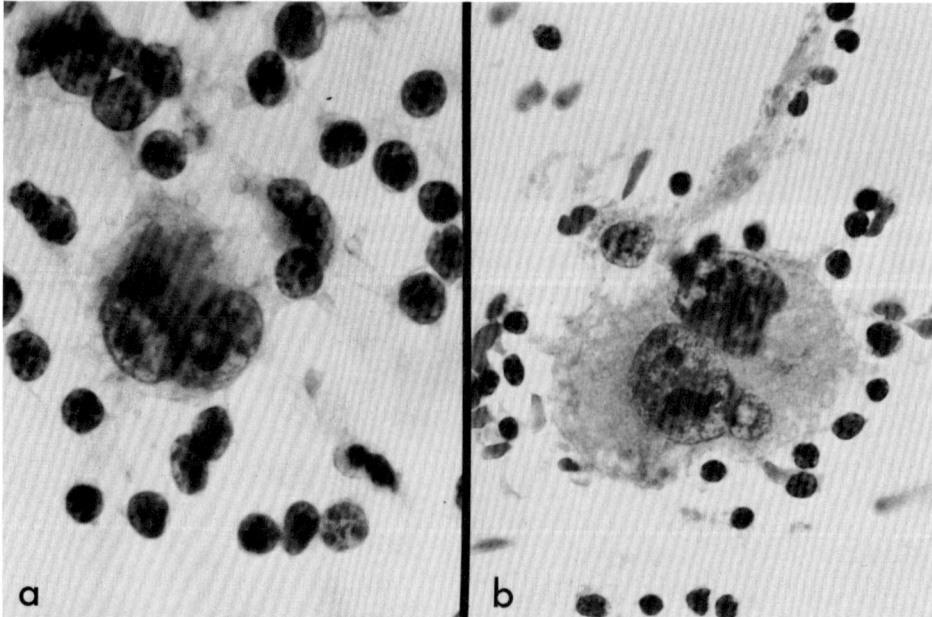

Fig. 15.9. A., B. Typical Reed-Sternberg cells from two cases of Hodgkin's lymphoma of cervical lymph nodes, clinically presented as thyroid nodules. Papanicolaou preparation. × 630.

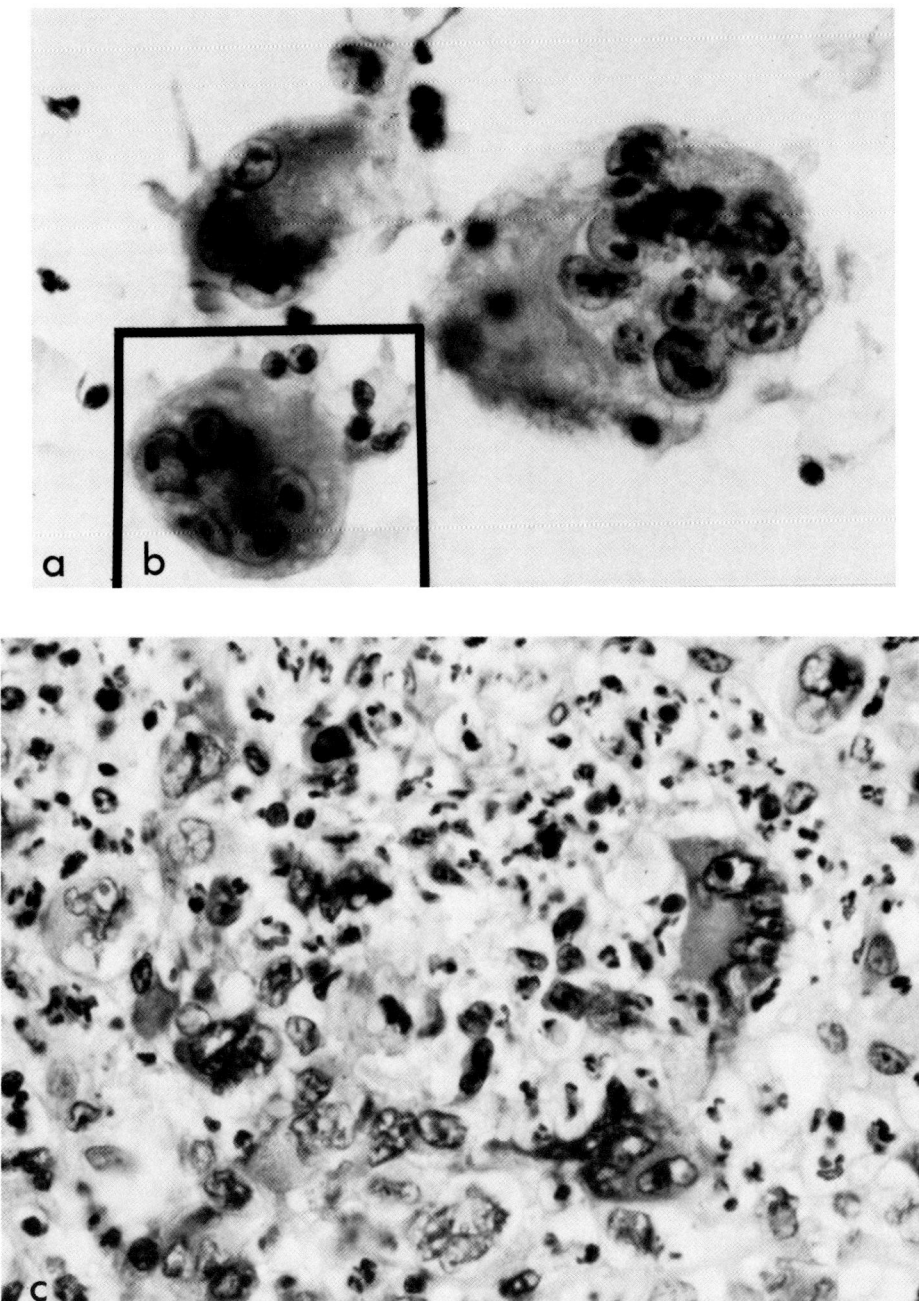

Fig. 15.10. A., B. Bizarre tumor giant cells, from aspirates of cervical lymph node involved by Hodgkin's disease, presenting as thyroid nodule. Papanicolaou preparation. × 630. **C.** Histologic section of the lymph node confirmed Hodgkin's disease. Hematoxylin and eosin preparation. × 630.

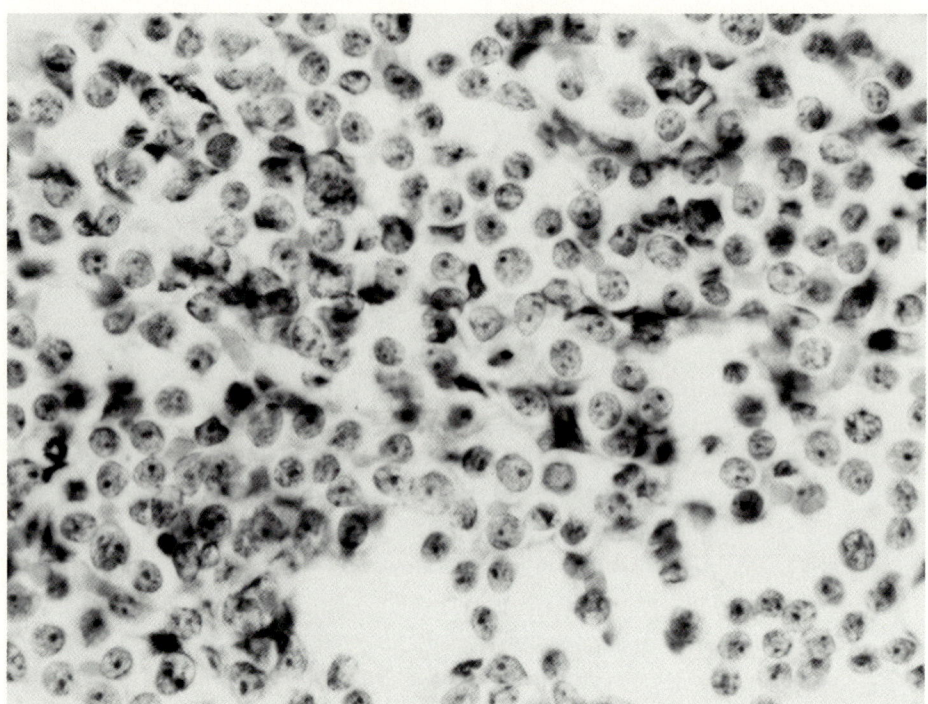

Fig. 15.11. Aspirate of mediastinal malignant lymphoma, poorly differentiated lymphocytic type, extending into the anterior neck and presenting as goiter. Papanicolaou preparation. × 630.

Cartilaginous Tumors of Larynx

Cartilaginous tumors of the larynx[26,56] are unusual lesions, and very few cases are reported in the literature. These are predominantly seen in patients in their fourth to sixth decades, and they are more common in men.

Clinical signs and symptoms are nonspecific and are related to poor voice, hoarseness, or dysphagia. About 25% of these tumors grow outward from the larynx and present as neck masses; they even masquerade as thyroid nodules. These tumors are either chondromas or chondrosarcomas, the latter reported to be more frequent. An aspirate of chondrosarcoma may be an unexpected finding (Fig. 15.12).

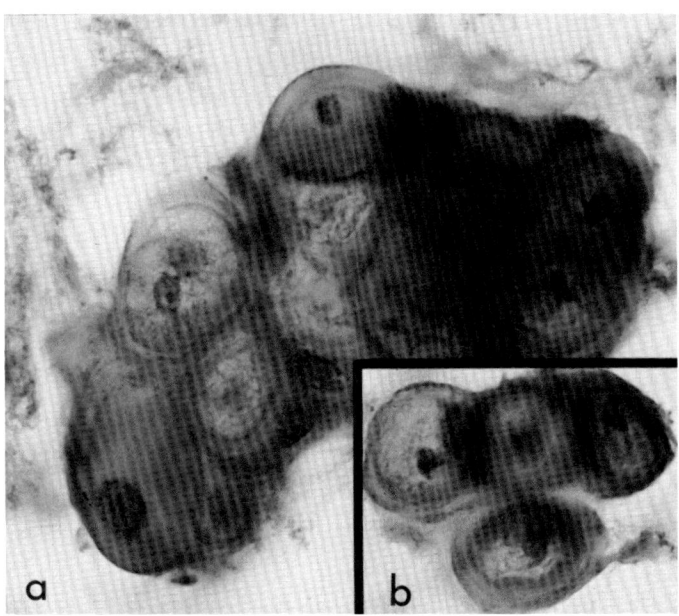

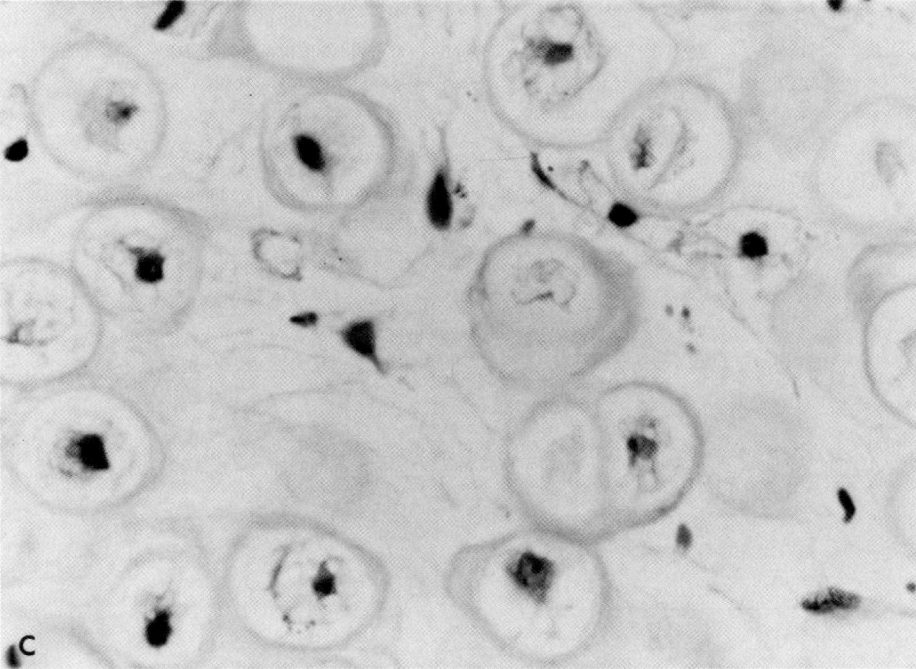

Fig. 15.12.   **A., B.** Aspirate of a "thyroid" nodule showing clusters of markedly enlarged neoplastic chondrocytes containing more than one nuclei. Papanicolaou preparation. × 630. **C.** Large-needle biopsy specimen identified the mass as chondrosarcoma. Hematoxylin and eosin preparation. × 160. A laryngectomy was performed for chondrosarcoma of the cricoid cartilage.

Parathyroid Lesions

Palpable parathyroid lesions may be clinically mistaken for thyroid nodules. Ultrasonography is often performed to identify these lesions, but both false-positive and false-negative results are common. A fine-needle biopsy may be performed to diagnose the lesion. The cytologic features of parathyroid adenoma are sometimes difficult to differentiate from follicular lesions. Friedman et al[17] reported a case of parathyroid adenoma cytologically diagnosed as papillary carcinoma of the thyroid. We have no experience with cytology of parathyroid lesions. Further information can be found in the literature.[10,17,20,46,54]

PAPILLARY CARCINOMA IN LATERAL NECK

Occult papillary thyroid carcinomas may clinically present with cervical node metastasis, and have also been reported to arise in the ectopic thyroid in the neck.[35] However, all papillary carcinomas so identified should not be considered as thyroidal in origin, although the thyroid is a common primary site.[60]

Carcinomas of lung or ovary may clinically manifest as cervical node metastasis (Fig. 15.13). Their cytologic and histologic pattern can be identical to that of papillary carcinoma of thyroid, especially if the follicular component with colloid is lacking. Imaging of thyroid may not identify the small occult cancer. In such instances, unnecessary thyroidectomies have been performed when the primary site was presumed to be thyroid. Immunoperoxidase stain for thyroglobulin will help identify the primary site as thyroid.

INFARCTION OR NECROSIS OF THYROID NODULES AFTER ASPIRATION BIOPSY

Necrosis along the needle track is not unusual following a cutting needle biopsy with Vim-Silvermann® or Tru-Cut® needles, whereas fine-gauged needles used for aspiration biopsy procedures are not generally traumatic and rarely induce necrosis. Jones et al[29] reported two cases of necrosis of thyroid nodules after fine-needle aspiration, one of which showed extensive necrosis and shrinkage of the tumor. Bauman and Strawbridge[4] reported one case of Hürthle cell tumor, diagnosed cytologically, which disappeared 5 weeks after diagnosis, and without treatment. It may be presumed that the tumor underwent infarction with subsequent involution. Such phenomena are rarely described in the literature. Davies and Webb,[14] however, reported a case of segmented infarction of the lymph node after fine-needle biopsy. They suggested that possible venous thrombosis after the biopsy procedure was the cause of infarction.

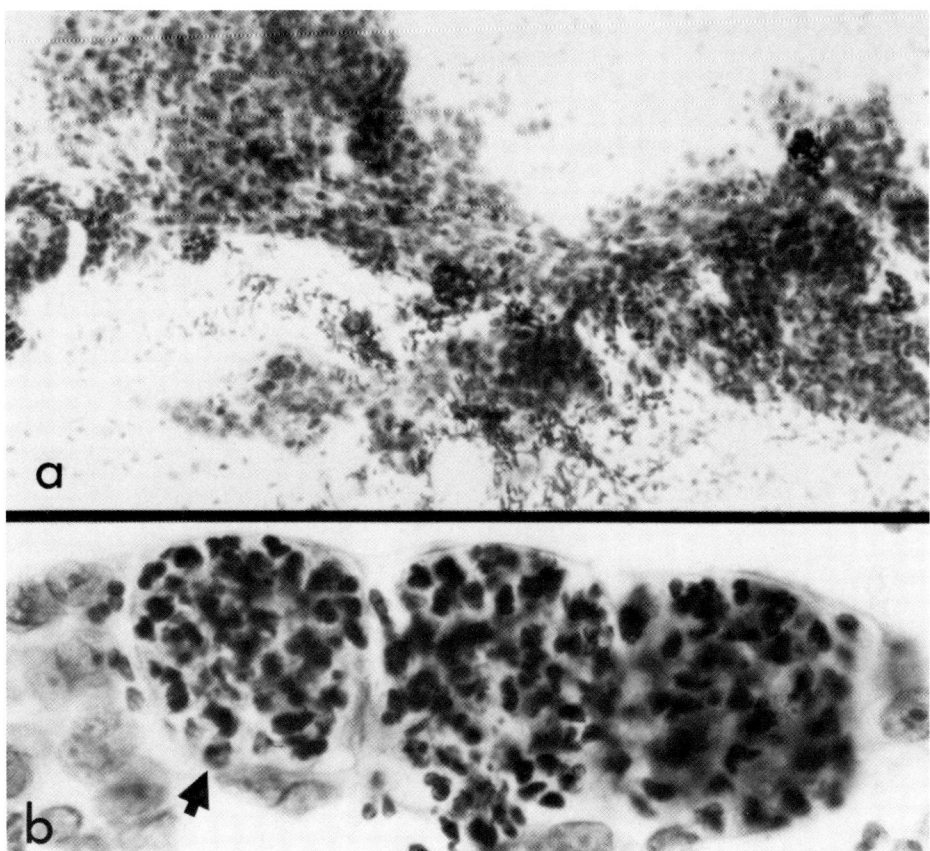

Fig. 15.13. **A.** Aspiration biopsy specimen of a lateral neck mass in a 67-year-old woman with a history of ovarian adenocarcinoma, showing large branching papillary tissue fragments. Papanicolaou preparation. × 63. **B.** Higher magnification of **A** showing secretory vacuoles in the cytoplasm filled with neutrophils *(arrow)*. This suggested a mucin-producing carcinoma, not originating in thyroid. Papanicolaou preparation. × 630.

We have seen 16 cases of near total infarction of neoplasm after aspiration biopsy procedures. For an unknown reason, this phenomenon was observed commonly in Hürthle cell tumors (12 of 16). The remaining four cases were papillary carcinomas.

In all cases, the neoplasm was present as a thin rim along the capsule. It was difficult to recognize without prior knowledge of the cytologic finding. Aspiration biopsy specimens in all these cases were cellular and characteristic of the lesions (Figs. 15.14 and 15.15).

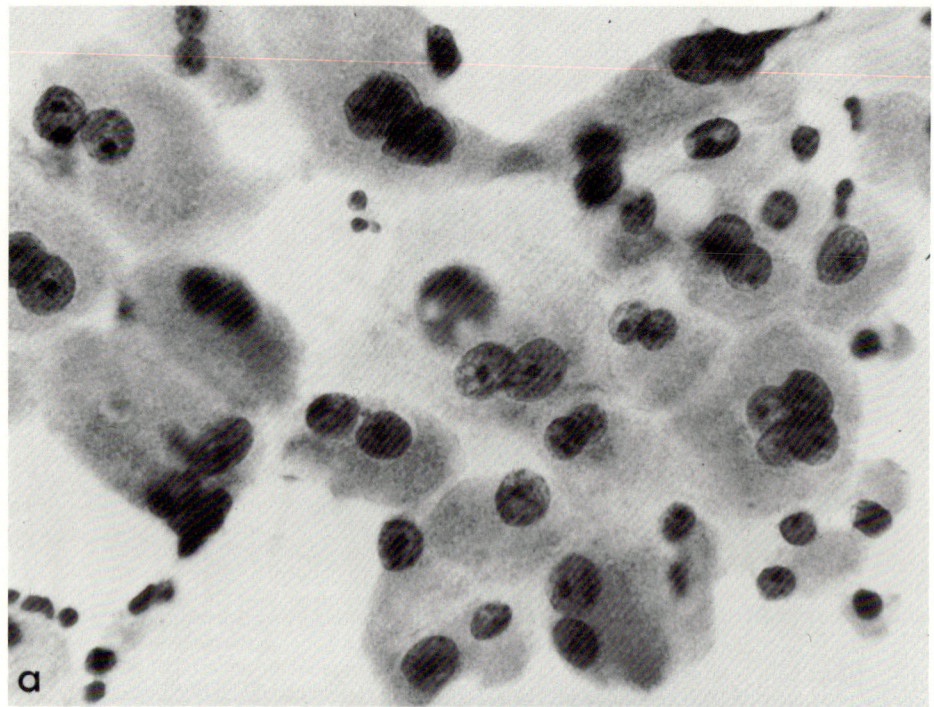

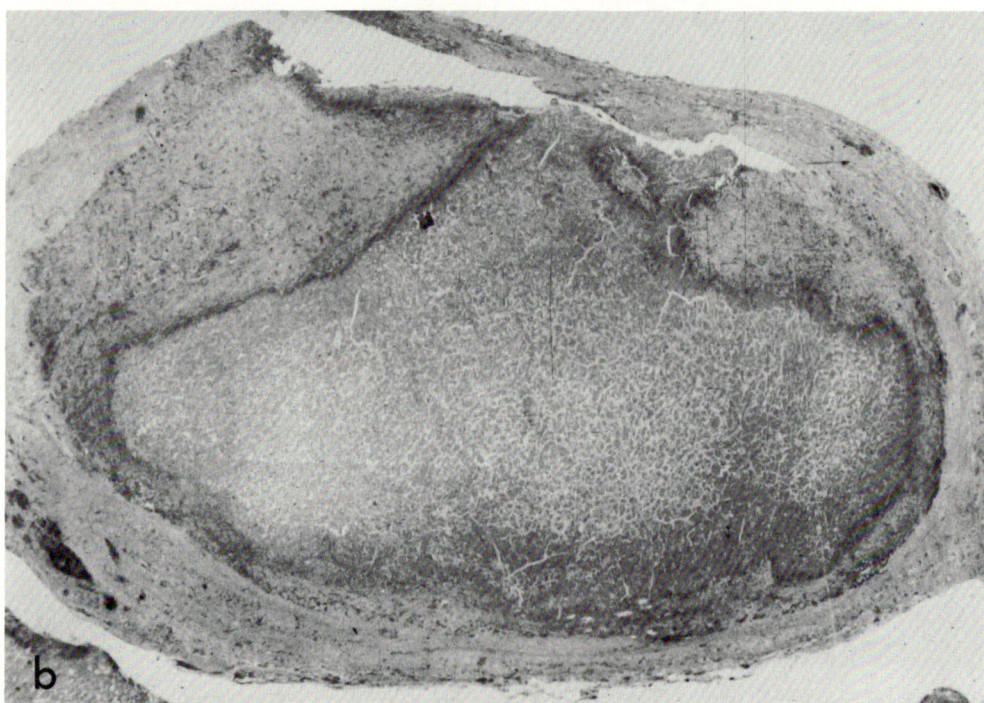

Fig. 15.14. A. This aspirate, characteristic of Hürthle cell neoplasm, shows large discrete Hürthle cells with eccentric nuclei and prominent macronucleoli. Papanicolaou preparation. × 630. **B.** A total thyroidectomy was performed. The 1.5-cm nodule showing only a thin rim Hematoxylin and eosin preparation. × 2.2.

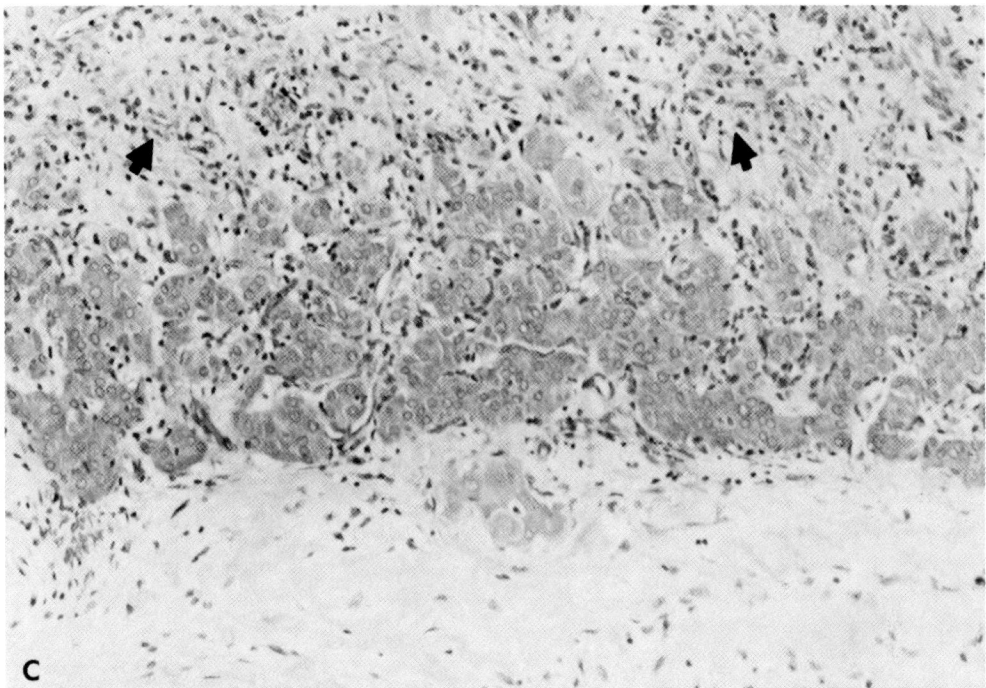

Fig. 15.14. C. Section of the nodule showing only a thin rim of Hürthle cells at the periphery bordering granulation tissue *(arrows)* around the infarcted tumor. Hematoxylin and eosin prepartion. × 160.

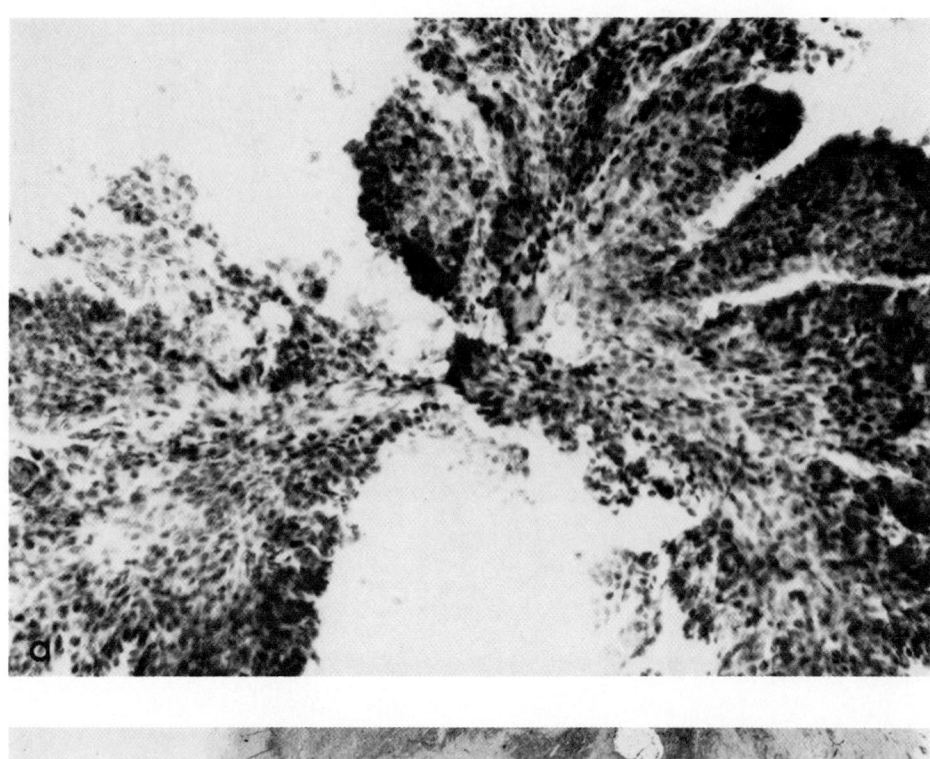

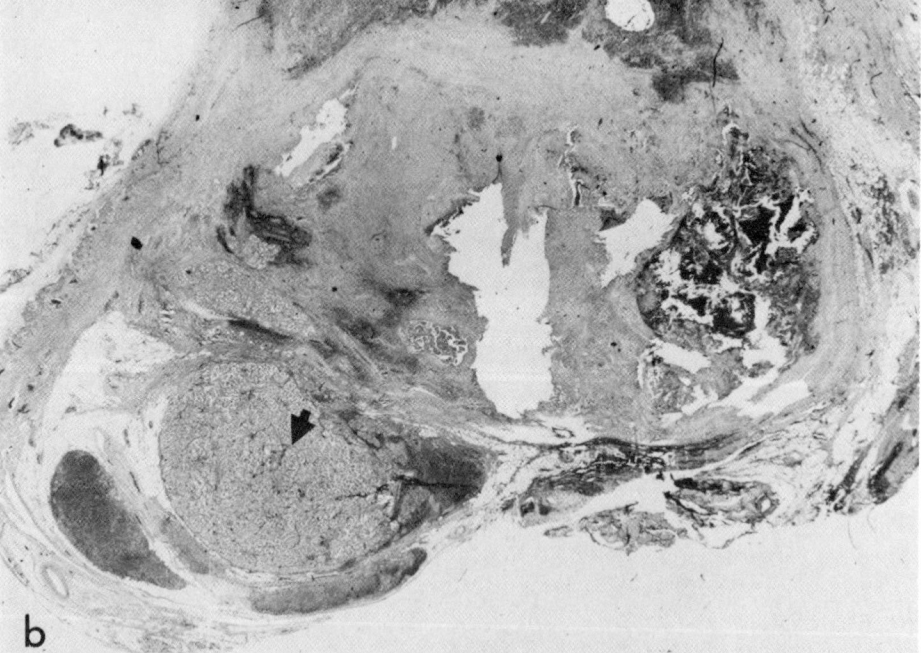

Fig. 15.15. A. Aspirate presenting the characteristic cytopathologic pattern of papillary carcinoma. Papanicolaou preparation. × 160. **B.** Total thyroidectomy showed almost totally infarcted hemorrhagic nodule, with viable tumor extending beyond the capsule *(arrow)*. Hematoxylin and eosin preparation. × 1.7.

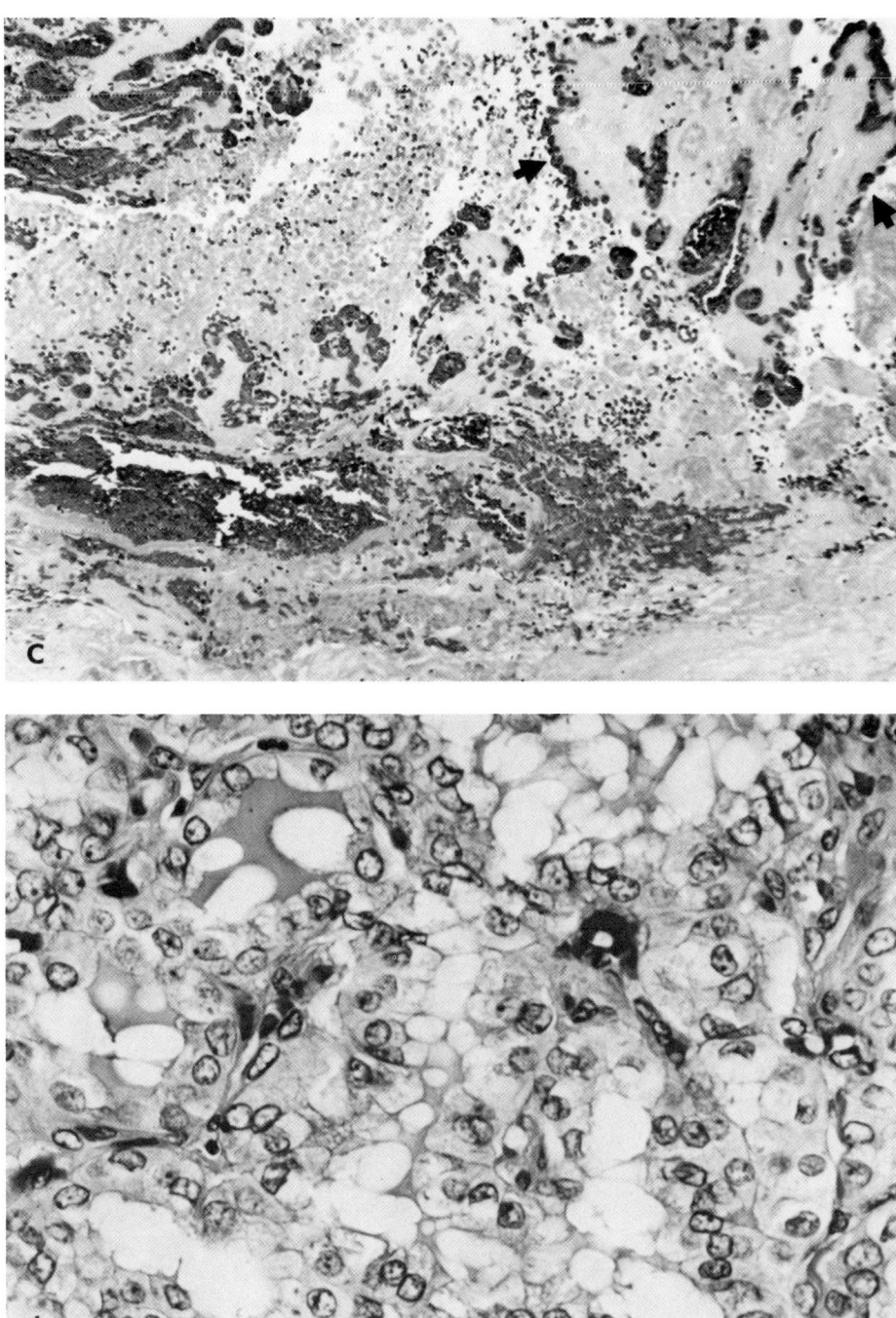

Fig. 15.15. C. Section of hemorrhagic nodule showing ghost appearance of papillary fronds *(arrow)*. Hematoxylin and eosin preparation. × 160. D. Section of tumor beyond the capsule, showing follicular variant of papillary carcinoma. Hematoxylin and eosin preparation. × 400.

COLD THYROID NODULES IN
CHILDREN AND ADOLESCENTS

Solitary cold nodules of thyroid are infrequent in the pediatric and adolescent age groups.[32] Rallison et al[45] reported 93 nodules in 5179 children aged 11–15 years, an incidence of 1.8%. This incidence could be higher if the age group is extended to 21 years.[11]

The management of the cold nodules in children is a subject of controversy. The incidence of cancer in solitary nodules in this age group is reported anywhere from 14.3% to 73%.[12,23,25,43,53,57,64] As in adults, clinical evaluation, laboratory data, or imaging techniques are not very helpful in differentiating non-neoplastic from neoplastic, and benign from malignant, nodules. Some authors suggest surgical removal of all solitary nodules, whereas Fisher[16] recommends a somewhat conservative approach, based on clinical, laboratory, and imaging data. Fine-needle biopsy, although a very useful, indispensable technique in the evaluation of cold nodules in adults, is not routinely used in pediatric patients. Large-needle biopsy has been used by some with success.[61]

Our experience with 175 children and adolescents, aged 9–21 years, with cold nodules indicated that fine-needle biopsy is as useful in this age group as it is in adults. Table 15.1 presents the different cytologic diagnoses. Nonsurgical diseases, such as nodular goiter or Hashimoto's thyroiditis, are readily identified by aspiration biopsy specimen. Table 15.2 lists the cytohistologic correlation of 69 patients who underwent surgery.

The incidence of neoplasm was 36% and that of malignancy was 25%. Papillary carcinomas were the most common malignant neoplasm. Of 45 papillary carcinomas, 18 (40%) were associated with lymphocytic thyroiditis (Hashimoto's disease) (see Chapter 11, Thyroiditis, for a discussion of the association between the two diseases). Mauras et al[37] recently reported three cases of papillary carcinoma with Hashimoto's disease in the pediatric age group.

TABLE 15.1. Cytologic Diagnoses of 175 Patients, Aged 9–21 Years, with Cold Nodules

Nodular goiter	64
Lymphocytic thyroiditis	21
Cellular follicular adenoma	14
Hürthle cell tumor	5
Papillary carcinoma	45
Suspected papillary carcinoma	2
Medullary carcinoma	1
Follicular carcinoma	1
Abcess	1
Unsatisfactory	21
Total	175

TABLE 15.2. Cytohistologic Correlation of 69 Patients with Cold Nodules

Cytologic Diagnosis	No. of Patients	Histologic Diagnosis					
		Nodular Goiter	Follicular Adenoma	Follicular Carcinoma	Hürthle Tumor	Papillary Carcinoma	Medullary Carcinoma of Thyroid
Nodular goiter	1	1					
Cellular adenoma	14		12	1		1	
Hürthle cell tumor	5				5		
Suspected papillary carcinoma	2	1				1	
Papillary carcinoma	45				1	44	
Follicular carcinoma	1	1					
Medullary carcinoma	1						1
Total	69						

CYTOPATHOLOGY OF METASTATIC THYROID CARCINOMA

The incidence of metastasis of thyroid carcinoma to different body sites varies among different types. Metastasis to distant body sites, such as lungs and bone, is more common in follicular, Hürthle cell, medullary, and anaplastic carcinomas.[2,7,9,24,28,62] Although lymph node involvement is more common in papillary and medullary carcinomas, these also metastasize to lung pleurae, bones, and liver.[9,24,27,28,48,49,62,65] Initial presentation of thyroid carcinomas, occult or otherwise, is infrequent at a distant site, and only a few cases have been reported.[7,49,55,65] Cytopathologic recognition of metastatic thyroid carcinomas is not always easy. Diagnostic difficulties may be encountered when (1) the thyroid cancer presents initially at a metastatic site; or (2) a primary thyroid carcinoma has been removed several years prior, and malignancy of an organ other than thyroid is also being considered.

Cytopathologic features characteristic of any particular type of thyroid carcinoma may not be very evident, especially when the metastatic carcinoma is poorly differentiated or undifferentiated (Figs. 15.16 and 15.17). Also, Albores-Saaveedra et al[1] reported weakly positive reaction to thyroglobulin in 10 of 14 cases of anaplastic thyroid carcinomas, and negative reaction in the remaining 4 cases.

Metastatic papillary thyroid carcinomas can be recognized only if a follicular component is present. This is easier histologically than cytologically. The presence of psammoma bodies is not pathognomonic of thyroid carcinomas alone, but is characteristic of papillary carcinomas in general. Cytologic diagnosis of papillary carcinoma in specimens from the respiratory tract, such as specimens from aspiration biopsies or endoscopic brushing and washings, must be differentiated from bronchiolo–alveolar carcinoma using immunocytochemistry or ultrastructural studies.[52]

Up to 19.7% of thyroid papillary carcinomas present with cervical lymph node metastasis.[9] Cystic degeneration is very frequent, and its identification is difficult due to degeneration and necrosis (Fig. 15.18).

Some difficulty is experienced in recognizing malignancy as thyroidal in origin from cells exfoliated in body cavity fluid. The fluid medium initiates regressive changes and marked cytoplasmic vacuolization, with considerable variation from usual cytopathologic patterns (Figs. 15.17 and 15.19).

Follicular or Hürthle cell carcinomas metastasize frequently to bone. A well-differentiated follicular carcinoma is easily recognized (Fig. 15.20). Hürthle cell carcinomas may be difficult to differentiate morphologically from liver cell carcinomas or malignant melanoma (Fig. 15.21). Medullary carcinomas, however, present the least diagnostic difficulties due to their characteristic cytologic presentation (Fig. 15.22).

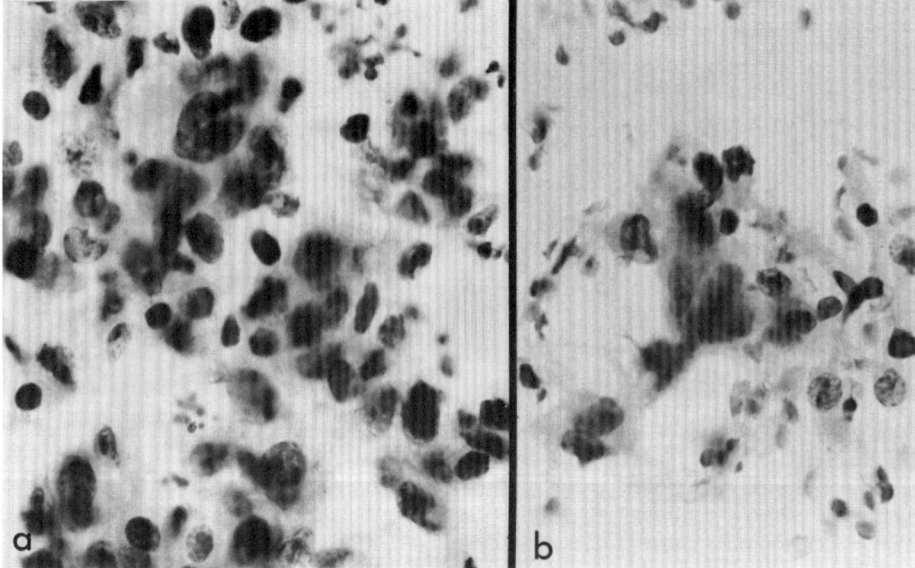

Fig. 15.16. A., B. Anaplastic carcinoma metastaatic to pleura. Carcinoma cells in pleural fluid show marked degenerative changes. Identification of these cells as primary thyroidal carcinoma is not possible. Papanicolaou preparation. × 630.

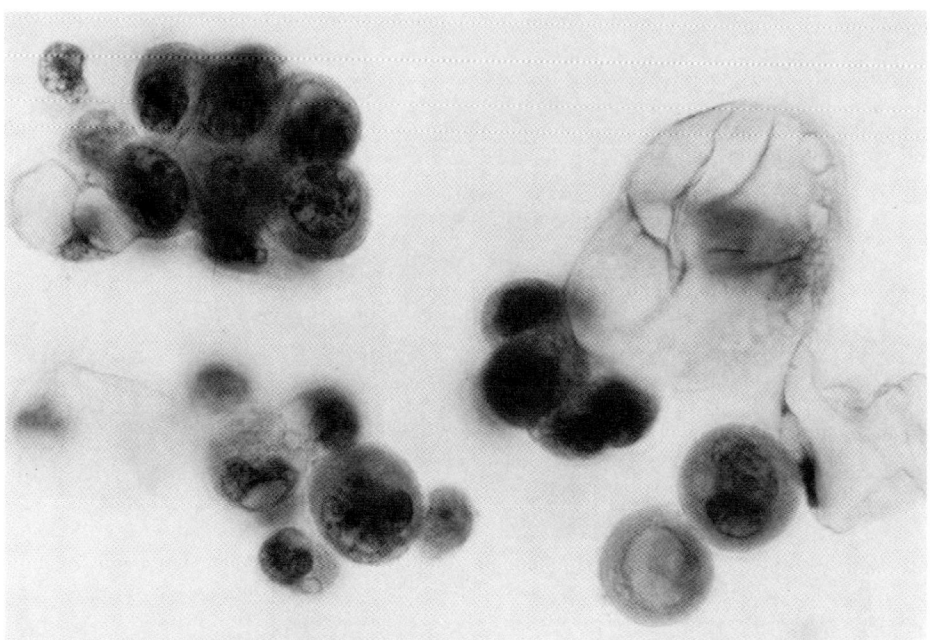

Fig. 15.17. Anaplastic giant cell carcinoma, metastatic to pleura. Carcinoma cells in pleural fluid have bizarre nuclei and marked cytoplasmic vacuolization resembling mucin-producing adenocarcinoma. Papanicolaou preparation. × 630.

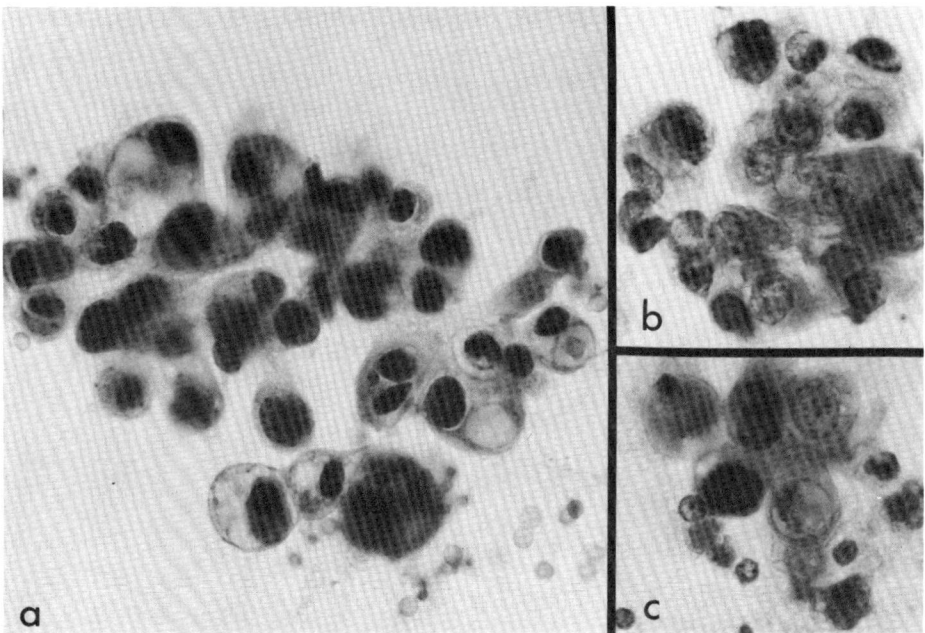

Fig. 15.18. A–C. Aspiration biopsy specimens from three cases of cystic papillary carcinoma in neck. Note regressive changes in nuclei and cytoplasm. Without sufficient criteria, papillary carcinoma is difficult to identify. Papanicolaou preparation. × 630.

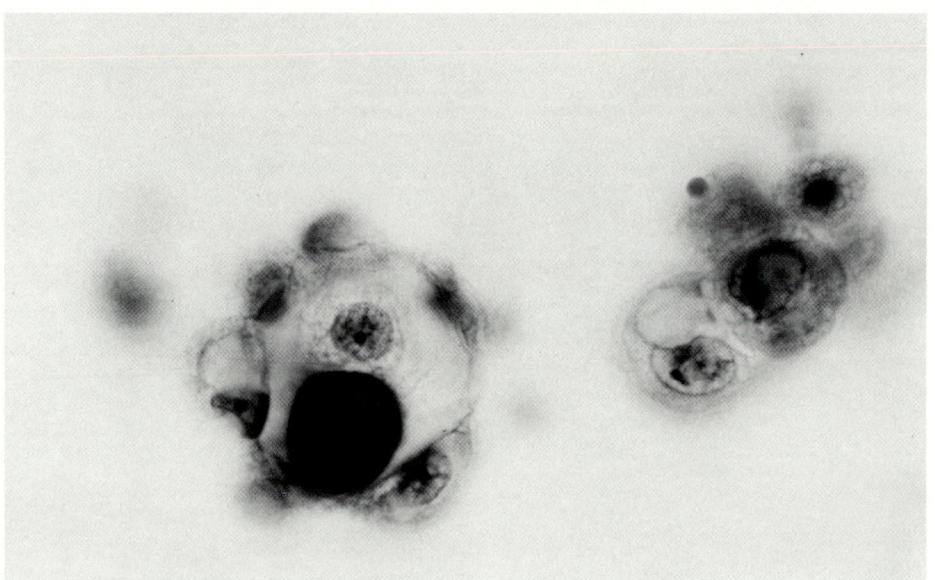

Fig. 15.19. Metastatic papillary carcinoma in pleural fluid from a patient with a history of thyroid carcinoma. Note psammoma body, marked cytoplasmic vacuolization, and intranuclear cytoplasmic inclusion. Cells did not demonstrate thyroglobulin by immunoperoxidase staining technique. Papanicolaou preparation. × 630.

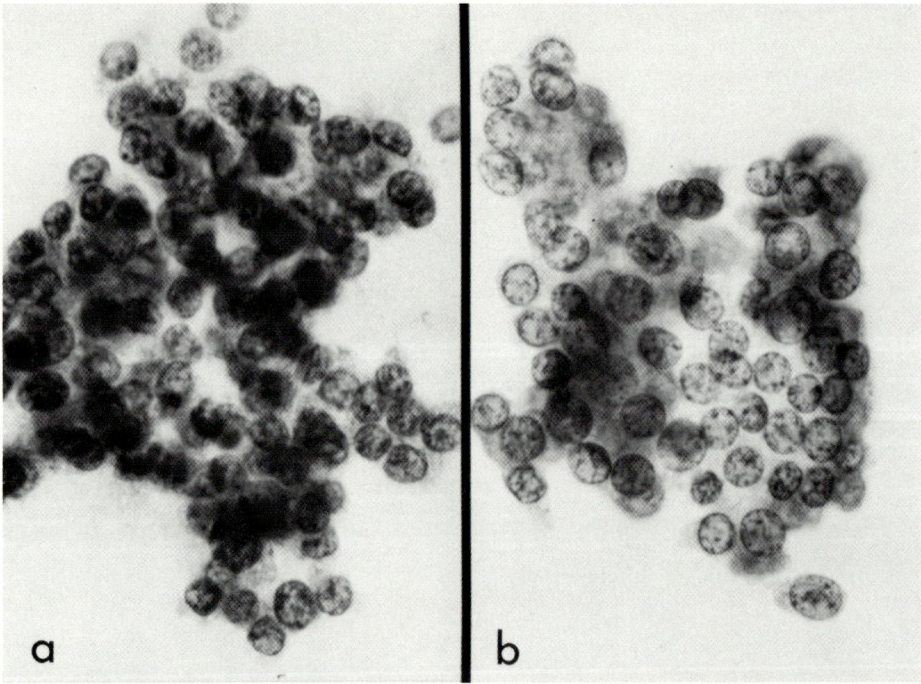

Fig. 15.20. Follicular carcinoma presenting as a pulsatile mass involving the sternum, in a 69-year-old woman. **A.** Imprint of the sternal mass showing syncytial type tissue fragment of follicular cells with enlarged crowded nuclei. Papanicolaou preparation. × 630. **B.** Aspiration biopsy specimen of thyroid nodule showing cells similar to those seen in **A.** Papanicolaou preparation. × 630.

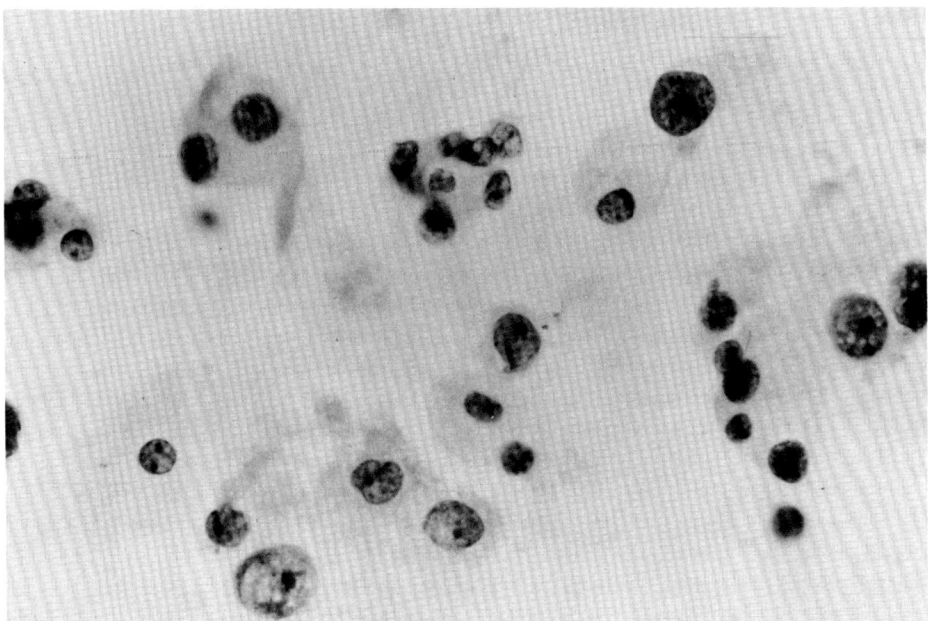

Fig. 15.21. Hürthle cell carcinoma presenting as lytic lesion of the vertebra and paraspinal mass. The carcinoma cells are mostly discrete and large, and some are in tissue fragments. The nuclei are pleomorphic and still contain macronucleoli. Morphology resembles that of malignant melanoma or liver cell carcinoma. Papanicolaou preparation. × 630.

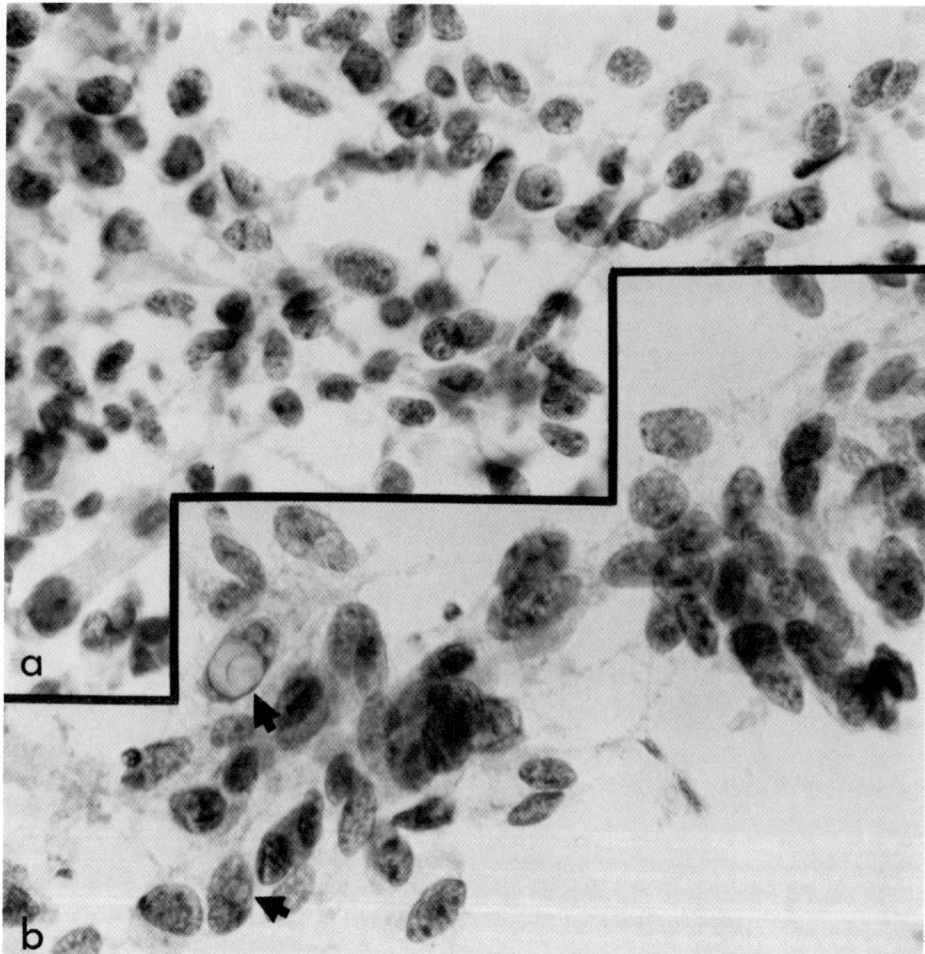

Fig. 15.22. A. Metastatic medullary thyroid carcinoma to cervical lymph node. Cervical lymphadenopathy was the initial presentation in this case. Papanicolaou preparation. × 630. **B.** Metastatic medullary thyroid carcinoma to mediastinal lymph nodes, several years after thyroidectomy in a 50-year-old man. Papanicolaou preparation. × 630. The cytomorphology in both **A** and **B** is very characteristic of medullary carcinoma. Note intranuclear cytoplasmic inclusions in **B** *(arrow)*.

REFERENCES

1. Albores-Saaveedra J, Nadji M, Civantos F, Morales AR: Thyroglobulin in carcinoma of the thyroid: an immunohistochemical study. *Hum Pathol* 14:62–66, 1983.

2. Aldinger KA, Samaan NA, Ibanez M, Hil-Stratton C Jr: Anaplastic carcinoma of the thyroid: a review of 84 cases of spindle and giant cell carcinoma of the thyroid. *Cancer* 41:2267–2275, 1978.

3. Ayala A, Sloane J, Woling FJ Jr: Coexistent lymphoma, adenocarcinoma, and struma lymphomatosa. *JAMA* 204:829–831, 1968.

4. Bauman A, Strawbridge HTG: Spontaneous disappearance of an atypical Hürthle cell adenoma. *Am J Clin Pathol* 80:399–402, 1983.

5. Berger SA, Zonszein J, Villamena P, Mittman N: Infectious diseases of the thyroid gland. *Rev Infect Dis* 5:108–122, 1983.

6. Block MA, Brush BE, Horn RC: The incidental carcinoma found in surgery for thyroid nodules. *AMA Archives Surg* 80:715–719, 1960.

7. Brodner RA, Berman AJ, Wisniewski M, Nakagawa H: Thyroid carcinoma presenting as epidural metastasis with spinal cord compression. *Mt Sinai J Med* 42:307–315, 1975.

8. Carcangiu ML, Steeper T, Zampi G, Rosai J: Anaplastic thyroid carcinoma. *Am J Clin Pathol* 83:135–158, 1985.

9. Carcangiu ML, Zampi G, Pupi A, Castagnoli A, Rosai J: Papillary carcinoma of the thyroid: a clinicopathologic study of 241 cases treated at the University of Florence, Italy. *Cancer* 55:805–828, 1985.

10. Clark OH, Grouding GAW, Ljung BM: Locating a parathyroid adenoma by ultrasonography and aspiration biopsy cytology. *West J Med* 135:154–158, 1981.

11. Committee on Adolescence, On the Terminology of Adolescent/Adolescence, 1977–1978, American Academy of Pediatrics. *Pediatrics* 62:838, 1978.

12. Crile G Jr: Carcinoma of the thyroid in children. *Am Surg* 150:959, 1959.

13. Dailey MZ, Lindsay S, Miller ER: Histologic lesions in the thyroid glands of patients receiving radioiodine for hyperthyroidism. *J Clin Endocrinol Metab* 13:1513–1529, 1953.

14. Davies JD, Webb AJ: Segmented lymph node infarction after fine needle aspiration. *J Clin Pathol* 35:855–857, 1982.

15. Droese M: *Cytological Aspiration Biopsy of the Thyroid Gland.* Stuttgart, Schattauer Verlag, 1980, pp. 55–62.

16. Fisher DA: Thyroid nodules in childhood and their management. *J Pediatr* 89:866–868, 1976.

17. Friedman M, Shimaoka K, Lopez C, Shedd D: Parathyroid adenoma diagnosed as papillary carcinoma of thyroid on needle aspiration smears. *Acta Cytol* 27:337–340, 1983.

18. Gay JD, Bjornsson J, Goellnner JR: Hematopoietic cells in thyroid fine needle aspirates for cytologic study: report of two cases. *Mayo Clin Proc* 60:123–124, 1985.

19. Gold RL: Primary squamous cell carcinoma of the thyroid gland: report of a case and review of the literature. *Am Surg* 30:247–252, 1964.

20. Grouding GAW, Clark OH, Stark D, Moss A, Montgomery C: Parathyroid aspiration biopsy under ultrasound guidance in the post-operative hyper-parathyroid patient. *Radiology* 155:193–196, 1985.

21. Halazun JF, Lukens JN: Thyrotoxicosis associated with aspergillus thyroiditis in chronic granulomatous disease. *J Pediatr* 80:106–108, 1971.

22. Harach RH, Day ES, Franssila RO: Thyroid spindle-cell tumor with mucous cysts: an intrathyroid thymoma? *Am J Surg Pathol* 9:525–530, 1985.

23. Hayles AB, Johnson ML, Beahrs OH, Woolner LB: Carcinoma of the thyroid in children. *Am J Surg* 106:735–743, 1965.

24. Heitz P, Moser H, Staub JJ: Thyroid cancer: a study of 573 thyroid tumors and 161 autopsy cases observed over a thirty-year period. *Cancer* 37:2329–2337, 1976.

25. Hung W, August GP, Randolph JG, Schisgall R, Chanchei R: Solitary thyroid nodules in children and adolescents. *J Pediatr Surg* 17:225–229, 1982.

26. Hyams VJ, Rabuzzi DD: Cartilaginous tumors of the larynx. *Laryngoscope* 80:755–767, 1970.

27. Hyman MP: Papillary and undifferentiated thyroid carcinoma presenting as a metastatic papillary serous effusion: a case report. *Acta Cytol* 23:483–486, 1979.

28. Ibanez ML: *Medullary carcinoma of the thyroid gland.* In Summers SC: *Pathology Annual*, vol. 9. New York, Appleton-Century-Crofts, 1974, pp. 263–290.

29. Jones JD, Pittman DL, Sanders LR: Necrosis of thyroid nodules after fine needle aspiration. *Acta Cytol* 29:29–32, 1985.

30. Joseph TJ, Komorowski RA: Thyroglossal duct carcinoma. *Hum Pathol* 6:717–728, 1975.

31. Kampsen EB, Jages N, Man MH: Squamous cell carcinoma of the thyroid: a report of two cases. *J Surg Oncol* 9:567–578, 1977.

32. Kirkland RT, Kirkland JL, Rosenberg HS, et al: Solitary thyroid nodules in 30 children and reports of a child with a thyroid abscess. *Pediatrics* 51:85–90, 1973.

33. Lamberg BA, Reissel P, Steman S, et al: Concurrent medullary and papillary thyroid carcinoma in the same thyroid lobe and in siblings. *Acta Med Scand* 209:421–424, 1981.

34. LiVolsi VA, Merino MJ: Squamous cells in the human thyroid gland. *Am J Surg Pathol* 2:133–140, 1978.

35. LiVolsi VA, Perzin KH, Savetsky L: Carcinoma arising in median ectopic thyroid. *Cancer* 34:1303–1315, 1974.

36. Lui AHF, Littler ER: Thyroid carcinoma originating in thyroglossal cyst: report of a case. *Am Surg* 36:546–548, 1970.

37. Mauras N, Zimmerman D, Goellner JR: Hashimoto's thyroiditis associated with thyroid cancer in adolescent patients. *J Pediatr* 106:895–899, 1985.

38. Meissner WA, Warren S: *Tumors of the Thyroid Gland.* Fascicle 4, Second Series, *Atlas of Tumor Pathology.* Washington, DC, Armed Forces Institute of Pathology, 1985, p. 111.

39. Miyavhi A, Kuma K, Matskzuka F, et al: Intrathyroidal epithelial thymoma: an entity distinct for squamous cell carcinoma of the thyroid. *World J Surg* 9:128–135, 1985.

40. Mobini J, Krouse TB, Klinghoffer JF: Squamous cell carcinoma arising in a thyroglossal duct cyst. *Am Surg* 40:290, 1974.

41. Motoyama T, Watanabe H: Simultaneous squamous cell carcinoma and papillary adenocarcinoma of the thyroid gland. *Hum Pathol* 14:1009–1010, 1983.

42. Murphy E, Zervantes C: Atypical changes in thyroid follicular cells secondary to radioiodine. *Am J Roentgenol* 109:724–728, 1970.

43. Nishiyama RH, Schmidt RW, Batsakis JG: Carcinoma of the thyroid gland in children and adolescents. *JAMA* 181:1036–1038, 1962.

44. O'Neill ME, Lomas FE: Medullary and papillary thyroid carcinoma. *Med J Aust* 140:747, 1984.

45. Rallison ML, Dobyns EM, Keating FR, Rall JE, Tyler FH: Thyroid nodularity in children. *JAMA* 233:1069–1072, 1975.

46. Rastad J, Johonson H, Lindgren PG, et al: Ultrasonic localization and cytologic identification of parathyroid tumors. *World J Surg* 8:501–508, 1984.

47. Rosai J: Invited commentary on intrathyroidal epithelial thymoma. *World J Surg* 9:134–135, 1985.

48. Rosai J, Zampi G, Carcangiu ML: Papillary carcinoma of the thyroid: a discussion of its several morphologic repressions with particular emphasis on the follicular variant. *Am J Surg Pathol* 7:809–817, 1983.

49. Sampson R, Olea H, Kay CR, Buncher CR, Iidima S: Metastasis from occult thyroid carcinoma: an autopsy study from Hiroshima and Nagasaki, Japan. *Cancer* 25:803–811, 1970.

50. Segal K, Sidl J, Abraham A, Konichezky M, Bessat M: Pure squamous carcinoma and mixed adenosquamous cell carcinoma of the thyroid gland. *Head Neck Surg* 6:1035–1042, 1984.

51. Shimaoka K, Tsukade Y: Squamous cell carcinoma and adenosquamous carcinomas originating from the thyroid gland. *Cancer* 46:1833–1842, 1980.

52. Silverman JF, Finley JL, Park KH, Novis TH, Strausbach PH: Psammoma bodies and optically clear nuclei in bronchioloalveolar cell carcinoma: diagnosis by fine needle aspiration biopsy with histologic and ultrastructural confirmation. *Diagn Cytopathol* 1:205–215, 1985.

53. Silverman SH, Nussbaum M, Rausen AR: Thyroid nodules in children: a ten-year experience at one institution. *Mt Sinai J Med* 46:460–463, 1979.

54. Solbiati L, Montali G, Grove E, et al: *Radiology* 148:793–797, 1983.

55. Strate SM, Lee EL, Childers JH: Occult papillary carcinoma of the thyroid with distant metastasis. *Cancer* 54:1093–1100, 1984.

56. Tardy EM Jr, Tenta LT: Non-thyroid mass in the thyroid area. *Trans Am Acad Ophthalmol Otolaryngol* 76:1373–1374, 1972.

57. Tawes RL, Delorimier AA: Thyroid carcinoma during youth. *J Pediatr Surg* 3:210, 1968.

58. Trail ML, Zeringue GP, Chicola JP: Carcinoma in the thyroglossal duct remnants. *Laryngoscope* 84:1685–1691, 1977.

59. Vickery AL Jr: Thyroid alterations due to irradiation. In Hazard BJ, Smith DE: *The Thyroid*. International Academy of Pathology Monograph No. 5. Baltimore, Williams and Wilkins, 1964, pp. 183–205.

60. Wallace MP, Betsill W: Papillary carcinoma of the thyroid gland seen as lateral neck cyst. *Arch Otolaryngol* 110:408–411, 1984.

61. Weitzman JJ, Ling SM, Kaplar SA, et al: Percutaneous needle biopsy of goiter in childhood. *J Pediatr Surg* 5:251–255, 1970.

62. Williams ED, Brown CL, Doniach I: Pathological and clinical finding in a series of 67 cases of medullary carcinoma of the thyroid. *J Clin Pathol* 19:103–113, 1966.

63. Winzelberg GG, Grose J, Yu D, Vagenakis AG, Braverman LE: Aspergillus flavus as a cause of thyroiditis in an immunosuppressed host. *Johns Hopkins Med J* 144:90–93, 1979.

64. Withers EH, Rosenfeld L, O'Neil J, Lyneli JB: Long-term experience with childhood thyroid carcinoma. *J Pediatr Surg* 14:3322–3325, 1979.

65. Woolner LB, Lemmon ML, Beahrs OH, Black BM, Kealing FR Jr: Occult papillary carcinoma of the thyroid gland: a study of 140 cases observed in a 30-year period. *J Clin Endocrinol* 20:89–105, 1960.

16

Application of Needle Biopsy Data to Management Decisions

J. Martin Miller, M.D.

The primary consideration in the application of needle biopsy data to the management of thyroid nodules is the perception of thyroid cancer by the responsible physician. When thyroid nodules were selected for lobectomy by noninvasive means, it was recognized that some cancers were missed. (Just how many were missed was not appreciated until we began doing thyroid biopsies.) The problem, however, was not failure to identify cancers that later proved lethal, but a plethora of operations for removal of benign disease. Simply stated, in the minds of most physicians, the consequences of observing some cancerous thyroid nodules did not justify the removal of all thyroid nodules. Consider this example of a translation of this perception of thyroid cancer into aspiration biopsy language: A cytologic diagnosis that admits to a small (10%) chance of a nodule being a mini-invasive thyroid cancer is not synonymous with a surgical mandate. Under certain circumstances, even a definite diagnosis of carcinoma might not be a surgical mandate. For example, a 65-year-old man with congestive heart failure, previous myocardial infarction, and a 1-cm isthmus nodule diagnosed as papillary carcinoma by fine-needle biopsy is probably not a surgical candidate.

The cytopathologist and thyroidologist must understand each other's objectives. The former has been justifiably trained never to miss a diagnosis of cancer. The thyroidologist, however, places maximum emphasis on being certain that the morbidity and mortality of the thyroid lesion in question exceeds that of the anesthesia and surgery for a particular patient. The cytopathologist appreciates that a diagnosis other than outright malignancy may represent a very small chance of a lethal cancer. When the cytopathologist perceives that the clinician favors conservative management, he or she is free to note the presence of small numbers of abnormal cells or to vacillate between a diagnosis of benign and adenoma without provoking early, and usually unnecessary, surgery. The clinician will respond to such a diagnosis by prescribing observation with thyroid-stimulating hormone suppression, repeat biopsy after 3–12 months, or a large-needle biopsy before considering lobectomy. For the clinician, a definitive diagnosis is not required. A needle biopsy diagnosis is needed that is more accurate on the average than that from non-invasive diagnostic methods. The needle biopsy diagnosis must identify all cancers with proximate lethal potential and, utilizing previous biopsy diagnoses correlated with surgical data, provide a statement of probability of a nodule being a less aggressive differentiated cancer. It must also reliably select nodules that may be safely observed; if this is at variance with clinical judgment, it must be almost 100% accurate selection. When clinical and biopsy data both suggest a diagnosis of benign disease, but both are in error, the delay in making a proper diagnosis should not prove catastrophic. When the physical description or behavior of a nodule suggests malignancy and the diagnosis by needle biopsy is benign, the tissue diagnosis must be correct, or a therapeutic opportunity may be lost. It is the responsibility of the physician who correlates the biopsy diagnosis and the clinical findings to make sure the biopsy diagnosis adequately explains the total clinical picture. This has been our guideline for 10 years of needle biopsy use. Abele and TR Miller[1] have expressed this philosophy very well.

The approach of many physicians to nodule management is quite simple. If the biopsy diagnosis is benign, observe it or treat it by thyroid-stimulating hormone suppression. If the biopsy diagnosis is anyting else (and, therefore, does not exclude cancer), remove the nodule. As clinicians, our opinion is that such a therapeutic philosophy results in too many diagnostic surgical lobectomies. If the pathologist member of the biopsy team is aware that all nodules diagnosed as nonbenign will be removed anyway, much of the incentive for attempting specific diagnoses has been eliminated. This applies mostly to follicular lesions for which the specificity of the diagnosis is less than that for papillary lesions. The specificity varies with the exact cytologic diagnosis made. Therefore, we encourage the cytopathologist to make as accurate a diagnosis as possible on all lesions and for selective removal to be employed. If the presence of cancer is highly probable, surgery is usually advised. If it is only possible, other factors are considered.

In our experience, 10–15% of fine-needle biopsy specimens are diagnosed as cellular adenoma. Perhaps 25% of these are false-positive results, as the correct pathologic diagnosis is nodular goiter. If the nodule is 2 cm or larger, a large-needle biopsy is done, and the histologic specimen often enables us to screen out the nodular goiters. If the fine-needle biopsy diagnosis of cellular adenoma is confirmed, or if the nodule is too small for large-needle biopsy, the decision for or against surgery is based on several factors. These include the length of time at risk (the patient's age), the presence of diseases that increase the operative risk, the perception of risk based on the cytopathology, and the perception of risk based on the clinical features of the nodule. It is important to note that follicular cancers identified by the diagnosis of cellular adenoma have consistently been mini-invasive in our experience. All aggressive cancers have been easily diagnosed as such.

Different cytopathologists have different classifications for fine-needle biopsy diagnoses based on different microscopic criteria. Therefore, decisions made by one biopsy team may not be applicable to the experience of another team. Consider the

TABLE 16.1. Percentage of Diagnoses by Diagnostic Classification at the Mayo Clinic and Henry Ford Hospital

Mayo Clinic	Percent	Henry Ford Hospital	Percent
Malignant	5	Malignant or suspected malignancy	15
Suspected	17	Abnormal; cellular adenoma or Hürthle cell adenoma	18
Benign	78	Benign	67

differences in diagnoses made on the first 2000 satisfactory fine-needle biopsy specimens interpreted at the Mayo Clinic,[2] in Rochester, Minnesota, and the first 2000 diagnoses made from a combination of fine- and large-needle biopsy specimen interpretations at the Henry Ford Hospital, in Detroit, Michigan. Table 16.1 summarizes the percentage of diagnoses in each diagnostic classification.

When the middle categories are compared, nonequivalence of microscopic criteria is suggested by the number and type of the cancers identified. At the Mayo Clinic, 253 of 333 patients were operated on who had a diagnosis of suspected malignancy. Of these, 60 cancers were found—32 papillary, 14 follicular, 4 medullary, 1 anaplastic, 2 metastatic, and 7 assorted cancers including malignant lymphoma. Among the Henry Ford Hospital group diagnosed as abnormal (possible cancer), 224 of 354 nodules underwent operation. Only 20 were cancer—8 Hürthle cell variant of follicular carcinoma, 6 follicular, 5 papillary, and 1 medullary carcinoma. It appears that the management of a diagnosis of suspected malignancy in Minnesota and a diagnosis of possible cancer in Michigan should not be the same.

It is appropriate to close the discussion of needle biopsy management of thyroid nodules with a restatement of the goals of such management. They are, first, to remove all potentially lethal thyroid cancers and, second, to remove as few benign nodules as possible in achieving the first goal. Continued refinement of diagnostic biopsy criteria is necessary for maximum approximation of these objectives.

REFERENCES

1. Abele JS, Miller TR: Fine needle aspiration of the thyroid nodule: clinical application. In Clark OH: *Endocrine Surgery of the Thyroid and Parathyroid Glands.* St. Louis, Mosby, 1985, p. 293.

2. Gharib H, Goellner JR, Zinsmeister AR, Grant CS, Van Heerden JA: Fine-needle aspiration biopsy of the thyroid: the problem of suspicious cytological findings. *Ann Intern Med* 101:25, 1984.

Appendix to Chapter 16

Observations on Pathophysiology of Thyroid

J. Martin Miller, M.D.

The raison d'être for needle biopsy of thyroid is the palpable nodule of uncertain nature. The term "nodule" is defined for our purposes as an area within or adjacent to a thyroid lobe that has a consistency other than that of normal thyroid tissue. Theoretically, a portion of a lobe different from the remaining tissue should be included only because of increased thickness. The palpatory differences may be related to the cellularity, vascularity, the amount of fluid or colloid, or any combination of these factors.

There is no perfect experimental model for studying the pathogenesis of thyroid nodules. Using the rat as an imperfect experimental model, it seems that most thyroid nodules appear as a result of thyroid-stimulating hormone or thyroid-growth immunoglobulin stimulation, remittent or intermittent. The nodule represents an area of hyperinvolution remaining after the remainder of the thyroid-stimulating hormone-stimulated hyperplastic tissue has returned to normal, or it begins as a group of follicles that partially or totally escapes from thyroid-stimulating hormone control and grows and/or functions independently of the trophic hormone. In many instances these nodules are multiple, although one may be dominant and palpable and the others small, or microscopic, and not felt.

The hyperinvolution hypothesis of nodule formation was well described by Marine[4] based on material from patients with endemic goiter. A diffuse enlargement of the gland preceded the formation of palpable nodules. Miller et al,[5] in 1967, observed by autoradiographic studies single follicles or groups of follicles that escaped thyroid-stimulating hormone control as the genesis for autonomous functioning nodules.

When a nodule enlarges to approximately 1 cm, an important classification can be made by radionuclide imaging. About 10% of nodules will appear to be functioning. On a second study, with the patient taking triiodothyronine to suppress thyroid-stimulating hormone, the nodule will continue to function, whereas the extranodular tissue will suppress and takes up less radionuclide. This identifies the nodule as a true functioning tumor of the thyroid. These tumors are composed of a spectrum of histologic structures ranging from large, colloid-filled follicles to small, hyperplastic follicles. The latter may have nuclear chromatin patterns that can be confused with those of malignant neoplasia. Of the many thousands of these tumors surgically removed, only two of those reported in the literature were probably well-differentiated carcinomas.[1,3] Most patients with thyroid nodules have radionuclide imaging before biopsy, and the autonomous functioning tumors are not evaluated cytologically. The possibility of interpretive error must be kept in mind when looking at the cytology of patients whose nodules have not been imaged.

On radionuclide image, 90% of thyroid nodules localize to an area of decreased function. At least two-thirds of these are involutional nodules, or have been diagnosed as nodular goiter rather than follicular adenoma (a true tumor), by a thyropathologist. The other one-third are usually grossly solitary tumors, with a well-defined capsule, composed of follicular cells of varying patterns. Autoradiographically, these nodules collect little radioactive iodine, which accounts for their appearance on scintiphoto.

As most nodules subject to biopsy do not trap or bind pertechnetate or iodine radionuclide, the epithelium that the pathologist calls "benign" or "nodular goiter" is composed of functionally inactive cells, as judged by iodine metabolism. Nuclei of normal follicles appear much more active. This difference might prove confusing except that normal thyroid follicles are rarely aspirated through a fine needle. The evidence for this is circumstantial. We routinely make six separate slides from each nodule using six different needles. In studies of over 6000 nodules, we have virtually never found tumor on one slide and diagnostic numbers of normal-appearing cells on another. As most of the 1–2-cm tumor nodules are at least partially surrounded by normal tissue, this is a remarkable observation. We have, however, diagnosed Hashimoto's thyroiditis on one slide and tumor on another when the paranodular tissue had features of autoimmune thyroiditis. We hypothesize, therefore, that we usually get an unsatisfactory aspirate and an acellular smear when the fine needle is placed in normal thyroid tissue. It is probable that the structural integrity of normal tissue is far greater than that of tumor. This is in keeping with the observation we have made on 16-gauge aspirations of follicular tumors: The ease of sample aspiration is inversely proportional to the follicular size.

Hashimoto's thyroiditis, generally recognized as an autoimmune process, is of concern in several different ways to the pathologist interpreting biopsies. If the cytotoxic antibodies destroy the follicular epithelium without producing a hyperplastic reaction, or if thyroid-stimulating-hormone–blocking antibodies prevent the formation of a goiter, the associated hypothyroidism is of concern only to the clinician. If compensatory hyperplasia of the damaged epithelium and lymphocytic infiltrate combine to produce palpable thyroid enlargement, then it is possible that the needle biopsy specimen will supply information of value for the physician making management decisions. Diffuse thyromegaly is not usually considered an indication for needle biopsy, but in the following instances, biopsy may follow a clinical diagnosis of Hashimoto's thyroiditis:

1. Thyromegaly does not regress with thyroid-stimulating hormone suppression.

2. Thyromegaly increases despite thyroid-stimulating hormone suppression, either in the intial treatment period or after a period of stable gland size.

3. Diffuse thyroid enlargement or abnormality is accompanied by an area different enough in size or consistency to be described as a nodule.

In each instance, the original diagnosis may be questioned as to correctness or completeness, ie: Is the enlargement either totally or partially from lymphocytic thyroiditis? If it is partial, what is the other pathologic entity?

Two diseases coexist in the thyroid with lymphocytic thyroiditis often enough to recommend their inclusion in its differential diagnosis. The first disease, papillary carcinoma. Carcinoma has been reported as occurring in as many as 3% of thyroids operated on for Hashimoto's thyroiditis.[8] The majority of these tumors are papillary. The tumor may present as a nodule, and may be palpable or may present with multiple microscopic foci throughout a lobe. These add to the lobe's size, but are not individually identifiable. Our series of 593 cancers did not include a follicular carcinoma in a palpable, diffusely abnormal gland of lymphocytic thyroiditis.

The second disease associated with lymphocytic thyroiditis is malignant lymphoma. We have noted in our practice an increase in the occurrence of malignant lymphoma of the thyroid.[6] Although malignant lymphoma is rare in patients with lymphocytic thyroiditis, about 75% of patients with malignant lymphoma have an underlying lymphocytic thyroiditis.[2] As malignant lymphoma of the thyroid is easily curable when diagnosed early, and almost incurable when diagnosed late, it behooves the clinician and the cytopathologist to have a high index of suspicion for this disease in patients with Hashimoto's thyroiditis. For the clinician, this means abandoning the picture of malignant lymphoma of the thyroid as a massive, rapidly enlarging goiter in an elderly female, and substituting any suspicious enlargement (or lack of regression) in patients with Hashimoto's thyroiditis, regardless of their age or sex. For the cytopathologist, this means reporting any suspected coexisting malignant lymphoma, and determining false-positive results by use of a histologic examination of a large needle biopsy specimen.

The occurrence of medullary carcinoma of thyroid has special significance for the physician interpreting or performing biopsies. This tumor may be sporadic (80%) or familial (20%). The familial variety may be associated with a parathyroid adenoma or pheochromocytoma, and the presence of either will alter surgical planning. Therefore, a specific biopsy diagnosis is of great importance. A good cytologic specimen should rarely be interpreted as other than cancer, and if there is any suspicion that this might be a medullary carcinoma, immunoperoxidase and serum calcitonin studies should be done. This will ensure proper determination of the presence or absence of ancillary tumors.

Most of the statistics concerning cancer metastatic to the thyroid are based on autopsy material. In our 10 years of biopsy experience, we have observed cancer of the lung, esophagus, colon, kidneys, sebaceous glands and breast as well as malignant melanoma presenting as thyroid nodule. Most were not the primary site of identification of the tumor, although the metastatic nature was sometimes unsuspected.

Undifferentiated cancer of thyroid may occur in an otherwise normal gland, and even modest growth makes the patient aware of its presence. (In such situations, dedifferentiation of a papillary or follicular cancer may be present, which might have been prevented by early biopsy, identification, and removal of the differentiated cancer.) Undifferentiated cancer of thyroid may also arise in a multinodular goiter that has been present for many years. This possibility presents two caveats for the biopsy physician. First, the physician must remember the very limited information provided by fine-needle biopsy of large multinodular goiters, and must perform repeat biopsy of any areas of anatomic change. Second, the physician must carefully avoid giving the patient the impression that carcinoma has been ruled out by a benign biopsy.

CYSTIC NODULES

The number of thyroid nodules that are partially or totally cystic at the time of presentation has been estimated to be about 20%.[7] The thin-walled veins in many nodules are susceptible to minor trauma with subsequent hemorrhage, tissue necrosis, and cyst formation. Potential for such change depends on the vascularity of the lesion. Most thyroid cancers are less vascular than benign lesions; this accounts for the unusual presentation of cancer as a cystic lesion. At the other end of the spectrum is the autonomous functioning thyroid nodule, which frequently presents with partial cystic change. The degree of vascularity apparently relates to the degree of metabolic activity. Judging from our experience[4] with cyst aspiration, hemorrhagic cysts present in two different ways. In one, following the bleeding, hemoglobin is absorbed. At initial aspiration, straw-colored fluid is found. In the other, it is hypothesized that partial reabsorbtion of the cyst contents decreases the pressure on the vein from which the original bleeding took place, and hemorrhage recurs. At initial aspiration, the cyst contents is always that of recent bleeding. Although cytologic examination of most cyst aspirates identifies only histiocytes, the recent bloody contents are more apt to contain viable follicular cells than straw-colored residue from bleeding that occurred at least 6 to 8 weeks previously.

Some thyroid cysts contain viscous, clear material that has the same appearance as aspirates from a tendon sheath cyst or ganglion. This material stains like colloid with Papanicolaou stain, and may well be colloid. Rare lesions of this sort that have been removed have been endothelial-lined cavities (simple cysts).

Hemorrhagic cysts are turgid and quite firm on palpation, as bleeding has been stopped by the pressure of the capsule. Cysts that are spongy or soft almost invariably contain water-clear or gray-opalescent fluid. These are parathyroid cysts, and their etiology is established by a level of cyst fluid parathormone at least three times that of blood serum.

We do not routinely examine cyst fluid for either thyroxine or parathormone, as neither contributes to management decisions. Patients with parathyroid cysts diagnosed from the above description are routinely checked for hyperparathyroidism.

Certain clinical observations are relevant for pathologists interpreting or performing thyroid biopsies. Even with palpable residual after initial aspiration, obtaining a satisfactory fine-needle biopsy specimen is difficult. Efforts made at the second or third aspirations are more apt to be rewarding. Partial or complete recurrence of the cyst is considered presumptive evidence of existence of part of the original nodule.

Aspiration biopsy may be attempted in the area suspected, as well as in palpable residual tissue. On second and third biopsies of nonpalpable or barely palpable residuals of small cysts, we have identified four papillary carcinomas.

REFERENCES

1. Abdel-Razzak M, Christie JH: Thyroid carcinoma in an autonomously functioning nodule. *J Nucl Med* 20:1001, 1979.

2. Hamburger JI, Miller JM, Kini SR: Lymphoma of the thyroid. *Ann Intern Med* 99:685–693, 1983.

3. Hopwood NJ, Carrol RG, Kinney FM, Foley TP: Functioning thyroid masses in children and adolescence. *J Pediatr* 89:710–718, 1976.

4. Marine D: Etiology and prevention of simple goiter. *Medicine* 3:453, 1924.

5. Miller JM, Horn RC, Bloch MA: The autonomous functioning thyroid nodule in the evolution of nodular goiter. *J Clin Endocrinol Metab* 27:1264, 1967.

6. Miller JM, Kini SR, Rebuck J, Hamburger JI: Is lymphoma of the thyroid a disease which is increasing in frequency? In Hamburger JI, Miller JM: Controversies in Clinical Thyroidology. New York, Springer-Verlag, 1981, pp. 267–297.

7. Miller JM, Zafar S, Karo JJ: The cystic nodule: recognition and management. *Radiology* 85:702–710, 1965.

8. Woolner LB, McConahey WM, Beahrs OH: Struma lymphomatosa (Hashimoto's thyroiditis) and related thyroid disorders. *J Clin Endocrinol Metab* 19:53, 1959.

Index

Page numbers in italics refer to illustrations.